Holistic Cancer Care

An Herbal Approach to Reducing Cancer Risk, Helping Patients Thrive during Treatment, and Minimizing Recurrence

CHANCHAL CABRERA

Storey Publishing

This book is dedicated to my sister, Dee Atkinson—
my best friend, my greatest inspiration.

The mission of Storey Publishing is to serve our customers by publishing practical information that encourages personal independence in harmony with the environment.

Edited by Carleen Madigan
Art direction and book design by Michaela Jebb
Text production by Jennifer Jepson Smith
Diagrams by Andrew Wang © Storey Publishing, LLC

Storey Publishing
210 MASS MoCA Way
North Adams, MA 01247
storey.com

Storey Publishing, LLC is an imprint of Workman Publishing Co., Inc., a subsidiary of Hachette Book Group, Inc., 1290 Avenue of the Americas, New York, NY 10104

ISBNs: 978-1-63586-373-4 (paperback); 978-1-63586-374-1 (ebook); 978-1-63586-648-3 (hardcover); 978-1-63586-655-1 (audio)

Printed in the United States by Lakeside Book Company (interior) and PC (case and cover)

10 9 8 7 6 5 4 3 2 1

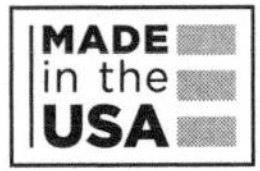

Library of Congress Cataloging-in-Publication Data on file

CONTENTS

iv Foreword by Christopher J. Etheridge, PhD, MCPP
1 Preface: Opening the Door to the Power of Herbs
2 An Introduction to Holistic Cancer Care

10 **Part 1: Holistic Strategies for Patients and Caregivers**

11 Chapter 1: Understanding Cancer

38 Chapter 2: Nutrition and Lifestyle Choices to Inhibit Cancer

87 Chapter 3: Preparing for Surgery and Enhancing Recovery

126 Chapter 4: Managing Pain with Botanicals

143 Chapter 5: Thriving during Chemotherapy and Radiation

237 Chapter 6: Materia Medica: A Directory of Herbs for Cancer

308 **Part 2: For the Practitioner and Herbal Prescriber**

309 Chapter 7: Herbal Formulating for Cancer Care

342 Chapter 8: Diagnosis and Treatment Planning in Collaborative Oncology

404 Chapter 9: Materia Medica for Managing Cancer: The Cytotoxic Herbs

450 Chapter 10: Case Histories

487 Acknowledgments
488 References and Background Reading
526 Glossary
529 Resources
534 Metric Conversions
535 List of Plants by Common Name
541 List of Plants by Latin Name
547 Index of Recipes and Formulas for Patient Care
548 Index

FOREWORD

Interest in holistic medicine has soared in recent years, along with an increase in quality research being published in this important area. There is now an opportunity for patients to work with holistic practitioners to reduce their risk of developing cancer, to obtain support during conventional cancer treatments, and to ensure their return to full health after completion of those treatments. There is a real need for a comprehensive handbook that equips readers with the information to understand and access targeted treatment strategies for holistic cancer care. I was therefore excited when I heard that Chanchal was writing this book.

I first met Chanchal at a conference in London in 2012, where she was presenting a talk on holistic cancer care, and I was impressed with the depth of her knowledge and understanding of the science behind the use of herbal medicine to support cancer patients. Chanchal has more than 35 years of clinical experience, giving her a keen insight into the pivotal role of herbal medicine in the treatment of cancer.

Understanding that patients and practitioners often need different levels of information, Chanchal has divided the book into two main sections. The first is focused on giving patients an understanding of how holistic care can help at every stage of the cancer treatment process—from reducing the side effects and improving outcomes of treatments like chemotherapy and radiotherapy, to managing pain, to enhancing recovery from surgery. Helpfully, she includes an in-depth discussion of some of the main herbs used for cancer support.

The second part of the book is specifically aimed at practitioners. Chanchal shows how to support cancer patients by formulating effective, balanced herbal prescriptions that employ key herbs in a synergistic way, at the correct dosage and in the right form for the individual patient. She highlights vital issues in herbal medicine safety and toxicology, including herb-drug interactions, and provides a comprehensive, fully referenced monograph for each of the cytotoxic herbs. Because she has been practicing in the world of holistic oncology for so long, she's able to include several case histories from her own patients that illustrate the effectiveness of the practices she recommends.

I have been greatly inspired by reading *Holistic Cancer Care* and am already applying its concepts to my own practice. Chanchal's enthusiasm, knowledge, and vast experience of the practice of herbal medicine in the cancer supportive setting is an excellent resource to have at your fingertips.

CHRISTOPHER J. ETHERIDGE, PHD, MCPP
Founder and Director of Integrated Cancer Healthcare
President of the College of Practitioners of Phytotherapy
President of the European Herbal & Traditional Medicine Practitioners Association
Chair of the British Herbal Medicine Association

PREFACE

Opening the Door to the Power of Herbs

As a newly graduated medical herbalist in the late 1980s, I will admit I felt somewhat hopeless and helpless when patients came in with a cancer diagnosis. The extent of their fear, the extent of the medical interventions they were undergoing, and the nature of the condition itself all served to make me feel that there was little I could offer. Even after 10 years of running a busy herbal medicine clinic, I could count just a handful of cancer patients whom I felt I had really helped in all that time.

It wasn't until I enrolled in the Master of Science in Herbal Medicine program at the University of Wales that I began to learn just how powerful herbs could be in cancer support. For my dissertation project, my colleague and friend Donald Yance invited me to conduct research in his herbal medicine practice in Oregon. Donnie had been focusing on cancer care for a few years by then and had just published a book about it (called *Herbal Medicine, Healing & Cancer*). He wanted research done into quality-of-life parameters in long-term breast cancer survivors in his practice.

The opportunity to be paid to do research that I could use for my degree was irresistible. I moved to Oregon in 2001 to conduct the research and to work alongside Donnie in his clinic, seeing patients and learning from him. It was a deep dive into a world of research I had never seen before and new ways of clinical practice. It was also an apprenticeship with a master. Much of the original inspiration for this book came from my decade of working closely with Donnie in his clinic, helping him create a 2-week professional training in herbal medicine for cancer, and from the research and writing we did together. After 2 years in Donnie's clinic, I had written my thesis ("Living with Breast Cancer"), received my master's degree, and seen beyond doubt that herbal medicine has extraordinary potential to help people survive and thrive through cancer. My clinical practice since that time has evolved to be largely cancer focused, and nothing I have subsequently learned about herbal medicine and cancer care has caused me to change my mind. Obviously, not all my patients survive and thrive past cancer; some come to natural medicine very late in their journey or have particularly aggressive cancers, and some are just too weak and compromised to overcome the disease. However, in every case, whatever the circumstances and wherever they are in their journey with cancer, there is a strong role for herbs, targeted nutrition, and other holistic practices that are useful to promote wellness.

An Introduction to Holistic Cancer Care

Herbal medicine and other natural therapies help people with cancer. They may not be the only thing that helps—in fact they rarely are—but there is no doubt that they have a role to play not only in caring for the long-term, chronic consequences of cancer and conventional treatment but also in the immediate interventions required with a new diagnosis and an active cancer case. People with cancer reading this book will find many recipes, formulas, and self-care ideas that can be implemented safely and easily. For the practitioner, there are guidelines, strategies, and a materia medica that I have honed through the last 20 years of cancer-focused clinical practice and through helping hundreds of patients with natural medicine. Many of the recommendations are for specific orthomolecular or targeted nutritional supplements as well as herbs. Nutritional, nutraceutical, and herbal therapies can be used in conjunction with other specific targeted drug therapies to offer a truly coherent strategy for cancer management.

My goal here is not to convince you that holistic medicine and natural therapies can help treat cancer. If you didn't already know that they work, you wouldn't have picked up this book. My effort here is to help you understand *how* they work, why it matters, and, most of all, how to use them safely and effectively. This is not a textbook with hundreds of references after each section, but I have given a representative sample of research and studies for those of you who like to look up the details.

The details do matter. I am a strong believer that in order to know how to fix something, you first need to know how it works and how it goes wrong. Understanding what cancer is and how cancer comes about makes it so much easier to understand how to apply useful interventions, be they herbs, drugs, or lifestyle choices. This book describes the mechanisms by which cancer initiates, proliferates, and progresses, and the steps and processes by which it can be addressed.

One of the biggest drawbacks to understanding how herbs and targeted nutrition can work in preventing and treating cancer is that, while we may have decades or even hundreds of years of evidence-based medicine to draw upon, and while there may be great congruence among natural medicine prescribers in how they use remedies, most of the research today is being done on isolates or super-concentrated extracts in test tubes or cell lines or animals—rarely in humans—and is far removed from traditional practices. This often means that contemporary approaches to herbal medicine risk being fragmented or watered down. Nevertheless, it's fascinating to understand at a cellular level how some of our herbs bring about their remarkable effects.

This dilemma of holism and reductionism, and the risks inherent in extrapolating from analytical research to clinical practice, compounded by the sheer inhumanity of the animal research, creates a treacherous minefield for clinicians and researchers trying to find the best and most useful information from among such a plethora of data. In researching studies for this book, I focused on human studies and human cell lines. I mention animal research only where it is particularly pertinent. This is not a perfect solution, I know. It is important for herbal practitioners to share their learning through case reviews (such as the patient case histories in Chapter 10), so that they can contribute to the knowledge base that current research does not always extend to.

How to Use This Book

My intention in writing this book is to provide a useful handbook for a person newly diagnosed with cancer and for their support team, to give practical guidelines and helpful strategies that can be realistically implemented, and to be a guide for safe and effective use of herbal medicine in cancer care by patients and by healthcare providers. The first part of the book discusses healthy lifestyle choices and how to maximize general health, strength, resilience, and resistance measures in your life using herbs and targeted nutrition. Preparation and recovery from surgery, optimizing chemotherapy, managing pain, and a wide materia medica listing of herbs used in cancer care are reviewed in Part 1.

In addition, this book is intended for the practitioner, the healthcare professional who wants to integrate herbal medicines into their clinical competencies. Part 2 of the book is for practitioners; it describes how to formulate with herbs, how to use the cytotoxic herbs, how to use herbs with chemotherapy, targeted nutrition for specific purposes, and case studies from my clinic. There are recipes and formulas as well as extensive resources for finding practitioners and products and a detailed glossary.

A wealth of research and decades of clinical experience have confirmed that there are multiple and overlapping ways to raise the odds in your favor, to support and encourage your body to resist a host of chronic, degenerative diseases, including cancer.

What Is Holistic Cancer Care?

This all-embracing approach to healthcare has classically been called "integrative" or "integrated" medicine. In 2017, cancer researcher Ken Witt and his colleagues defined *integrative oncology* in the following words:

> A patient-centered, evidence-informed field of cancer care that utilizes mind and body practices, natural products, and/or lifestyle modifications from different traditions, alongside conventional cancer treatments. Integrative oncology aims to optimize health, quality of life, and clinical outcomes across the cancer care continuum and to empower people to prevent cancer and become active participants before, during, and beyond cancer treatment.

Sounds great, doesn't it? I can agree with all that. But here are some reasons why this term and others commonly used to describe this approach to treatment aren't necessarily the best.

Alternative medicine. This term implies a requirement to choose one or the other, conventional or holistic, a dichotomy that is not useful or appropriate for patients most of the time.

Complementary medicine. This implies a second tier of treatment that is somewhat subordinate to the mainstream conventional therapies, that complements them. This demeans the value of the natural medicines. Notwithstanding these legitimate concerns of etymology, the term *CAM*, or complementary and alternative medicine, is still widely used and occurs in much of the literature on the subject.

Integrative or integrated medicine. These were the terms I used for many years, on the premise that I was attempting to meld the best of Western biomedical understanding of the body and disease with a deeply rooted holistic materia medica and methodologies, integrating old and new thinking to reach a state of dynamic equilibrium in the clinical practice. Sometimes this requires wearing a more "medical" hat, and other times it means using nutrition or herbal remedies as the main platform of treatment. It worked for me for a number of years, and there were (and still are) a good number of established clinics that refer to themselves as "integrative."

However, more than 10 years ago, my friend Dr. Pierre Haddad from the University of Montreal alerted me to the semantics of these terms and suggested a new way of describing the work. He told me about his ethnobotanical research in First Nations communities of northern Québec, where the Indigenous peoples objected to the term *integrated* to describe how some of their healing practices could be used and applied in contemporary times. *Integration* to them had connotations of loss—loss of cultural identity and loss of traditional knowledge, homogenization and weakening of societal bonds.

When asked to come up with a better term, they suggested *collaborative*. This seems to me to capture the intention of my work in supporting patients through cancer. It values, validates, and respects all the protagonists: The doctors and medical specialists, the nutritionist, the counselor, the herbalist, and most importantly the patient are all heard and recognized. Collaborative medicine is a holistic model, and holistic oncology is one area of medicine where this approach or practice of medicine is extremely beneficial to the patient.

Holistic Oncology

Holistic oncology represents an entirely new approach to cancer intervention. It promotes a synergy of traditional healing and wellness concepts, as well as modern science, innovative drug therapies, and unique botanical and nutritional formulations. Working with patients in this model is like fitting together the various pieces of a puzzle; it is interwoven, synergistic, and most of all successful. It does not throw out the old simply because it is old, nor does it neglect effective conventional or allopathic therapies simply because they are not old.

The key word here is *effective*. A treatment plan should be crafted based on which strategies will be most effective for a particular patient. To that end, practitioners should perform a thorough investigative intake interview and review relevant blood and pathology reports before putting a plan in place. How you measure wellness and how much emphasis you place on quality versus extension of life will be critical factors in deciding how to proceed with treatment, whether herbal or conventional. Treatment choices may change over time as the health picture changes, perhaps starting out with stronger targeted treatments to set back the cancer and progressing to a long-term health maintenance plan over time. The protocol is not something permanent; it must be continually changed, reflecting changes in the individual. It starts from foundation building and sustaining the "vital force," and then various layers and more specific compounds are added.

Conventional Cancer Care vs. Holistic Oncology

Conventional cancer care has historically been a tumor-based model, in which the patient is a passive recipient of oncology care, of invasive and risky surgeries, drugs, and radiotherapy, without much ability to influence or control the situation; holistic wellness support is offered as an afterthought, if at all. This is changing rapidly as evidence of the benefits of a more holistic approach mounts. As such, it is important to seek out the most open-minded, forward-thinking oncology professionals—those who are willing to work with a care team that includes natural medicine providers.

Holistic or collaborative oncology puts the patient at the center of the equation. It considers all health, social, and interpersonal influences that may have bearing on wellness outcomes, including individual tolerance and success of conventional therapies, with due regard for quality of life, not just duration or longevity. It is practiced over a continuum of care, from prevention to palliative care. And it is, by definition, a team effort with members who represent fields of expertise appropriate to the needs of the individual, with everyone providing their best input for the patient. This is my wish for cancer patients, for their caregivers and loved ones, and for all the practitioners who seek to support them.

Tumor-Centered Approach

- Surgery (outcomes improved by minimally invasive techniques)
- Chemotherapy (outcomes improved by predictive testing for sensitivity/resistance and with newer, targeted immunotherapies)
- Radiation (sometimes necessary but not curative, outcomes improved by predictive testing for sensitivity/resistance)
- Symptom management

Patient-Centered Approach

- Healthy diet and appropriate supplements
- Healthy lifestyle and exercise, plus avoidance of toxins
- Liver support
- Immune support
- Stress management
- Emotional support (family, friends, spiritual)
- Tumor profile (blood work and primary pathology tests on biopsy slides)
- Assessment of pharmacogenomics (specialized biopsy slide testing)
- Sensitivity/resistance testing (fresh biopsy)
- Surgery
- Chemotherapy
- Radiation
- Symptom management

First Steps after Receiving a Diagnosis

The world of cancer is a scary one. Even though 50–70 percent of us can expect to get this diagnosis in our lifetime, it still comes as a shock when the reality of the situation must be faced. When a cancer diagnosis is received, the ensuing stress and adrenaline impair our ability to make clearheaded and well-considered decisions. The stress hormones cause us to make spur-of-the-moment, survivalist decisions. On top of that, the conventional model is rushed, so there is pressure to start treatment quickly, and any delays are discouraged. Last, but not least, is the fear-based thinking of family and friends who are anxious or distressed if we choose to delay treatment. One of the most challenging issues for the cancer patient can be the well-meaning, well-intentioned person offering unsolicited and ill-informed advice.

Confronting cancer can be a daunting prospect for both the patient and the practitioner. Making sense of treatment options, both conventional and nonconventional, can be even more overwhelming. Few people are prepared to untangle the web of medical jargon and complicated decision-making that accompanies a diagnosis and a long-term understanding of the disease they may have. People want to do "whatever it takes" to "get rid of the cancer," regardless of the consequences and without a true understanding of the impact on their quality or quantity of life. Clear answers are often in short supply.

Take the Time to Consider Your Options

The first step upon receiving a cancer diagnosis is to slow down and take the time to research options and their consequences, consider best practices, and prepare yourself, physically and mentally, to receive treatment. In many circumstances, time is of the essence. However, it's important not to make quick decisions that may have negative outcomes.

The decision about how fast to begin treatment is determined by the biopsy; the higher the stage and grade, the more progressed the cancer is and the more urgent the situation. With the exception of some of the acute cancers like leukemia, by the time a malignancy is diagnosed, it has probably been growing for several years at least. Indeed, some cancers are notably slow growing, for example low-grade prostate cancer, ductal carcinoma in situ (DCIS) and low-grade breast cancer, low-grade thyroid cancer, and most nonmelanoma skin cancers; these are extremely unlikely to metastasize and cause systemic harm.

I encourage patients to take at least 2 weeks, or even a month, to sort out their best options for targeted treatment and to pursue additional testing. For example, I may recommend additional tests to evaluate the likely sensitivity of cells to the treatment before patients consider chemotherapy or radiation. Whether or not conventional treatments are chosen, there is much information to be sought—from reading and researching to meeting doctors and other practitioners—and it is important to weigh the pros and cons of different approaches. While this is underway, patients can begin a regimen of restorative, rejuvenating, and balancing therapies.

> Health is more than simply the absence of illness. It is the active state of physical, emotional, mental, and social well-being.
>
> WORLD HEALTH ORGANIZATION

Get Organized and Empower Yourself

One of the first things I ask my patients to do is to gather all the information I will need to help them make an informed choice about treatment strategies. This will mean asking medical offices for all records and files since your diagnosis and keeping copies of all test results and reports conducted in the future.

You will need to create some system to keep track of all your medical records. A spreadsheet of blood work results documented over time is convenient if you want to share records with different medical providers. Indeed, your holistic practitioner may be able to provide you with a spreadsheet to start with.

If you prefer not to do this on a computer, then I recommend using a simple three-ring binder with divider pages and tabs, so that you can separate out the written pathology reports from the blood work and other diagnostic reports, and then sort and file them by date: one tab for blood work, one tab for scans, and so on, arranged chronologically. Another tab will be used for the herbal or supplement prescriptions your holistic practitioner will write. In this way, you can build your own health file and have a full record that is easily referenced across time to see your progress.

Doing it this way may sound old-fashioned, but it is often more practical than using a spreadsheet. You may be attending several different medical specialists who all use different online portals, which can be complicated to keep track of. They are also likely to give you paper copies of reports and records when you visit, so a binder is a practical way to keep everything organized in one place and in chronological order.

Develop a Treatment Plan with a Holistic Practitioner

If you are reading this as a cancer patient, then I strongly recommend you seek out an experienced healthcare professional to help you navigate the difficult decisions that come with the process of pursuing cancer treatment. In addition to an oncologist, who will make a diagnosis and suggest conventional treatment options, you can work with a medical herbalist who can prescribe you cytotoxic herbs, given in carefully calculated doses and targeted to disable cancer cells. Naturopaths, nutritionists, a health coach, or other wellness professionals can also assist you in building optimal health. See Resources on page 529 for links to referral directories of professional herbalists worldwide.

Start a Preparation Plan

A preparation plan can begin the day you receive your diagnosis. No matter what type or stage or grade of cancer, and no matter what treatment options you are offered, you'll want to implement certain core practices in order to improve your circumstances overall. Not all of these are feasible for everyone, though, so don't beat yourself up for what you can't do; just make incremental steps in the right direction and know that it all helps.

Many of these are explored in more detail in Chapter 2, but you can start by doing the following:

- Clean out the kitchen cupboards and discard anything packaged, processed, sweetened, or artificially flavored or colored.
- Avoid fast food, takeout, and snack foods. If it is processed, packaged, or prepared in advance, then it is lacking nutritional value.
- Clean out the garage or garden shed and dispose of all noxious chemicals and solvents.
- Commit to buying organic foods and natural body care and household cleaning products.
- Eat at least three servings of leafy greens and one serving of dark berries daily.
- Drink 2–3 cups of green tea daily (and finish consuming them by 4 p.m.).
- Get plenty of sleep.
- Find ways to manage stress effectively.
- Get regular exercise.
- Avoid alcohol, except for the occasional glass of red wine.
- Drink 3–6 big glasses of pure water daily.
- Spend time with friends and loved ones. Be outside in nature. Laugh often.
- Use herbs for liver support, immune building, and antioxidant effects while waiting on test results, gathering information, and making decisions and choices about next steps.
- Use adaptogen herbs for managing stress.

PART 1

Holistic Strategies for Patients and Caregivers

CHAPTER 1

Understanding Cancer

There are myriad ways in which cancer expresses itself. Both symptoms and prognosis can vary dramatically among individuals and among types of cancer. However, at the heart of the matter, in the infinite intricacy of the cellular metabolic processes, there are more or less always the same core (dys)functions expressing themselves.

CHAPTER 1 CONTENTS

12 **It All Starts with a Gene Mutation**
15 What Causes Genetic Mutations

15 **Cancer as a Systemic Disease**
17 Warning Signs of Cancer

18 **Understanding Your Diagnosis**
18 Classification of Tumors
20 Critical Differences between Dysplasia and Cancer
20 Measuring the Extent of Cancer
22 Poor Differentiation of Cells

23 **Factors That Contribute to the Initiation of Cancer**
23 Where You Live
24 Exposure to Toxins
26 The Relationship between Hormones and Cancer
28 Viral and Bacterial Infections
30 Stress, Distress, Anxiety, and Loneliness
32 Dietary Influences
33 Brighter Days Tea
34 Inflammation
36 UV Radiation Exposure

It All Starts with a Gene Mutation

Every cancer is unique, with its own particular predispositions and triggers, and hence "the cure" for cancer is an illusion that will never be found. However, in contrast to this uniqueness, every cancer also expresses certain behaviors and metabolic pathways in common, the first of which is that cancer commences with an oncogenic, or tumor-causing, gene mutation that survives and replicates. There are different schools of thought about how these principal or primary mutations happen, but fundamentally that is where it all starts.

Genes act like the letters of an alphabet to encode the molecular instructions by which a cell can make specific proteins. Those proteins are either structural (such as muscle fiber or cell wall) or functional (such as enzymes that activate all the metabolic processes of cells). Some proteins the cell makes may be both structural and functional, as is the case with receptor sites embedded in and spanning the cell wall. These are a structural part of the cell wall or cell membrane, but they are also so-called kinase enzymes (from *kinesis,* which means "to move"). They adjust their shape when a ligand—a hormone, a cell-derived growth factor, or another trigger molecule—binds to them. This movement of the protein initiates a message that travels from the cell surface to the nucleus inside to instruct it which proteins to make next. The movement of that message through the cell cytoplasm by way of a cascade of enzyme reactions is called signal transduction; when the message reaches the nucleus, it causes signal transcription, or the reading of the message and activation of the appropriate genes.

If a gene has mutated, it will code for proteins that are dysfunctional. These proteins may include cell surface or intracellular receptor sites and their associated enzyme series, as well as transcription factors, and this dysfunction will lead to disordered binding of trigger molecules (ligands like estrogen or cortisol) and deranged signal transduction and signal transcription. Early mutations in many cancers also lead to disruption of cell adhesion molecules, which are made of glycoproteins and normally facilitate proper cell-to-cell communication. Without proper cell adhesion molecule activity, the damaged cells become isolated and evade the immune system, and normal regulation of cell growth and reproduction fails.

Mutated tumor suppressor genes. Genes can mutate for many reasons; sometimes, it's simply random. Other times, mutation is the result of ionizing radiation, oxidative stress, or pollutants. Most often, cancer starts as a mutation of a tumor suppressor gene; this is a gene that controls how quickly cells replicate and when they die. One example is the p53 gene mutation, which occurs in as many as 50 percent of all cancers. The p53 protein, coded for by the p53 gene, acts as a sort of quality control mechanism to determine if the copied DNA is accurate and the cell can divide, or if it's faulty, in which case replication should be inhibited, the error corrected, or the cell forced into apoptosis (programmed cell death). When p53 is mutated, it fails to recognize these errors, and the cell continues to thrive until it dominates the local environment and becomes what we recognize as cancer.

Mutated oncogenes. These are genes that code for proteins that promote and drive cell division or that inhibit apoptosis (cell death). In healthy cells, these procancer genes are necessary but tightly regulated to allow for natural cell senescence (irreversible cell cycle arrest), cell death, and replacement. When they mutate, they promote procancerous cell behaviors and cells become immortal. Examples of cancer-promoting oncogenes include genes

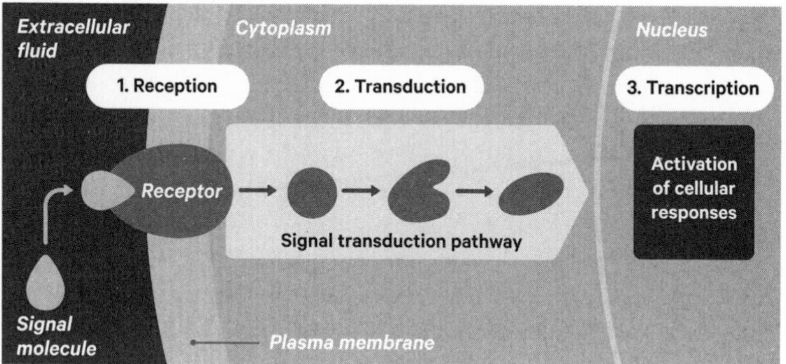

Cancer originates with gene mutations that disrupt communication from the cell surface to the nucleus (a process called signal transduction). When this process becomes dysfunctional, abnormal cells are created that can divide quickly, avoid dying, and evade the immune system.

coding for growth factors and their kinase receptors, for the cyclin-dependent kinases, and for Ras proteins.

Lack of contact inhibition. Normal body cells need to know when to copy or replicate and when to stop; for example, skin cells multiply to heal a cut, then stop when the wound is healed. This process is called contact inhibition, meaning excess cell replication is inhibited by contact on all sides with other cells. Malignant tumor cells can tune out contact inhibition, so they can just keep on replicating and migrating without any natural checks. Healthy normal cells have close communication with their neighbors through cell adhesion molecules that keep them in contact and through gap junctions that allow the exchange of information across cell walls. Cancer cells mutate the cell adhesion molecules and thus disable cell-to-cell communication. Eventually, a malignant cell becomes isolated from external control mechanisms and is able to develop at will. This is the process of oncogenesis, the development of cancer.

Cells that won't die. Each normal cell is programmed to die when it reaches the end of its functional life or when there is sufficient metabolic derangement to trigger senescence and apoptosis. Cancerous cells are able to keep thriving, multiplying, and spreading throughout the body because they disable the mechanisms that cause cell death. Cancer cells mutate early on, fail to undergo cell death properly, and become persistent and aggressive.

In cancer cells, when the DNA mutates, they code for erroneous proteins and the enzymes they make may be dysfunctional and defective. Because the natural systems of checks and balances are disrupted, it isn't usually long before the cell starts exhibiting abnormal behavior. This can quickly become a downward spiral, as each subsequent mutation codes for progressively more dysfunctional cell behavior. As the cells of the malignant tumor replicate and the cancerous growth expands, it competes with normal tissue for space and nutrients. Eventually, the normal tissue is subsumed into the tumor.

There is no single cause of cancer; the probability of developing it is influenced by a variety of factors. There may be one deciding factor in every case, one final insult or injury that tips the balance, but it is probably a different combination or set of circumstances in each person. What is the same in each case are the fundamental molecular effects—misreading of DNA and failure to check the damage. These effects are the core of the problem.

> Eating a vegetarian diet, walking (exercising) every day, and meditating is considered radical. Allowing someone to slice your chest open and graft your leg veins in your heart is considered normal and conservative.
>
> DR. DEAN ORNISH, CLINICAL PROFESSOR OF MEDICINE AT THE UNIVERSITY OF CALIFORNIA, SAN FRANCISCO

What Causes Genetic Mutations

Although this progression may appear to be a formidable list of missteps and mistakes, of genetic errors and their downstream consequences, in fact they are all driven by essentially the same set of circumstances and triggers—principally, oxidative stress and disturbances of metabolic control systems fueled by excess sugar intake and micronutrient deficiency, as well as physical, physiological, and psychological stressors. The ways the body can "go wrong" are legion, but the fundamental strategies of natural treatment are remarkably simple.

This is to our advantage; it means there are ways we can play an active role in our own healing. Reducing or eliminating tobacco use and alcohol consumption, eating more nutrient-dense foods, and minimizing stress are all part of preventing cancer and may play some role in treating cancer too. Eating whole foods and taking supplements that contain major antioxidant polyphenolic compounds from plants are also key. Plants need antioxidants to live just as much as humans do; thus, all the nutritious fruits and vegetables we eat and the herbs we take contain antioxidant molecules. Although it's best to eat whole foods wherever possible, rather than take isolated constituents as supplements, it's not always feasible to consume the amounts of whole foods that might be required to ward off or treat serious disease. Supplements include such natural agents as green tea catechins, apigenin and luteolin from chamomile, essential fatty acids (omega-3 fish oil), sulforaphanes from broccoli, and curcumin from turmeric. These and numerous others can affect multiple metabolic pathways, all of them helping to knock the cancer back in multiple ways.

Cancer as a Systemic Disease

Cancer is not some sort of alien beast—something that has arrived in the body and taken up residence. It is inherently of the host, your own cells run amok, and this contributes to some of the challenges of overcoming it. The immune system is programmed not to react to self, and so it fails to recognize the danger of cancer until it's too late. Cancer is not primarily a problem of overly rapid cell cycling, although that is part of the problem. Cancer is primarily a metabolic disturbance that arises from DNA mutations, in which cells lose the ability to communicate with each other and with the rest of the body and become autonomous and immortal.

In conventional allopathic medicine, cancer is viewed as clones of cells that have outgrown their environmental constraints and control mechanisms. These cells have abnormal behaviors and are considered to be foreign to the body. The main philosophy of conventional cancer treatment is direct annihilation of the cancer cells using aggressive and destructive therapies.

In the holistic approach to oncology, the development of cancer is viewed as a part of a complex syndrome representing an imbalance of the entire body-mind-spirit network. In other words, cancer is a systemic disease from the start, and the terrain is considered to be as important as the tumor itself. Holistic medicine purports that if one can strengthen and rebalance the body-mind-spirit network—if we can become "whole" again—then normal patterns will be restored, and the body may be able to resolve the cancer. It is worth pointing out here that it does not require eradicating every single cancer cell for cancer to be resolved. People can survive and even thrive with cancer, and herbs may contribute to that; healing is not the same as curing.

Addressing Cancer through Metabolic Pathways

Many holistic treatments slow the growth of cancer by inhibiting or encouraging certain metabolic pathways. Metabolic pathways are a series of sequential processes or functions in the body, controlled by enzymes, that catalyze a series of chemical reactions in a cell. They may be anabolic (building up), usually requiring energy and nutrient input, or catabolic (breaking down), usually releasing energy in the process. Some of these include the core or central functions of sugar metabolism (glycolysis and the Krebs cycle), fat metabolism (the pentose phosphate pathway), and the detoxification processes in the liver.

Key Steps in the Progression from Normal Cell to Malignant Tumor

- Terrain vulnerability and physiological derangement; predisposing factors include tobacco and alcohol use, a nutritionally deficient diet, environmental pollution, certain pharmaceuticals, ionizing radiation, chronic stress, and heredity
- Mutations of genes leading to abnormal expression of cells and the proteins they code for (faulty structural or functional proteins)
- Upregulation (stimulation) or downregulation (suppression) of signal transduction (movement of messages from the cell surface to the nucleus) and of signal transcription (reading of message by nucleus), leading to suppression of control proteins that would normally regulate cell replication and promotion of oncogenic cell behaviors, such as excessive production of growth factors and evasion or suppression of the immune system
- Weakening of the gel matrix that all cells are embedded into, and through which all nutrients, metabolic waste, and medicines must transit in order to enter or exit the cell
- Breakdown of cell adhesion and failure of cell-to-cell communication (failure of contact inhibition)

- Inhibition of mitochondrial activity (Krebs cycle), which also shuts down the mechanisms of apoptosis (cell death)
- High demand for glucose to fuel cancer cell activities, and high rate of glycolysis (the process by which sugar is metabolized), also called the Warburg effect and glycolytic shift
- Low cellular requirement for oxygen, meaning the cell can grow even in a low-oxygen (hypoxic) environment, which allows cancer to grow faster than the blood supply can keep up with
- Production of lactic acid from aerobic glycolysis, which contributes to a local inflammatory environment and promotes angiogenesis (new blood vessel growth)
- Loss of control of cell cycling, leading to rapid cell replication and tumor growth
- Crowding and eventual recruitment of adjacent cells
- Metastasis and invasion (the cancer cells spread from the original site)
- Increased platelets/coagulopathies (blood clotting)

Warning Signs of Cancer

Although there are exciting new tests on the horizon, there are currently no readily available or reliable blood tests to diagnose cancer, except for some of the blood cell cancers, such as leukemia or lymphoma. Cancer markers from solid tumors may be seen in the blood as cancer progresses and may be useful for tracking changes after treatment. There are some effective prognostic tests, such as Pap smears for cervical cancer or fecal occult blood tests for colon cancer, but by the time cancer is diagnosed it will have already been present for several months or even years. This, of course, is why prevention is so essential—by the time you know about it, the damage is done. In the beginning, most cancers grow very slowly and need to have doubled and doubled again many times to reach a size that is sufficient for symptoms to be noted or for them to be palpated.

AMERICAN CANCER SOCIETY'S LIST OF EARLY WARNING SIGNS

Below are some of the key early warning symptoms that warrant closer investigation. To this list we can add persistent headaches or dizziness, unexplained loss of weight and appetite, and persistent unexplained tiredness.

C—change in bowel or bladder habit
A—a sore that does not heal
U—unusual bleeding or discharge
T—thickening or extension of a lump
I—indigestion or difficulty swallowing (dysphagia)
O—obvious change in a wart or mole
N—nagging cough or hoarseness

Physical Effects of Cancer

Cancer may start out small and localized, but if left unchecked it will infiltrate or invade local tissues and then travel through the blood supply, in lymph, and even along nerves to adjacent organs or to distant sites as metastatic growth. In an advanced state it can begin to disrupt metabolic processes and cause widespread or systematic symptoms.

Local Effects

- Lumps, lesions, or obstructions
- Infiltration of cancer into adjacent tissues leading to local pain
- Tissue death leading to bleeding and/or infections and pain

Metastatic Effects

- Swollen regional lymph nodes (downstream from tumor)
- Shortness of breath (lung metastases)
- Jaundice (liver metastases)
- Fractures (bone metastases)
- Seizures (brain metastases)

Systemic Effects

- Fever, night sweats (especially in lymphoma)
- Blood disorders, including anemia
- Hormonal and metabolic disorders
- Cachexia (general physical wasting)

Understanding Your Diagnosis

A pathology report—the actual document that defines your cancer—is going to be full of technical jargon and possibly quite confusing to read. The following section is a summary of some of the key information that may be covered and what it means.

Classification of Tumors

A new growth of tissue in the body (a neoplasm) may be classified in four different ways. This information is very significant for treatment planning and prognosis:

- Site or location—where it occurs
- Histogenesis (tissue of origin)—where it began or where it came from (metastases may be distant from the original tumor but still recognizably that tissue)
- Behavior (benign or malignant)—the key question for a diagnosis of cancer
- Primary tumor (growing in the tissue of origin) or secondary/metastatic tumor (growing in a distant site)

Appearance and Behavior of a Tumor

Benign Tumor

- Local
- Well-differentiated cohesive cells
- Usually contained within a fibrous capsule
- Grows from its center outward, with well-defined edges; smooth, rounded, and soft
- Slow growing
- Does not metastasize
- Only dangerous if causing symptoms or compromising vital organs (such as bleeding from a uterine fibroid or difficulty swallowing from a thyroid goiter)
- High oxygen requirement, low glucose requirement; metabolizes efficiently to make 38 units of ATP (the energy currency of the cell) per unit of sugar processed; can readily derive energy from fats as well
- Communicates with neighboring cells; contact inhibition reduces cell growth
- Angiogenesis (new blood vessel growth) occurs only after injury
- Undergoes apoptosis (cell death) when appropriate

Malignant Tumor (Cancer, High-Grade Cancer)

- Rough, irregular, and hard
- Incohesive and disorganized cells; poorly differentiated
- Evasion of immune surveillance
- Fails to undergo apoptosis (cell death); cells become "immortal"
- Rapid and continued growth; insensitivity to inhibitory signals
- Direct invasion of edges into neighboring tissues
- Metastasizes readily; cancer is a "systemic" disease, with approximately 50 percent of patients going on to develop metastatic disease
- Often outgrows blood supply; cell death from lack of oxygenation (known as ischemic necrosis)
- Low oxygen requirement, high glucose requirement; metabolizes inefficiently to make just 2 units of ATP (the energy currency of the cell) per unit of sugar processed; can use fat and protein for energy, but not first choice
- Poor cell-to-cell communication; failure of contact inhibition

Low-Grade Malignant Tumor (Low-Grade Cancer, Indolent Cancer)

- Subclinical tumors that often cannot be felt or noticed by the patient (only by imaging or blood tests)
- Fewer and less severe mutations than high-grade cancer
- Somewhat disorganized cells; moderately differentiated
- Fails to undergo apoptosis (cell death)
- Moderate continued growth, not unlimited and not rapid
- Usually noninvasive and nonmetastatic

CLASSIFICATION BY TISSUE OF ORIGIN		
Type of Tissue	**Benign**	**Malignant**
Germ cells (ovary or testes)	Dermoid cyst	Teratoma
Surface epithelium (skin)	Papilloma	Carcinoma
Glandular epithelium (lining cells)	Adenoma	Adenocarcinoma
Fibrous connective tissue (muscle)	Fibroma	Fibrosarcoma
Fatty connective tissue	Lipoma	Liposarcoma
Vascular tissue	Angioma	Angiosarcoma
Lymph nodes	Lymphadenopathy	Lymphoma

Other cancer types include osteosarcoma in bone, leiomyosarcoma in smooth muscle, leukemia in white blood cells, and myeloma in bone marrow.

Critical Differences between Dysplasia and Cancer

The presence of abnormal cells in tissues is classified as dysplasia. There are some key differences between dysplasia and cancer. Dysplasia is noninvasive, but it exists on a continuum where it readily progresses to *carcinoma in situ*—a localized cancer. Dysplastic cells don't spread deeply and surgical removal is usually curative, although terrain and overall health and well-being will need attention to prevent recurrence. This is why regular Pap smears to identify dysplastic cells in the cervix are so helpful. These are readily treated before they become cervical cancer, which is quite resistant to treatment. Of course, even better is preventing cervical dysplasia in the first place; it's usually caused by certain strains of human papilloma virus (HPV), also known as genital warts.

Cellular and Tissue Changes Associated with Malignant Transformation

- Dysplasia—abnormal cells, abnormal tissue architecture, noninvasive, partially reversible
- Anaplasia—abnormal cells, abnormal tissue architecture, invasive, not reversible without treatment

Measuring the Extent of Cancer

One established way of measuring cancer is to assess the doubling rate of cells. Left to its own devices, cancer would show exponential growth; cells would divide without constraint and continue to double indefinitely. This is the case in early tumor growth, but limitations in availability of nutrients, oxygen, and space mean that exponential growth is tempered by inhibiting factors. Growth varies depending on the type of cancer, as well as by the individual patient. Estimates are made of the average doubling rates for specific types of cancers, and these are used to assess prognosis, but they are always somewhat inaccurate due to the range of individual patient factors.

CANCERS THAT GROW SLOWLY OR QUICKLY

Medicine is a constantly evolving art, and nowhere is this seen more readily than in oncology. The dividing line between an indolent cancer and an active or aggressive cancer is one such moving target, and it is by no means inevitable that a slow-growing cancer will progress to be an aggressive cancer. This has immense implications in treatment planning, and even the classifications of some types of prostate cancer and breast cancer are being questioned now. For example, a woman diagnosed with ductal carcinoma in situ (DCIS) 10 years ago would have been subjected to the full gamut of surgery, chemotherapy, and radiation, whereas today the treatment strategy is much more conservative.

Some cancers, such as prostate cancer, can grow so slowly that "watchful waiting" is often recommended for an early-stage diagnosis, on the basis that active treatment may be worse than letting the disease play out slowly. Indeed, if you are a man over the age of 70 who is diagnosed with prostate cancer, there is a high probability that your cancer will never progress to a severe state. Unfortunately, watchful waiting in the conventional medical model means sitting back and doing nothing, which for the holistic practitioner and for most patients is untenable. This situation is actually a very good opportunity for a holistic practitioner to instigate an active management plan to keep the cancer from growing and developing, if not to reverse it entirely.

On the other hand, patients with a high stage or grade of cancer or with a rapidly doubling cancer are likely to be rushed into aggressive medical treatments with no time to spare, and will then use natural therapies for recovery from surgery, chemotherapy, or radiation before being able to address lifestyle issues or deeper constitutional imbalances.

STAGING AND GRADING

The *stage* refers to the extent to which cancer has spread in the body. The *grade* refers to the extent to which the cancer cells resemble their tissue of origin. The higher the stage or grade, the worse the prognosis.

Stages

- Stage 0: early lesion or cellular abnormality, not yet a measurable tumor
- Stage 1: in situ (localized, not spread)
- Stage 2: invading adjacent tissues
- Stage 3: distant metastases

Grades

- Grade 1: well differentiated
- Grade 2: moderately differentiated
- Grade 3: slightly differentiated
- Grade 4: poorly differentiated

TNM (TUMOR, NODE, AND METASTASES) CLASSIFICATION

Each tumor is given a number from 1 to 4 to indicate its severity. Gradations of T1a, b, c, and so on describe the nuances of a specific cancer. Gradations of N describe the degree to which the cancer has spread to lymph nodes. Gradations of M describe the degree to which the cancer has spread outside of the original location (other than to lymph nodes).

For example:

- T1, N0, M0—localized tumor, no lymph node involvement, no metastases
- T4, N4, M3—highly graded and staged tumor, considerable lymph node involvement, marked metastases

This classification is sometimes also written as pT, N, M, indicating the diagnosis was made based on pathology slides, or cT, N, M, indicating it was made based on clinical findings and scans with no slides. Each type of cancer may have its own unique subclassification criteria as well, such as the Gleason score in prostate cancer or the FIGO staging for uterine cancer.

Poor Differentiation of Cells

One of the key features of a progressed cancer is that the cells are high grade, meaning that they are poorly differentiated and no longer closely resemble the tissue of origin, and they do not necessarily behave as the original tissue might have. The less the degree of differentiation, the higher the grade of the cancer, so a grade 1 cancer still resembles the tissue of origin while a grade 4 cancer is barely recognizable as any specific tissue.

It is not unknown for a patient to present with a late-stage cancer and multiple metastases where the primary tumor location is never identified because differentiation is so degraded that the original tissue can no longer be determined.

Critical to overcoming cancer is the capacity of cells to properly differentiate as they replicate, so that they resemble and behave like the tissue of origin and are more likely to respond to cellular controls. It is worth noting here that differentiation occurs immediately after cell division, and therefore agents that promote differentiation are likely to be most active in those cells that are actively dividing—ironically, in the more aggressive cancers. This does not mean that supporting differentiation isn't helpful in an earlier stage, because any cell can become malignant anytime it copies. However, it is possible that these agents may offer greater benefits in more de-differentiated aggressive cancer.

Factors That Contribute to the Initiation of Cancer

In addition to inherited genetic predispositions or gene defects, the onset of cancer may be triggered by any of the following contributing factors: tobacco and alcohol; viruses, parasites, and infections; environmental toxins; hormones and xenoestrogens; stress, distress, anxiety, and loneliness; disturbed sleep; poor diet, insufficient exercise, and chronic inflammation; and ionizing radiation. These many and variable factors may all play a role in causing gene mutations.

Worldwide, tobacco and alcohol contribute to the most cancer diagnoses. Tobacco smoking doesn't just cause lung cancer; it contributes to or causes cancers all over the body, including in the mouth, throat, kidneys, cervix, liver, bladder, pancreas, stomach, colon, rectum, and even blood. There is a similar long list for cancers caused by alcohol consumption. There may be many dietary and lifestyle recommendations for supporting health and resisting cancer, but it's likely that none of them are as important as quitting tobacco and alcohol.

By the time of diagnosis, it's too late to avoid the triggers of a lifetime, but positive changes in lifestyle are still encouraged. Even after apparently successful treatment, cancer cells may persist and grow again, sometimes many years later. Recurrence can occur near the site of the original cancer (local recurrence); this may be inhibited by radiotherapy after the original diagnosis. Cancer can also recur in lymph nodes near the original site (regional recurrence) or elsewhere in the body (distant recurrence or metastasis). Eating a varied and nutrient-dense diet with little or no refined sugars, practicing stress management, ensuring good sleep quality, avoiding toxin exposure, quitting smoking, restricting alcohol intake, and getting regular exercise are all self-care strategies that may help resist recurrence as much as they may help resist cancer development in the first place.

Research suggests that anywhere from 45 to 65 percent of cancers could be avoided through diet and lifestyle changes, and the percentage may be even higher if we could avoid all environmental toxins as well. Because diet and exercise also benefit overall metabolic health, an added benefit would be less heart disease, less obesity, and less diabetes—all the biggest killers of the developed world.

Where You Live

Where you live affects your chances of getting certain types of cancer. Some cancers are directly linked to particular locations. For example, there is an increased risk of lung cancer with prolonged exposure to radon, so people who live in areas with a lot of granite (which emits high levels of radon) may be at a higher risk. Although there are no hard-and-fast rules, and there are innumerable factors that can influence an individual's chances of developing cancer, there may also be differences in types of cancer from one part of the world to another attributable to regional cultural practices or dietary habits. Cancers of the cervix, mouth, throat, esophagus, and liver are more prevalent in developing countries, possibly due to foodborne toxins and carcinogens such as aflatoxins (molds) on seeds and grains, as well as exposure to endemic viruses or parasites. In Europe and North America, cancers of the lung, breast, colon, prostate, and uterus predominate, possibly caused by high intake of animal fats, excessive xenoestrogen exposures, and a low-fiber diet. In Australia, skin cancer is vastly more common in the white population than in Aboriginal peoples, clearly indicating sun exposure and skin burning as a causative factor.

Researchers who follow ethnic groups that migrate often note that they tend to take on the cancer incidence pattern of the host country within one to two generations. For example, breast cancer is relatively uncommon in women in Japan, but within two generations of emigration to the United States, their descendants will exhibit almost the same incidence as American-born women who are not of Japanese descent. Again, this points to the importance of lifestyle or environmental factors in initiating cancer. These are the so-called epigenetic factors that can determine whether procancer or anticancer genes are switched on or off.

Exposure to Toxins

Cancer has been described in medical literature for thousands of years, but the first type that was recognized as associated with a specific toxic agent was scrotal skin cancer found in young chimney sweeps in Victorian England. In that case, exposure to soot was a trigger for cancer. This risk has only increased with increasing industrialization. For example, a study published as long ago as 1997 in *The Lancet* revealed that patients who contracted non-Hodgkin's lymphoma had dramatically higher blood levels of polychlorinated biphenyls (PCBs)—toxic chemicals widely used in industry—than did others who were demographically similar but remained cancer-free. Childhood leukemias have been linked to toxin exposure, and children have an increased risk of cancer if they live within a few miles of certain kinds of industries, especially those involving large-scale use of petroleum or chemical solvents.

DETOXIFICATION

For the last few hundred years, it has been a common folk medicine belief that cancer occurs in the body where toxins accumulate, and that cellular wastes, whether from the environment or from metabolic activities of the cells, could contribute to a cancer-promoting environment in the body. It is still common today for natural health practitioners to approach cancer with detoxification

SOME INDUSTRIAL TOXINS AND THE CANCERS THEY CAN CAUSE	
Toxin	**Cancer Type**
Arsenic	Bladder, lung, and skin
Asbestos	Mesothelioma
Chlorination by-products, such as trihalomethanes	Bladder
Industrial solvents	Leukemia and non-Hodgkin's lymphoma (caused by benzene); bladder (caused by tetrachloroethylene)
Pesticides	Leukemia and non-Hodgkin's lymphoma
Petrochemicals, including motor vehicle exhaust	Bladder, lung, and skin

programs and liver support programs. Some of these programs can be quite demanding, involving extensive juice fasting and daily enemas, and definitely are not suited to all patients. Other detox programs are more moderate, but all involve some degree of diet limitation and cellular/organ detoxification practices.

The principle behind these programs is to limit ingestion of macronutrients (carbohydrates, fats, and proteins) but to maintain good provision of essential phytochemicals and micronutrients that are critical for metabolic processes, as well as to manage or increase intake of fiber, probiotics, and noncaloric fluids. Natural health practitioners may prescribe green plant juices with minimal to no fruits or root vegetables, plain green salads, supplements that promote phase I and II detox pathways in the liver, and herbs that promote bowel functions, as needed. The idea is that the liver can rest from processing macronutrients, while liver detoxification enzymes are supported by the micronutrients and phytonutrients. (This principle is addressed further in the section on liver support; see page 49.)

Natural health practitioners have been promoting the principles of detoxification in treating cancer for more than a hundred years, and there is a wealth of anecdotal evidence and case reports supporting its benefits. There is, however, scant evidence of robust or reproducible research to validate the process or the outcomes. That is not to say that detoxification doesn't help. However, it is unlikely that a 2- or 3-week detoxification plan—even if followed by a healthy, well-balanced diet—will overcome an existing cancer. A more realistic expectation is for a detoxification plan to enhance the health and resilience of the overall terrain, improve tolerance of chemotherapy and reduce its symptoms and side effects, and possibly promote resistance of recurrence. In addition, many of the popular detox treatments could have all kinds of beneficial effects that have nothing to do with the liver. For example, eating a diet that is very high in fruit and vegetables provides all kinds of micronutrients and can take the place of harmful foods, whether or not it actually helps remove carcinogens from the body.

The Relationship between Hormones and Cancer

Many cancers (including breast, bone, brain, melanoma, uterus, prostate, and lung cancer) may be promoted by proliferative hormones—notably estrogen, as well as testosterone and cortisol, which mediate stress responses and the immune system.

Increased exposure to estrogen. Lifetime estrogen exposure for women is higher today compared to in the time of our ancestors, due to better childhood nutrition leading to a younger age of puberty and menarche (onset of menses), having fewer children, experiencing menopause later, using estrogen replacement therapy, and being obese (abdominal fat has aromatase enzymes that make estrogen from testosterone). Exposure to estrogen decreases with the number of pregnancies and with prolonged breast feeding, which reduces total estrogen production. The risk for endometrial cancer increases with lifetime exposure to estrogen, particularly when the estrogen is unopposed by progesterone, and this is also likely to be a contributing factor in other estrogen-responsive cancers such as lung, bone, and brain, as well as breast cancer.

In modern times, breast cancer is the leading cancer diagnosed in women. Women today have a substantially greater degree of body fat compared to women in times past, leading to earlier menarche and later menopause, and hence a prolonged exposure to ovarian estrogens and progesterone. Women today have a higher risk of estrogen-driven cancers than they have historically because of both modern reproductive choices (such as having fewer children) and exposure to synthetic estrogens. In times past, a woman was usually married shortly after menarche and was mostly pregnant or breastfeeding for the next 15–20 years, possibly having only 30–50 menstrual periods in her lifetime. Hence, she had an overall low estrogen exposure. (I am not actually advocating for women to have more children, but there is no denying that pregnancies and breastfeeding give cumulative protection against breast cancer.) In the treatment of estrogen-driven breast cancer, estrogen receptors are targeted by drugs such as tamoxifen, which blocks alpha-receptors in the breast, and the newer aromatase inhibitor drugs that downregulate estrogen production in fat cells.

Synthetic hormones. Xenoestrogens (synthetic estrogens from outside the body) are found in ordinary substances such as detergents, cosmetics, plastics, pesticides, and herbicides. These mimic a woman's own estrogen signaling and have endocrine-disrupting properties that may cause long-lasting repercussions on reproductive health and contribute to estrogen-sensitive cancers. This is also a concern for men, because estrogens contribute to bone, brain, and prostate cancer, among others, and men's exposures to xenoestrogens are just as great as women's.

Phytoestrogens. These are plant compounds that are either steroidal or isoflavone in nature. They act as selective estrogen receptor modifiers (SERMs), and thus they are agonist (stimulating) or antagonist (inhibiting) to estrogen receptors. Overall, they tend to modulate and balance estrogen responses. This neatly illustrates the conundrum of the SERMs, whereby phytoestrogens can actually be dual acting under different circumstances or in different environments and can actually balance and normalize hormones. These phytoestrogens include isoflavones from soybeans, lentils, and other legumes; coumestans from legume sprouts; prenylflavonoids from hops; and lignans from whole grains, flax, fruits, and vegetables. The isoflavones from soy have been especially well researched in this regard; the isoflavones from fermented soy (such as tempeh or miso) are effective in downregulating, and therefore inhibiting, many cancer-promoting cell pathways.

Intriguing evidence suggests that the normal bacteria in a person's colon make a huge difference in whether phytoestrogens are active in the person's body. The phytoestrogens in food can be thought of as precursors, and they require certain colon bacteria to convert them into forms that are well absorbed and active in the body. Studies suggest that one overlooked, long-term adverse effect of antibiotic overuse is increasing cancer risk by interfering with the colon flora and reducing the degree to which these healthy molecules are formed. Many phytoestrogenic chemicals also have specific anticancer effects, in addition to their effects on estrogen receptors.

Ways to Avoid Environmental Estrogens

- Avoid using hormone replacement therapy (HRT) for menopause, and if you must use it, avoid unopposed estrogen (that is, estrogen taken without progesterone).
- Don't use plastic film wrap for foods, especially for anything oily like cheese or butter.
- Don't use plastic food containers or water bottles, especially those that might go into a microwave.
- Eat only organic foods whenever possible.

NUTRIENTS FOR ASSISTING IN REMOVAL OF ESTROGENS

The following micronutrients are essential cofactors in catalyzing some of the enzyme reactions involved in liver detox pathways. They can be taken as supplements for a high dose and a fast response, and they can be included in dietary form for a longer-term benefit.

Calcium-D-glucarate. This is found in many fruits and vegetables, especially oranges, grapefruit, apples, and cruciferous vegetables (cabbage and its cousins). Taken as a supplement, it can inhibit beta-glucuronidase, an enzyme produced by colonic microflora. Calcium-D-glucarate is also a cofactor in phase II liver detoxification. It may reduce the risk of certain hormone-dependent cancers such as breast, prostate, and colon cancer.

Choline. This is found in meat, poultry, fish, dairy products, and eggs, as well as cruciferous vegetables and many beans, nuts, seeds, and whole grains. It is a source of methyl groups used in many metabolic steps, including replicating DNA correctly, as well as promoting liver detox pathways. It is required to make acetylcholine, the primary neurotransmitter of the parasympathetic nervous system, which activates metabolism, stimulates digestion, and promotes relaxation.

3,3'-diindolylmethane (DIM). This is a metabolite of indole-3-carbinol (I3C), found in cruciferous vegetables. It is an anti-inflammatory with liver-protective and anticancer properties. It promotes phase I detox in the liver. Some practitioners prefer to use I3C supplements, but this is an unstable molecule with low oral bioavailability, and use of DIM may give more consistent responses. In a dietary (food) form, however, I3C is antimicrobial, antioxidant, antiviral, and anti-inflammatory and has anticancer activities.

Folate. This is another methyl donor, found in leafy greens.

L-methionine or S-adenosylmethionine (SAMe). These are methyl donors. Methionine is found in meat, fish, dairy products, nuts, and grains; SAMe is made in the body from methionine. SAMe is also used as a supplement for chronic fatigue and brain fog, memory enhancement, and cognitive impairment.

Magnesium. This is a key micronutrient for proper liver function, found in whole grains, dark green leafy vegetables, beans and other legumes, nuts, milk, and yogurt.

N-acetylcysteine (NAC). This is a supplement manufactured from the amino acid cysteine. Cysteine can also be found in foods; poultry, yogurt, eggs, and garlic have especially high levels of it. It is used to make glutathione (an antioxidant produced in the liver) and is protective to the lungs as well.

Selenium, vitamin B6, and vitamin B12. These micronutrients all promote detox pathways by acting as cofactors with specific enzyme series. They are found in Brazil nuts (selenium) and in whole grains and beans (B6) and meat (B12).

Viral and Bacterial Infections

Viruses may contribute to more than 10 percent of all cancers worldwide, including human papillomavirus (HPV), which causes genital warts and triggers cervical and anorectal cancer; hepatitis C virus, which causes liver cancer; and the Epstein Barr virus, which contributes to Burkitt's lymphoma and

Hodgkin's disease. Bacteria may also be a culprit; for example, *Helicobacter pylori* bacteria may contribute to gastric cancer through chronic gastric inflammation.

Viral infections may take many years to trigger cancer. For example, it can take up to 20 years after contracting hepatitis C for liver cancer to be diagnosed. This is like a smoldering fire in the immune system that can cause chronic, subclinical inflammation, so identifying viral infections and addressing them with an active herbal and/or pharmaceutical plan is important as a cancer-prevention strategy. For example, there are drugs that can cure hepatitis C and thus prevent progression to liver cancer, but this is not something we can realistically expect from herbs alone. If the virus cannot be eliminated (as is the case with Epstein Barr virus), then active management is required long term. Some of the herbs that can be used to fight viruses are quite generic in action; for example, taheebo works throughout the body. Others are more targeted to specific tissues or organs; for example, greater celandine tends to work in the subdiaphragmatic areas, and andrographis has particular focus in the liver and gallbladder. Some of these herbs have active anticancer effects as well.

Herbs with Antiviral Properties

Not every herb targets every virus. Some are very specific to certain viruses, such as St. John's wort for Epstein Barr virus or licorice for hepatitis C. For this reason, it is important to consult with your natural health practitioner when deciding if one of these herbs could be right for you, or to confirm that the herb chosen addresses the problematic pathogen.

- Andrographis
- Baikal skullcap
- Bupleurum
- Garlic
- Greater celandine
- Japanese knotweed
- Licorice
- Oregon grape
- Kutki

Cytotoxic Herbs

These moderately potent herbs are also antiviral or antibacterial. They are safe for topical use but should be used internally only under advisement of a qualified practitioner.

- Bloodroot
- Chaparral
- Pokeroot
- Thuja

Stress, Distress, Anxiety, and Loneliness

For more than 2,000 years, since the time of Galen (the Roman doctor who codified a system of medicine based on the four qualities of hot, cold, wet, and dry, and the four humors that arose from them), it has been understood that people with a "melancholic" disposition were more susceptible to cancer than "sanguine" people. Modern research has clearly demonstrated that mood and mindset, outlook, and constitution are factors in well-being, and that persistent activation of the hypothalamic-pituitary-adrenal (HPA) axis, as a result of chronic stress, is a key contributor to cancer.

The HPA axis is the pathway from the brain to the pituitary gland to the adrenal glands, and it controls adrenal cortex functions. The adrenal glands should produce cortisol under stress, but this production was never intended to be continuous, and the glands become increasingly large and overactive with chronic stress. The process of pouring out more and more cortisol over time trying to deal with stress will ultimately be destructive to the body. Unresolved stress and persistently high cortisol contribute to depression, impair immune responses, and promote development and progression of some types of cancer. (In fact, there is a whole discipline, called psychoneuroimmunology, that studies the interplay between mental states and immunology.)

Herbs that modulate stress responses are called adaptogens; these are explored in more detail in Chapter 2. Adaptogenic herbs build vital force (healing capacity, resilience, and immune resistance in the body), sustain energy outputs and support recuperation and restoration after exertion, normalize mitochondrial energy production, support resistance to disease, promote healing, and retard cellular aging. Adaptogens can also normalize the HPA axis and the hypothalamic-pituitary-thyroid (HPT) axis, meaning they can stabilize metabolic demands and energy utilization.

> A sad soul can kill you quicker, far quicker, than a germ.
>
> JOHN STEINBECK, *TRAVELS WITH CHARLEY*

STRESS AND TRAUMA

Chronic stress or distress adversely influences neurochemical, hormonal, and immunological functioning and, if left unresolved will eventually cause chronic low-grade inflammation, which can promote cancer. Studies in mice suggest that chronic stress causes elevated levels of stress hormones, greater tumor burden, and an invasive pattern of ovarian cancer growth, as well as increased tumor blood vessel growth. Stress hormones promote enzymes that weaken connective tissue and facilitate cancer spread. Stress also increases growth factors that promote angiogenesis (production of new blood vessels). Both stress and depression are associated with decreased cytotoxic T cell and

NK cell activities, impairing immune responses and immune surveillance and promoting gene instability.

Stress contributes to the onset of cancer and also plays a significant role in the body's defense or management of cancer. Breast cancer patients with elevated levels of cortisol appear to be at higher risk for metastasis. A study of women with breast cancer showed that those who had abnormal cortisol rhythms survived an average of 3.2 years, while those with normal rhythms survived an average of 4.5 years. Suppression of NK cell count and NK function in these women appeared to be a mediator or a marker of more rapid disease progression.

There is a strong association between prolonged stress and a pro-inflammatory tissue state conducive to both the onset of cancer and the progression of cancer. Psychological stress may also mediate immunosuppression by altering the expression of transcription factors in the nucleus of the cell. In a study of past experiences of traumatic life events among 94 women with metastatic or recurrent breast cancer, there was a significantly longer disease-free interval among women who had reported no traumatic or stressful life events (median = 62 months) compared to those who had experienced one or more stressful or traumatic life events (combined median = 31 months). These findings confirm that life stress can have long-lasting effects on stress response systems such as the HPA axis.

SOCIAL ISOLATION

Wellness can be defined as physical, emotional, spiritual, and intellectual vitality—cultivating emotions and engaging in activities that enhance our quality of life. A true state of being "well" is not merely a condition of the individual. Our wellness exists when it is interrelated with the wellness of family, community, and environment. Disease can manifest physically, emotionally, psychologically, and spiritually and often involves many or all of these. Ultimately, to be well, I believe, you must give love, receive love, and feel a true sense of belonging and purpose. Having strong family ties and a sense of community is protective against cancer, and conversely, feeling lonely and isolated increases risk. Higher levels of social embeddedness and support are associated with better survival from breast, colorectal, and lung cancer.

In a study of women with ovarian carcinoma, those who reported higher levels of social interaction and well-being had lower levels of vascular endothelial growth factor (VEGF), a protein produced by cancer that encourages new blood vessel growth. Elevated levels of VEGF are associated with shortened survival. Greater support from friends and neighbors and less geographic distance from friends were aspects of social well-being associated with lower VEGF levels. Individuals who reported greater helplessness or worthlessness had higher VEGF levels, but depression as a whole was not related to VEGF levels.

This speaks to the great importance of emotional well-being in fighting back against cancer. If anxiety, depression, and fear are predominant emotions for you, then seeking out counseling or other forms of therapy may be critical to your healing journey, and building or rebuilding meaningful relationships with people you love may be some of the work you need to do.

Dietary Influences

Physical activity, lifestyle, and diet play a crucial role in promoting cancer. The five most important risk factors for developing cancer are high body mass index, low intake of fruit and vegetables, lack of physical activity, use of alcohol, and smoking. An increase in body mass index is associated with an up to 50 percent increased risk of several cancers and involves several mechanisms, including increased estrogens and testosterone, hyperinsulinemia (high levels of insulin in blood) and insulin resistance (type II diabetes), increased inflammation, and depressed immune function.

Randomized clinical trials have shown that physical activity and diet interventions can change biomarkers of cancer risk. Thus, adoption of lifestyle changes may have a large impact on the future incidence of cancer. The Western diet is typically low in fiber and high in red meat, calories, animal fats, trans fats, refined carbohydrates, and sugar. All of these factors tend to increase inflammation, which promotes gut microbiome disturbance and may alter intestinal immunity and contribute to leaky gut syndrome. Inappropriate passage of proteins from the gut to the bloodstream will cause persistent low-grade systemic inflammation and a high level of oxidative stress, all of which promote cancer. The types of cancer that are particularly associated with excess weight include endometrial, gallbladder, renal, rectal, breast, pancreatic, thyroid, colon, and esophageal cancers; leukemia; multiple myeloma; non-Hodgkin's lymphoma; and melanoma.

In my clinical practice, I try not to prescribe rigid diet plans. Telling someone they cannot have things they love rarely works—no to this and no to that, and no fun at all. Rather, I try to highlight all the delicious foods they *can* have. Laying out the principles and giving flexibility, leeway, and choices are usually more successful all around. That might mean a day off a week from all diet restrictions, or it might mean a "sweets allowance"—whatever it takes to get buy-in the rest of the time. My patients will often start with the Clean and Green Detox Diet (page 41) as a sort of jumping-off point or a fresh start to make a renewed commitment to overall healthier diet habits. Allowing some organic meat, fish, fermented dairy, and eggs at the beginning enables people to graduate into it, getting stricter as they go, until they can do the full month, then to work their way back out of it to a healthy maintenance eating plan. The long-term diet is a version of the Mediterranean diet, with allowances

Brighter Days Tea

This tea may be helpful for patients and their families and caregivers who are struggling with grief, sadness, or despair.

DECOCTION BLEND

+ 25 g milky oats (seed)
+ 25 g ashwagandha
+ 25 g silk tree bark
+ 15 g eleuthero root
+ 10 g rhodiola root

INFUSION BLEND

+ 25 g St. John's wort
+ 15 g tulsi tops
+ 15 g hawthorn flower
+ 15 g damiana tops
+ 15 g blue vervain tops
+ 15 g rose petals

Put 1 heaping teaspoon of the decoction blend in a pan with 3–4 cups cold water, cover with a lid, and bring to a boil. Turn the heat down and simmer very low for 15 minutes. Take off the heat and add 2 heaping teaspoons of the infusion blend. Replace the lid and steep for 10 minutes. Drink 2–4 cups daily.

Hawthorn flower, rhodiola root, and rose petals. These are all indicated where there is crushing grief, heartbreak, despondency, and despair. Rhodiola can be astringent (drying in the mouth), so some people prefer a capsule product.

Tulsi, damiana, and silk tree. These are particularly indicated for depression; they lift the dark clouds and bring a sense of hope and possibilities. They are all considered *thymoleptic*, meaning "to raise the spirits" (from the Greek word *thymos*, meaning "temper" or "emotion"). Tulsi is very easy to grow and dry to use in teas year-round.

Milky oats. This is restorative and nutritive to the nervous system, used for hypersensitivity and emotional fragility, and often added to a formula to help us feel more grounded and in touch with the world. Though more commonly seen in a tincture made from fresh unripe (green) seed heads, the dried unripe heads are also popular in teas.

Eleuthero and ashwagandha. These are adaptogens (stress-modulating herbs) for building resilience, resistance, and stress tolerance.

Blue vervain. This is a cooling, calming, bitter herb known to support the emotional body as well as the physical body. It is for people who are having a hard time accepting a situation, blaming themselves or being hard on themselves for things done or undone, and holding themselves to an unreasonably high standard. It is also one of the Bach Flower Remedies, where it has similar properties.

made for personal preferences and choices and periodic repeats of the Clean and Green Detox Diet.

The Mediterranean diet allows unlimited consumption of vegetables, fruits, and legumes, with smaller amounts of nuts, fish, lean meat, whole grains, and some dairy (preferably raw or fermented) and low intake of saturated animal fats. Coupled with some form of intermittent fasting (see page 53), this will provide the dense nutrition required without excess calories and will keep blood sugar at a healthy level.

The Principles of an Anticancer Diet

The key features of an anticancer diet are as follows:

- Regular intake of fruits and vegetables (especially garlic, onions, other alliums, and cruciferous vegetables, such as cabbage, broccoli, Brussels sprouts, and wasabi), with an emphasis on those with dark purple pigments, such as plums, purple carrots and potatoes, and red cabbage
- High dietary intake of selenium, folic acid, vitamins, minerals, and antioxidant phytonutrients such as carotenoids and lycopene
- Plenty of plant fiber (such as whole grains, legumes, and leafy greens)
- Low intake of (preferably fermented) milk and dairy
- Cold-water, oily fish once or twice weekly
- Modest intake of meat and animal products (two to four times weekly); animal fats and oils should not be cooked at high temperatures. Chicken and turkey skin should be avoided, as they are high in carcinogenic heterocyclic amines—even more so if crisped or charred.
- Limited sweets. The best sweet treat is cocoa or very dark chocolate.

Inflammation

Chronic systemic inflammation is a key contributor to all stages of cancer development. Increasing levels of inflammation are seen in the blood by measuring C-reactive protein (CRP) levels and erythrocyte sedimentation rate (ESR or sed rate). These are not routinely done in cancer care but can be requested.

In individuals who experience chronically high levels of subjective social isolation (loneliness), there is impaired transcription of glucocorticoid-response (anti-inflammatory) genes and increased activity of pro-inflammatory genes, which may provide a functional genomic explanation for their elevated risk of cancer. In both human and animal studies, as mentioned above, chronic stress has been shown to cause decreased immunity, leading to hyperinflammatory states (autoimmune conditions), poor production of NK cells and diminished T cell response, and an overall diminished resistance to cancer.

HERBS AND SUPPLEMENTS THAT MODULATE INFLAMMATION

Inflammation-mediating herbs may contain a range of saponins, both steroidal and triterpene, that mimic cortisol (the body's natural anti-inflammatory); these are called "adrenal sparing" herbs, as they may reduce the amount of cortisol overstimulated adrenals make. They have many other mechanisms of action relevant to stress and cancer, including modulating the immune system.

Other herbs may contain salicylates and resins that inhibit cyclooxygenase (COX) and lipoxygenase (LOX) enzymes to reduce inflammatory prostaglandin production. Herbs and supplements that may modulate inflammation include the following.

- **Triterpenes:** bupleurum, licorice, sarsaparilla, wild yam, yucca
- **Resins:** ginger, Indian frankincense
- **Flavonoids:** turmeric
- **Essential fatty acids:** omega-3 fish oil (EPA and DHA)
- **Polyphenols and essential oils:** rosemary, spearmint
- **Salicylates:** willow, meadowsweet, balsam poplar

HERBS WITH HIGH LEVELS OF RESINS AND TRITERPENES

Ginger. This helpful herb should be eaten often. The resins need a solvent—extracting it by sautéing it in cooking oil is effective.

Indian frankincense. Also known as boswellia, this herb contains a resin full of anti-inflammatory triterpene acids called boswellic acid (BA) and its derivatives.

Yucca, licorice, wild yam, sarsaparilla, and bupleurum. These all have triterpene or steroidal saponins with cortisol-like action, are adrenal sparing, and inhibit inflammation.

HERBS WITH HIGH LEVELS OF SALICYLATES

Meadowsweet and willow. Meadowsweet leaves and flowers and willow bark are rich in salicylic acid, which plants produce as part of their defense system against diseases, insects, bacteria, and environmental stress. To properly metabolize and activate plant salicylates for human use, we first have to subject them to fermentation by the gut microbiome. Thus, it is recommended to take prebiotics and probiotics alongside salicylate-rich herbs to optimize activation of constituents.

HERBS WITH HIGH LEVELS OF POLYPHENOLS

Turmeric. This is one of the most intensively studied herbs, and one of the best-selling natural medicines in the US, Canada, and Europe, as well as in India, where it is actually from. Known for its complex of flavonoids and its powerful anti-inflammatory actions across many tissue types, it is used for inflammation of joints, muscles, and soft tissues; of the liver, gallbladder, and large intestine; and of the skin when applied topically. Curcumin extracted from turmeric has now been extensively studied in innumerable cancer cell lines, animal studies, and human studies and has demonstrated anticancer activity through multiple pathways, mostly mediated through inhibition of cyclooxygenase-2.

Rosemary. Rosemary is rich in rosmarinic acid (RA), a caffeic acid ester (a natural polyphenol) notably found in several plants from the mint family, including rosemary, spearmint, and perilla. It has been widely studied as a feed additive in animal husbandry for promoting growth and fertility, lowering oxidative stress states, and enhancing immune profiles. RA acts as an antimicrobial, immunomodulatory, antidiabetic, antiallergic, anti-inflammatory, and liver- and kidney-protective agent. Specifically in cancer, it significantly inhibits an enzyme called microtubule affinity regulating kinase 4 (MARK4) that controls the first steps of cell division. In vitro studies have shown that treatment of cancer cells with RA significantly controls cell growth and subsequently induces apoptosis (cell death).

UV Radiation Exposure

The incidence of skin cancers has been increasing rapidly over the last 50 years or so, especially in fair-skinned people around the world, and it has been attributed to excess sun exposure. An entire industry has built up around sunscreens and sun avoidance, but this has possibly been making the problem worse. Vitamin D is essential for a healthy immune system, especially T cell activation, priming T cells to kill virally infected and cancerous cells, as well as many other critical functions in the body. Because it is made when we have sunlight on our skin, strict sun avoidance or overassiduous use of sunblocks may actually lower vitamin D and compromise immune functions.

There are two types of ultraviolet rays that affect humans: UVA and UVB. UVA rays contribute to the direct damage of DNA and impair the removal of ultraviolet photoproducts. Fair skin and nevi (strawberry birth marks) are major risk factors for melanoma, probably because they both contain large amounts of pheomelanin and its early precursor molecules that absorb UVA1 radiation, which drives mutations.

Ironically, sunscreen formulations usually decrease only UVB doses and successfully prevent sunburn on the surface and the reddening and heat that indicate time to go indoors. This possibly leads to prolonged sun exposure and greater exposure to UVA rays, contributing to increased skin cancers in a dose-dependent manner. Additionally, outdoor sunshine has both UVA and UVB radiation, while sun coming through windows has only UVA radiation (unlike UVB, it can pass through glass). So, if you are indoors a lot to avoid sun exposure but sit near windows, you may not be as protected as you seem.

A 2017 comprehensive worldwide analysis of melanoma incidences and UVB doses for males and females with all six Fitzpatrick skin types (skin phototyping, based on a person's tendency to sunburn and ability to tan) showed no evidence for a significant trend or correlation between the increasing incidences of melanoma and increasing personal UVB dose for males or females of any age group or skin type anywhere in the world. In fact, in Europe, there was a significant correlation between decreasing UVB doses and increasing melanoma for fair-skinned, skin type I to III females over 29 years old. In other words, reduced UVB exposure increases the risk of melanoma; sunlight has a protective effect.

How to Be Safe in the Sun

The best protection is a light tan. Given the understanding that sunscreen lotions can play a role in blocking UVB rays and hindering production of vitamin D, how can we experience the benefits of sunlight without the cancer risk? The best protection against sunburn is judicious exposure early in the season, and early in the day before the sun is strong, to build a base tan. No burning should ever occur; when the skin is just beginning to feel warm to the touch or to look slightly pink, you should move to a shaded area. To calculate how much sun exposure you need to get adequate vitamin D production, as well as your maximum safe sun exposure before burning, follow the link at the end of the references and readings for this chapter, on page 491.

CHAPTER 2

Nutrition and Lifestyle Choices to Inhibit Cancer

It is certainly true that we can't control all the variables that may contribute to cancer. Background radiation, childhood sunburns, and exposure to environmental toxins are some of the burdens on the immune system that we may have to contend with. However, there is no question that personal choices about food, activity, sleep practices, and stress management are critical and impactful on our health and well-being. Even the National Institutes of Health in the US, generally a conservative authority, has suggested that 60–65 percent of cancers could be prevented by better diet and lifestyle.

The advice and suggestions in this chapter are intended for prevention in people who are not diagnosed with cancer, as well as for inhibition of cancer and as a part of a treatment plan for cancer patients. These are the same sort of healthy outlines that I would give in my clinical practice to patients with other chronic degenerative diseases.

CHAPTER 2 CONTENTS

40 Healthy Eating to Restore Vitality

41 The Clean and Green Detox Diet Plan

45 Soy: Anticancer or Procancer?

48 The Role of the Liver in Detoxification

49 Herbs That Protect and Support the Liver

50 Alteratives

51 Essiac Formula

53 Intermittent Fasting

53 Types of Fasting Regimens

54 Restore Bowel Health and Boost the Microbiome

54 Functions of the Gut Microbiome

55 Weeding, Seeding, and Feeding

56 "Weeding" Protocol

58 Support the Immune System

58 Immune Boot Camp

59 Immunostimulating Tincture Formula

60 Immune Boot Camp Nutritional Breakfast Smoothie

61 Deep Immune Tonic Herbs

63 Managing Stress

64 Systemic Effects of Chronic Stress

64 General Adaptation Syndrome

66 Effects of Unresolved Stress

66 Using Adaptogens to Support the Vital Force

67 Benefits of Adaptogens

69 How to Choose Adaptogens

69 Stimulating Adaptogens

71 Restorative and Balancing Adaptogens

74 Nature Therapy for Improved Mental Health

74 Shinrin Yoku: The Practice of Forest Bathing

75 Coping with Grief

76 Herbs for Grief and Sadness

80 The Role of Hallucinogens

80 Promoting Deep and Restful Sleep

81 Circadian Rhythms

81 Good Sleep Hygiene

82 Herbs and Supplements for Better Sleep

84 Melatonin

85 Exercise

Healthy Eating to Restore Vitality

When I first began clinical practice in the late 1980s in Glasgow, Scotland, recommending that people do detox diets and avoid sugar, soda pop, and junk food was definitely an uphill battle. I still remember my amazement and despair one day after spending 15 minutes trying to explain to someone that there truly is such a thing as brown rice and that it is not hard to cook. We've come a long way since then! Today, my conversation is more likely to be about special diets (paleo, keto, macrobiotic, vegan), fermenting, and fasting.

In general, I prefer to have patients focus on developing healthy eating habits, rather than following a specific diet—which can make it seem as if eating well were some sort of penance. The trick to making this work in the long term is to find foods you really like that are actually good for you, and to train your taste buds to like the healthy foods better than those that are sugar laden, salt laden, processed, or fried. However, some people need a jump start or simply want to do a periodic reset. If you are just getting started or if you need to reboot your good intentions, then a month of the Clean and Green Detox Diet (page 41) can give you a useful set of guidelines and a realistic end point.

Choose organic produce. An important part of any healthy diet is choosing organic produce. According to the Environmental Working Group (EWG), a US not-for-profit organization, nearly 70 percent of the nonorganic fresh produce sold in the US contains residues of potentially harmful chemicals, including carcinogenic and neurotoxic fungicides, pesticides, and herbicides routinely sprayed on food crops. Every year EWG analyzes test data from the US Department of Agriculture and publishes an updated list of Dirty Dozen and Clean Fifteen foods; these are the foods that are most important to buy organic and those that are less harmful, based on the number of different chemical residues they contain. I recommend purchasing only organic foods if possible; when your budget does not allow for that, check these lists to make the best choices you can.

Guidelines for Eating to Promote Good Digestion

- Ensure that you are relaxed when you eat. Take 2 minutes of quiet time before diving into your food, light a candle, close your eyes, say a prayer, or speak some words of gratitude for the meal. This helps switch from adrenaline-driven activity mode (sympathetic nervous system) to acetylcholine-driven relaxation mode (parasympathetic nervous system) and is critical to good digestion.
- Always put your food on a plate and sit to eat, even for a snack; don't stand in the kitchen and eat from saucepans.
- Avoid watching the news or scary shows while eating, and avoid distressing conversations at the table. Don't eat in a hurry or if you are upset—better to miss a meal.
- Take bitter herbs or eat a green salad with unsweetened dressing before the main meal.

- If the bitters are unpalatable, then 10 minutes before your meal, chew slowly on two paper-thin slices of fresh gingerroot with a sliver of fresh lime (including the skin), a pinch of cayenne, and a grain of sea salt on each. This promotes salivation and kick-starts the digestive process.
- Use the Stomach Settler Seed Sprinkle (page 201) as a tasty carminative digestive aid.
- Drink lemon balm, lemongrass, lemon verbena, chamomile, linden, or mint tea after a meal.

The Clean and Green Detox Diet Plan

I usually ask patients to follow this strict plan for 2 nonconsecutive days per week for 4 weeks, to ease themselves into it, then to do it for 1 whole week. After that, they can revert to 2 nonconsecutive days per week for another month. For a longer-term maintenance plan, I suggest repeating it 1 day per week and 1 weekend per month for as long as they want to keep it up.

Generally, I recommend eating whole vegetables and fruits, not juicing them and losing the fiber. However, for a short-term detox plan, maximizing the other phytonutrients is important, so juicing is suggested for a few days to get a high volume of plant extract.

Do not do this type of restrictive diet if you are pregnant or breastfeeding or if you are notably debilitated, depleted, and weak. If you have high or low blood sugar or high or low blood pressure, you should undertake a program like this only under the supervision of a qualified healthcare professional. Also note that this diet is relatively high in oxalates, so it may not be recommended for people with kidney stones or with interstitial cystitis.

Keep in mind that there are limitations to what we can expect from detoxification or tissue cleansing; fasting will not cure cancer. And while weight loss may be recommended for some people, in others the concern of cachexia, or general physical wasting, requires feeding, not starving. However, if nothing else, this diet plan serves as a good benchmark for kicking off some generally healthier eating habits and bringing more awareness to how you eat and how you feel when you eat.

What to Eat on the Strictest Days

- Unlimited green juices: cucumber, celery, parsley, spinach, cabbage, fennel, kale, watercress, and other green vegetables
- Smaller amounts of beet greens, Swiss chard, and wild greens if you can gather them from unpolluted places, including dandelion, chickweed, miner's lettuce, purslane, sheep sorrel, and nettle
- One or two servings daily of jicama, green apple, carrot, or beet to sweeten the green juice

- Unlimited steamed leafy vegetables: broccoli, savoy or red cabbage, bok choy, spinach, Brussels sprouts, kale, collards, turnip greens, red chard, or beet greens
- One serving daily of whole grain: quinoa, millet, brown rice, amaranth, buckwheat (kasha), oats, or corn
- Dress grains and leafy greens with lemon juice, balsamic vinegar, liquid aminos sauce, or soy sauce, as well as seaweed sprinkle, nutritional yeast, or fresh herbs as desired; no oil
- Two servings daily of fresh or frozen fruit; best are blueberries, blackberries, raspberries, purple plums, cherries, apples, or pears

What to Add the Rest of the Time

- Add one or two more servings of whole grain daily, or a starchy vegetable like carrot, beet, potato, sweet potato, or squash.
- For fats, use cultured butter, ghee, small amounts of full-fat dairy if tolerated, olive oil, or coconut oil.
- Aim for 60–70 grams of protein daily, including nuts, seeds, and nut butters; beans/pulses, tempeh, occasional tofu, or animal products if desired. If you want meat, make it organic, free-range chicken and turkey two or three times weekly; organic grass-fed lamb, venison, or other lean wild meats one or two times a week; and North Sea or cold-water fish such as salmon, sardines, herring, halibut, and mackerel two or three times a week. Avoid farmed fish altogether.
- Sweet tropical fruits such as banana, mango, pineapple, and papaya can be an occasional treat.

ADDITIONAL RECOMMENDATIONS

Choose good oils. Use only high-quality, organic, cold-pressed vegetable oils. The best oil for cooking is olive oil as it oxidizes the least when heated. Some butter is okay so long as it is organic and from grass-fed cows, which will ensure that it contains conjugated linoleic acid, a fatty acid that is anabolic (builds muscle) and helps manage cachexia (general physical wasting). It also contains butyric acid, which has direct anticancer effects in the bowel. Coconut oil is another good choice for cooking; it contains antiviral and antifungal fatty acids (although whether they survive extraction, cooking, and digestion is uncertain). Nut oils and nut butters can be used as condiments on food but should not be cooked.

Eat colorful fruits and vegetables. Emphasize orange, red, and purple fruits; citrus fruits; and berries for their polyphenols and flavonoids that are antioxidant.

Steam cabbage and its cousins. Broccoli, cauliflower, Brussels sprouts, cabbage, kale, and other members of the cabbage family are especially rich in sulfur-containing isothiocyanates that help the liver generate glutathione, an important detoxification compound. For this reason, they should be eaten frequently, but it is best if they are lightly steamed or otherwise cooked because they can slow the thyroid if eaten raw too often. Eat plenty of garlic, leeks, shallots, and onions—these are also rich in sulfur compounds.

Add mushrooms. All edible mushrooms are good: shiitake, oyster, portobello, lion's mane. Cook them well to access their immunomodulating beta-glucans.

Top dishes with dried seaweed and miso paste. Seaweed and miso (fermented soybean paste) can be eaten regularly. They supply vitamins, minerals, and trace elements and add great taste to food. Be sure to get seaweeds from suppliers that are testing for heavy metals, as they can concentrate in seaweed and accumulate in the body.

Eat for maximum nutrition. In ancient times our hunter-gatherer ancestors sought out the foods that provided the most caloric value for the least effort, as this could be a matter of life or death. This is still seen in our primate relatives, who will take fruits and sweet foods over leaves and roots if given the choice. This tendency to choose food for sugar and caloric value is explained by the "thrifty gene hypothesis," which suggests that craving sweet foods is an inborn instinctual behavior to achieve maximum calorie input for minimal effort.

Unfortunately, in the modern world, we have largely stripped the phytonutrients, vitamins, minerals, and other nutritional factors out of the sugary foods, and hence we see an apparently uncontrollable epidemic of obesity and diabetes, heart disease, and cancers, as people are unconsciously driven by their primitive survival genes to seek out calorie-rich foods (assisted and enabled by the sugar and fast-food industry, but that is a different discussion).

> To cure permanently any case of cancer, we must have good digestion to make good blood; and if we can make good blood, we first can fortify the system against the inroads of cancer.
>
> ELI JONES (1850–1933), MEDICAL DOCTOR AND CANCER SPECIALIST

The Role of Sugar in the Progression of Cancer

In addition to the dysbiosis it causes, sugar also plays a role in actively helping cancer grow and spread. Cancer cells require a lot of energy to fuel their fast metabolism, but they are extremely inefficient at making it, and as a result, cancer cells are always hungry for more sugar to fuel their growth. This metabolic process produces a lot of lactic acid and creates a low pH that benefits the growth of cancer. These metabolic derangements are behind the traditional recommendations of avoiding sugar in cancer and eating lots of fruits and vegetables that can help with detoxification of acid wastes. For more information on this phenomenon (called "glycolytic shift"), see page 366.

Recent research into the gut microbiome has suggested that eating sugary foods will feed certain strains of bacteria that then crave sugary foods for themselves, and because of the close link between the gut and the brain through a range of neurotransmitters, this dysbiosis (microbial imbalance) may become a self-perpetuating feedback loop that causes overeating, weight gain, and all the attendant problems therein.

If you want to treat, avoid, prevent, or reduce your risk of cancer, then choosing only nutrient-dense foods is one of the best ways to go about it. You don't need to avoid all sweet foods entirely, but there is a wealth of research now confirming how complex carbohydrates and whole-plant sugars may be beneficial in the microbiome of the colon and may have cancer-inhibiting action. In one widespread epidemiological study, complex carbohydrate intake was inversely associated with the risk of several types of cancer. Avoid added sugars, refined carbohydrates, and manufactured foods. These are "empty calories." It takes vitamins, minerals, and other cofactors to process and metabolize sugar into energy, and if these are absent from the food, as is the case with refined sugar, the vitamins, minerals, and other cofactors may be drawn from body reserves. Enjoy fresh fruits, whole grains (especially sprouted grains), and sweeter vegetables such as corn, squash, and carrots.

Eat 60–70 grams of good protein daily to support muscle strength and immune functions; 8–10 servings of fruits and vegetables daily; 50 grams daily of dietary fiber in the form of green vegetables, whole grains, and beans; cold-water fish several times weekly to give you good omega-3 intake; and organic food as much as possible. To boost protein intake, especially if your appetite is low, use an undenatured, cold-processed, microfiltered whey protein powder with immunoglobulins, or use a hemp protein powder as a vegan option. Note that the hemp does not give the same immune fractions that the whey can offer.

Active Anticancer Compounds in Foods

- Allicin, diallyl disulfide, and related compounds from garlic
- Beta-glucans from mushrooms, oats, onions, and nutritional yeast
- Calcium-D-glucarate from apples, grapefruit, grapes, bean sprouts, cauliflower, and cabbage
- Carotenoids from carrots, kale, yams, sweet potatoes, and red peppers
- Curcuminoids from turmeric, ginger, and galangal
- Fiber from whole grains, beans, fruits, and vegetables
- Ellagic acid from strawberries, raspberries, cranberries, loganberries, and marionberries
- Epigallocatechin gallate (EGCG) from black tea and green tea
- Isothiocyanates from cabbage, broccoli, kale, beet greens, turnip greens and root, kohlrabi, mustard greens, Brussels sprouts, and collards
- Isoflavones from fermented soy (miso, natto, tamari), clover, and alfalfa sprouts
- Limonene from citrus juice and peel, especially tangerine, as well as cannabis
- Lycopene from tomatoes, watermelon, and other red fruits and vegetables
- Omega-3 fatty acids from fish, flax oil, and walnuts
- Polyphenols from black tea, green tea, rooibos tea, dark purple/black berries, coffee, cacao, and red wine
- Selenium from shiitake and maitake mushrooms, Brazil nuts, and garlic
- Sulfur from garlic, onions, leeks, shallots, chives, and cabbage-family vegetables (wasabi sprouts, broccoli sprouts)

Soy: Anticancer or Procancer?

Soy has attracted much attention as a potential chemoprotective agent because of its high rate of consumption in Asian countries, such as Japan and China, where the incidence of breast and prostate cancers (among others) is notably lower than in Western populations. In reality, epidemiological and migrant studies have suggested that *multiple* factors—including lifestyle, diet, and fat or fiber intake—may play a role in the etiology of these cancers. In Asia, soy is traditionally consumed as fermented soy foods (tempeh, miso, and natto) as well as nonfermented soy foods (tofu, soybeans, and soy milk), and the average intake is 25–50 mg of isoflavones per day from early childhood. In Europe and North America, daily intake is usually less than 1 mg, mostly from soy flour and soy protein isolates that are found in most processed and prepared foods. It is worth noting here that all legumes have similar chemistry to soy, and that some beans have more of various isoflavones than even soy does. While we don't have as much research on other beans, they still seem to be at least preventive against a range of cancers.

SOY AS A SELECTIVE ESTROGEN RESPONSE MODIFIER (SERM)

Overall, soy has a hormone-balancing effect on the body. The isoflavones in soy, daidzein and genistein, are considered to be phytoestrogens because they function as selective estrogen response modifiers (SERMs), fitting into estrogen receptor sites on cells and acting as partial agonists ("on" switches). The soy isoflavones mainly occur in the plant bound to sugars, which must be removed by bacterial fermentation in the gut before absorption. This indicates that the functional health of the gut is significant in determining the bioavailability and utility of ingested phytoestrogens, and it points to the need for pre- and probiotics in the diet and as supplements. Soy protein isolates used in body-building powders and in power bars are a source of amino acids for nutrition but are not a good source of bioavailable isoflavones, and they are unlikely to have much or any influence on hormones in the body.

Daidzein and genistein are two of the most researched of the isoflavones in soy and other legumes. They are metabolized to compounds called equol and 5-hydroxyequol (respectively) if people have the right gut bacteria. Only these molecules get into the body in amounts significant enough to be active (not the daidzein and genistein themselves). Though equols are not very similar to the structure of estrogens, they activate the same receptors. They can bind reversibly into estrogen receptor sites and have a weakly agonist (stimulating) effect, but significantly less than your own estrogen might offer. However, now the receptor site is occupied, at least temporarily, and your own stronger estrogen cannot dock. This results in an overall lowering of estrogen influence in the body, but the bonding of the phytoestrogens is also readily adjusted by the body in a way that allows agonist/antagonist effects and creates a balance of hormonal influence. These compounds also have been shown to have other anticancer effects unrelated to estrogen receptors.

SOY AND CANCER PREVENTION

Soy isoflavones have antiproliferative, antiangiogenic (reducing the growth of new blood vessels), antioxidative, and anti-inflammatory properties against the cancers that are influenced by estrogens. Multiple studies over many years have confirmed an inverse association between total soy intake and the incidence of breast cancer, especially in premenopausal women. Increased mammographic density is associated with a four- to sixfold increased risk of breast cancer, and higher soy intakes are associated with reduction in breast tissue density in women aged 56–65 compared to age-matched controls.

Soy intake in youth, in particular, reduces the risk for breast cancer development or progression. Animal studies indicate that early life exposure to genistein, the major isoflavone in soy, confers a protective effect against chemically induced breast tumors, and human studies with whole soy foods have confirmed this. Age at exposure is a strong codeterminant of risk, with earlier exposure conferring greater benefit. Women who were high-soy consumers during adolescence demonstrated a 23 percent risk reduction compared to matched controls, and continuing to consume soy in adult life as well increases the risk reduction to 47 percent. Eating little soy in adolescence but more in adult life does not confer any marked advantage. This is clinically significant because it promotes the use of soy as an early preventive but it challenges the overall usefulness of soy products to treat breast cancer in women who have not grown up eating such foods.

One possible mechanism explaining this phenomenon is that eating soy foods in younger life is known to lead to the flourishing of specific gut flora able to metabolize the compounds in the soy, and these microbes are less prevalent in people introducing soy foods later in life.

IS THERE A CASE AGAINST SOY?

There has been some suggestion that the proliferation rate of histologically normal breast tissue in premenopausal women was increased in women taking soy, which suggests that short-term dietary soy supplementation may induce proliferation in breast tissue of premenopausal women. However, this is countered with epidemiologic data showing no studies with an increased breast cancer risk associated with soy consumption.

THE IMPORTANCE OF FERMENTATION

Some studies suggest that soy isoflavones are more bioavailable in food if present as aglycones (as in fermented soy products like tempeh) than when present as glycosides (as in unfermented soy products like soy milk and tofu). This is likely due mostly to differences in gut flora capacities. The gut microbiome can ferment soy to its active isoflavones, but this is not assured or consistent, especially if you did not eat soy in your youth.

Fermentation also neutralizes the antitrypsin, antichymotrypsin, and anti-alpha-amylase digestive inhibitor substances found abundantly in soybeans. These enzymes normally inhibit digestion and promote allergic reactions. Soaking, sprouting, and fermenting the beans reduces these negative nutrients, promotes digestibility, and enhances the availability of isoflavone compounds. Just to add to the confusion around soy, however, some trypsin inhibitors themselves may have anticancer properties. The Bowman-Birk protease inhibitor from soybeans is particularly effective in suppressing carcinogenesis.

TO USE OR NOT TO USE SOY?

Research into the health benefits of soy foods and soy extracts and isolates is contradictory and confusing. Early consumption of soy foods may confer reduced susceptibility to breast cancer later on. Soy isoflavones (genistein and daidzein) markedly counteract the formation of tumors. Soy foods reduce breast density (and hence cancer risk). However, the value of soy supplementation after adolescence is dubious.

There is no easy answer to this apparent conundrum. No doubt as more and more research is conducted, the details will be revealed. In the meantime, I do prescribe soy foods to my patients for estrogen modulation in menopause or in estrogen-dependent cancers, and for bone health. I suggest mostly tempeh and some tofu, soy milk, and soybeans. In cases where I specifically want therapeutic doses of the isoflavones, I also prescribe a fermented soy powder supplement product that is rich in the therapeutically active compounds.

TAKING SOY TO SUPPORT BONE DENSITY

One of the most useful attributes of soy isoflavones can be in supporting bone density, which not only reduces fractures but also resists bone metastases from cancer. Capsule supplements of genistein and daidzein are available in health food stores or from practitioners. A daily dose in the range of 80–120 mg may be sufficient to support bone density and resist development of metastases. A higher dose of up to 250 mg daily may be used for treating osteoporosis or in cases of existing bone metastases.

Doctors in China have created a proprietary fermented soy formula called Haelan 951 that is rich in nitrogen, polysaccharides, protease inhibitors, saponins, phytosterols, and inositol hexaphosphate, as well as the fermentation metabolites of isoflavones, genistein, and daidzein. Robust clinical trials have not been done yet; the product is the subject of current research and results so far are inconclusive.

For people avoiding soy foods, it is also worth noting that kudzu (*Pueraria lobata*) is from the same pea family as soybean and works in a similar fashion to soy. Kudzu inhibits angiogenesis (new blood vessel growth), induces the p53 gene and apoptosis (cell death), increases the binding of testosterone to sex hormone binding globulin (SHBG) protein, and acts as a partial antagonist (inhibitor) to estrogen receptors.

The Role of the Liver in Detoxification

The liver is one of the largest organs in the body, and all liver cells are capable of doing all the same work, thus providing lots of spare capacity to manage unexpected toxin exposure, for example from ingesting a poison. Approximately 25 percent of the blood in your body is held in the liver at any given moment, where it is being filtered and biochemically modified before being released back to the heart for systemic distribution. Everything you eat, drink, breathe in, or get on your skin is going to end up in your liver. Dissolved compounds will transit across the liver cell membrane into the hepatocytes for metabolic processing and then back across that membrane to return to the blood for distribution around the body or to the bile for elimination. Those movements across the hepatocyte membrane create oxidative stress, so when we use detoxification practices to move toxins from tissue through lymph and blood to the liver and out of the body, it literally stresses the liver. This is where milk thistle plays a key role as an antioxidant to protect the cell membrane.

Herbs That Protect and Support the Liver

Use bitter foods where possible to promote digestive functions (enzymes, peristalsis), including watercress, radish, daikon, dandelion greens, kale, and cabbage, and take bitter herbs before meals.

Supporting good liver function is a key part of the detox process. The following herbs are safe at all stages of health and disease and will not interfere with chemotherapy. They act as tonic and restorative agents in the liver, and they may be useful at any stage of treatment as well as in preventive programs.

MILK THISTLE (*SILYBUM MARIANUM*)

Milk thistle seed contains specific flavonoid compounds, collectively called silymarin, that strongly protect the liver from oxidative stress. The liver has a sophisticated antioxidant system that uses glutathione peroxidase, which it can recycle several times before enzymes become depleted and deficient. Milk thistle supports the recycling of glutathione, so that the antioxidant effect is prolonged and oxidative stress is consequently diminished. In acute liver toxicity, such as mushroom poisoning, really high doses of up to 5 grams daily of silymarin, or even intravenous milk thistle, can be lifesaving.

During chemotherapy or in the aftermath of treatment, milk thistle can substantially improve liver function. In 2009, the American Cancer Society reported that children with acute lymphoblastic leukemia (ALL) and liver toxicity from the chemotherapies they received, who also took milk thistle, showed significant reductions in liver toxicity. The herb did not counteract the effects of chemotherapy agents used for the treatment of ALL and was found to be safe and effective.

In addition to supporting liver function, milk thistle protects the kidneys, which may be quite damaged by certain chemotherapies. Animal studies have shown that using doses of silymarin at 100 mg/kg for 8 weeks provided significant protection against the toxic effects of lead in the kidneys.

SCHISANDRA (*SCHISANDRA CHINENSIS*)

Schisandra berry has a long tradition of use in Asian medicine for restoring liver functions and cooling inflammation. Research supports its use in various liver diseases, including liver cancer, high cholesterol (LDL), and toxin-induced liver injury. It contains immune-activating and stress-resisting lignans, antioxidant and tissue-repairing anthocyanins, and anti-inflammatory terpenes. Additionally, schisandra berry extract has a mild phytoestrogenic effect, allowing it to function as a SERM to normalize estrogen effects in the tissues.

In studies, the fruit extract—and especially the seed extract—has shown significant blood-thinning action. Although these were only in vitro studies, they suggest a degree of caution in people taking prescription anticoagulants.

Alteratives

Alteratives are herbs that have traditionally been used to enhance cellular and lymphatic detoxification systems, promote uptake of metabolic wastes from cells into lymph, promote movement of lymph out of tissues, and, most especially, support liver functions and detoxification pathways. Although few of these herbs have been subjected to rigorous clinical studies, there is a long history of using them as blood purifiers, and they are often prescribed for eruptive conditions at the surface of the body, such as cystic acne, psoriasis, chronic infections, suppurations, and poorly healing sores, as well as for cancer.

Many alteratives are bitter herbs with particular liver action, being choleretic (bile producing) or cholagogue (bile releasing). Some promote lymphatic flow, and some also move the bowel to promote elimination of toxins.

Different alteratives may be recommended based on the principles of tissue specificity, a somewhat difficult-to-explain practice based on hundreds of years of experience that suggests that certain herbs will preferentially influence certain tissues or organs. Thus, an experienced practitioner may be able to promote alterative actions in particular areas of greater need. Although these metabolic and physiological changes may be hard to measure objectively, the historic experience of patients and practitioners supports their use in this way.

Choleretics

These herbs promote bile production.

- Artichoke leaf
- Greater celandine
- Boldo
- Dandelion root and leaf
- Barberry, Oregon grape, goldenseal

Cholagogues

These herbs promote bile secretion and gallbladder emptying.

- Fringe tree bark
- Fumitory
- Turmeric
- Greater celandine

Alteratives for the Skin

- Burdock
- Cleavers
- Figwort
- Fumitory
- Red clover
- Sarsaparilla
- Stinging nettle leaf
- Wild pansy
- Yellow dock

Alteratives for the Ovaries and Peritoneum

- White or yellow pond lily
- Thuja
- Wild indigo
- Pokeroot

Alteratives for the Prostate

- Hydrangea
- Goldenrod
- Thuja

Alteratives for the Kidneys and Bladder

- Goldenrod
- Stinging nettle seed
- Stinging nettle leaf
- Corn silk
- Couch grass

Alteratives for the Lymphatic and Immune Systems

- Pokeroot
- Red root
- Cleavers
- Calendula
- Thuja
- Wild indigo

Essiac Formula

Essiac Formula is a traditional Canadian recipe for bowel health that dates back 100 years or more and is still in popular use today. It was first popularized in Ontario in the 1920s and 1930s by a nurse named Rene Caisse (Essiac is her name spelled backward), who apparently was given the recipe by an older First Nations patient she was caring for (though not all the herbs are native to North America, so the origins could be debated). Caisse spent the rest of her life promoting it and providing it to patients with cancer, many of whom claimed good results.

In my clinic, I prescribe Essiac Formula quite often, usually mixed with other herbs specific to an individual patient. I have seen Essiac be very effective in slowly normalizing bowel movements so that they are regular and comfortable. It is gentle but effective. The slippery elm and the burdock root provide slow but persistent bowel support, with fructo-oligosaccharides as prebiotics and a stool bulking, softening, and moistening action; it is not a stimulant like other traditional laxative formulas.

Isolates of the herbs in the formula show promise in lab research, and there is almost 100 years of continuous use by thousands of people, but well-designed clinical trials are lacking. One study assessing differences in health-related quality of life between women who were new Essiac users (since breast cancer diagnosis) and those who had never used Essiac—including differences in depression, anxiety, fatigue, and rate of adverse events during standard breast cancer treatment—had ambiguous results. Numerous women reported beneficial effects of Essiac. Only two reported adverse effects, but their scores on some of the objective assessments were actually worse than women not taking Essiac. More research remains to be done on the formula itself, but certainly there are studies supporting the use of each of the individual herbs.

Essiac Formula

- Slippery elm inner bark powder
- Burdock root powder
- Sheep sorrel root powder
- Rhubarb root powder

Start by mixing 2 parts each of the slippery elm, burdock, and sheep sorrel, and 1 part of rhubarb. Proportions may vary, but generally lower amounts of rhubarb are used because it can have a stronger laxative effect. Adjust the amount of rhubarb up or down, as the bowel tolerates.

For a low dose, simply make an infusion with 1½ teaspoons of herb powder mix per cup. Be prepared for a thick texture and strong flavor. It may be more palatable used as a base in a blend with other herbs added to customize it for the individual.

The best way to take this formula is as a thin paste or gruel. Simmer 2 tablespoons of finely chopped roots (rather than powder) of sheep sorrel, burdock, and rhubarb in 2 cups of water in a covered pan for 10 minutes; allow to cool and then strain off the tea. Use ¼–½ cup of this decoction to moisten 1–3 teaspoons of powdered slippery elm to make a thin paste. Flavor the tea by adding peppermint, cardamom, or other herbs or 1 drop of high-grade essential oil (peppermint, clove, cardamom, orange, or fennel).

Slippery elm bark. This contains complex fructo-oligosaccharides (large sugar molecules) that act as prebiotics or a substrate for beneficial gut flora. It is an endangered species in the wild, but sustainably cultivated bark can be purchased.

Rhubarb and sheep sorrel root. Emodin, the most abundant anthraquinone of rhubarb and sheep sorrel root, induces apoptosis (cell death), inhibits cellular proliferation, and prevents metastasis in cell line and animal studies. This is achieved through modulation of numerous signaling cascades in the cell. Aloe-emodin is another major component in rhubarb that has been found to have antitumor properties through the p53 gene and its downstream p21 pathway (an inhibitor of cyclin-dependent kinases, enzymes required for cell cycle progression).

Burdock root. This is a traditional detoxifying blood cleanser, a gentle laxative, without the bowel-stimulating anthraquinones but providing more of a nutritive, tonic effect; it is mild but effective, well tolerated, and safe. Research also supports the use of the seeds, which are particularly high in lignans and considered to be even more effective as alteratives and detoxifiers than the root. There is no specific upper dose of burdock and it can even be a vegetable—the cultivated variety is called gobo and is popular in Japanese cuisine. As a medicine it is considered to be slow acting, requiring 2–4 weeks of use before effects are observed, and safe to continue for several months at least. Burdock root can be taken in a slow decoction as part of a soup mix, combined with astragalus and mushrooms, used in making a blood-building bone broth.

Intermittent Fasting

Fasting itself won't cure cancer, but calorie limitation and intermittent fasting can be helpful for preventing cancer and maintaining good blood sugar and blood fat measurements. Fasting can be good for almost anyone; however, if you are underweight, have cachexia (general physical wasting), or are debilitated, run down, or depleted, it may be necessary to start by eating blood-building and energy-dense foods to build up strength before embarking on a stringent calorie-restriction program. Even in those situations, though, it's still worthwhile to try having at least 10 hours in every 24 when you do not eat. This means not eating after 6 or 7 pm—no late-night snacking.

A significant amount of research over many years has demonstrated that modified fasting regimens promote weight loss, improve metabolic health, and resist cancer. In particular, avoiding nighttime eating and prolonging the nightly fasting interval, so that the majority of calories are consumed in an 8-hour window with 16 hours of fasting, can trigger a metabolic switch from glucose-based to ketone-based energy. This can result in increased stress resistance, increased longevity, and a decreased incidence of metabolic diseases, including cancer and obesity. In one study using rats who were restricted to no food on alternate days, or on every third or fourth day, interspersed with days of normal eating, there was increased longevity by 15–20 percent and reduced mammary tumor growth by 65–90 percent compared with those allowed to eat as desired. Reductions were proportional to the number of days of fasting per week and the amount of weight reduction.

Types of Fasting Regimens

There are several fasting regimens that can be helpful. The main principles are that you are trying to reduce overall calorie intake while maintaining maximal nourishment, and that alternating or intermittent restrictions are more successful than daily limitation of calories; it is the on/off fasting aspect that is critical, rather than overall calorie restriction, as it mimics the feast and famine cycles our ancestors evolved with. It's also more manageable than everyday restrictions.

The 16/8 Method. Also called the "Leangains method," this involves fasting for 16 hours a day and eating all your calories within an 8-hour window. This is possibly the easiest to implement and sustain and is the model I suggest to my patients. Eat a good breakfast, then eat lunch 4 hours later and dinner 4 hours after that, with no snacks in between.

Modified Alternate-Day Fasting. This calls for modified fasting every other day but eating "normally" on nonfasting days. You are allowed to consume 20–25 percent of your usual calorie intake (about 500 calories) on a fasting day.

Five-Two Diet. Five days of the week are normal eating days, with 2 nonconsecutive days of restricted calories (500–600 per day). This is actually more of an eating pattern than a diet. There are no specific requirements about which foods to eat; the focus is on when you should eat, rather than which foods to eat.

Crescendo Method. Fast for 12–16 hours for 2–3 days a week. Fasting days should be nonconsecutive and spaced evenly across the week (for example, Monday, Wednesday, and Friday).

Eat-Stop-Eat. Also called the 24-hour protocol, this is a 24-hour full fast once or twice a week (maximum of two times a week, nonconsecutive). Start with 14- to 16-hour fasts and gradually build up.

Restore Bowel Health and Boost the Microbiome

The complex microbiome of the large intestine plays a pivotal role in the regulation of metabolic, endocrine, and immune functions. It is involved in the modulation of multiple neurochemical pathways through the highly interconnected gut-brain axis and is the source of the majority of the serotonin our bodies use to govern our mood and mind.

Cancer patients need to pay careful attention to bowel microbiome health because the plethora of drugs they are likely to be given, including routine antibiotics, will cause some significant disruption.

In the last decade there has been an explosion of research into the microbiome and its role in health and disease. One result of this research has been the increased use of fecal transplants; it is now standard of care to provide fecal transplants in cases of *Clostridium difficile* infection. In just one of many studies of relevance in cancer care, a report published in 2021 showed how, in melanoma, resistance to the new checkpoint inhibitor immunotherapy drugs can be overcome by changing the gut microbiota with fecal transplants.

Functions of the Gut Microbiome

A healthy gut microbiome improves overall health in a variety of ways. It produces vitamin K, which can help with blood clotting and is critical to tissue repair after surgery. It neutralizes and removes toxins and potential carcinogens. Importantly, the short-chain fatty acids produced by the bacterial fermentation of plant fibers in the gut also reduce fecal pH, which is a marker of colonic health and reduced risk of colon cancer. A healthy gut also activates health-promoting dietary compounds. For example, cruciferous vegetables (such as kale, cabbage, and broccoli) contain glucosinolates that ferment in the gut into isothiocyanates, sulfur-rich compounds that are strongly anticancer and support liver detoxification of various carcinogens. Willow and meadowsweet contain salicylates that partially ferment in the gut into salicylic acid, which has anti-inflammatory and pain-relieving effects.

The short-chain fatty acids produced by bacterial fermentation in the gut—chiefly butyric, proprionic, and acetic acids—provide fuel for cells lining the colon. They also stimulate colonic blood flow, increase muscle activity of the gut, and reverse the atrophy associated with fiber-poor diets. This is an essential fuel for cells lining the colon and is one reason why low-fiber foods can contribute to colon cancer. Butyrate, in particular, may affect gene expression and induce apoptosis (cell death), which further decreases the risk of developing colon cancer.

It all seems to come down to bacteria. My husband, a former microbiologist, says bacteria rule the world and farm us for their optimal benefit. He may well be right. Bacteria that crave sugar can cause you to crave and eat it, which feeds the dysbiosis. Some of these bacteria ferment sugars and make alcohol—a tiny drip feed continuously dumping alcohol into the bloodstream. This makes its way to the liver for removal and leads to fatty liver disease (nonalcoholic steatohepatitis, also referred to as NASH) and fatty pancreas disease (nonalcoholic steateopancreatitis). This creates obesity, insulin resistance, and increased blood sugar, which create the chronic low-grade inflammatory state that underpins heart disease, cancer, and chronic degenerative diseases of modern times.

Weeding, Seeding, and Feeding

Herbalist Kerry Bone has coined the phrase "weeding, seeding, and feeding" to describe the holistic approach to optimizing the microbiome. This means removing disease-causing bacteria or yeasts, replenishing the beneficial bacteria and yeasts, and then providing appropriate "food" for them to flourish and thrive. Whether or not an individual has actual bowel parasites, it is highly probable that most people have some degree of imbalance in their gut bacteria (also known as dysbiosis) from a lifetime of eating foods low in fiber and taking antibiotics.

Weeding. This means reducing the population of abnormal and pathogenic intestinal microorganisms. If there are symptoms of possible parasitic bowel infection (diarrhea, abdominal cramping, smelly gas, gurgling, or rectal itching), then a stool test should be done to assess for ova and parasites. Testing may need to be repeated more than once before a positive response comes back. If intestinal parasites are diagnosed, then repeating the 2-week cycles of the "Weeding" Protocol (page 56) may be required for 2–4 months. If actual parasites are not diagnosed, then this bowel-balancing formula can be taken for 1–2 weeks prior to surgery, as a proactive and preventive practice as part of a prehabilitation plan, ahead of antibiotics you'll almost inevitably be prescribed. Garlic can be eaten freely in the diet. The other herbs are best taken in capsule form; there are numerous effective proprietary formulas in health food stores.

"Weeding" Protocol

A typical "weeding" protocol might include the following powdered herbs.

+ 25 g olive leaf
+ 15 g barberry root
+ 10 g black walnut
+ 10 g garlic
+ 10 g goldenseal
+ 15 g neem
+ 5 g andrographis
+ 5 g clove
+ 5 g wormwood

Mix the powders well and fill 500 mg capsules. Take three capsules once or twice a day, on an empty stomach. Intestinal parasites have life cycles that include phases when they are vulnerable to treatment, and at other times they are encysted and unreachable, so the treatment needs to be repeated a few times in cycles of 2 weeks on and 2 weeks off for 2 months or until there are no discernable parasites found in a stool test.

*An additional option: Take 500 mg each of nigella seed oil and oregano oil, in capsules, daily. These are both powerful antimicrobials.

Seeding. This enhances the population of beneficial intestinal microorganisms by encouraging growth of the population already existing in the body and providing a supplemental population if necessary. This can be initiated before or after surgery and will not adversely affect blood clotting risk or surgical outcomes. The following are ways to introduce and support beneficial bacteria in the gut.

- Probiotic fermented foods, such as sauerkraut, kimchi, salsa, miso, natto, and tempeh; probiotic fermented beverages, such as kombucha, jun, kefir, and other fermented nonalcoholic drinks; unpasteurized (live) apple cider vinegar; and live yogurt
- Probiotic supplements. Aim for 50 billion live bacteria twice daily. The exact range of species recommended may be informed by stool analysis that can look for the dozen or so strains that are predominant, but there are at least several hundred in real life, and only a handful are actually available in a capsule. For this reason, I often simply recommend as wide a range of species as possible, and a fairly high dose, and also a beneficial commensal yeast supplement, such as *Saccharomyces boulardii*.

Feeding. This provides the complex polysaccharides and high-fiber diet that is food for beneficial gut flora, supporting fermentation pathways and making short-chain fatty acids (notably butyric acid). Include the following.

- Prebiotics and fructo-oligosaccharides found in starchy (roots) and non-starchy vegetables and certain fruits such as organic berries (unless you have a problem digesting fructose)
- Resistant starch. This type of starch—found in high quantities in rice, corn, oats, pearl barley, potatoes, green bananas (plantains), and most lentils, beans, and legumes—is not digested into small sugars for absorption as other carbohydrates are. Instead, it passes through the small intestines without being broken down, until it reaches the large intestine, where it is used as fuel by the bacteria of the microbiome for fermentation. Resistant starch can also contribute to feelings of fullness and satiety and thus limit calorie intake. Start with small amounts and build up over time.

Some herbs specifically indicated to promote an optimal bowel environment and microbiome balance include garlic, burdock root, turmeric, artichoke leaf, and dandelion root. Interestingly, garlic, which we know as a potent antibiotic for infections, is also a probiotic in the gut, probably because of the large amount of fructans that ferment to feed the beneficial gut flora, but also contribute to gas when we eat a lot of it.

More about Resistant Starch

Resistant starch—fiber that passes through the colon without being broken down and absorbed by the body—increases fecal weight, treats and prevents constipation, and lowers the risk of colon cancer, due to healthier colonocytes and possibly because of decreased contact between the potential carcinogens and the colon wall. There's no official recommended daily allowance or other standardized recommendation for the intake of resistant starch. Most Americans eat around 5 g each day, Europeans get 3 to 6 g, and people in China average almost 15 g. Because resistant starch is fermented quite slowly, it can be taken at reasonably high doses if you work up to it, and with less gas production than other fibers. In studies, doses of 20–40 g have been well tolerated.

A strange quirk of resistant starch is that it becomes even less digestible, and hence even better for the microbiome, after being cooked and cooled. Upon cooling, there is a process of rehydration that causes the starch to thicken and set (think cold pasta or oatmeal) and makes the fibers even more resistant. Reheating the food is fine, meaning you can cook enough for 2 or 3 days in one pot and reheat it as needed each day.

Support the Immune System

Underlying all cancer in the body is some failure of the immune cells to recognize the pathogen in its midst and to deal effectively with it. Cancer starts as a DNA defect in a cell that the p53 protein, or a similar mutated tumor suppressor gene, fails to eradicate or correct. It may replicate quite slowly for months or even years before progressing to be a tumor that the immune system must engage with to quell the abnormal growth. The ability of cancer to hide out, to evade immune surveillance, is a key part of its growth in the body.

Immune Boot Camp

While you are gathering information, assessing options, and putting other pieces of your treatment plan in place, you can start an Immune Boot Camp (a name coined by medical herbalist Jonathan Treasure). This up-front immune upregulation (stimulation) regimen is good preparation for conventional cancer treatment. Ideally, you would follow this for 2–4 weeks before conventional treatment commenced. After surgery, chemotherapy, or radiation is over, immune boosting should recommence for another 3–6 weeks. During active conventional treatment (chemotherapy and radiation), it may be necessary to scale it back a bit, but if you are able to tolerate it all, then keep it up.

The immune system deficiencies and depletion seen in cancer are usually significantly worsened by chemotherapy and radiation, and when those procedures are completed, the immune system will recover. It can take months, though, and herbs and nutritional support can speed recovery. Below is an outline of the kind of immune-boosting plan I would prescribe to a new patient in my clinic.

Suggestions for the Immune Boot Camp Protocol

- Clean and Green Detox Diet (page 41) and intermittent fasting
- Bone broths and good protein intake to build immune cells (especially whey protein with immunoglobulins)
- Liver support and alteratives as needed
- Support for the microbiome and bowel health (prebiotics, probiotics, fiber, and bowel stimulants or laxatives if needed for constipation)
- Thymic protein supplement, 4 mcg daily (activates T cells in immune system)
- High-dose medicinal mushrooms. Actual doses depend on the type of mushroom and the potency of the product (whether it is a concentrated extract or a simple powdered dried mushroom). Optimally, they can be eaten freely in the diet, 2–4 ounces of fresh mushrooms daily, cooked long and slow. Because this isn't always possible, at least not daily, when I prescribe medicinal mushrooms in the clinic, I usually use a proprietary branded formula of five or seven mushrooms made into a concentrated

Immunostimulating Tincture Formula

This herbal tincture formula is a powerful alterative and detoxifier with immunomodulating and anticancer properties. This formula would be used in the week before and the week or two after surgery, or if there is any infection that occurs from surgery or chemotherapy. The pokeroot and mistletoe are cytotoxics, given in a substantial dose, and intended to kick-start the nonspecific immune system and lymphatic and lymphocyte activities. They are available only from qualified herbalists, not health food stores. If you can't obtain them, then increase the amounts of Oregon grape and wild indigo. All the herbs listed below are in tincture form, made at 1:2 strength—1 part dried herb (in grams) to 2 parts alcohol (in milliliters)—except where indicated. These amounts add up to 100 mL, which is about a week's supply at the dosage indicated below.

+ 20 mL calendula
+ 15 mL echinacea
+ 15 mL red clover
+ 10 mL Oregon grape
+ 10 mL wild indigo
+ 10 mL stillingia
+ 10 mL mistletoe (1:10)
+ 5 mL propolis
+ 5 mL pokeroot (1:10)

Combine all tinctures. The recommended dose is 7.5 mL (1½ tsp.) twice daily in hot water before meals.

Wild indigo was a favorite of the Eclectic herbal doctors for "bad blood," as a deep detoxifier, and is often used alongside echinacea. Oregon grape is a bitter liver detoxifier, and it also downregulates (suppresses) multidrug resistance so it helps keep chemotherapy or cytotoxic herbs in target cells. Red clover and calendula are gentle alteratives. Other deeply alterative herbs that could be considered include red root or blue flag.

extract and then powdered for encapsulation. This allows someone to take three to five capsules daily and get a substantial daily dose.

- Larch arabinogalactan. This immunomodulating sugar from *Larix laricina* and *L. occidentalis* enhances natural killer cell and macrophage activity and regulates secretion of pro-inflammatory cytokines. Studies suggest that it interacts with the immune system either indirectly through fermentation, which produces short-chain fatty acids that control inflammatory responses via modulation of white cell functions, or directly through the capacity of specific intestinal lining cells (called M-cells) that can transfer intact arabinogalactan through the intestinal barrier, delivering it to immune cells in the blood. Doses can range from 1.5–4.5 g daily, taken for several weeks.

Immune Boot Camp Nutritional Breakfast Smoothie

+ ½–1 teaspoon buffered vitamin C powder (1 teaspoon = 2,500 mg)
+ 25,000 IU liquid beta-carotene
+ 5,000–10,000 IU liquid vitamin D3
+ 1–3 teaspoons (5–15 g) glutamine powder
+ 1 cup fresh or frozen berries (blueberries, raspberries, blackberries)
+ ½ cup plain or flavored unsweetened live yogurt (or nondairy substitute)
+ 1 tablespoon nut butter, for good fats and protein and to add creaminess
+ 2 dates, figs, or prunes, soaked in water overnight
+ 1–2 cups liquid (such as unsweetened nut milk or raw, organic cow or goat milk) to achieve desired consistency
+ 1–2 scoops whey protein powder (cold processed, cross filtered, with immunoglobulins), to provide at least 20 g protein

Blend together all ingredients, adding the whey to the smoothie at the last minute. Additional supplement tablets and capsules can be added to the smoothie as well (which is especially helpful when the patient has difficulty swallowing). Crush the tablets before adding them; puncture gelcaps and squeeze their contents into the smoothie. Be sure to check for taste—don't add so many supplements that the smoothie becomes inedible.

Glutamine. This is an amino acid taken as a supplement for a host of benefits. It is important in intestinal cells as a precursor to promote the synthesis of glutathione, a critically significant antioxidant. Glutamine supports the immune system, stabilizes blood-sugar levels, improves brain function, decreases muscle soreness and fatigue, and increases muscle mass. Many commercially available supplements use L-glutamine, which is unstable in heat or acid and is poorly absorbed, so be careful of the brand you buy.

Whey protein powder. This is a milk-processing by-product made up of several immune-enhancing proteins—lactoferrin, beta-lactoglobulin, alpha-lactalbumin, glycomacropeptide, and immunoglobulins. These proteins have hypotensive (blood pressure–lowering), antitumor, hypolipidemic (cholesterol-lowering), antiviral, and antibacterial actions, mostly by intracellular conversion of cysteine to glutathione, a potent intracellular antioxidant. Not all whey protein is sufficiently high quality for cancer patients. Some are just protein supplements for body building; those are not what you want. A good product is cold processed, microfiltered, and undenatured and sold with a stipulated amount of immunoglobulins. It is easy to add as a powder to a smoothie or onto oatmeal or cereal.

Optional extras. Other ingredients you might consider adding include half an avocado (for good fat); one other fruit, such as half a mango, 1 slice of melon, or 1 kiwi; green superfood powder; mushroom extract powder; coconut powder (for calories and flavor); raw cocoa powder to taste; and other spices or herbs for flavor, such as vanilla, stevia, cinnamon, cardamom, or fennel.

- Turmeric extract, 1,500–2,000 mg daily, standardized at 94% curcumin
- Quercetin, 1,500–2,000 mg, and bromelain, 2,000 GDU, daily
- Broad-spectrum antioxidant/redox-regulating supplement formula (e.g., zinc, coenzyme Q10, alpha-lipoic acid, selenium, flavonoids, resveratrol, and oligomeric proanthocyanidins)
- B-vitamin complex dosed at 50–100 mg of the main vitamins daily
- Adaptogen formula and stress support herbs, such as ashwagandha, eleuthero, ginseng, codonopsis, licorice, rhodiola, and tulsi
- Immunostimulating, alterative, and lymph-restorative herbs

Deep Immune Tonic Herbs

Many herbs are considered nutritive, stimulating, and restorative to the whole body and especially to the immune system, and they can be made into strong infusions (leaves and flowers) or decoctions (roots, barks, and seeds) to add to green juices or bone broth soups. Some of these include the following.

- Ashwagandha
- Astragalus
- Codonopsis
- Goji berry
- Leuzea
- Mushrooms
- Rehmannia (prepared)
- Schisandra

MUSHROOMS

All edible mushrooms have medicinal qualities, though some are better researched and understood than others. They support and nourish the bone marrow to optimize immune functions and to activate the immune system to fight disease. Some have a tissue specificity, such as cordyceps, which helps with gaseous exchange in the lungs, or lion's mane, which is a particular brain tonic. Even grocery-store mushrooms are helpful; oyster, shiitake, crimini, and portobello mushrooms are all medicinal and can be easily incorporated into the diet. You can also cook mushrooms to a slurry, dehydrate and powder them, then put them in capsules, if you have the time. However you prepare them, they do need to be cooked long and slow in water in order to extract the immune-active beta-glucans.

In his research, Christopher Hobbs, a true mushroom expert, has found that turkey tail and reishi have the highest amounts of beta-glucans for immune support. He recommends at least 6 grams daily of cooked and dried mushroom powder. He also suggests switching species every 3 months and cycling through other powerful immunomodulating mushrooms.

ASTRAGALUS (*ASTRAGALUS MEMBRANACEUS*)

In Traditional Chinese Medicine, this root is classified as a warm, sweet herb that enhances the functioning of the spleen and lung and is a qi tonic (energy or vitality booster). It is recommended for general strengthening, treating excessive perspiration, eliminating toxins, and promoting the healing of damaged tissues. In addition, it is used for the treatment of edema (buildup of fluids), night sweats, skin ulcerations, and abscesses. It is considered inherently safe in doses up to 30 grams per day by decoction.

Astragalus has water-soluble polysaccharides that are immunomodulating, as well as stress-reducing and stress-modulating triterpene saponins that require alcohol or another solvent. In order to get the best out of this herb, you may want to simmer the chopped root in water, then use that liquid as the water phase, mixed with alcohol (approximately 30–35 percent water and 65–70 percent alcohol) and poured over more herbal material to make a tincture. This maximizes the extraction of water-, fat-, and alcohol-soluble constituents. Another method I sometimes recommend is to make a mix of tough or woody mushrooms (reishi, turkey tails) with astragalus root in a cotton bag or a clean, thin sock tied off at the top and add it to the soup pot. If you started by sautéing onions and then adding stock, the oil and water will act as a dual solvent for the herb. When it is all well cooked, remove the bag of herbs. Another method is to make a strong decoction of those herbs, strain it off and use it as the base for the stock, and put the wet herb mash into a cotton bag to simmer in the soup in order to extract all of the oil-soluble compounds.

Anticancer Actions of Astragalus

- Strengthens the body's natural defenses (immunity)
- Increases the number of macrophages and increases phagocytosis (white blood cell activity)
- Induces the production of interferon by white blood cells (heightening antiviral defenses)
- Antiangiogenic (reducing the growth of new blood cells)
- Enhances effectiveness and reduces toxicity of chemotherapy
- Increases the cleaning rate of toxins through the liver
- Protects vital organs (liver, kidney, heart)
- Increases the life span and quality of life of cancer patients

The Neuroendocrine System: Organs and the Hormones They Make

- **Adrenals.** The cortex (outer layer) produces pregnenolone, which goes on to make cortisol and androstenedione, ultimately forming testosterone and estrogens, as well as aldosterone, the hormone that holds salt and hence water in the bloodstream and sustains blood volume. The medulla (inner core) makes epinephrine (adrenaline) and norepinephrine (noradrenaline) for governing the sympathetic nervous system.
- **Adipose tissue.** Fat cells make leptin, which is a strong appetite suppressant. It is often deficient in depressed people and this contributes to overeating and early-onset obesity.
- **Gonads.** Ovaries and testes produce estrogens, progesterone, and testosterone to control reproduction. Estrogens also promote cell proliferation and fuel some cancers.
- **Pancreas.** This organ produces insulin and glucagon, which control blood-sugar uptake as well as sugar storage and release.
- **Pineal.** This gland produces melatonin in response to daylight exposure, which sets diurnal rhythms of metabolism.
- **Pituitary.** This "master gland" produces and secretes control hormones: thyroid-stimulating hormone, adrenocorticotropic hormone, growth hormone, follicle-stimulating hormone, luteinizing hormone, prolactin, antidiuretic hormone, and oxytocin.
- **Thymus.** This gland primes the T lymphocytes, regulates Th1/Th2 balance (lymphocytes and immunoglobulins), and also supports the deep immune system.
- **Thyroid.** This gland produces mostly inactive T4 and a small amount of active T3 thyroid hormone.

Managing Stress

Stress, distress, social isolation, and chronic anxiety can all be contributing factors to a terrain that is conducive to the development of cancer. This is not quite the same as saying that stress causes cancer, but it is not all that big of a stretch to imagine that is true. Adaptogenic, stress-reducing herbs have a role to play here, especially where stressors are unremitting or unavoidable. Avoid the more stimulating adaptogens such as ginseng or leuzea, as they may be too strong, and don't fall into the trap of using adaptogens to compensate for poor lifestyle choices (getting more sleep will always trump taking any herbs).

> I am an old man now, and I have known a great many problems in my life . . . most of which never happened.
>
> MARK TWAIN

Systemic Effects of Chronic Stress

Chronic cortisol elevation from chronic stress leads to a whole host of systemic disturbances, many of which are cancer promoting, including the following.

- Disturbance of insulin and deranged blood-sugar management—insulin resistance and fluctuating blood sugar
- Disturbance of leptins (hormones that control fat metabolism)—gain in adipose (fat) tissue, increased estrogen sensitivity
- Increased production of insulin-like growth factor 1 (IGF-1), a protein that facilitates cellular uptake of sugar, leading to increased cell stimulation
- Impaired cellular utilization of glucose—promotion of glycolysis and generation of lactic acid
- Diminished lymphocyte numbers and function
- Increased protein breakdown and decreased protein synthesis that can lead to muscle wasting
- Demineralization of bone that can lead to osteoporosis
- Impaired skin regeneration and healing
- Atrophy of thymus, leading to diminished immunocompetence
- Lessening of SIgA (secretory antibody productions), a key part of the enteric (digestive) immune system that protects against ingested toxins
- Widespread immune system suppression that may lead to increased susceptibility to allergies, infections, and degenerative disease

The Stress Response

The neuroendocrine network is an interlinked mesh of influences and counterinfluences that are intended to sustain us through allostasis and help us attain balance in our cells and in ourselves. Allostasis is a constant adjustment between anabolic (building and replenishing) and catabolic (breaking down and eliminating) forces in the body. It involves careful and continuous calibration of hormones in response to stimulus received by the nervous system and can be seen as an integrated network of control and regulation across the whole body.

The process of physiological enhancement in cancer care is mostly directed at stabilizing and regulating this allostatic stress response and ensuring the pendulum swings of anabolic and catabolic activities are properly balanced.

General Adaptation Syndrome

The idea of stress as a medical state was first articulated by Canadian endocrinologist Hans Selye, who famously said, "Stress is the nonspecific response of the body to any demand made upon it," and pointed out that all types of stress bring about similar physiological and endocrine effects. It is immaterial whether the stress stimulus is pleasant or unpleasant; all that matters is the frequency, intensity, and duration. Selye came up with his theory of a general adaptation syndrome in 1936, suggesting that stress responses in the body fall into three broad categories, with progressively worse symptoms and outcomes, and that they are progressively harder to recuperate from.

Stage 1: Alarm. Catecholamines (adrenaline/epinephrine) are released quickly in the nervous system in response to sudden stress and cause activation of the neuroendocrine system that leads to increased heart rate and respiration, increased blood pressure, gluconeogenesis, and increased insulin. This should entail a short-lived and rapidly resolved anabolic surge to repair damage. In the modern world, the stressors are so persistent that recovery and restoration after an alarm may not occur properly or sufficiently, in which case the metabolism moves on to stage 2.

Stage 2: Resistance. Activation of the hypothalamic-pituitary-adrenal (HPA) axis causes adrenal hypertrophy (increased size) within a few weeks, which leads to increased cortisol, thymic and lymphoid atrophy (wasting), and immune disturbance. An initial increase in immune responses is unsustainable, leading to eventual reduced natural killer cell function, lowered T cells and reduced antibody responsiveness, overactivity of inflammatory cytokines, and oxidative stress.

Stage 3: Exhaustion. The adrenal glands can't meet the persistent demand, leading to failure of the feedback loop, reduced hypothalamic responses and endocrine depletion, disturbances of cortisol, causing chronic inflammation, and disturbances of DHEA, causing menstrual and fertility issues.

It has to be said that some of Selye's assertions are no longer entirely supported by research; in particular, the adrenal glands don't exactly become exhausted (stage 3). However, they do cease to be adequately responsive to demand, and the result is system-wide depletion, debility, and failure to recuperate after exertion. True adrenal failure is a medical emergency requiring hospitalization and strong steroid drug therapies.

With all of that said, it is worth pointing out that stress is natural and normal. It cannot be avoided, but stressors can be avoided and recuperation is possible. Most people hover up and down the scale of adrenal resistance or stage 2 in the general adaptation syndrome. This is sustainable in the short term, but over the long term, the immune system becomes deficient and chronic ill health ensues.

Stressors contribute to constitutional weakness, and how we interpret and respond to stress may make all the difference in who thrives with cancer and who succumbs. The neuroendocrine system is the master system that sets the tone for all metabolic processes in the body, whether anabolic (building up) or catabolic (breaking down). The neuroendocrine system involves an array of mechanisms that are minutely calibrated through numerous hormones and feedback loops, and forcing any one of these endocrine processes with pharmaceuticals will lead to imbalance in the others. On the other hand, using adaptogens (stress-reducing drugs or herbs), even those with some tissue specificities, will be supportive, regenerative, and healing to the system as a whole.

Effects of Unresolved Stress

The issue, as described above, is not so much that stressors occur, which is inevitable in life, but that persistent and relentless stressors keep the body in a state of sympathetic dominance. This tends to drive catabolic states and becomes debilitating and depleting over time, and it inhibits cell repair, tissue repair, and organ repair systems.

Excess cortisol from chronic unresolved stress:

- Diminishes cellular utilization of glucose, which increases glycolysis and oxidative stress in the cell
- Diminishes lymphocyte numbers and functions
- Increases blood-sugar levels
- Decreases protein synthesis
- Increases protein breakdown, which can lead to muscle wasting
- Causes demineralization of bone that can lead to osteoporosis
- Interferes with skin regeneration and healing
- Causes shrinking of lymphatic tissue

HPA axis activation from excess cortisol leads to:

- Increased C-reactive protein—a marker of inflammation
- Increased PGE2, COX, and LOX—markers of inflammation
- Increased creatine kinase—a marker of muscle breakdown
- Increased IL6, IL10, and TNF-α—markers of inflammation
- Impaired function of 5-diodinase (reduced conversion of T4 to T3)—reduced thyroid hormone, slower metabolism
- Reduced free T3 and increased reverse T3—markers of inflammation of the thyroid
- Reduced lymphocytes, NK response, IL2, and IL12—weakened immune response

Using Adaptogens to Support the Vital Force

Adaptogen is a term coined in Russia by Nicolai Lazarev in the mid-twentieth century. Today it's used as a broad term that includes the herbs that nourish and support the vital force, promote healing and restoration in the body, resist oxidative stress, and normalize cell behaviors. These herbs may have a range of active constituents, including polyphenols and lignans, but most especially, many of them have steroidal and triterpene derivatives that are active in cortisol pathways and consequently may have downstream benefits on immunomodulation and on tissue repair and regeneration.

Over time, we physically age as the catabolic processes of cellular breakdown and tissue oxidation overtake the anabolic growth processes of youth. Some situations or conditions that promote catabolic states and rapid aging include surgery, chemotherapy, radiation, physical or mental trauma, severe illness, endurance exercise (such as running marathons), statin drugs, chronic stress, and inflammatory diseases and infections.

Benefits of Adaptogens

Adaptogenic herbs aim to slow this catabolic state of cellular breakdown and prolong functionality and healing. These are the herbs that build and restore vital force, protect against stress (by enhancing our capacity to adapt to stressors), sustain energy, support resistance to disease, promote healing, normalize the HPA axis and the hypothalamic-pituitary-thyroid (HPT) axis, mediate inflammation, normalize mitochondrial energy transfer, promote redox regulation, promote anabolic metabolism without promoting malignancy, and more. They show antifatigue effects, enhance learning, and increase memory, physical endurance, work, and exercise capacity. Adaptogens can improve oxygen uptake; have generally supportive effects; stimulate protein synthesis in the pancreas, liver, adrenal cortex, and throughout the body; support optimum endocrine response; and regulate blood-sugar levels.

Due to their normalizing and stabilizing effects, often brought about by redox regulation and immunomodulation, the adaptogens are used in the background, in the foundation or base of a formula, to give a solidity or inner strength to the patient facing the challenge of cancer. Some constituents of adaptogenic herbs, given in isolation, may have cytotoxic effects, but they are not prescribed specifically for that purpose. The adaptogens are used as a broad-acting, nonspecific physiological enhancement strategy, reducing risk from multiple predisposing factors and offering a very low-risk profile.

Adaptogens in Oncology

- Build and sustain the vital force
- Build bone marrow and optimize immune responses; restore immune surveillance and increase nonspecific immune resistance (biological response modification)
- Improve recovery and healing
- Reduce levels of cortisol
- Increase anabolic activity and inhibit catabolic activity—resist cachexia (general physical wasting), normalize blood sugar
- Increase the tumor toxicity of chemotherapy and radiation

- Inhibit cancer invasion and metastases
- Inhibit multidrug resistance
- Protect organs from toxins and oxidative stress due to chemotherapy and radiotherapy

Cortisol, the main inflammatory mediator of the body, is produced from a steroid skeleton in the adrenal cortex. Interestingly, it has structural similarity to several plant compounds, also derived from steroids, enabling the body to use these herbs to support the body's hormones in various ways, and these cortisol analogues in plants contribute to the adaptogenic action in many herbs. Not all adaptogens have these steroidal compounds (rhodiola and schisandra do not, for example), but adaptogens overall have an adrenal-sparing effect and downregulate the HPA axis. They are considered nerve restoratives, broadly safe for most people most of the time, but should not be used long term (that is, for weeks or months) without consideration of the cause and source of the stress as well.

A FEW KEY CONSTITUENTS AND TARGET ORGANS OF ADAPTOGENS

Adaptogenic Herb*	Key Constituent Group	Main Target Organ/System
Ashwagandha	Withanolides (triterpenes)	Brain, adrenals
Astragalus	Astragalosides (triterpenes)	Immune system
Codonopsis	Polyacetylenes, alkaloids, phenylpropanoids, triterpenoids, and polysaccharides	General restorative and energy-boosting herb
Eleuthero	Eleutheroside A (saponin and sterol glycoside) Eleutheroside B (phenylpropanoid glycoside)	Adrenals
Licorice	Glycyrrhizin (saponin)	Adrenals
Tulsi	Oleanolic acid and ursolic acid (triterpenes) Rosmarinic acid (polyphenol)	Brain
Ginseng (American and Asian species)	Ginsenosides (triterpenes)	Adrenals
Leuzea	Phytoecdysterones (triterpenes)	Adrenals
Rhodiola	Salidroside (glucoside of tyrosol) Rosavin (cinnamyl alcohol glycoside)	Heart
Schisandra	Lignans	Liver

**There are numerous other herbs that may have some adaptogenic qualities of calming and tonifying (restoring) the nervous system, but without the same adrenal- and energy-boosting and immune-supportive effects as the primary adaptogens listed above. These may include gotu kola, blue vervain, damiana, and milky oats.*

How to Choose Adaptogens

Different adaptogens have their own specificities—astragalus for the immune system, tulsi for mood elevation, schisandra for the liver, and rhodiola for the heart. Be cautious of Asian ginseng—it can be a little stimulating, and American ginseng may be preferable in some cases. Rhodiola, ashwagandha root, eleuthero, licorice, or codonopsis may be gentler and safer. Codonopsis is a Traditional Chinese Medicine for replenishing qi (energy) deficiency, strengthening the immune system, decreasing blood pressure, and improving poor gastrointestinal function, gastric ulcer, and appetite, and it is sometimes used as a substitute for ginseng but is less anabolic. Licorice is loved by some and hated by some, so herbal practitioners should ask the patient before including it, especially in teas. In Traditional Chinese Medicine, licorice is often used as a synergistic herb in blends, assisting the other herbs and supporting their actions.

Stimulating Adaptogens

These herbs should be used occasionally or intermittently for a specific reason, to give extra support and energy after a particular stress—such as before and after surgery or chemotherapy. They should not be used without good cause and should not be continued for longer than 6–8 weeks without a break.

LEUZEA (*RHAPONTICUM CARTHAMOIDES*)

This is a member of the thistle family without the prickles, and it looks like a small globe artichoke as it grows. The root is the medicine. It grows wild only in alpine and subalpine zones of southern Siberia, and nowhere else, but it is easy to grow in your garden. The root is rich in phytoecdysteroids, especially ecdysterone and turkesterone, as well as a full spectrum of potent flavonoids, glycosides, organic acids, carotenoids, tannins, and resins. In the insect world, ecdysteroids act as hormones that govern molting and formation of the new exoskeleton; hence, they are very anabolic, as the insect or invertebrate is literally growing under their influence. They are the most powerful anabolic compounds in nature, and the phytoecdysteroids of leuzea are the strongest anabolic compounds in the plant world. This herb is best used with really good nutritional support and plenty of sleep and rest to counterbalance its stimulant nature. Leuzea should be used in pulse doses: 2 to 3 weeks on it, then the same amount of time off, then repeat. It is contraindicated during active chemotherapy and in people who are very weak, run down, or debilitated; patients need some inner strength to get the best out of this herb. It is useful after surgery or chemotherapy in the restorative phase.

Main Actions of Leuzea

- Adaptogenic, accelerates recovery
- Anabolic (increased protein synthesis throughout the body)
- Anticancer
- Antidiabetic, insulinotropic
- Antifatigue (mental and physical)
- Antimicrobial
- Cardiovascular protective
- Cerebral protective
- Chemotherapy protective
- Decreased platelet aggregation
- Immune system enhancement
- Redox cycling (antioxidative)

ASIAN GINSENG (*PANAX GINSENG*)

This is considered the archetypal adaptogen, a broad-spectrum adaptogen without particular tissue specificity. Asian ginseng and its active compounds, mostly the Rb and Rg ginsenosides, possess profound anticancer activity. A study of 1,500 breast cancer patients followed for up to 6 years found that the regular use of ginseng prolonged life, reduced recurrences, and increased the quality of life compared with those who did not take ginseng.

How Ginseng Suppresses Cancer

- Angiogenesis adaptation (promotes the formation and differentiation of new blood vessels for healing after surgery while inhibiting cancer-induced new blood vessel growth)
- Endocrine system enhancement/regulation (insulinotropic, protective against cortisol-induced immune suppression)
- Enhances immunosurveillance, including antibody response, natural killer cell activity, production of interferon, proliferation and phagocytic ability of leukocytes and activates dendritic cells; promotes gap junction intracellular communication
- Induction of apoptosis, or cell death (downregulates NF-κB, COX-2, AP-1)
- Inhibition of cell proliferation (G1/S phase)
- Promotes DNA repair
- Reduces oxidation and rate of mutation
- Regulates inflammation (COX-2, NF-κB, AP-1 inhibition)
- Selectively modulates new blood vessel growth and differentiation

RHODIOLA (*RHODIOLA ROSEA*)

This plant is from the northern zones—Scandinavia, Siberia, Mongolia—and is well adapted to withstand significant environmental stressors. The resilience and robustness in the plant is imparted to the medicine, and it has long been used as an adaptogen. It is traditionally recommended for enhancing oxygen exchange and promoting cellular respiration—for this reason it may be included in the mitochondrial rescue protocol described in Chapter 8. It has some specificity toward the heart, strengthening and nourishing the cardiac muscles, increasing the force of the contraction and the cardiac output, while not increasing oxygen demand by the cells. It is slightly stimulating to heart function and is not recommended for people with palpitations or arrhythmias.

Restorative and Balancing Adaptogens

These are the archetypal adaptogens—they have nutritive, tonic, and supportive actions across the whole body and are inherently safe for almost everyone under almost every circumstance. They can be used over many months to build resilience.

ELEUTHERO (*ELEUTHEROCOCCUS SENTICOSUS*)

This herb used to be called Siberian ginseng, but botanists have subsequently moved it into a different genus and further removed it in the evolutionary tree from classic Asian ginseng (*Panax ginseng*). However, eleutheroside A (saponin and sterol glycoside) and eleutheroside B (phenylpropanoid glycoside) exhibit potent stress-reducing effects, equivalent to those of ginseng. In fact, in Russia where it grows wild, this herb is called the King Adaptogen and is considered to be less growth-promoting and less stimulating than Asian ginseng, and therefore more suitable for longer-term use.

Overall Actions of Eleuthero

- Antifatigue; enhances endurance, work capacity, and mental acuity
- Antiviral and immunomodulating
- Enhances learning and memory
- Free radical scavenging (antioxidant)
- Improves oxygen uptake by cells
- Improves the overall health of the patient—reducing fatigue, enhancing organ health
- Increases the body's immune response
- Increases tolerability and effectiveness of chemotherapy and biological therapy, improving immune system recovery; protects and enhances the general condition (appetite, sleep, energy)
- Increases toleration of radiation treatment, preventing radiation sickness; protects and enhances effectiveness of radiation
- Protects against environmental toxins
- Protein sparing (insulinotropic)
- Retards the development of cancer and metastases

ASHWAGANDHA (*WITHANIA SOMNIFERA*)

This herb from India is most well known for its restorative and tonic (nutritive or normalizing) effects and has traditionally been used as part of a "rasayana" program of tonification in Ayurvedic medicine. It is prescribed to help people strengthen their immune system after an illness and for enhanced sexual potency for both men and women. It is a stress-reducing and restorative herb.

The root is rich in two main classes of compounds. At least 12 steroidal alkaloids and 35 steroidal lactones (withanolides) have been identified, which contributes to its broad range of beneficial effects. Much of ashwagandha's pharmacological activity has been attributed to two primary triterpene withanolides, withaferin A and withanolide D.

Actions of Ashwagandha

- Antioxidant properties—ability to scavenge free radicals
- Combats the effects of stress
- Improves learning, memory, and reaction time
- Reduces anxiety and depression without causing drowsiness
- Stabilizes blood sugar, lowers cholesterol
- Reduces brain cell degeneration
- Anti-inflammatory

Tests on human tumor cell lines revealed that ashwagandha may slow the growth of lung, breast, and colon cancer cells and that it may inhibit tumor growth without harming normal cells. The usual recommended dose is 600–1,000 mg of dried root powder twice daily. For people who suffer from insomnia and anxiety, having a cup of hot milk that contains ½ teaspoon of powdered ashwagandha before bedtime is beneficial. Its Latin name, *Withania somnifera*, refers to the known effect of this herb for inducing deep and restful sleep. Indeed, deep sleep (delta or phase 4 sleep) is a critical part of the normal circadian rhythm in the body that enables our immune system to repair itself and optimizes immune responses. So the sleep-inducing effects of ashwagandha are in fact an intricate and integral part of the adaptogenic influence of the herb.

LICORICE (*GLYCYRRHIZA GLABRA*)

This is one of the most widely used adaptogens; it is sweet and pleasant tasting and well tolerated by most people. It is considered an adrenal restorative and is a mucilaginous, moistening, and cooling herb with estrogen-normalizing and some antiviral properties. Licorice is often used as a harmonizer or a synergist in a formula; one of my teachers referred to it as the herb that helps draw all the loose ends of the formula together. Licorice contains triterpenes, including glycyrrhizin and its aglycone glycyrrhizic acid, as well as isoflavones and polysaccharides with immunomodulating effects. Licorice supports the HPA axis, is cortisol sparing, replenishes vital force, and is restorative, rejuvenating, and regenerating. Some people are especially sensitive to the steroids in licorice and may experience an aldosterone-like effect whereby they hold back sodium in the kidneys so that they conserve water in the bloodstream and blood pressure may rise. If you take licorice regularly, it is a good idea to check your blood pressure every couple of weeks. Licorice should be avoided in people with high blood pressure or edema (buildup of fluids).

TULSI (*OCIMUM SANCTUM*)

This is an aromatic member of the mint family that is easy to grow and harvest for yourself. It is pleasant in teas, although the flavor is strong, and for this reason it may be easier to use capsules or tinctures to achieve a higher therapeutic dose. It is mood elevating and uplifting and promotes mental clarity and cognitive functions, while also calming the mind and alleviating anxiety.

Adaptogenic Herbs for Morning Use

For someone who is tired and sluggish:

- Licorice
- Eleuthero
- Ginseng
- Rhodiola
- Leuzea
- Maca

For someone who is anxious, with a high startle reflex:

- Licorice
- Eleuthero
- Tulsi

Adaptogenic Herbs for Use in the Afternoon and Evening

For someone who is not rested or refreshed by sleep:

- Licorice
- Ashwagandha
- Eleuthero
- Tulsi

Nature Therapy for Improved Mental Health

It almost goes without saying that good mental health is crucial to preventing, resisting, coping with, and healing from cancer. This may involve counseling and psychotherapy to enable identification of blocks and fears that hold us back from living in the moment, and it may include mindfulness practices, art therapy, equine therapy, and many other ways of tapping into self-love, acceptance, and joy.

An overwhelming amount of research now exists to support the universal human experience of deriving health benefits as well as pleasure from green and natural environments. Whether it is hiking in the mountains, strolling through an urban park, or simply sitting on a garden bench, people are drawn to plants and natural scenes. Being in nature allows your heart rate and blood pressure to drop and your mood to lift. The ozone and negative ions in fresh forest air have long been recognized as one of the factors that cause the uplifted mood and energizing, calm feelings we have when we spend time in nature. In addition, volatile terpenoids, called phytoncides, emitted by trees (especially evergreens) actively stimulate immune responses.

Research supports claims that being in conifer forests will do the following:

- Lower salivary cortisol
- Lower subjective stress levels
- Lower pro-inflammatory markers
- Reduce oxidative stress

Nature therapy can be as simple as taking a walk in the woods or a park. It can be self-prescribed and self-administered. It is safe, has no side effects, and can be one of the most affordable self-care practices available to cancer patients. Even sitting outside on a balcony or beside an open window looking into a garden will be beneficial. Research suggests it takes about 20 minutes for cortisol levels to drop and deep relaxation to begin.

Shinrin Yoku: The Practice of Forest Bathing

Shinrin Yoku ("forest bathing therapy") has been a part of Japanese medical practice since the 1980s. You can actually get a prescription from your doctor to go to the woods for healing. There are more than 60 designated forest bathing therapy sites in Japan, and it is a recognized therapeutic medical modality. Many other countries (Korea, China, Taiwan, Malaysia, Australia, UK, US, Norway, Sweden, Germany, Austria, and Switzerland) are now developing forest therapy programs to complement conventional healthcare. In British Columbia, the provincial parks department has teamed up with the health department to launch a program called the Park Prescription, and they are supporting physicians with client-care programs and resources to encourage people to get outside.

Shinrin Yoku is akin to a meditation or a mindfulness practice. It is usually done very slowly, very consciously, with great awareness of the environment—sounds, colors, and smells. The participant learns to hold an awareness of the big picture (looking up, looking out) while also maintaining an attention to details (looking down, looking around, listening closely, smelling, touching). The participant practices an immersion in *being* not *doing* (breath awareness) and cultivates a feeling of integration, ideally taking this calm state onward into the rest of the day after the walk is over.

How to Practice Forest Bathing

Getting Ready to Walk, Setting the Intention

- Prepare yourself to receive peace and healing from the forest. Release the road and shake off the dust of the day. Start to shake your body, beginning with your hands, then your arms, legs, torso, and head, gently at first, then as much as you need for a minute or two to release any tension or resistance.
- Put one hand on your heart and one hand on your abdomen and take a few deep, slow breaths to slow your breathing down after the shaking.
- Practice an attitude of gratitude; give thanks to the forest.

Mindfulness Meditation in a Forest

- Practice close gazing and sky gazing. Walking slowly allows you to look up and around as well as to notice small details of nature as you go.
- Walk like an animal—Mouse treads silently, not breaking a twig; Fox has the sharpest ears, never missing a sound; and Deer has the biggest eyes and can see all around. Use your senses of sight, smell, hearing, and touch to deepen your experience in nature.
- Practice contemplative walking—very slowly, silently, paying close attention to nature.
- Sit in silence in the forest. Listen deeply.
- Hug trees and feel and smell bark, leaves, moss, and soil.
- Practice being present in nature.

Coping with Grief

Grief and a sense of loss or bereavement are as much a part of patients' experience of cancer as they are for the families and loved ones watching those patients go through it. These are natural emotions, and there are many simple and safe healing strategies that may be valuable to support this process. Loss is part of the human experience, be it loss of a loved one or loss of your trust in the future after a catastrophic diagnosis. In 1969 Elisabeth Kübler-Ross described five stages of grief, the emotional roller coaster of responses to significant loss or bereavement: denial, anger, bargaining, depression, and acceptance. Although they may be generalizations, they also reflect the lived experience for many people. An individual may experience more than one of these at any time and may cycle through them all more than once. A slightly more nuanced seven stages are recognized today, and they can apply to a cancer diagnosis as easily as a bereavement.

Shock and denial. A state of disbelief and numbed feelings. "This can't be true; it must be a bad dream."

Pain and guilt. "What did I do wrong? What did I fail to do? What could I have done more or done less of, or done better? Why me?"

Anger and bargaining. A state of resistance and resentment. "If I change this or do that, it will all go away and everything will be okay again."

Depression. A state of despair. A belief that nothing is working; a feeling of being doomed and destroyed.

The upward turn. When you hit the bottom there is nowhere else to go but in; seeing yourself and your own truth stripped bare allows a freedom from attachment that lifts you back up.

Reconstruction and working through. Striving to live your best life.

Acceptance and hope. Peace in your heart, tranquility in your mind, and ease in your body.

Herbs for Grief and Sadness

Herbal medicine can be prescribed for all sorts of physical ailments, including cancer, but it can also offer succor at a deep, psychospiritual level. Plants can embody emotional states and can gently influence us in positive ways, sometimes without us even ingesting the medicine. The practice of Shinrin Yoku is one such "medicine" that we receive, through the experience of being in the forest and through breathing forest air. Below are a few other ways in which I work with herbs in my practice.

Flower essences. The original Bach Flower Remedies were developed over a 30-plus-year period by Dr. Edward Bach, a medical practitioner and homeopath in the early twentieth century, and have been in continuous use for almost 90 years. They have been empirically proven, over and over, to be effective and completely safe. There are other collections of flower essences available, under other brand names, but they do not have the history and duration of Dr. Bach's remedies.

Dr. Bach identified seven key types of mental negativity that his remedies can alleviate: fear, uncertainty, insufficient interest in present circumstances, loneliness, oversensitivity to influences and ideas, despondency and despair, and overconcern for others (see the chart on pages 78–79).

The Bach Flower Remedies are made by floating fresh-picked blooms in pure water in the sun for a number of hours, or sometimes simmering woodier plants, and preserving the fluid with brandy. Remedies are taken by the drop, sometimes individually or sometimes as three to five remedies combined to address complex states.

The Bach Flower Remedies are subtle, vibrational medicines, but nonetheless powerful agents, if only by placebo or suggestion. I sometimes dispense them in a dropper bottle to take as a lone remedy with a deliberate process of self-awareness, thinking about the meaning of the remedy and why the patient needs it, and sometimes I add them to a tincture formula for simplicity and compliance. They are exceptionally helpful for allowing people to see their way more clearly, to better understand themselves and their responses and reactions, and to help manage negative emotions that can sabotage their mental peace.

Get to know rose (the herb of the heart). The heart is considered to hold the emotions of love and grief or sorrow, which is reflected in words such as *heartfelt, heartsore, heartache,* and *heartbreak.* Roses have a long association with love and the heart, and this is seen in cultural traditions such as giving red roses for Valentine's Day and anniversaries. Rose can be invoked to help soften sadness into something we can accept and live with. I use rose petal tincture in my formulas, and I use rose petals in tea blends. I also encourage people to wear pink, use rose-scented soaps, wear rose or geranium essential oil as a perfume, buy roses for the house, and put out bowls of dried rosebuds with rose or geranium essential oil to spike the scent. Rose quartz crystal is said to be helpful to facilitate heartfelt or heart-to-heart communication; patients can hold it in their hand as a reminder of this when they want to speak from the heart.

Encourage patients to plant a rosebush in the garden, or even grow just one miniature rose in a pot on a balcony, and spend time tending it and caring for it. They could find a local rose garden and volunteer some time there, or just sit on a bench and enjoy the flowers. Patients may want to harvest rose petals for nature arts and crafts, such as pressed-flower pictures, rose petal potpourri, or rose beads (the original rosary beads were pressed rose petals). Rose petals also make excellent simple syrup, which can then be diluted with sparkling water and a squeeze of lemon to make a refreshing summer drink. All of these ways of engaging with rose allow grief and sadness to be tempered by beauty and creativity.

Plant a memory garden. This may be a container on a patio, a bed of flowers in a garden, or even an indoor planter with specific plants that have special significance for the patient. They may be flowers that were favorites from the patient's garden (lavender, miniature roses, marigolds, and snapdragons), flowers that were in their wedding bouquet (lily of the valley, orchids), flowers that remind them of happier times (cactus from a holiday at the Grand Canyon), or a favorite color theme with yellow or pink or white flowers. The planning, planting, and tending of this memory garden is a profound horticultural therapy opportunity, and not only will the patient benefit, but family, friends, or caregivers who see the finished product will also have a living memorial to their loved one after they are gone.

BACH ESSENCES FOR SPECIFIC EMOTIONS		
	Essence	**Type of Behavior**
FEAR	Rock rose	Extreme fear, nightmares, terror, feeling frozen, hypersensitivity, hyperawareness
	Mimulus	Fear of known cause, nervous tension, spasms and tics, restlessness and agitation
	Cherry plum	Fear of losing control, suicidal thoughts or risk-taking behaviors, loss of belief in the future
	Aspen	Apprehension, anxiety, fears of the unknown, withdrawal and self-isolating
	Red chestnut	Fear for others, overconcern and controlling, micromanaging, and obsessing over details
UNCERTAINTY	Cerato	Lack of faith in one's own judgment, questioning and second-guessing, doubting self
	Scleranthus	Indecision, inability to choose, feeling unbalanced in life, torn between extremes
	Gentian	Despondency, disappointment, lack of faith, crushed and set back, let down by others
	Gorse	Hopelessness, despair, desperation, can't see a way out of the situation, trapped by self
	Hornbeam	Mental tiredness, procrastination, putting off the inevitable, resigned but resentful
	Wild oat	Inability to see one's direction, unclear about the future, questioning and feeling uncertain
INSUFFICIENT INTEREST IN PRESENT CIRCUMSTANCES	Clematis	Dreamy, absent-minded, distracted, inattentive, living in a fantasy world
	Honeysuckle	Living in the past, homesickness, nostalgia and regrets, wishing for different outcomes of past choices
	Wild rose	Apathy, lack of enthusiasm, lethargic, "can't be bothered," lack of interest in others, lack of curiosity
	Olive	Physical and mental tiredness, exhaustion, depleted and debilitated, worn down and worn out
	White chestnut	Persistent unwanted thoughts, repetitive thinking and perseveration
	Mustard	Gloom, depression for no apparent reason, black cloud descending, pessimistic
	Chestnut bud	Inability to learn one's lessons, repeating mistakes, arrogance and inflexibility

BACH ESSENCES FOR SPECIFIC EMOTIONS		
	Essence	**Type of Behavior**
OVERCONCERN FOR THE WELFARE OF OTHERS	Chicory	Possessive, controlling, domineering, demanding attention and obedience
	Vervain	Overenthusiasm, perfectionism, own hardest judge, driven to do better
	Vine	Clinging and needy, fearful and fragile, tearful, low self-worth, self-deprecating
	Beech	Overcritical, never satisfied, always wants more or better, cravings and obsessions
	Rock water	Resistance, denial, refusal to accept a situation, insistent, isolated
LONELINESS	Water violet	Proud, righteous, opinionated, lecturing others how to be
	Impatiens	Impatience, irritability, intolerant, demanding, bossy, and insistent
	Heather	Overtalkative, not listening or hearing other people, narcissistic
OVERSENSITIVE TO INFLUENCES & IDEAS	Agrimony	Hiding worries behind a false smile, putting on a brave face, walling off feelings
	Centaury	Weak willed, subservient, feels undeserving, easily swayed by others
	Walnut	Change, need for adaptability, protection when feeling vulnerable, opening to new ideas
	Holly	Anger, jealousy, suspicion, imagining problems, making trouble
DESPONDENCY & DESPAIR	Larch	Lack of confidence, inability to take risks, fearful, and constrained
	Pine	Feelings of guilt, unworthiness, lack of self-regard
	Elm	Overwhelmed by responsibility, can't carry the burden any longer, giving up
	Sweet chestnut	Extreme anguish, dismay, despair, hopelessness
	Star of Bethlehem	Shock, trauma, accidents, fear for your life
	Willow	Stubbornness and inflexibility, rigid thinking, needing to find ease and grace in a situation, inability to work around obstacles
	Oak	Feeling buffeted and battered by vicissitudes of life, needing to learn to stand up strong with deep roots and take what comes
	Crabapple	Feelings of shame, unworthiness, uncleanliness, needing to be renewed and refreshed, physically and mentally

The Role of Hallucinogens

In response to psychospiritual and psycho-emotional conflicts, patients today are seeking out hallucinogenic plants and psychedelic experiences as part of their healing journey. This is no longer the taboo subject in academia and scientific literature that it was for so many decades. In the past 10 years, there has been an explosion of research in numerous reputable medical centers that has documented the immense value of these shamanic practices, done with great care regarding the set and setting, and with careful guidance before and after the "trip."

This treatment is usually reserved in the research for the terminally ill; after these experiences people report a great alleviation of the natural stress, fear, and anxiety they feel as they face their demise. For anybody wishing to explore these realms, I would urge considerable caution—not so much about the plant medicines themselves as about the people who offer their services to guide you through the process. Some of them may be entirely genuine and well intentioned, and some of them are unskilled and potentially unhelpful. The setting and context are critical, and when the experience is done right it can be life (and death) changing.

This treatment is certainly not a thing to do in a casual manner without appropriate care and consideration of what you are getting into. If it is something you wish to pursue, I suggest first reading the *Manual for Psychedelic Guides*, self-published by Mark Haden, from the Multidisciplinary Association for Psychedelic Studies, which describes in detail the process of supporting someone who is using a psychedelic for therapeutic or spiritual purposes. This sets a standard and provides a road map for how to get the best from the whole experience.

Promoting Deep and Restful Sleep

Not getting enough sleep at night gradually changes the brain and the neuroendocrine system in a similar way to that seen in stress-related disorders such as depression. Lack of sleep directly or indirectly causes increases in HPA activity and cortisol release. By acting on stress systems, insufficient sleep may sensitize individuals to stress-related disorders. This can easily become a self-perpetuating cycle, in which reduced sleep predisposes you to stress responses and the stress responses impact sleep quality.

Lack of sleep is also associated with an increased risk of developing breast cancer. A study involving 35,000 women over 11 years found that women who slept an average of 9 hours per day had a two-thirds reduced risk of getting breast cancer, compared to women who slept 6 hours or less. The longer sleep cohort also had an average of 42 percent higher levels of melatonin—a hormone that is synthesized in the brain in response to duration and intensity of daylight and is released from the pineal gland during the dark of the night. It is estimated that nearly 50 percent of the adult population in the US is sleep deprived, so it's reasonable to assume that this is contributing to some significant health risk.

Circadian Rhythms

Disruption of circadian rhythms (sleep–wake cycles) by shift work, regular travel across time zones, or lifestyle choices (such as staying up late or falling asleep with the TV or lights on) leads to an increased risk of breast cancer. This may be partly attributed to the fact that light exposure at night suppresses the nocturnal production of melatonin that inhibits breast cancer growth.

In a groundbreaking study of circadian rhythms, researchers at the University of Haifa in Israel overlaid satellite images of Earth onto cancer registries and found that women who live in neighborhoods with large amounts of nighttime illumination, where melatonin is disrupted, are more likely to get breast cancer than those who live in areas where nocturnal darkness prevails, even after controlling for other factors such as pollution in a city.

Epidemiological studies of nurses, flight attendants, and others who work at night have found breast cancer rates up to 60 percent above normal, even when other factors, such as differences in diet, are accounted for. On the basis of such studies, the International Agency for Research on Cancer now classifies shift work, especially a swing shift, as a "probable carcinogen." That puts night-shift work in the same health-risk category as exposure to toxic chemicals such as trichloroethylene, vinyl chloride, and polychlorinated biphenyls (PCBs).

Good Sleep Hygiene

Here are a few tips to help you establish a good sleep routine.

Unwind. Schedule an hour at the end of the evening for bedtime preparation. This will allow you time to unwind, relax, and get yourself in the mood for sleep. Have a warm bath with lavender, light a candle, listen to soft music; make it a ritual. Avoid watching TV for a couple of hours before bed and don't read thrillers or scary books in the evenings. Don't do vigorous exercise within 3 hours of bedtime, as it is stimulating and invigorating and will keep you awake.

Set a regular bedtime. As much as possible, go to bed and wake up at the same time every day. Up to 30 minutes variance can be okay, but try not to deviate by more than that. The body usually responds well to a routine like this. It doesn't preclude the occasional party, but know that you will probably pay for it the next day and will need a few days to reestablish the routine.

Ensure that your bed is really comfortable. Sleep in the biggest bed you can, so that you never feel crowded. Get a good mattress and box spring. The mattress should be firm; you can top it with an egg-crate foam pad or a sheepskin cover, if you have sensitive places that press in the night. Use cotton flannel sheets for immediate warmth when you get in at night. Use a hot-water bottle if you are chilly (not an electric blanket because of electromagnetic frequencies). Make sure you have the best pillow you can buy; try the contoured ones that are available from chiropractors or medical stores. Use a long, firm pillow between your knees when you lie on your side, or under your knees when you lie on your back. This supports and protects the sacroiliac joints.

Stay cool. Keep the bedroom cool, with some fresh air but no drafts. Consider using a humidifier if you live in a dry climate. Use aromatherapy to scent the room; lavender, orange blossom, and rosewood are especially relaxing.

Turn down the lights and listen to soothing sounds. Prepare to sleep by turning out all the electric lights and using candles for the last hour before you go to bed. This will slowly adjust the brain chemistry to night mode. Be sure to sleep in absolute darkness. Use heavy curtains or wear an eye mask. Do not use digital bedside clocks and avoid night lights. If you must have a night light to see the way to the bathroom, position it low on the ground and do not look at it when you get up in the night. If there is a lot of noise, wear earplugs or listen to soft, instrumental music or sounds of nature.

Move your clock. If possible, don't keep a clock in the bedroom. If you must see the time in the morning, or be woken by the alarm, then keep your clock in a place where you can't see it from the bed. Resist the urge to check the time when you wake in the night and can't go back to sleep. This just creates stress and tension.

Visualize. Use the time waiting for sleep for a meditation practice, guided visualization, imagining pleasant and happy things, or any other thoughts that are positive and creative. Try not to use the time to rehash the day or plan tomorrow; avoid worrying and fretting, as it doesn't help.

Make your bedroom a sacred space. Reserve the bedroom for sleeping and lovemaking. Try to make it a sacred space that is tranquil and calm. Don't use it for watching TV, reading, working, making phone calls, and so on.

Don't snooze in the morning. When you first wake in the morning, try to stay awake. Don't hit the snooze button on the alarm clock. Drifting in and out of sleep in the morning will disrupt the wakening cue and make you groggy. Get up, go outside, and look up into the morning sky for a minute, with no windows, glasses, or contact lenses to filter the light. This will switch off the melatonin production and start the daytime boost of serotonin.

Herbs and Supplements for Better Sleep

Herbal remedies are very useful for aiding sleep, preferably in tincture or capsule form to avoid a large fluid intake shortly before bed. Some of these herbs also relieve pain, so if pain is part of the cause of poor sleep, these will be particularly effective.

Mild Sedatives and Relaxants

These herbs are suitable for teas in the day to calm agitation or anxiety, or in higher doses in capsules and tinctures at night before bed.

- Catnip
- Chamomile
- Lemon balm
- Linden
- Milky oats
- Skullcap
- St. John's wort

Medium Strength

These are best in tinctures or capsules, as water will not extract them so well. Use caution, as they may induce drowsiness in higher doses, so you should avoid operating machinery or driving after taking them.

- California poppy
- Hops (also good in a traditional sachet to tuck into a pillow and inhale the volatile oils all night)
- Kava
- Passionflower
- Wild lettuce

Strong Sedatives

These herbs are best used in tincture for precise dose calibration. They may cause grogginess the next day. Consider premeasuring a dose before bed to have ready to take if you wake in the night. They won't knock you out like a pharmaceutical sleeping aid will, but they will quiet the mind and ease rest.

- Corydalis
- Jamaican dogwood (there are some sustainability concerns with this herb, so only purchase cultivated plant material, not wild harvested)
- Valerian

Supplements for Better Sleep

- 5-HTP (5-hydroxytryptophan)—makes melatonin
- Calcium citrate—muscle relaxant
- Cannabidiol (CBD)—nonpsychoactive extract from cannabis
- GABA (gamma-aminobutyric acid)—an inhibitory neurotransmitter
- Glycine—sweet-tasting amino acid that calms the mind
- L-theanine—calming and relaxing amino acid from green tea
- Magnesium glycinate/bisglycinate—muscle relaxant
- Vitamin B6—nervine

Melatonin

Melatonin is a hormone that has multiple actions in the body, including regulation of circadian sleep–wake cycles and of seasonal rhythms and antioxidant and anti-inflammatory effects. Melatonin also regulates immune responses as well as cell proliferation and immune mediators. In the immune system, melatonin acts as a buffer; it acts as an immunostimulant or an anti-inflammatory as needed to support healing. This makes melatonin a sort of "adaptogen" for the immune system that optimizes responses and normalizes cell behaviors.

MELATONIN AND CANCER

Melatonin has anticancer action through several mechanisms. It is primarily considered a preventive agent but also has specific use in managing cancer. It is an antiestrogen that suppresses genes coding for estrogen receptors. It inhibits cell proliferation, and it impairs the metastatic capacity of breast cancer cells. Melatonin also decreases the formation of estrogens from androgens via aromatase inhibition.

Makes cancer cells more susceptible to chemotherapy. Because many cancers (such as brain, bone, melanoma, cervical, prostate, and lung cancer) are sensitive to estrogen, melatonin has also been investigated as a treatment option in some of these as well. In one study of non–small cell lung cancer, the conventional chemotherapy drugs cisplatin and etoposide were given alongside 20 milligrams of melatonin nightly. This study of 100 patients was randomized so they received either chemotherapy alone or chemotherapy and melatonin. Results showed overall tumor regression rate and the 5-year survival results were significantly higher in patients treated with melatonin alongside chemotherapy. Chemotherapy was better tolerated in patients treated with melatonin, and this may have been a contributing factor to the improved outcomes, as patients were better able to complete the prescribed drug regimen. In addition, coadministration of melatonin with chemotherapy agents may also deactivate cell pathways that allow for development of drug resistance and resensitize cancer to drugs that have ceased to work.

Improves healing and inhibits metastasis. Other nonspecific benefits of taking melatonin concurrent with chemotherapy include protection of gastrointestinal mucosa against chemotherapy and radiation injury, improved wound healing after surgery, and reduced tissue damage, pain sensation, and weakness. Melatonin also inhibits metastasis by limiting the entrance of cancer cells into the vascular system and preventing them from establishing secondary growths at distant sites.

Melatonin limits uptake of linoleic acid, an omega-6 dietary fat that promotes cell proliferation and growth. Melatonin inhibits the activity of telomerase, an enzyme that is essential for the synthesis of specialized ribonuclear proteins (the telomeres) that extend the ends of chromosomes. These molecular extensions are required for stabilizing chromosomal structure, and they shorten with each cell division in normal cells, eventually weakening the chromosomal structure and triggering senescence (irreversible cell cycle arrest) or apoptosis (cell death). In cancer cells, there is upregulation of telomerase activity that allows the cancerous cells to maintain DNA stability and contributes to their immortality despite repeated cell division. Melatonin is helpful to downregulate this activity.

SUPPLEMENTING WITH MELATONIN

Melatonin is readily available as a dietary supplement in Canada and the US. It is a hormone, so some caution is warranted, but millions of doses over a couple of decades in North America have certainly shown it to be safe. A healthy adult would normally make approximately 0.5 mg +/− within 24 hours. Very young children and older seniors make less melatonin, partly explaining why they sleep in fits and starts, on and off in short bursts not governed by day–night cycles.

A suitable supplement dose for most individuals can be calibrated by dream tolerance. Melatonin is a tryptamine-derived molecule that contributes in the brain to the visual content of your dream life (similar to how dimethyltryptamines in psilocybe mushrooms can give you hallucinations), and doses higher than your individual tolerance will tend to cause busy, vivid, or even disturbing dreams. Much of the research in cancer therapy has been with high doses of 10, 20, or even up to 40 mg, but these higher doses may not be well tolerated in some cases. Dose from 1–20 mg, according to dream tolerance. (See page 402 for dosing guidelines.)

Exercise

A substantial body of evidence indicates that physical activity and exercise offer significant benefits in resisting, preventing, and even treating cancer. Physically active individuals are less likely to develop breast, colon, prostate, bladder, and some gynecologic cancers. Breast cancer patients who are physically active may have up to 40% lower risk of dying from their cancer than case-matched patients who are largely sedentary. Maintaining physical activity after a colorectal cancer diagnosis is associated with a 30% lower risk of death from colorectal cancer, while maintaining physical activity after a prostate cancer diagnosis gives 33% less risk of death from prostate cancer and 45% less risk of death from any cause. Similarly, the risk of bladder cancer is up to 15% lower for individuals with high levels of physical activity than for those with the lowest level of activity. Exercise training can lead to improvements in aerobic fitness, muscular strength, quality of life, and levels of fatigue, as well as change the tumor microenvironment and trigger stronger antitumor activity in the immune system.

Some Benefits of Exercise on Cancer Development or Progression

- Reduced body fat (adipose tissue) leading to lower levels of sex hormones, such as estrogen, and lower levels of growth factors that are associated with cancer development and progression
- Reduced serum insulin, insulin resistance, and blood sugar
- Reduced inflammation, enhanced lymphatic flow, lessening of edema (buildup of fluids) and of stagnation
- Improved immune system function
- Better bone density to resist metastasis
- Enhanced sleep quality

Physical activity can include walking, dancing, biking, performing vigorous household or garden chores, and engaging in sports activities. Physical activity should include at least 150 minutes (2½ hours) per week of moderate-intensity activity or 90 minutes of vigorous-intensity activity every week. This should include resistance training (weight lifting, resistance bands) for building muscle strength and bone density, regular stretching and balance exercises for flexibility and agility, and aerobic activities for cardiac health and weight management.

CHAPTER 3

Preparing for Surgery and Enhancing Recovery

Chances are you will need to have surgery at some point in your cancer journey—if only as part of the diagnostic process. There are a few cancers that may be diagnosed by blood work (such as leukemias) or sputum (some lung cancers), but in almost every cancer case there will be a biopsy to obtain a diagnosis, and very likely some follow-up surgery to remove the primary tumor as well, either before or after chemotherapy. Natural therapies can help you prepare for and heal more quickly from surgery.

CHAPTER 3 CONTENTS

89 **Considering the Risks of Surgery**

90 Does Surgery Contribute to Cancer Spread?

91 Tumor Shrinkage as a Measure of Chemotherapy Response

93 **Enhanced Recovery after Surgery (ERAS)**

93 Better Recovery Starts before the Surgery

94 **Preparing for Surgery**

94 Ask Questions and Understand the Process

95 Informed Consent

96 One to Two Months before Surgery

98 Four Days before Surgery

99 The Day before Surgery

100 **Recovery from Surgery**

100 Manage Pain

101 Prevent Blood Clots

102 Prevent Postoperative Cognitive Impairment

105 Let Go Liniment

105 Counteracting Immunosuppression

106 **Herbs for Enhanced Recovery after Surgery**

106 Brain Tonic Herbs and Mental Stimulants

111 Herbs That Regulate Inflammation

112 Tonic Herbs to Support the Nervous System after Surgery

113 **Avoiding Complications of Healing**

113 Phases of Wound Healing

114 Control Local Infection

115 Tumor Spray

115 Support the Immune System and Manage Inflammation

116 Promote and Support Connective Tissue

118 Topical Treatments to Reduce Scarring

120 Scar Oil

120 **Dietary Supplements to Support Healing after Surgery**

120 B-Complex Vitamins

121 Zinc

122 Vitamin C

122 Chlorella (*Chlorella* spp.)

124 Healing and Recuperation Tincture

Considering the Risks of Surgery

Given that wound healing and new blood vessel growth (angiogenesis) share so many metabolic pathways and control systems—in other words, the biological processes that help wounds heal are the same ones that can help cancer spread—it may seem counterintuitive to undergo surgery, which then creates a perfect environment for growth of any cells left behind. There is ongoing debate about the relative safety and merits of surgery during cancer treatment. Even a needle biopsy, such as is utilized in sampling many breast or prostate lumps, may leave a trail of potentially malignant cells dropping off the needle tip as it is withdrawn, to say nothing of the inflammation and aggravation of poking and piercing the tumor itself. There may even be an argument here for excisional biopsy, removing the entire tumor and then getting the detailed pathology report on it, entailing only one surgery, albeit a bigger one than a fine needle aspiration biopsy.

All surgeries have risks, and complications of surgery may delay recovery and make it more challenging to treat the underlying cancer; crisis intervention may trump chronic care and deep-healing strategies. In principle, avoiding surgery would be ideal, but in reality, you're likely to have surgery at some point. Because of that, it's most practical to focus on ways to better manage your preparation for and recovery from surgery, in order to mitigate the risks and to regulate the inflammation and repair pathways that are necessary for recovery from surgery but that could also drive cancer behaviors in cells.

Some of the complications associated with surgery (such as clotting and bleeding) are medical emergencies and require hospitalization or changes to prescription drugs and cannot be managed by natural medicines alone. However, cognitive and memory decline, scarring and adhesions, infection, and pain can all be significantly and safely aided by herbal medicine, and it is these that we shall discuss here.

Possible Complications of Surgery

- Blood clots (myocardial infarction or heart attack, stroke, pulmonary embolism, thromboembolism)
- Bleeding or infection
- Pain (acute and chronic)
- Adverse drug reactions
- Cognitive and memory decline
- Scarring and adhesions
- Disablement
- Poor self-image afterward
- Dysbiosis (both from antibiotics given before/during surgery and from the stress of the surgery) and higher risk of leaky gut

Also keep in mind that surgery by itself may not remove the cancer. I often use the analogy of a mushroom when explaining this to patients: You can harvest all the fruiting bodies aboveground that you want (the mushrooms), but when the next rains come the mushrooms will grow back because the "roots" are still there and the terrain is conducive. In this way, surgery without attention to diet, lifestyle, and health habits is unlikely to be sufficient. For example, a woman with cervical dysplasia (an indication of potential cervical cancer) who has a colposcopy and LEEP (loop electrosurgical excision procedure) to remove affected cells should consider quitting smoking and eating more vegetables to reduce the risk of recurrence.

Does Surgery Contribute to Cancer Spread?

Eli Jones' statement below was made more than 100 years ago, in 1894, and obviously the experience of surgery is very different today, with much better pain and sepsis control, as well as more generally conservative techniques and procedures. However, his comments about the possible spread of cancer cells systemically and the effects of that on outcomes are no less relevant for the passage of time.

There may be several mechanisms by which cancer is encouraged to grow after surgery. One of the common behaviors of cells to injury (including surgery) is to grow new blood vessels. This is something that serves a tumor as well and is one way in which surgery for cancer may possibly drive growth of any cells left behind from the surgery.

Surgery stimulates new blood vessel growth by upregulating (stimulating) several cell-derived growth factors as well as inflammatory pathways such as cyclooxygenase-2 (COX-2) and 5-lipoxygenase (5-LOX), and this illustrates an intrinsic contradiction with strategies for managing cancer such as reducing inflammation and inhibiting the growth of new blood vessels. Stress-induced suppression of natural killer cell activity also contributes to increased susceptibility to tumor development, so stress management and effective pain management can downregulate (suppress) and reduce blood vessel growth induced by surgery.

> A surgeon can only cut out what is seen and felt under the knife, while millions of cancer cells grow and multiply in the blood, the nuclei of future cancer. Another fact that the surgeon forgets is that every operation is a shock to the nervous system, it lowers the nerve power, weakens the power of resistance to disease and thus encourages the invasion of cancer.
>
> ELI JONES, *CANCER—ITS CAUSES, SYMPTOMS, AND TREATMENTS*

SURGERY-INDUCED ANGIOGENESIS

For a few types of cancer, studies have indicated a correlation between surgical removal of a primary tumor and increased growth in metastatic tumors. In approximately 20 percent of premenopausal breast cancer patients, surgery is estimated to initiate blood vessel growth (angiogenesis) of dormant cells in distant sites and contribute to involvement of lymph nodes. It is suggested that surgery may induce this angiogenesis and accelerate disease by a median of 2 years in these patients.

In colorectal cancer with spread to the liver, studies have correlated the continued presence of a primary tumor with decreased vascularization (blood vessel distribution) of its distant metastases. Surgical removal of the primary tumor resulted in increased growth of new blood vessels to metastatic tumors. Also in studies involving colorectal cancer, a decrease in circulating antiangiogenic factors (angiostatin and endostatin, which reduce the growth of new blood vessels) after surgical removal of primary colorectal carcinoma coincided with increased metabolic activity of liver metastases. In a study of gastric cancer, removal of a primary tumor resulted in increased metabolic activity in liver metastasis. All these studies suggest that the presence of the primary tumor suppresses angiogenesis in its distant metastasis, and that removal of the primary lesion causes a flare-up in new blood vessel formation.

For more detailed information, see Further Mechanisms behind Surgery-Induced Angiogenesis on page 124.

Tumor Shrinkage as a Measure of Chemotherapy Response

If the primary tumor has been removed, then cancer markers may go up at first as an immune response, and there is no tumor to observe or palpate, both of which can make it harder to assess the success of chemotherapy or cytotoxic herbs. If a cancer is assessed as stage 1 and grade 1—if it is caught early and is relatively small, localized, and well differentiated—then it is often left in place while chemotherapy and/or natural remedies are used first. If these approaches are effective, then seeing a tumor shrink on repeated scans or cancer markers in the blood go down may be a useful gauge of success.

Measuring overall survival in response to cancer treatments takes years to give reliable and robust results, while tumor shrinkage is rapid and readily visualized. Tumor size is used for treatment planning and is considered a convenient, readily measurable surrogate end point for measuring success of a treatment. However, even this seemingly objective measurement is open to challenge, and contradictory studies suggest that tumor shrinkage may not be a useful gauge of treatment success after all. A 2019 study of data from 20 randomized clinical trials reported that the time to nadir (time to shrinkage) and depth of nadir (extent of shrinkage) were found to have only weak or moderate associations with overall survival.

Even more significantly, a 2020 article reported on the well-known clinical phenomenon where initial tumor shrinkage to undetectable levels is followed by an aggressive tumor recurrence. The author suggested that any residual cancer cells present at the end of treatment or at the start of a treatment break may evolve independently and become rapidly proliferative in the tumor microenvironment of a degrading cancer. Where chemotherapy fails to eliminate or stabilize the disease, treatment holidays may provide an opportunity for surviving cancer cell populations to proliferate, due to a greater supply of space, nutrients, oxygen, and growth factors as weaker cells die off. This may be an argument for the metronomic dosing schedule described in Chapter 5, where the drugs are supplied in low dose continuously instead of in the maximum tolerated dose with breaks. Significantly, it appears that more tumor shrinkage promotes multiplication of resistant cells. Thus, use of tumor shrinkage as a surrogate end point in clinical trials is unreliable.

There is also an issue of inaccuracy in measuring tumor shrinkage. For example, in a review of breast-imaging modalities (mammography, ultrasound, and tomosynthesis), tumor size was correctly estimated in less than half of the cases. Similarly, a 2021 report in the *Journal of Urology* highlighted how MRI scans frequently underestimated prostate cancer tumor size, and the authors recommended a larger ablation margin (a wider radiotherapy field) to compensate for this.

All this is to say that while there may be merit in delaying surgery to assess the effects of chemotherapy and to reduce potential risks of local proliferation or distant metastases, tumor shrinkage may not be a reliable way to assess outcomes, and contradictory research also suggests that early removal of tumor burden has merit as well. Surgical decisions need to be made with care and consideration for all these factors.

Certainly, if a tumor is compromising function in some way, such as by obstructing the esophagus or bowel or compressing a nerve or a major blood vessel, then surgery is clearly indicated. However, if surgery is elective, then there may be considerable value in preparing the body in advance by modulating inflammation and new blood vessel growth to promote healing while inhibiting any stray cancer cells that have evaded the knife. This preparation might be for 1–2 weeks or a month or more, depending on how far in advance surgery is scheduled, but even just a few days may have clinical benefit.

Enhanced Recovery after Surgery (ERAS)

As medicine has evolved, with improved infection control, safer obstetrics, better accident and emergency care, and lifesaving drugs, so have people lived longer and longer. The average person born in the US in 2000 can expect to live almost twice as long as the person born in 1900 (the actual difference is 73 to 46 years for men and 79 to 48 years for women). One consequence of this evolution is that ever-older people are undergoing extensive surgeries, and a new branch of research into mitigating the harm and damage from these surgeries has developed. Although much of the research is in seniors, with an eye to reducing the onset or worsening of dementia, there are many useful concepts and strategies here that anyone having surgery could adopt.

Better Recovery Starts before the Surgery

The idea of ERAS can be credited to Henrik Kehlet, a Danish doctor who has specialized in managing supportive care for surgery. In the early 1990s, he proposed an innovative program, or protocol, for recovery that was functional and proactive rather than symptomatic and reactive. The principle is to bring about an accelerated recovery by preparing the body in advance and by assisting the recuperation phase. Among the main surgical principles he identified were restrictive intravenous fluid therapy, use of laparoscopy in combination with appropriate anesthesia, appropriate and effective pain management, early return to proper feeding and digestion, and early postoperative mobilization. Benefits include lessening of perioperative neuroendocrine stress response, maintenance of organ function, and an accelerated return of gut function. The proactive and preventive preoperative ERAS program also addresses chronic illnesses to achieve best possible physical status (including exercise, nutritional supplementation, and health education, such as in regard to alcohol cessation, for 1–2 months prior to major surgery), a program the researchers called "prehabilitation."

A formal clinical program of prehabilitation and subsequent postsurgical rehabilitation is the medical ideal, addressing lifestyle and overall wellness in advance of a significant stressor, and following up in a custom plan for recuperation. This is a great opportunity for herbal and nutritional medicine to be put front and center of the plan. The healthier and stronger the person is before undergoing surgery, the better the recovery. When it is possible to take a few weeks to optimize health, there may be value in postponing surgery in order to do so.

Preparing for Surgery

How you prepare for surgery can make a significant difference in how quickly you recover from it and in how effective the surgery is. Electing to have surgery may be one of the most significant decisions in your cancer journey, and it deserves careful consideration and preparation for best outcomes.

Here is a suggested list of actions to take and plans to make if surgery is expected.

- Find out all you can about the proposed procedure—what will be done, what the expected recovery stage will be like, what kinds of outcomes you can expect (see the next page for a list of questions to ask the surgeon).
- Make a good plan for hospital visitors to bring you home-cooked food, fresh juices, smoothies, soups, and so forth every day.
- Make a whole lot of ready meals for the freezer that are nourishing, high protein, easy to prepare, and easy to digest; bone broths, stocks, soups, and stews are ideal.
- Plan for home care when you leave the hospital—this includes a home care nurse if needed, someone to cook, clean, run errands, and do other tasks including childcare/eldercare. If finances are a problem, then discuss your needs with the designated hospital social worker, who can help you access services and resources.
- Organize herbs and supplements for the recovery phase so you have them all counted out and ready before the procedure.
- Ensure you have physiotherapy/occupational therapy arranged for recovery, and consider rehabilitation yoga or Pilates for regaining physical strength.
- Arrange a hospital bed at home that allows easy in and out with adjustable height, as well as a special mattress for preventing bedsores if you end up bedbound for a couple of weeks or more. Consider a commode as well if getting to the bathroom may be difficult.

Ask Questions and Understand the Process

When you commit to surgery, it is vitally important that you understand what you are signing up for and why you are doing it. It is an irreversible decision and needs to be based ideally in research and information and not in fear. Knowing what to expect will help you set up a good self-care plan and manage the whole experience better.

General Questions

- Why am I having this operation? What are the chances of its success?
- Is there any other way to treat my disease?
- Aside from my disease, am I healthy enough to go through the stress of surgery and the drugs used to do it (anesthesia)?

Questions for Your Surgeon

- Are you certified by the American Board of Surgery and/or a specialty surgery board?
- How many operations like this have you done? What is your success rate? Are you experienced in operating on my kind of disease?
- Exactly what will you be doing in this operation? What will you be taking out? Why?
- What other surgical options are there?
- Will any implants or devices be left inside my body after the surgery?
- How frequently is a second or other surgery needed in people who undergo this procedure? What are the causes of or reasons for these additional procedures?
- How do we know the procedure will have the results you say? (What is the medical evidence supporting the idea that this is the best procedure?)
- How long will the surgery take?
- Will I need blood transfusions? If so, can I donate blood now?
- What can I expect afterward? Will I be in a lot of pain? Will I have drains or catheters? How long will I need to be in the hospital?
- How will my body be affected by the surgery? Will it work differently or look different? Will any of the effects be permanent?
- How long will it take for me to go back to my usual activities?
- What are the possible risks and side effects of this operation? What is the risk of death or disability?
- What will happen if I choose not to have the operation?
- What are the chances that the surgery will cure my disease?
- What drugs will I need to take before or after the surgery?
- If you were in my situation, is this the treatment you would undergo?
- Who is the best surgeon for doing this procedure in this country? In the world? Should I seek care from them?

Informed Consent

When you sign the consent form at the hospital for the surgery, you are saying that you have received all required information about risks and benefits and that you are willing to have the surgery. It's important that you read the consent form and understand each of the possible risks before signing it. The details may vary from state to state, but the informed consent form usually says that your doctor has explained the following things:

- Your condition and why surgery is the best option
- The goal of the surgery
- How the surgery is to be done
- How it may benefit you
- What your risks are

- What side effects to expect
- What other treatment options you have instead of, or as well as, surgery

If you specifically do not want a certain procedure, then you must write that into the informed-consent document and have it witnessed. You must also take responsibility to make sure the surgeon acknowledges it. For example, if you are undergoing mastectomy, you may decline in advance to have a lymph bed dissection but give permission for sentinel node biopsy.

One to Two Months before Surgery

Start the Clean and Green Detox Diet. Beginning up to 8 weeks before surgery, start the Clean and Green Detox Diet (page 41). This will help with eliminating dietary toxins and burden on the liver.

Supplement with milk thistle. The flavano-lignan complex called silymarin protects the liver, inhibiting oxidative stress and supporting toxin clearance. According to herbalist Kerry Bone, based on many years of clinical experience, 200 mg of silymarin three times daily is recommended for 2 weeks before and 2–4 weeks after surgery, with higher doses and longer duration of use after longer surgeries (approximately 2 weeks of use for every hour of anesthesia). Importantly, innumerable studies document the safety and benefits of milk thistle extract in all stages of cancer care, from prevention to acute intervention.

Boost nonspecific immune function. Take astragalus and medicinal mushrooms several times a week at least, and daily in the last 2 weeks before surgery. Consider taking thymic protein powder and the Immune Boot Camp Nutritional Breakfast Smoothie (page 60).

Restore bowel health and boost microbiome. Signing up for surgery, as with signing up for chemotherapy, comes with a raft of pharmaceuticals that are recommended, if not required. Muscle relaxants and opioids for pain can contribute to flaccid constipation, hospital food is generally lacking in fiber and micronutrients required for proper digestive function, and antibiotics are routinely prescribed as a prophylactic. For all these reasons it may be useful, both before and after surgery, to work to optimize microbiome health and bowel function.

Herbal and Nutritional Strategies to Prepare for Surgery

The herbs and supplements listed below can be mixed and matched to suit an individual as needed. Layering the herbs and nutrients in this way is the art and science of formulating that is explored in Chapters 7 and 8.

- **Optimize the immune system.** Use immune tonics (restoratives) and stimulants, such as echinacea, cat's claw, taheebo, pokeroot, mushrooms, astragalus, vitamin A, vitamin C, vitamin D, zinc, and selenium.
- **Reduce systemic inflammation.** Use turmeric, Indian frankincense, licorice, fish oil (omega-3), sarsaparilla, yucca, bupleurum, and phytosterols.
- **Balance blood sugar.** Include the minerals vanadium and chromium, the Ayurvedic herbs gurmar and bitter melon, and goat's rue and licorice to bring down blood sugar and support the pancreas.
- **Support liver detox pathways.** Include vitamin B12, vitamin B6, folate from leafy green vegetables, sulforaphanes from the cabbage family, and diindolylmethane (DIM) to promote phase I liver detox pathways; calcium-D-glucarate to promote phase II liver detox pathways; and dandelion root, burdock, greater celandine, barberry, and andrographis to promote bile flow and gallbladder release.
- **Ensure optimal bowel function.** Follow the "weeding, seeding, and feeding" protocol (page 55). Use herbal laxatives (aperients) as required, as well as herbs that promote bile production (choleretics), herbs that promote bile release (cholagogues), and herbs that alleviate gas and cramping or colic (carminatives).
- **Utilize nutritive and blood-building botanicals.** Cook herbs like stinging nettle leaf, seaweeds, red clover, alfalfa, yellow dock, millettia, chlorella, leuzea, rehmannia (prepared), codonopsis, and burdock into bone broths.
- **Develop a stress-management plan.** Practice mindfulness, meditation, Shinrin Yoku, and other techniques as desired. See page 74 for more information.
- **Use stress-reducing adaptogen herbs as adrenal boosters.** Good choices are rhodiola, ginseng, licorice, eleuthero, ashwagandha, and leuzea.
- **Lose weight.** Anesthetic gases are stored in fat tissue and released slowly over several weeks, if not months, after the procedure. This may contribute to postoperative cognitive impairment, although the overall risk of postsurgical complications in obese patients is not dissimilar to that for normal-weight patients.
- **Consider using magnolia bark extract (honokiol).** This offers neuroprotection, anticancer, pain-relieving, anti-inflammatory, and antianxiety effects, which are helpful before and after surgery.

Four Days before Surgery

The biggest concern around using herbs at the time of surgery is probably the risk of inadvertently contributing to blood stasis or a clot or, conversely, promoting anticoagulant effects and risking hemorrhage. Blood clots form almost immediately in response to breaching of a vessel, such as occurs during surgery. Platelets or thrombocytes are white blood cells that conduct the first response to a damaged vessel, where they rush to try and fill the gap and glue themselves together to make a patch. Because this first response is weak and unstable, it is quickly reinforced by a true clot, where fibrinogen protein made in the liver is converted by enzymes at the site of the injury to make cross-linked fibrin strands that form a mesh over the platelet plug to strengthen and stabilize the clot.

Platelets carry clotting factors in granules that are released into the blood plasma when they are activated at a wound site, including serotonin, platelet-activating factor (PAF) clotting factors, and the pro-inflammatory omega-6-derived thromboxane A_2 (TXA_2). These, in turn, activate additional platelets and induce local immune responses for tissue repair. Any disruption to this intricate dance of coagulation controls can result in problems with bleeding or hemorrhage, subcutaneous bleeding (bruising), or clots that can block downstream blood supply (thrombosis).

Antithrombotic agents can be antiplatelets (agents that stop platelet adhesion or aggregation, such as ginkgo, ginger, berberine, and hawthorn), anticoagulants (agents that prevent fibrin formation, such as turmeric and garlic), or fibrinolytics (agents that cause fibrin degradation, such as pomegranate, amla, or proteolytic enzymes).

Although some of the research on blood-thinning herbs is quite strong (especially for turmeric, ginkgo, and fish oils), unfortunately most of the research is from in vitro experiments, animal studies, and individual clinical case reports (such as the research on chamomile and cranberry). Some herbal effects are also speculative, based on extrapolations from research in cell lines or using isolated constituents. These are interesting and important, but not always clinically significant. For example, drinking just two cups of green tea per day can measurably reduce the level of fibrinogen in healthy adults, but there is no suggestion that people in Asia with a high green tea intake are experiencing more bleeding episodes (e.g., nosebleeds, prolonged menses, easy bruising) than people from other nations who don't drink it at all.

There is even research suggesting an actively beneficial role for ginkgo in the perioperative phase (before and after surgery). While some might worry about ginkgo causing excessive bleeding, there is really little to no robust research (including multiple studies in surgery) to document significant bleeding instances, and there are multiple studies showing ginkgo is not only safe but actively helpful in people undergoing surgery, including for cancer.

Surgeons may not understand these nuances and will usually strongly advise patients to cease any herbs and supplements prior to surgery. Natural practitioners may feel differently. Out of an abundance of caution, although none of the following supplements is expected to cause notable bleeding, it is still prudent to stop taking any herbs or supplements that may possibly thin the blood or may prevent clotting. Stop their use 4 days before surgery and recommence 4 days after surgery.

Herbs and Supplements to Stop Using 4 Days before Surgery

- Cayenne
- Chamomile
- Cranberry juice
- Curcumin
- Dong quai
- Evening primrose oil
- Flaxseed oil
- Garlic
- Ginger
- Ginkgo
- Grapefruit
- Green tea
- Omega-3 fish oil
- Proteolytic enzymes
- St. John's wort
- Turmeric
- Vitamin E (including tocopherols and tocotrienols)

The Day before Surgery

In the past, fasting guidelines prior to surgery were quite long, up to 24 hours in some cases, to allow safe general anesthesia without the increased risk of pulmonary aspiration (inhalation) of stomach contents. However, this can cause anxiety and discomfort to some people, so avoiding solids for 6–10 hours and clear liquids for 2–3 hours is now considered acceptable. Oral carbohydrate preloading is recommended, usually meaning you drink a clear carbohydrate beverage such as Ensure the night before the surgery and again 3 hours prior to surgery. Herbalists and natural health practitioners would not generally recommend a sugar-laden and artificially flavored drink like this, but it is useful in this circumstance to give a measured dose. Carbohydrate preloading avoids dehydration; reduces the neuroendocrine stress response, catabolism (cellular breakdown), and insulin resistance; and improves recovery.

Commercial clear carbohydrate drinks contain maltodextrins, which are complex sugars that empty readily and predictably from the stomach (unlike glucose or milk). A first dose containing 100 g of carbohydrate is taken around 12 hours before surgery (usually the night before) and the second dose of 50 g of carbohydrate is taken 2–3 hours before surgery (or the morning of surgery) for maximum benefit. A review of all of the ERAS elements determined that oral preload had a significant effect on reducing complications and improving well-being. The review also found that excessive intravenous fluid given on the day of surgery increased the incidence of complications. Oral carbohydrate preloading reduces the need for intravenous fluid.

If abdominal surgery is planned, it is necessary for the bowel to be as empty as possible; strong pharmaceutical laxatives may be taken the day before the procedure. A more natural alternative would be 250–400 mg of magnesium oxide at bedtime, with 0.5–1 g of cascara bark, or a colonic irrigation the day before.

Other useful immunonutrients for the perioperative phase include omega-3 polyunsaturated fatty acids and the amino acids glutamine and arginine to improve wound healing and reduce inflammation. It is important to ensure plentiful nitric oxide within muscles for optimal metabolism and efficiency. This can be produced by metabolism of arginine or from nitrites and nitrates, which can be increased in muscle by foods and supplements containing inorganic nitrates (such as beets and spinach—Popeye had the right idea!).

Recovery from Surgery

Each person will respond to surgery differently. Some people seem to sail through and others have infections, brain fog, pain, and other complications that can get in the way of pursuing proper or effective cancer treatments. As always in medicine, prevention is better than cure, and the ERAS protocols are intended to prepare you for surgery in hopes of minimizing complications and promoting recovery. In the immediate aftermath of surgery, holistic management strategies can be commenced right away.

As soon as you are sitting up, able to take solid or semisolid foods, and able to have a bowel movement, herbal and nutritional support can be introduced. Highly nutritious green juices, bone broths with restorative and blood-building herbs, teas, tinctures, and liquid supplements can be taken as soon as solid foods are allowed. Powders can be introduced next; add capsule products slowly, increasing by a couple more per day to reach full dosing over a week or two. Supplements and herbs can be taken as concentrated powders if capsules or tinctures are challenging. These may be easiest to take if you make a strongly flavored tea, like mint or chai spice, and stir in the powder to make a thin gruel or paste. Add a pinch of cardamom, cinnamon, or stevia to sweeten as desired.

Manage Pain

Any surgery involves some considerable pain in the recovery period, but pain can be a significant hindrance to healing and recuperation, and it is certainly a good target for herbal medicines. There is, in fact, so much to say about using herbs for managing pain that the whole of Chapter 4 is devoted just to that. Whether pain is a natural part of healing from surgery, a side effect of treatment, or due to progression of the cancer, it may be approached through similar strategies and formulations.

Prevent Blood Clots

After surgery, it's important to take steps to prevent blood clots. Your doctor may recommend the use of an intermittent pneumatic compression device—a set of inflatable sleeves for your legs—and compression stockings to encourage lymph flow and prevent blood clots. Getting back up and moving is key to a good recovery. Keep the feet elevated when seated to promote venous return and consider a 2-inch-thick plank of wood under the foot of the bed for a gentle gravity assist at night. Occupational or other rehabilitation therapy can be useful to regain function; horticultural therapy is especially useful.

Some doctors recommend 81 milligrams of aspirin (also known as baby aspirin) as a daily low-dose blood thinner. I prefer to see patients take a potent proteolytic enzyme like nattokinase or lumbrokinase to reduce inflammation and the risk of blood clots. The herbs and supplements that I recommend stopping before surgery, because they could theoretically contribute to bleeding, should be recommenced as soon as possible after surgery to reduce the risk of clotting. Again, these herbs may not be sufficient to treat a clot, but they can at least have mild preventive actions.

If you are taking anticoagulant drugs, then blood tests should be done for prothrombin time, international normalized ratio, fibrinogen, and D-dimer readings that can assess clotting rate and relative risk. Once these factors as well as platelet count are known, then an herbalist may recommend antithrombotic herbs be introduced and blood levels carefully monitored. When the clotting markers show decreasing risk, then it is time to consider reducing the drug dose and maintaining or increasing the herbs.

ANTITHROMBOTIC ENZYMES TO THIN THE BLOOD

Although extensive clinical trials have not yet been done, the following agents are prescribed by natural practitioners and can be purchased over the counter in health food stores. They are indicated in lower doses as a preventive or preemptive against the risk of clots, but they can also be used in higher doses if there is elevation of blood clotting factors or an actual clotting event. Pharmaceutical treatments that break up clots have adverse and dangerous side effects, including severe bleeding and hemorrhage; those side effects are not seen with these natural agents. The enzymes below are listed from mildest to strongest.

Papain and bromelain. These are plant derived, mild, and very safe. If taken with food, they act as "primers" for protein digestion in food and can help in cases of protein maldigestion leading to food allergies. If taken between meals, they are attracted to sites of low pH, as is seen in inflammation and cancer, and they assist in the removal of metabolic debris from tissue damage and repair.

Serrapeptase and nattokinase. Serrapeptase is a proteolytic enzyme from silkworms, and nattokinase is from fermented soy and fish paste. Both are useful in cases of impaired circulation to the arms and hands or the legs and feet (peripheral ischemia) or in managing acute inflammation after injury.

Lumbrokinase. This is a proteolytic enzyme from earthworms, used in Traditional Chinese Medicine for supporting healthy blood circulation. Lumbrokinase acts as a potent fibrinolytic (clot-busting) agent and can be used to treat phlebitis (inflammation of veins and thrombosis).

Lumbrokinase targets excess clot material (fibrin) and can be safely used for dissolving clots, lowering whole blood viscosity, and reducing platelet aggregation (clumping or clotting). It does not cause excessive bleeding and has not shown any adverse effects. It is widely used in China as a thrombolytic agent to treat cerebral infarction, coronary heart disease, pulmonary heart disease, deep vein thrombosis, angina pectoris, and diabetes.

Prevent Postoperative Cognitive Impairment

Many patients exhibit cognitive impairment, including memory deficits, after surgery and anesthesia. Called postoperative cognitive impairment (POCI), this condition may affect orientation, attention, perception, consciousness, and judgment. It is estimated that some degree of POCI is seen after surgery in more than 35% of young adults and more than 40% of elderly patients at hospital discharge and in 6% of young adults and 13% of elderly patients at 3 months after surgery. Symptoms of POCI may persist for days or weeks and are correlated to the duration of anesthesia (the longer you're under anesthesia, the greater your chances of developing POCI).

POCI is essentially a reaction of the sympathetic nervous system, which releases adrenaline (the hormone of fright, flight, or fight) and subsequently cortisol in response to a stressor and which reacts to the inflammation and trauma of surgery by causing blood vessels to constrict, blood pressure to rise, heart rate to increase, and muscles to spasm. This, in turn, affects blood flow to the brain and directs flow to core survival centers—away from advanced intellectual thinking processes—and this is experienced as POCI. To prevent and to heal from this response, supporting the parasympathetic nervous system (rest and relaxation state) is key.

This idea of brain protection by promotion of parasympathetic support is entirely in keeping with the old and well-established idea extolling the healing value of rest and of deep rejuvenation and restoration practices. The "rest cure" at a sanatorium in the mountains was a great prescription in the past for nervous exhaustion, and prostration and recuperating from surgery in the countryside, with fresh air and nature all around, is ideal. The use of stress-reducing and adrenal-supportive herbs is also warranted here (see the section on stress management on page 63).

Does the Kind of Anesthesia and the Type of Surgery Play a Role in POCI?

Research suggests that as well as the depth and duration of anesthesia, the molecular size of the drugs may play a role in POCI. Smaller-size anesthetic agents such as isoflurane and desflurane may cause greater beta-amyloid oligomerization (complex binding patterns) and neuroinflammation. Sevoflurane, desflurane, intravenous thiopental, and propofol infusion are larger molecules and may exhibit shorter half-life and less neuroinflammation. Consider asking your surgeon to review the options with you.

The least-invasive surgeries and the shortest time under anesthesia are better tolerated with less complications, so lumpectomies are preferred over mastectomies, laparoscopic surgeries are preferred to open abdominal surgeries, epidural analgesia supplementation is recommended where possible, and sentinel node biopsies are preferred over lymph bed dissections. Insertion of drains and nasogastric tubes should be avoided if possible to help early mobilization of patients. Supplemental oxygen is shown to reduce postoperative nausea and vomiting.

PREVENTING POCI WITH LOBELIA (*LOBELIA INFLATA*)

Lobelia may be helpful during the postoperative period to reduce the risk of POCI. One of its most active and most researched constituents, lobeline, acts on the parasympathetic nervous system in much the same way nicotine does to induce feelings of calm. In fact, lobelia has been used by herbalists to support people quitting smoking, and also as a smooth and skeletal muscle relaxant, both topically (by poultice, infused oil, or tincture) and internally. It is prescribed in respiratory deficiencies like asthma and chronic obstructive pulmonary disease (COPD), where it acts as a bronchodilator to deepen breathing and increase gaseous exchange capacity. After surgery, this improved blood flow—and increased flow of oxygen to the brain—can help improve cognitive functioning and prevent POCI.

The genus *Lobelia* comprises almost 400 species worldwide, but *Lobelia inflata*, used in herbal medicine, is a small flowering plant found naturally in woodland clearings and meadows across the eastern part of North America. The root of this plant was historically used by the Iroquois to treat ulcers and leg sores, and the leaves were mashed and applied as a poultice to treat abscesses. The Cherokee mashed the roots of lobelia and used them as a poultice for body aches, and the leaves were rubbed on sores, aches, and stiff necks.

In modern herbal medicine the aerial parts (leaves and especially seeds) are preferred, but all parts of the plant have been shown to contain active constituents. Tests like high-performance liquid chromatography and mass spectrometry have demonstrated that at least 52 alkaloids, primarily of the piperidine/pyridine family, are found in all parts of the plant. Lobeline is one of the alkaloids, and it acts in the parasympathetic nervous system as a nicotinic receptor agonist/antagonist (stimulates or inhibits the receptor sites of the parasympathetic nervous system under varying circumstances) and a neurotransmitter transporter inhibitor. Lobeline occupies nicotinic receptors in the brain, stimulating many of the parasympathetic responses that tobacco does, but also acting to reduce tobacco cravings.

The value of lobelia in the postoperative period is largely due to inhibition of drug-induced respiratory depression (DIRD), thus suppporting oxygenation of the brain. This may be in part by parasympathetic-induced bronchodilation, but lobeline also sensitizes the carotid and aortic chemoreceptors that register oxygen and carbon dioxide levels and trigger compensatory reflexes of breathing deeper when oxygen declines. However, achieving a therapeutic dose of lobelia may be challenging due to the fact that most DIRD is due to the use of opioids, drugs that often induce vomiting, as does lobelia, and the summative effect may not be tolerated. Topical applications, such as a chest rub or liniment, may be better tolerated than oral ingestion.

Animal research suggests a positive benefit from lobeline on learning and memory tasks in which nicotine-induced enhancement of performance has previously been demonstrated, but this has not been researched in human clinical trials. Certainly learning and memory are enhanced under parasympathetic dominance, and this indicates that lobelia may have a role to play in promoting cognitive functions after surgery.

Dosing: A single dose of 100–400 mg of lobelia is considered safe and effective. In the UK it is a restricted (Schedule 20) herb, and the dosage guidelines suggest a tincture made at 1:8 strength and a weekly maximum dose of 32 mL. This would suggest an average daily dose of 4.5 mL; at 1:8 strength, that is equivalent to 562 mg of dried herb.

The dose-limiting factor with lobelia is the emesis (vomiting) it causes. This is unlikely to be an issue with topical use, although hands should be washed well after applying it so you don't inadvertently get it in your mouth from your fingers. Tinctures should be taken in drop doses until individual tolerance is established.

Topical applications in the form of poultices or liniments are a traditional way to use this herb. If you have access to the fresh herb, make a poultice of mashed stems, leaves, and flowers folded into a piece of cheesecloth. With a hot-water bottle or a heating pad on top, it will penetrate deeply into a cramped muscle and ease spasming. If the fresh herb is not available, the dried herb can be moistened with hot water and applied in the same way. A liniment may be easier to apply and more practical.

Let Go Liniment

In the postoperative recovery phase, Let Go Liniment is useful over the chest and upper back to introduce lobelia through the skin, where it can have a local action without risk of nausea, and over any muscles that are cramping or spasming.

+ 20 mL lobelia tincture (1:8)
+ 10 drops each essential oils of niaouli, marjoram, benzoin, lavender
+ 30 mL cramp bark tincture (1:5)
+ 10 mL cayenne tincture (1:5)
+ 20 mL juniper-infused oil
+ 20 mL pokeroot-infused oil

Add the essential oils to the tinctures and shake well, then add the infused oils. Shake before use. Apply liberally as needed. Wash hands well after use.

This recipe was inspired by a patient in my student training days—a gentleman who had severe bronchitis and emphysema and could not get enough air to speak easily in the consultation. He was trying so hard, using all the accessory muscles of respiration, with his shoulders up by his ears and gasping. On the instructions of my tutor, I went to the dispensary and poured out 5 mL each of lobelia and cramp bark tinctures and 5 mL of almond oil. I warmed the mixture in my hands and massaged it into his neck, shoulders, and upper back. I felt his muscles relax even as I was doing it. Within minutes he could take a deeper, more effective breath and speak a little easier. I have been making this in my dispensary and giving it to patients ever since. It's useful not only for asthma and chest restriction but also for abdominal cramping or colic, menstrual cramping, skeletal muscle cramping, and tension headaches (when rubbed on the back of the neck).

Counteracting Immunosuppression

Cancer drives immunosuppression through various metabolic processes, and this may promote the opportunity for metastases to grow after surgery. This immunosuppression is partly ascribed to the neuroendocrine responses to stress. If the hypothalamic-pituitary-adrenal (HPA) pathway that responds to stress is blocked with specific spinal blockade anesthesia during surgery, then metastasis is inhibited. This suggests that stopping pain alone isn't enough to prevent new blood vessel growth; there is also a need to stop the stress responses in the body. Clearly, managing stress is critically important, and this can be a good time to consider using stress-reducing and tonic herbs. Perioperative immunonutrition is aimed at modulating immunological and metabolic functions in the context of major surgery and includes supplementation of essential substrates such as glutamine, arginine, omega-3 fatty acids, or specific botanicals given 5–7 days before and again after the intervention.

Herbs for Enhanced Recovery after Surgery

The list of herbs that can be used to enhance recovery after surgery could be quite extensive, but by identifying certain key desirable actions, an herbal practitioner will formulate individual protocols for different symptoms in each person. These may be prescribed for a relatively short period of time, usually 3–6 weeks or a bit longer if symptoms persist; they should not be needed for the long term.

Brain Tonic Herbs and Mental Stimulants

One way to improve mental sharpness, cognitive functions, and memory is to take herbs that improve cerebral circulation and blood perfusion to the brain and hence delivery of oxygen and glucose to fuel the brain functions. In humans, around 25 percent of our daily energy quotient is spent on brain function, and when you are run down, depleted, or debilitated you may not have sufficient energy available. Fatigue, mental dullness, and depression may result.

Ginkgo, gotu kola, and rosemary are all supportive of optimal blood flow to the brain, with redox-regulating and anti-inflammatory effects. Gotu kola also has supportive effects for connective tissue, which especially support the brain and central nervous system.

While the herbs below have not all been studied in POCI specifically, they are generally recognized as offering benefits in depression, memory loss, and cognitive decline of the elderly, and it is reasonable to expect similar benefits in the postoperative period. Lobelia is included as an oxygenator.

Botanicals for Enhanced Mental Sharpness

- Ginkgo
- Gotu kola
- Rosemary
- Periwinkle
- Huperzia
- Rhodiola
- Lobelia
- Basil, peppermint, and rosemary essential oils

GINKGO (*GINKGO BILOBA*)

Ginkgo is probably one of the best-researched herbal medicines available, with more than 400 scientific studies conducted on proprietary standardized extracts of ginkgo leaf in the past 30 years, according to the American Botanical Council. Interestingly, Traditional Chinese Medicine uses the fruit for lung health, not the leaf. Widespread screening of plants for active compounds identified a series of flavonol glycosides (based on flavones like quercetin, kaempferol, and isorhamnetin) and terpene lactones (ginkgolides and bilobalide) in the leaf that are pharmacologically active. Ginkgo extract must be standardized in order to deliver the intended benefits; there is no evidence of efficacy with other dosage forms of crude ginkgo leaf or low-concentration extracts made from the leaf. The dry extract is pharmaceutically prepared to a super concentrate, in a ratio of anywhere from 35–65 parts herb in 1 part finished product and usually standardized to 24 percent ginkgo flavonol glycosides and 6 percent terpene lactones.

Ginkgo is prescribed for its neuroprotective properties and ability to aid circulatory problems, especially cerebral insufficiency and consequent cognitive effects, and for peripheral circulatory impairment, particularly intermittent claudication (poor circulation to the lower legs), vertigo, and tinnitus, as well as for protection against altitude sickness and to manage erectile dysfunction in men.

Dosing: 3–4 mL daily of a concentrated 2:1 extract, with at least 9.6 g/mL of ginkgo flavone glycosides and standardized at 6–8% terpenes. Ginkgo is generally considered safe and effective at daily doses of 120–240 mg of standardized extract. Crude extracts of ginkgo leaf contain ginkgolic acids that are quite similar to the urushiol found in poison ivy and potentially harmful if handled extensively or if ingested—another reason to use a standardized botanical pharmaceutical product.

Because of some in vitro studies of isolated compounds, an idea (almost a myth) in herbal medicine has developed that ginkgo is a powerful anticoagulant and can cause bleeding. This is not supported in the research, although the herb does have some inhibitory functions on platelet-activating factor and may normalize platelet activity. In extrapolating from research to practice that it is perhaps more anticoagulant than it truly is, there has arisen an understandable but unjustified concern that it is also riskier to use than it truly is.

Actions of Ginkgo in the Postoperative Period

- Improves brain tolerance of low oxygen states
- Inhibits development of cerebral edema (buildup of fluids) after a head trauma or toxic overload and accelerates its regression
- Reduces symptoms of retinal edema
- Increases memory performance and learning capacity
- Inactivates toxic oxygen radicals (flavonoids)
- Serves as antagonist of the platelet-activating factor (ginkgolides)—lessens the stickiness of the blood
- Improves blood flow, particularly in the microcirculation
- Has neuroprotective effect (ginkgolides A and B, bilobalide)

GOTU KOLA (*CENTELLA ASIATICA*)

Gotu kola is one of the most interesting herbs in managing cancer care. It is the herb I prescribe the most in my clinical practice (right up there with turmeric). It is a cerebral circulatory stimulant and also a calming anxiolytic (reduces anxiety). It was the preferred herbal remedy in times past for meditating priests in India who wanted to be totally alert and focused but also relaxed. In India today, gotu kola is commonly eaten as a green leafy vegetable. It is a connective-tissue restorative that nourishes, strengthens, and supports the extracellular matrix (ECM) all cells are held in. The ECM is a gel that comprises sugar-protein complexes (such as chondroitin and hyaluronic acid), along with water and embedded fibers (including collagen and elastin). In this way it also has antimetastatic and anti-invasive properties. Research supports its use as a nerve-regenerating, immunomodulatory, antidepressant, memory-enhancing, gastroprotective, cardioprotective, radioprotective, anticancer, and wound-healing agent.

Dosing: 3–6 mL daily of a 1:2 tincture made with 60% ethyl alcohol, equivalent to 1.5–3 g of dried herb. It is an inherently safe herb and doses of up to 8–10 g daily are acceptable and sometimes useful.

Juicing the fresh plant is also an option if it is available; the juice can be frozen in ice cubes trays for later use. You can also make pesto or dips with it.

ROSEMARY (*ROSMARINUS OFFICINALIS*)

Rosemary, with its beautiful blue flowers and singular scent, is one of the most recognizable Mediterranean herbs. It is well known in the kitchen, where it is used in many dishes, and it is also valuable as a medicine. Due to its effect of directing blood to the head, it is known as an herb for memory and recall, and even Shakespeare referenced those properties in *Hamlet*, in which the character Ophelia speaks of rosemary "for remembrance."

Rosemary is a gentle, cooling, bitter herb and a notable antioxidant and antibacterial that is helpful in treating gastroesophageal disease (GERD) and acid reflux, gallbladder insufficiency and chronic indigestion, and small intestine bacterial overgrowth (SIBO) or colon microbiome dysbiosis.

Dosing: 2–5 mL daily of a 1:2 tincture, equivalent to 1–2.5 g of dried herb. Rosemary may occasionally be overstimulating to the heart, so avoid combining it with rhodiola; also avoid rosemary if you have high blood pressure.

PERIWINKLE (*VINCA MAJOR, VINCA MINOR*)

Periwinkle extract is used to increase the uptake of oxygen and glucose in the brain and is prescribed by herbalists for attention-deficit/hyperactivity disorder, dizziness, memory loss, senility, head trauma recovery, stroke recovery, and cognitive decline, among other things, like POCI and depression. All of these benefits make it an ideal herb for an ERAS protocol. The leaves, buds, and flowers are used, yielding up to 1 percent by dry weight of total alkaloids comprising around 10 percent vincamine plus 30 other indole alkaloids and derivatives.

The leaves also contain a high amount of tannin and exert an astringent action. They are traditionally used in a mouthwash for bleeding gums, mouth ulcers, or sore throats. Leaves are also taken internally for bowel looseness or bowel bleeding (colitis or diarrhea)—periwinkle can reduce the loss of fluid or blood while toning the membranes—and for heavy uterine bleeding (menorrhagia or metrorrhagia).

Dosing: 5–10 mL daily of 1:5 tincture made with 45% ethyl alcohol.

Contraindications: Isolated vincamine alkaloids from periwinkle are contraindicated in cases of cerebral tumors with intracranial hypertension and should be avoided in people with cardiac arrhythmia. This is unlikely to be a concern in whole herb extracts taken in formulas.

HUPERZIA (*HUPERZIA SERRATA*)

This ancient club moss first occurred more than 400 million years ago and is featured in Traditional Chinese Medicine as qian ceng ta, used for cooling fevers and reducing inflammation. Research suggests that one of its main alkaloids, huperzine-A, protects the brain cells from toxins and improves memory. In one double-blind study on the effectiveness of huperzine-A capsules on memory and learning performance in adolescent students, a dose of 100 mcg huperzine-A twice daily significantly enhanced memory and learning performance with no side effects.

Huperzia serrata prevents cognitive dysfunction through its inhibitory effects on an enzyme called acetylcholinesterase, which allows prolonged bioavailability of acetylcholine, the major neurotransmitter of the parasympathetic nervous system. This relaxed state enhances cognitive functions; anyone who has blanked out in an exam, where the stress of the situation has emptied their mind, can attest to the cognitive dysfunction brought on by stress.

Mice treated with *Huperzia serrata* at an oral dose of 100 mg/kg showed improved cognitive functions and decreased lipid peroxidation in the brain with no side effects.

Dosing: Huperzine-A in pure form has shown efficacy at doses of 0.2–0.4 mg/day for Alzheimer's disease. In one study of people with schizophrenia, 0.3 mg/day for 12 weeks was used with no adverse effects. More than 100 years ago, Finley Ellingwood, an Eclectic practitioner from the 1800s, suggested a 1:1 tincture from the green sporophyte phase and dosed it from 1–15 minims. For context, 1 minim = 0.0616115 mL and 15 minims = 0.924172798829 mL (almost 1 mL). So approximately 1 mL/day or 1 g/day is the upper limit for the sporophyte extract.

Historic Use of Huperzia

Historically, the spores of this ancient (nonflowering) plant were considered medicinal. According to *King's American Dispensatory* of 1898, huperzia is especially recommended for intractable fevers, intermittent with afternoon exacerbations; dark urine or red, sandy deposits in the urine; spasmodic retention of urine with painful urination; constipation, indigestion, and colic or cramps with digestive gurgling (borborygmus) and esophageal reflux; cough with bloody mucus; congestive headache; and dizziness. According to John Milton Scudder, another Eclectic practitioner, lycopodium (huperzia) is adapted to disorders showing "extreme sensitiveness of the surface; sensitiveness of a part and care to prevent it being touched; slow, painful boils; nodes or swellings; external sensitivity of the organs of special sense, with pale, livid, or dirty complexion."

RHODIOLA (*RHODIOLA ROSEA*)

Also known as Arctic rose, rhodiola is not actually a rose but rather a lovely northern saxifrage. It has fleshy and colorful leaves like a succulent but is able to withstand the harshest winters. The root has a rosy scent and is harvested and extracted for constituents that stimulate the nervous system, reduce anxiety, enhance work performance, relieve fatigue, improve learning and memory function, and prevent high-altitude sickness. It is prescribed for antiaging, anti-inflammation, DNA repair, and anticancer effects. Paradoxically, it is able to promote tissue healing while downregulating, or suppressing, cancer. Its multitude of actions and effects puts it in the category of herbal adaptogen (stress reducer) and systemic stabilizer.

Dosing: 200 mg twice daily (400 mg/day) is a safe dose. Clinical doses are commonly 200–600 mg daily.

BASIL, PEPPERMINT, AND ROSEMARY ESSENTIAL OILS

These scents are all fresh, bright, uplifting, refreshing, and invigorating. They can be used as a blend in a room spray, on a plug-in or a tea candle diffuser, or even on a handkerchief tucked in your top pocket where your body warmth evaporates the oils and they rise for you to breathe them. These oils are affordable, safe, and effective, although people with high blood pressure or who are prone to throbbing headaches should avoid the rosemary.

OTHER USEFUL AGENTS FOR BRAIN SUPPORT

Phosphatidyl choline. Also known as lecithin, this is a major fatty compound in the brain. Supplementing with up to 5 g or more daily is recommended. This can be taken in the form of granules added to the diet.

Fish oil. Omega-3 fats in fish oil can significantly influence brain functions with eicosapentaenoic acid (EPA) being excitatory or stimulating and docosahexaenoic acid (DHA) being depressive or calming. A daily dose of 500–1,000 mg EPA and around half that of DHA is recommended.

Lion's mane mushroom. Although all the medicinal mushrooms have incredible benefits in preventing, treating, and recovering from cancer, the particular role of lion's mane is to heal the brain from tumors, chemotherapy, or surgical and radiotherapy damage. It is suggested for preventing dementia, to lessen mild symptoms of anxiety and depression, and to promote nerve tissue repair. It is anti-inflammatory, antioxidant, and immune boosting.

Herbs That Regulate Inflammation

After surgery, the body enters an acute inflammatory state. It needs inflammation to repair tissues and resolve injuries, but it also needs a downregulating control system to end the inflammation at the appropriate time. Inflammatory pathways in the body tend to be driven by omega-6 fats, while anti-inflammatory pathways are largely controlled by omega-3 fats. To promote anti-inflammatory pathways, it's important to restrict omega-6 fats (those found in grains and dairy foods) and increase consumption of omega-3 fats from cold-water fish.

Herbs that are known to regulate inflammatory pathways, such as turmeric, licorice, sarsaparilla, Indian frankincense, and yucca, all have a role to play here.

SEA BUCKTHORN (*HIPPOPHAE RHAMNOIDES*)

For centuries, Greeks, Romans, Russians, Tibetans, and Chinese have used sea buckthorn berry in traditional medicine as a source of nutrients for skin care remedies and a cosmetic aid with nourishing, revitalizing, and restorative action. It has high nutritional and medicinal value, likely due to its high content of essential fatty acids, carotenoids, vitamin E, and phytosterols, all of which are critically important for proper wound repair with minimal inflammation.

A hardy shrub with yellow or orange berries, sea buckthorn is easy to grow and commonly used as an ornamental hedging plant with thorns to keep animals out. In a study of best harvesting practices, berries were collected at several stages during a complete planting and harvesting cycle. Whole berries were analyzed for physical characteristics, and fruit and seed fractions were analyzed for bioactive content. Late-season berries yielded the highest values for berry sizes.

Dosing: This plant has no standard dosing, as it is considered a food medicine. A daily dose of 10–20 berries would be reasonable. A pleasant and refreshing tea can be made from the leaves, and berries can be added to smoothies, breakfast bowls, and salads.

A heavy orange oil can be expressed from the fruit and seed with the right industrial equipment. This is not something you can do at home, but the oil is readily available to purchase. It is used in skin care products for its intensely moisturizing, nourishing, and skin-repairing qualities.

Tonic Herbs to Support the Nervous System after Surgery

If the body has undergone a significant stress, in this case surgery but also, for example, a severe injury, then it may draw upon all reserves to drive the healing process. It is common after surgery to feel debilitated and depleted, and the convalescent period should be managed carefully. A light but nourishing diet is recommended—one that is nutrient dense but easy to digest, such as the one described as part of the daily self-care routine for managing chemotherapy on page 161.

ST. JOHN'S WORT (*HYPERICUM PERFORATUM*)

St. John's wort's flowering tops are used for treating melancholy, low mood, despondency, or depression; to promote liver functions and bile production; and as a tonic, uplifting, and calming nervine. These actions are intimately linked in traditional, energetic, Western medicine models in which the element earth, the humor of black bile, and the melancholic temperament are all associated with accumulation of "morbid waste." This waste could include cellular and physiological metabolites, food waste matter, and even morbid thoughts or dysfunctional mental processes. These all are associated with low mood and gloomy or bleak outlook and may be counteracted by supporting the liver—literally the organ that distills the good and useful from the bad and unwanted. A liver that isn't processing wastes effectively may manifest as dark mood, dark thoughts, and feelings of congestion or stagnation in personal situations (professional or relational) as well as physical states (tonic constipation, dryness, bloating, indigestion, atrophy, and withering). This herb exemplifies the opportunity to raise the spirits and lift the mood by promoting proper detoxification pathways. These actions are especially indicated after surgery when the anesthetic gases, pain medications, and medical experience as a whole can conspire to burden the liver and depress mood.

Dosing: 2–6 mL daily of a 1:2 tincture, equivalent to 1–3 g of herb. A standardized product should contain around 3–5% hyperforin.

For more information about St. John's wort, see page 288.

OTHER HERBS FOR NERVOUS SYSTEM SUPPORT

Horsetail and oat straw (*Equisetum arvense* and *Avena sativa*). These two herbs are often used together for connective tissue stimulation and nutrition. Horsetail is mineral-rich and provides a substrate for healthy extracellular matrix. Histologically, nervous tissue is considered to be connective tissue, and these herbs support structure and strength. Oat straw is a traditional synergist with horsetail, although research suggests it actually has quite low mineral content itself.

Milky oat seed (*Avena sativa*). This is an herb that, like St. John's wort, can be stimulating and uplifting as well as calming and relaxing at the same time. It is harvested when the seed head is young and green and a milky fluid comes out when it is squeezed. Classically it is considered to be a "nerve food" and restorative and balancing for all mental functions.

Sage (*Salvia* spp.). A meta-analysis of human clinical trials in 2014 suggested that *S. officinalis* and *S. lavandulifolia* both enhance cognitive performance in healthy subjects and patients with dementia or cognitive impairment and are safe for this indication. Improved cognitive outcomes are attributed to the terpenes, which inhibit the enzyme anticholinesterase that breaks down the calming neurotransmitter acetylcholine, hence prolonging its availability. Terpenes also activate receptors for gamma-aminobutyric acid (GABA), which is another relaxing neurotransmitter. The phenolic constituents also affect brain function, through increased brain-derived neurotrophic factor (BDNF), which regulates and supports tissue repair, and antioxidant and anti-inflammatory actions in nerve cells.

Avoiding Complications of Healing

Wound healing after surgery can cause significant complications, including infection, scarring, and disfigurement, if not disability. Chemotherapy and radiation may depress immune responses, making infection more likely or longer lasting. Radiation can also damage the tissue repair mechanisms, so that new tissue is weak and poorly constructed, vulnerable to repeated tearing. Once a wound has healed, there may be further complications from scarring.

Wound healing is a complex and dynamic process of removing and replacing damaged and dead cells and rebuilding the layers of the dermis or the structure of the organ affected. It is a set of biochemical events layered in a closely organized cascade to repair the damaged tissue and restore function. Wound repair requires some degree of inflammation, which triggers the healing responses, but it also needs to be managed and controlled so it is not too acute, and it needs to stop when the job is done.

Phases of Wound Healing

The process of wound healing involves several sequential steps.

Phase 1: Hemostasis. Blood vessels constrict and platelets aggregate to immediately stop bleeding from a breached vessel. A local fibrin clot forms to contain the injury and resist local collateral damage.

Phase 2: Defense/Inflammation. Blood vessels dilate to transport white blood cells and phagocytes (cells that consume bacteria) to the wound site, resulting in inflammation characterized by heat, redness, and swelling. This is followed by "granulation," in which fibroblasts form a bed of collagen in the wound and new capillaries are produced. During the "wound contraction" part of this phase, myofibroblasts decrease the size of the wound by drawing the wound edges together and contracting, using a mechanism that resembles that of smooth muscle cell contraction.

Phase 3: Proliferation/Epithelialization. During this stage, epithelial (skin) cells proliferate and cover over the newly forming tissue (in the form of a scab).

Phase 4: Maturation/Remodeling. Over the next several months, the dermis produces collagen and matrix proteins in an attempt to return to its pre-injury form and function. There is also apoptosis (cell death) of excess or superfluous cells.

Control Local Infection

During the wound-healing process, herbal medicines can help control infection. Herbs such as goldenseal, garlic, taheebo, Oregon grape, thyme, and usnea and plants with volatile oils—especially evergreens like fir, pine, thuja, eucalyptus, oregano, thyme, and tea tree—provide antibacterial functions. Willow and honey can be used for debridement (removal of damaged tissue and foreign material) and wound cleansing.

PROTOCOL FOR TREATING LOCAL INFECTION

Once primary dressings are removed and you can get access to skin:

- Wash with a strong tea of thuja or fir needles or thyme or oregano leaves. These are all rich in volatile oils with known antimicrobial actions. (Safety note: Do not apply the undiluted essential oils from these herbs directly to the skin or to a wound or lesion; a tea applied topically is safe.) To every liter of tea, add 1 teaspoon goldenseal powder or 25 mL of goldenseal tincture (1:5, made with 45–65% ethyl alcohol). Goldenseal, with its berberine alkaloids, acts like an antibiotic, killing bacteria on contact by disrupting bacterial metabolism, disabling bacterial defense mechanisms, and dispersing biofilms.
- Rinse with a solution of 10 ppm colloidal silver.
- Apply manuka honey with 10 drops of lavender essential oil added per teaspoon.
- Dress with a light gauze.
- Repeat two or three times daily until stitches are removed or resorbed and infection is resolved.

Tumor Spray

This mixture creates a cooling, soothing, anti-itch, anti-inflammatory, antimicrobial spray that can be applied directly to a tumor if the lesion is open to the surface and the cancer is accessible. The same formula and method, without the cytotoxic blend, can be used for a radiation burn but not actual cancer at the surface. It is also useful as a treatment for incisions after surgery, before you are able to touch the area.

- 25 g chamomile
- 5 g lavender
- 25 mL aloe vera gel
- 15 mL calendula juice
- 5 mL colloidal silver
- 5 mL cytotoxic tincture blend*
- 20 drops essential oil of lavender
- 20 drops essential oil of thuja

Bring two cups of water to a boil in a pan. Remove from heat, add the chamomile and lavender, cover, and let steep for 10 minutes. Strain the herbs through cheesecloth and allow to cool. Mix the rest of the ingredients with ¼ cup of the filtered infusion. Spray the mixture onto the tumor several times daily, or spray it onto a pad and use the pad to lightly bandage over the tumor.

*A cytotoxic blend from a qualified herbalist could contain some combination of annual wormwood, mistletoe, thuja, pawpaw, Pacific yew, pokeroot, bloodroot, or chaparral.

Support the Immune System and Manage Inflammation

In addition to echinacea, discussed below, other herbs and supplements that help modulate inflammation include turmeric, fish oils, vitamin E, licorice, and plant sterols.

ECHINACEA (*ECHINACEA* SPP.)

Echinacea angustifolia and *E. pallida* are the more immunostimulating species, but *E. purpurea* may be more common in commercial products, as it is easier to grow. This herb is particularly helpful right after surgery. Not only does it enhance immune resistance to infection through upregulation, or stimulation, of neutrophil and macrophage activities, but it also gains its traditional reputation for treating snakebite due to its ability to inhibit hyaluronidase, a proteolytic enzyme that breaks down hyaluronic acid in connective tissue and weakens the extracellular matrix. In the case of snakebite, hyaluronidase facilitates transit of venom through the limb, and in cancer it allows increase in size, ease of angiogenesis (new blood vessel growth), and ease of metastases.

Echinacea inhibits hyaluronidase and protects the extracellular matrix from degradation.

Dosing: Up to 6 mL daily of a 1:2 extract, equivalent to 3 g of dried herb (root, leaf, or flowering tops).

Promote and Support Connective Tissue

Connective tissue includes muscle, tendon fascia, and skin, all of which must be repaired after surgery. Once stitches are removed and the wound is no longer open, and once infection is resolved, then it is time to apply cicatrant herbs (astringents that knit up the edges of a wound) and vulnerary herbs (those with constituents that promote granulation, epithelialization, remodeling, and skin repair). These are often applied in the form of poultices and ointments.

CICATRANT HERBS FOR WOUND CLEANSING

Aftercare for surgery may require cleansing the incision. A visiting nurse may need to do this in the beginning, but as soon as stitches are removed or dissolved and you can take care of yourself, then you can use herbs to speed the healing. Make a strong tea from the herbs (½ oz. or 15 g of dried herbs in 2 cups water) and add tinctures of propolis, pine tips, cedar tips, frankincense, or myrrh to the tea. Use clean cotton swabs or a natural sponge to apply the tea topically, and boil them or discard after each use. After bathing the area, apply a healing cream or spray and a clean dressing.

Alder bark (*Alnus glutinosa*). This is a strongly astringent herb. An extract of the fresh catkins and dried bark has an antibiotic activity against many strains of bacteria, including methicillin-resistant *Staphylococcus aureus* and *Pseudomonas aeruginosa*. These are a real and present danger after surgery, so this herb can do double duty as an astringent and an antimicrobial. Widely distributed in northern countries, it's easy to harvest by removing a small branch and stripping the thin outer layer to reveal the inner bark—the green cambium or living tissue that is the medicine. Alder bark was used by Indigenous people as a soak to harden their feet, before the days of protective footwear. The fresh leaves were also placed in moccasins during a long journey. In modern research, the inner bark of alder has demonstrated antioxidant and cell protective effects, inhibiting nuclear factor-kappa B (NF-κB) activation and nitric oxide and tumor necrosis factor-alpha (TNF-α) production, and also showed liver-protective activity.

Thuja (*Thuja* spp.). Like other evergreens recommended for Shinrin Yoku, thuja has terpene phytoncides in its needles, and they are markedly antimicrobial. A pan of water simmering on a woodstove or warming on a radiator can have thuja twigs in it that will release their volatile compounds into the air. Green thuja branches are used in sweat lodges to cast the water onto the hot rocks to make the steam, releasing volatile oils to purify the air. If thuja is not available, then other evergreen boughs from pine, fir, and spruce will also be effective, used in the same ways.

Yarrow (*Achillea millefolium*). The leaf has tannins that make it drying, with astringent (tightening) properties; the flower has volatile oils rich in anti-inflammatory sesquiterpenes. Both used together over a wound as a wash or compress creates a powerful wound-healing effect.

Myrrh and frankincense (*Boswellia* spp.). True frankincense (*Boswellia carteri*), Indian frankincense (*B. serrata*), and myrrh are rich in resins and volatile terpenes. They have drying, toning, and tightening actions—especially on epithelia—and also are antiseptic, reduce bleeding from wounds, and are anti-inflammatory. Some species are endangered; only certified sustainably harvested resin should be used.

Propolis. Also known as beehive resin, propolis is strongly healing for wounds and is also antimicrobial and anti-inflammatory, and the caffeic acid phenethyl ester (CAPE) it contains inhibits many oncogenic pathways.

VULNERARY HERBS

The word *vulnerary* comes from the Latin *vulnerare*, meaning "to wound," and from *vulnerarius*, meaning "a plaster or dressing for healing wounds." It refers to the ability of herbs to promote tissue healing and wound repair. This may include herbs rich in tannins that bind the wound together and reduce bleeding and entry of pathogens, in antimicrobial essential oils, in triterpenes and saponins that promote connective tissue repair, or in polysaccharides that promote debridement and sloughing of dead tissues.

Aloe (*Aloe vera*). The inner gel of the aloe plant is softening and soothing. It relieves itching and inflammation as a wound heals and is moisturizing to the skin cells.

Comfrey (*Symphytum officinale*). The allantoin found in comfrey is a unique type of alkaloid that is cell proliferant (increases rate of cell turnover) and promotes granulation, a primary aspect of wound repair. Unlike most alkaloids, allantoin is water soluble, so a comfrey tea is effective. It also extracts into oil, so liniments and salves can be made with comfrey extract for topical use.

Corn silk (*Zea mays*). The allantoin found in corn silk is specific to the kidneys and urinary tract. Corn silk (actually the female part of the corn flower) is sweet tasting and ideal as a tea. The silks also have complex sugars that are soothing and mucilaginous in the urinary tract. This herb is ideal for inflammation and irritation in the kidneys and bladder from platinum-based chemotherapy or from bladder infusions of chemotherapy.

Gotu kola (*Centella asiatica*). Gotu kola leaves contain triterpenes that promote connective tissue repair by modulating the metabolism of alanine and proline, amino acids that stabilize connective tissue. This herb can promote healing and reduce scarring.

Calendula (*Calendula officinalis*). Calendula is antimicrobial and anti-inflammatory. It can be used in a strong tea as a wash, soak, or compress and can be incorporated into salves and lotions for a lasting application.

Plantain and self-heal (*Plantago* spp. and *Prunella vulgaris*). Plantain and self-heal are both astringent (cause tightening of soft tissues) and emollient (moistening and soothing) herbs that promote connective tissue repair.

Complications of Wound Healing

Even after the lips of a wound have closed and any local infection is resolved, there may still be complications of healing, sometimes lasting weeks or months. The use of cicatrants and vulneraries and diligent practice of rehabilitation activities (such as physiotherapy or occupational therapy) are all intended to reduce the risk of the following:

- **Scarring.** Thickening and shortening of the new collagen fibers
- **Keloid.** Extreme form of scarring, more common in people of African heritage
- **Traumatic neuroma.** Extreme and prolonged sensitivity of the injured area; may end up causing reflex sympathetic dystrophy, also known as complex regional pain syndrome (CRPS) type 1
- **Incisional hernia.** Outpouching of tissue through the site of an injury
- **Stricture.** Scarring within a tube, which has the effect of narrowing the lumen
- **Adhesions.** Scars that form on the internal organs and cause them to stick together (e.g., sections of the colon may attach to the uterus in endometriosis)

Topical Treatments to Reduce Scarring

Scarring is always a feature of tissue repair after surgery and may sometimes be quite disabling or disfiguring. Internal scarring is called adhesions, and if it is pronounced it can cause serious complications, including strictures or narrowing of the intestine, or otherwise compromise the function of internal organs. Some herbs are known to promote proper tissue healing by correcting the alignment of collagen, fibrin, and other fibers in the connective tissue for optimal remodeling (such as gotu kola), to enhance oxygen delivery to the tissue (such as prickly ash and cayenne), or to promote removal of wastes (such as castor oil and pokeroot).

CASTOR OIL PACKS

Castor oil is extracted from the castor plant (*Ricinus communis*). It has been used since ancient Egyptian times internally as a cathartic (stimulating laxative) and to induce labor, but it causes severe gastrointestinal cramping and is no longer recommended to be used in this way. However, it is safe if applied topically. It penetrates skin and muscle to reach right into underlying tissue and assists in decongestion and breakdown of inflammatory material through enhancing blood flow and lymphatic flow in the area. This also helps in the removal of toxins and the elimination of wastes. Castor oil is also warming to the tissues, and this eases stiffness and pain.

The main active constituent in castor oil appears to be ricinoleic acid (RA), which comprises 80–90 percent of the total fatty acids; other fatty acids include oleic acid and linoleic acid. RA has similar pain-relieving and anti-inflammatory effects as capsaicin, menthol, and piperine, and it binds through the same receptors in skin. Absorption of castor oil into the skin triggers local T lymphocytes, causing them to activate a local and/or generalized immune reaction that will lead to resolution of the injury and cessation of inflammation in due course.

How to Make and Use a Castor Oil Pack

1. Select a piece of flannel or toweling that is large enough to cover the area to be treated. Fold it three or four times.
2. Pour castor oil over it until it is thoroughly soaked.
3. Place the soaked flannel over the incision site and cover it all with a large piece of plastic wrap to reduce messy dripping.
4. Cover this all with a heating pad or hot-water bottle and leave in place for 1–2 hours.
5. After use, wrap the pack in plastic and store it in the refrigerator. Bring it back to room temperature before the next use. You may wish to add a little more castor oil with each use. The pack should be discarded after a few uses.

Notes: Frequency of application will depend on individual need. Usually a castor oil pack is used three to six times weekly until no more swelling or congestion is felt and the area appears normal.

Adverse effects are not expected with topical use, except occasional cases of temporary skin irritation from allergic contact dermatitis. If this occurs, wash the area well with soap and water, then apply a paste of baking soda and water. Repeat as needed until the irritation clears.

Scar Oil

This rich and nourishing anti-inflammatory oil promotes proper architecture of connective tissue and reduces scarring, swelling, and itching. It penetrates well because of the castor oil.

+ 20 mL rose hip seed oil
+ 20 mL jojoba oil
+ 20 mL pokeroot-infused oil
+ 20 mL calendula-infused oil
+ 20 mL comfrey leaf–infused oil
+ 20 mL gotu kola–infused oil
+ 10 mL sea buckthorn oil
+ 10 mL vitamin E oil
+ 5 mL castor oil
+ 1 mL each essential oils of helichrysum, benzoin, frankincense, and Peru balsam

Mix all the oils and apply frequently, as soon as the wound is clean and sealed.

Dietary Supplements to Support Healing after Surgery

In principle, it's always better to eat as well as possible rather than rely on pills and capsules for extra nutrition. As I tell my patients, these agents are called supplements for a reason; they should be thought of as supplemental to a good diet. However, in cancer care, including in the immediate aftermath of surgery, it may be hard to get a sufficient dose of some nutrients simply from normal eating, and especially if the appetite is diminished, if the patient experiences nausea, vomiting, or diarrhea, or if the surgery removed a section of the digestive system. In many cases it is helpful to seek out supplements that are liquids or powders, or possibly to open capsules and crush tablets so they can be taken off a spoon with water, and swallowed quickly if they taste bad.

B-Complex Vitamins

There are eight B vitamins: B1 (thiamine), B2 (riboflavin), B3 (niacin), B5 (pantothenic acid), B6 (pyridoxine), B7 (biotin), B9 (folate), and B12 (cobalamin), with a wide variety of functions in the human body. The B vitamins are critical for optimal function of the nervous system, and when taken together, vitamins B1, B6, and B12 interact synergistically to improve neuropathic pain. Stressors such as surgery or infection can deplete B vitamins.

Animals cannot synthesize B vitamins on their own; they must ingest them in sufficient quantities through their diet. Vitamin B12 is not produced by plants but by bacteria that colonize the foregut of ruminants or the colon of humans. Thus, it can only be found in animal products such as liver, fish, eggs, or dairy products.

Dosing. B vitamins are water soluble, so overdosing is implausible. Far more likely is a low-grade B vitamin deficiency, especially as foods are ever more refined and with the modern trend to eat fewer grains overall. Cancer patients should be aiming for the upper level of the daily doses recommended by the National Institutes of Health Office of Dietary Supplements. Clinical nutritionists might advise much higher doses in some cases, and there is no actual risk to higher doses as they are all water soluble and will be eliminated from the body if not used.

Recommended Dosage of B Vitamins for Cancer Patients

All doses should be given twice daily.

- B1 (thiamine or benfotiamine), 30–80 mg
- B2 (riboflavin), 10–15 mg*
- B3 (niacin), 50–100 mg
- B5 (pantothenic acid), 30–80 mg
- B6 (pyridoxine), 50–100 mg
- B7 (biotin), 20–40 mg
- B9 (folate), 200–400 mcg**
- B12 (cobalamin), 200–400 mcg

* Maximum daily intestinal absorption is approximately 20–25 mg

** Higher doses may mask functional B12 deficiency

Zinc

When taken 1–2 months before surgery, zinc reduces wound-healing time, rapidly reduces wound size, and supports immune functions to help ward off infection. Topical zinc, such as calamine lotion, also inhibits bacterial growth on the surface of skin, helping to prevent infection.

Dosing. Many people in the developed world have a low-level zinc deficiency because of the prevalence of processed foods in their diet. As such, a supplement of 5–10 mg daily is often recommended. If your blood work shows zinc levels below 25 percent of normal range, consider higher doses of 30–50 mg daily for a month. After a month, retest your levels and incrementally reduce the dose.

Zinc should always be taken in divided doses and with food. Taking zinc on an empty stomach induces severe and protracted nausea.

Vitamin C

Vitamin C is an essential vitamin required to make collagen, to strengthen scar tissue and give it tensile strength, and to strengthen the immune system and fight off infection. Levels of vitamin C drop in burn victims, in postoperative patients, and in people who have suffered physical trauma. Vitamin C is a free radical scavenger, removing reactive oxygen species that damage delicate tissues and cells, and it promotes immune functions, thus strengthening resistance to disease. High doses of vitamin C, and even ultra-high doses given intravenously, have demonstrated beneficial effects in many types of cancer.

Actions of Vitamin C against Cancer

- Antioxidant
- Strengthens the walls of the blood vessels
- Maintains the integrity of the skin, tissues, and bones
- Enhances resistance to carcinogens
- Increases the absorption of calcium and other minerals
- Inhibits the formation of atheroma plaques in the blood vessels

Dosing. Vitamin C is safe; any excess is eliminated from the bowel (and too much will cause diarrhea). Take 1 g of vitamin C daily for a week. Powder, capsules, or tablets are fine so long as the vitamin content is from a natural source, such as acerola cherry, with flavonoids.

After a week, increase the dose by 500 mg (0.5 g) per day, preferably in divided doses (two or three times daily). At a certain point you will notice a looseness in the stools. Don't go as far as diarrhea—just until you start to experience more frequent or looser stools. At this point, cut back the dose of vitamin C by 500 mg; your bowel habits should normalize. This constitutes your optimum dose at this present time.

Remember that your requirement will change over time, so keep playing up and down the scale, always keeping just within bowel tolerance. Even if your normal dose is around 3–4 g per day, if you are coming down with a bad cold or have some other acute condition, then your requirement may go as high as 10 g or more per day!

Caution. If you are pregnant, do not take more than 5 g of vitamin C per day.

Chlorella (*Chlorella* spp.)

Chlorella is a single-celled, freshwater cyanobacteria (photosynthetic bacteria) that contains macro- and micronutrients including proteins, omega-3 polyunsaturated fatty acids, complex sugars, vitamins including D2 and B12, and various minerals, although bioavailability is relatively low. There are more than 30 known species, of which two, *Chlorella vulgaris* and *Chlorella pyrenoidosa*, are the most commonly used as dietary supplements. Chlorella is traditionally used as a food product, to treat hyperlipidemia and hyperglycemia, to improve gaseous exchange in chronic obstructive pulmonary disease (COPD), and to protect against oxidative stress and risk of cancer. It may also be used to improve total cholesterol levels, reducing low-density lipoprotein levels, but not triglycerides or high-density lipoprotein levels.

Japanese studies have found chlorella growth factor (CGF) to be especially effective in speeding up cell growth, a major factor in the natural repair of wounds. Other studies reveal that CGF helps heal ulcers and promotes bone and muscle growth. When taken internally, it also acts as an immune booster. Topically, it functions as a protective cleansing compound for skin.

Studies in animals have suggested that chlorella taken orally can decrease the half-life of some toxins, promoting clearance pathways and reducing exposures. It also mitigates oxidative stress by reducing reactive oxygen production and increasing antioxidative processes. Chlorella contains an appreciable amount of protein by dry weight, and it exerts a hypoglycemic effect (decreasing sugar in the blood) through improved insulin sensitivity. Carotenoids in chlorella reduce serum lipid risk factors, mainly triglycerides and total cholesterol, in patients with high cholesterol levels.

Dosing. 1–2 g of the powder, twice daily.

Supplements for Meals and Bedtime

Supplements to Take with Meals

These can be purchased in most health food stores or from an herbalist. See page 399 for dosing guidelines.

- High-potency adaptogen blend (see pages 66–73)
- Turmeric, green tea, flavonoids, alpha-lipoic acid, CoQ10, zinc, selenium—antioxidant, anti-inflammatory
- Whey protein with immunoglobulins (1–2 scoops daily)—immune building
- Vitamin E succinate (800 IU)—antioxidant, antiscarring
- Omega-3 fats from fish oil (1,200–1,500 mg EPA, 600–800 mg DHA)—anti-inflammatory
- Glucosamine sulfate and methylsulfonylmethane (1,500 mg GLS, 3,000 mg MSM)—heals connective tissue
- Liquid chlorophyll (2 tablespoons twice daily)—pulls residues of anesthesia and pain medications from the cells

Supplements to Take at Bedtime

- Milk thistle (600 mg of silymarin twice daily)—protects the liver
- Serrapeptase/nattokinase/lumbrokinase—anti-inflammatory
- N-acetylcysteine (750–1,000 mg)—supports liver function
- Probiotic blend (50–100 billion bacteria)—supports bowel health

Healing and Recuperation Tincture

Begin to take this tincture mixture alongside any pain formula and then continue for 2 months after surgery to promote tissue repair and healing. All tinctures are made at 1:2 strength from dried herbs.

+ 20 mL gotu kola
+ 15 mL horsetail
+ 15 mL licorice
+ 15 mL meadowsweet
+ 10 mL rosemary
+ 10 mL yarrow leaf and flower
+ 5 mL cinnamon
+ 10 mL milk thistle

Mix all tinctures. Take 1 teaspoon twice daily in hot water.

Other Useful Agents for Postoperative Recovery

- Rescue Remedy (Bach Flower Remedy) for shock
- Arnica cream for bruising and soreness
- Peppermint or ginger tea and/or acupressure wrist bands for nausea
- Chamomile and skullcap for anxiety
- Silica to heal connective tissue
- Sunlight to accelerate wound healing by producing vitamin D in the skin (patients who are exposed to sunlight heal far faster than those who are not)

For the Practitioner

Further Mechanisms behind Surgery-Induced Angiogenesis

VASCULAR ENDOTHELIAL GROWTH FACTOR (VEGF)

VEGF is a potent inducer of angiogenesis, produced by injured cells and necessary for wound healing, but also hijacked by cancer cells to induce enhanced tumor growth. Plasma levels of VEGF increase after major surgery, and such elevations may contribute to tumor growth.

NM (NONMETASTATIC) 23 GENE

This is a family of at least eight related genes, found predominantly in primary tumors and acting to inhibit metastatic cancer. When nm23 is lost, the cell loses its ability to stay in one place and may start moving throughout the body. Mutated nm23 genes are found in a variety of tumors, including breast, colon, and pancreatic cancers, and their presence may promote metastases. Nm23 genes are lost when primary tumors are removed, and this eliminates the metastatic-inhibitory factors from the primary tumor. For example, in a 5-year study of colorectal cancer, both mutated p53 and mutated nm23-H(1) seemed to be independent and important prognostic factors. In another study, the presence of nm23 protein was a good marker for predicting resistance to metastases of salivary gland cancer.

Curcumin from turmeric may enhance the expression of nm23, as well as upregulating antimetastatic proteins, tissue inhibitor metalloproteinase-2 (TIMP-2), and E-cadherin, all of which serve to contain and control cancer growth.

MANAGING SURGERY-INDUCED ANGIOGENESIS

Ginseng exhibits apparently paradoxical effects, as it is both wound healing and antiangiogenic with opposing activities on the vascular system. A mass spectrometry analysis of American, Chinese, Korean, and Vietnamese ginseng revealed distinct "sterol ginsenoside" fingerprints, especially in the ratio between the protopanaxatriol Rg1 and the protopanaxadiol Rb1, which are the most prevalent ginsenoside constituents. Dominance of Triol Rg1 leads to angiogenesis, while Diol Rb1 exerts an opposing effect. Rg1 promoted neovascularization as well as the proliferation of endothelial cells in vitro, mediated through expression of nitric oxide synthase and the PI3K/Akt pathway. Rb1 inhibits the earliest step in angiogenesis, the chemo-invasion of endothelial cells.

This study explained the complexity of ginseng in vascular pathophysiology based on the existence of opposing active constituents in the extract, and the researchers suggested that Rg1 could be a prototype for a novel group of nonpeptide molecules that can induce therapeutic angiogenesis, such as in wound healing.

In the case of rhodiola, the root contains phenylpropanoid glycosides, notably salidroside and rosavin, rosin, and rosarin. Both the whole root extract and salidroside isolate exhibit paradoxical or contradictory actions on angiogenesis. Hypoxia-inducible factor (HIF) is a signal transcription regulator that plays a key role in many aspects of oxygen homeostasis. In cancer cells, rhodiola and salidroside inhibit the mTOR (signal transduction) pathway and reduce angiogenesis through downregulation of HIF. In normal (noncancer) tissues that have undergone surgery, however, rhodiola and salidroside activate the mTOR pathway and promote neovascularization. This paradoxical action may allow the plant medicine to promote tissue healing while downregulating cancer.

Salidroside specifically is a cardiac tonic and oxygenator, and overall the mechanisms of rhodiola are mediated through antioxidant, cholinergic-regulating, anti-apoptotic, anti-inflammatory effects that improve coronary blood flow and cerebral metabolism.

CHAPTER 4

Managing Pain with Botanicals

Cancer patients may experience pain for any number of reasons, including surgery, infection, a port-a-cath inserted for delivery of chemotherapy or other drugs, the chemotherapy drugs that burn the vessels as they go in, and the tumor itself, which may be pressing on a nerve or compromising blood or lymph flow. Pain management represents a whole subspecialty in oncology, up to and including palliative care and end-of-life support.

Strong prescription opioid painkillers (such as morphine and hydromorphone) have a soporific and depressing effect on the brain and mood, and this can have significant adverse effects on quality of life. In some parts of this continuum of care, herbal medicine has great value to offer as an alternative to opioid painkillers; for example, belladonna and corydalis can be used for spasmodic abdominal pain, willow for inflammatory pain, and California poppy, Jamaican dogwood, wild lettuce, and yellow jasmine for crushing pain or pain that keeps you from sleeping.

Prescription drugs have their place, but as soon as possible, I encourage patients to wean off them and replace them with herbs as needed. At no time, though, should a patient have to suffer unnecessarily on a point of principle—either theirs or the practitioner's. If the herbs don't work, or aren't enough, pharmaceuticals should be employed, and the herbalist can continue to offer supportive care alongside the drugs.

CHAPTER 4 CONTENTS

127 **Pain Management: Where to Begin**

127 Dosing Herbs to Manage Pain

129 **Botanicals for Mild to Moderate Pain**

129 California Poppy and Corydalis

131 Cannabis (*Cannabis* spp.)

135 Jamaican Dogwood (*Piscidia piscipula*)

136 Wild Lettuce (*Lactuca virosa*)

137 Palmitoylethanolamide (PEA)

138 **Herbs for Topical Use in Pain**

138 Monkshood (*Aconitum napellus*)

138 Arnica (*Arnica montana*)

140 Cayenne (*Capsicum minimum* and other species)

Pain Management: Where to Begin

Herbs work in multiple ways to alleviate pain. They can work at the peripheral or tissue level to reduce inflammation, relax muscle spasms, promote circulation, and inhibit transmission of pain impulses. These herbs tend to be relatively safe and have low risk, and they may sometimes be applied topically in a liniment, lotion, or patch. In contrast, the stronger herbal painkillers, such as corydalis and Jamaican dogwood, act on the central nervous system and are usually more potent and have more side effects, including sometimes quite marked sedation. Most herbs that are effective painkillers will cause sleepiness and may be best used in the evenings and through the night for deeper, more restorative sleep, rather than during the day. Salicylates, resins, muscle relaxants, and vasodilators (herbs that widen blood vessels) are not sedative and may be more appropriate for daytime use.

Some herbs—such as California poppy and corydalis—work in a similar way as prescription opioids, interacting with your own opioid receptors, but they are not addictive and don't have the same side effect of causing constipation. These may be used to lessen the need for opioids and in some cases to reduce cravings and addiction.

There are also a few herbs, such as yellow jasmine and deadly nightshade, that are very effective for pain management but have such a narrow therapeutic window that they are not suitable for self-prescribing, and these are explored in the section for practitioners.

Dosing Herbs to Manage Pain

When commencing the use of herbs for pain management, it is always advisable to start with the lowest dose of the milder herbs first and assess the response, gradually increasing the dose or the frequency, and then stepping up the potency of the herbs as necessary. This will preclude the risk of overprescribing, which could cause excessive sleepiness, impaired cognition, or impaired coordination and motor control.

For acute pain, it may be useful to take a standardized capsule product where the dose can be precisely calibrated. There is a temptation, if pain is really severe, to take more medicine and then more again. The more precise the dosing, the easier it can be to regulate and control the intake to a safe level while still being effective. Another option for herbalists is to include in a pain formula a small amount of lobelia, where it serves not only as a parasympathomimetic (parasympathetic nervous system) muscle relaxant and tissue oxygenator, but also as an emetic (which in large doses would bring on vomiting); this prevents overdosing on potent pain-relieving herbs such as yellow jasmine or belladonna.

I learned this the hard way, very early on in my practice, when a patient in desperate pain took so much yellow jasmine (3 days' supply in one dose!) that he was unable to speak properly or get out of bed for 4 days afterward. That would have been bad enough, but he also lived in the Haida Gwaii, remote islands between British Columbia and Alaska, 6 hours by ferry to a small hospital. His breath rate was 9 or 10 breaths per minute for almost 24 hours and I had his wife ready to call the air ambulance if it went down to 8. She called me hourly around the clock to report, I prayed to every god I knew, and miraculously he survived. He was very chastened, and I learned that desperate people don't always make good decisions. Ever since then I include a tiny bit of lobelia to keep patients safe.

Herbs and a Few Supplements for Pain

Mild Pain

- Anti-inflammatories: willow, turmeric, ginger, Indian frankincense, meadowsweet, licorice, plant sterols, fish oil (omega-3)
- Muscle relaxants: cramp bark, kava, lobelia, magnesium bisglycinate, magnesium sulfate (Epsom salts) flakes in a salve or 1 cup dissolved in a hot bath
- Relaxing nervines: skullcap, passionflower, hops
- Mild general pain reliever: capsaicin (topical)

Mild to Moderate Pain

- California poppy
- Cannabis
- Corydalis
- Jamaican dogwood
- Wild lettuce
- PEA (palmitoylethanolamide)

Severe Pain*

- Belladonna
- Jimson weed
- Henbane
- Yellow jasmine

*Practitioner intervention required

Herbs for Topical Use Only (toxic if taken internally)

- Aconite
- Arnica

Botanicals for Mild to Moderate Pain

These herbs may be safely used for most types of pain. Risk of overdose is low, although you may experience some side effects, including a morning-after headache, or some grogginess on waking, after high doses. With the possible exception of chronic use of cannabis, these herbs are not habit-forming.

California Poppy and Corydalis

These two poppies, from countries that are oceans apart, nonetheless need to be discussed together, as they represent a sort of continuum where the gentle (baby-safe) California poppy is used first and corydalis is held back until it is determined that the first herb is not enough. Corydalis therefore operates as a bridge from the milder to the strongest herbs.

Poppies generally are rich in benzylisoquinoline alkaloids, a large group of plant chemicals that includes protopines, protoberberines, and papaverine, occurring most notably in opium poppy (used to manufacture morphine and codeine) as well as in trace amounts in California poppy and corydalis. Papaverine relaxes smooth muscle fibers, reducing their tone or tension; thus, it is antispasmodic, especially to the gut, gall ducts, ureters, and arteries.

CALIFORNIA POPPY (*ESCHSCHOLZIA CALIFORNICA*)

This lovely bright orange flower that self-seeds in so many gardens has a long history of use for pain and spasms as a sedative and antitussive (cough-suppressing) agent. Aerial parts (flowering tops) are considered gentle but effective muscle relaxants, calming and sedative, and mild to moderate pain relievers, and they are hypnotic but not narcotic. Some practitioners today dispute California poppy's effectiveness, but traditional indications include insomnia, anxiety, agitation, melancholia, depression, headache, and nerve pain. Modern research shows that the protopine alkaloids increase the binding of gamma-aminobutyric acid (GABA) to neuroreceptors, which calms the nervous system. Sedative effects may occur at higher doses, whereas anti-anxiety effects are predominant at lower dose ranges.

Dosing. The dried herb (seedpods, aerial parts, or whole plant) may be taken at doses of 500–2,000 mg in divided doses throughout the day. Larger doses could promote light sedation and drowsiness. This herb tastes extremely bitter and is not recommended as a tea.

Cautions. Potential drug interactions include enhanced hypnotic effects of barbiturates (possibly due to enhanced binding of GABA receptors); increased effects of certain antidepressants, including monoamine oxidase inhibitors (MAOIs); and increased sedative effects of antipsychotic and antianxiety medications. These are all additive or synergistic effects that increase drug responses and may allow for lowering the drug dosing carefully.

CORYDALIS (*CORYDALIS AMBIGUA*)

This is a type of poppy from China with protoberberine alkaloids in the root that have potent painkilling, sedative, and tranquilizing effects. Corydalis is used in Traditional Chinese Medicine for pain relief and to "invigorate blood." Frying the root in vinegar is said to help increase the pain-relieving properties. It's also used in traditional combinations with other herbs to alleviate stuck qi (energy) and blood stagnation (manifesting as congestion, swelling, and buildup of fluids in the tissues). Overall, corydalis demonstrates analgesic, antiseptic, antihemorrhagic, and antispasmodic effects, largely attributed to the protoberberine alkaloids. Corydalis inhibits acute neuropathic pain, without causing tolerance. It also inhibits inflammatory pain.

In addition to its use in treating pain, corydalis may be helpful in reducing the risk of blood clotting—a common consequence of cancer and some of the drugs used to treat it. At least two clinical trials showed that a tetrahydropalmatine (dl-THP) isolated alkaloid extract from corydalis prevented platelet aggregation both in vitro and in vivo in rabbits and rats. In addition, dl-THP has been shown to both decrease the stickiness of blood platelets and protect against stroke, as well as lower blood pressure and heart rate in animal studies. Corydalis also exerts an antiarrhythmic action on the heart and is an anticonvulsant. All of these modern studies corroborate and confirm the traditional indications for blood stasis.

Another alkaloid in corydalis, called dehydrocorybulbine (DHCB), reduces sensations of inflammatory pain and injury-induced neuropathic pain by blocking pain signals from reaching the brain. DHCB induces potent dose-dependent pain relief without causing sedation and is independent of opioid receptors, so it does not induce tolerance with repeated use, as opioids do.

Actions and Uses of Corydalis

- Antispasmodic, promoting smooth and skeletal muscle relaxation
- Inhibits cyclooxygenase and lipoxygenase enzymes (COX-2 and 5-, 12-, and 15-LOX), which control inflammatory prostaglandins, and reduces inflammation
- Reduces blood stagnation (is blood moving)
- Reduces clot formation and breaks up clots; reduces swelling of tissues
- Invigorates blood and builds red blood cells and hemoglobin
- Synergistic with chemotherapy and radiation therapy, improving both white and red blood cell counts as well as hemoglobin and platelet counts
- May suppress further cancer development and/or metastasis

Dosing. Traditional doses of the whole herb are 3–9 g daily, equivalent to 6–18 mL of a 1:2 tincture made with 45–65% ethyl alcohol. Start low and build up as needed. This herb is a strong sedative and can make you feel hungover after higher doses. The alkaloids in this herb act synergistically with barbiturates. Overdose leads to excessive muscle relaxation and a narcotic effect.

Corydalis and Opioid Drugs

The alkaloids of corydalis bind into kappa opioid receptors in the nervous system, where they have a stimulating effect and may be responsible for reducing cravings in opioid drug addiction and relapse. Coadministration of corydalis with opioids may reduce the drug dose needed while maintaining pain-relief effects and may delay development of drug tolerance and need for increasing doses with concomitant increasing risks.

Cannabis (*Cannabis* spp.)

Cannabis leaf and especially the female flower bud contain a wide range of terpenes and cannabinoids that interact with receptors all over the body and regulate mood, pain pathways, and hunger, among other effects. The cannabinoids have been the most extensively researched, but there is some suggestion that the wide range of terpenes in this plant are at least as clinically significant. Indigenous to northern Asia (India), cannabis is now widely grown all over the world and almost as widely used as other (legal) mood- and appetite-altering drugs, such as coffee and tobacco.

Although cannabis is now legal in many countries, it is still a crime punishable with severe sentencing in some countries, so be sure to check local laws before using this medicine. In Canada, where I practice, it is legal for recreational and medical use, and 43 percent of people aged 15 years and older have used cannabis in their lifetime. The most common reason reported for use of medical cannabis, in up to 84 percent of medical marijuana users, is chronic pain. Other reasons include mental health concerns (such as anxiety), sleep disorders, and spasticity in multiple sclerosis (MS). Traditional uses of cannabis include pain-relieving, muscle-relaxing, mood-elevating, appetite-inducing, and euphoric effects. Excessive use may cause stupor and vomiting.

Cannabis presents challenges to the conventional research model, not the least of which is the impossibility of creating a blind study—if THC is present, the patient will know which arm of the study they are in. Despite this, there is good evidence to support the use of cannabis for chronic pain (neuropathic pain and refractory pain in palliative care), nausea and vomiting during chemotherapy, and muscle spasticity (MS and spinal cord injury). Clinical use also supports cannabis for relieving the symptoms of epilepsy (though it is not curative).

UNDERSTANDING CBD AND THC CONTENT

There are more than 400 identified compounds in female cannabis flowers, of which at least 100 are classified as cannabinoids. The precise proportions change through the lifetime of the plant as well as through morning/evening times and sun/shade exposures. Current research supports the fact that CBD (cannabidiol) and THC (tetrahydrocannabinol—the stuff that gets you high) are the most prevalent, and most of the medical and psychoactive claims are made for these compounds. However, these are just two of many compounds, the ones that have been best researched, and in the future many more may be studied and found effective. In addition, the application of heat (smoking or cooking it) modifies cannabinoids, activating some and deactivating others. Finally, we cannot forget the so-called entourage effect of the synergy and interactions of the various phytochemicals in the plant.

THE ENDOCANNABINOID SYSTEM

Cannabinoids may be made by the body (these are the "endocannabinoids," such as anandamide and palmitoylethanolamide [PEA]); they also may be derived from plants (such as THC and CBD) or they may be synthetic (such as nabilone, which is used to treat nausea and vomiting after chemotherapy). The compounds found in cannabis buds alleviate pain by targeting receptors in the endocannabinoid system—the collective term for receptors throughout the body whose main purpose is to regulate and manage cell activities, as well as being involved in many other complex regulatory processes. Cannabinoid receptors are found in almost all living creatures, even in very primitive organisms, and these receptors are almost identical across all organisms, implying that they have evolved over eons of time and are therefore presumed to confer survival advantages to the organism.

Cannabinoid receptors are involved in neurotransmitter activity and are also important for fat metabolism, modulating inflammation, enhancing insulin sensitivity, and immune regulation. Endocannabinoids modulate many interrelated and overlapping functions, most of which are explicitly helpful in managing cancer, including the following:

- Modulation of the hypothalamic-pituitary-adrenal (HPA) axis, which governs stress responses and the immune system
- Calming activity in the parasympathetic nervous system (likely contributing to the nausea-suppressing effects)
- Increased heart rate and strength of the heartbeat
- Vasodilation (widening of blood vessels) leading to reduced hypertension (high blood pressure)
- Protects the heart during angina (insufficient oxygen reaching the heart) or during a heart attack

- Promotes the formation of new brain cells in the case of injury or trauma to the brain
- Reduced seizure activity and lessening of brain damage caused by stroke

Endocannabinoid activity in the brain is involved with short-term memory, cognition, mood and emotion, motor function, and nociception (the perception of pain). In fact, the human body responds to injury by increasing cannabinoid receptors in peripheral nerves so that the body is able to accept greater levels of cannabinoids and is better able to mitigate pain.

Endocannabinoids play an important neuroprotective role (especially after injury) and promote neuroplasticity, including neurogenesis (formation of new brain cells). *Neuroplasticity* refers to the ability of the brain to form new neural connections throughout life, to allow the brain to compensate for injury and disease, and to help neurons in the brain adjust in response to new situations, such as adaptive learning (like relearning how to walk after a stroke).

WHICH SPECIES TO USE

Cannabis aficionados speak of the differences between *Cannabis sativa* and *C. indica*, as well as the various strains or varieties (hybrids developed to intensify specific characteristics of the plant, for marketing claims, or to make it more effective as a drug). In principle, *C. sativa* is energizing and more psychoactive, giving you more of a "head high," whereas *C. indica* gives more of a "body high," a physical effect that helps alleviate pain and can be sedative, although as Dr. Ethan Russo has pointed out, many or most commercial strains now are a blend of both species and may be indistinguishable from one another. For most strains available, the distinction between them is probably in the terpenoid makeup and levels, not the CBD and THC levels (though of course these can also vary).

> There are biochemically distinct strains of cannabis, but the *sativa/indica* distinction as commonly applied in the lay literature is total nonsense and an exercise in futility. One cannot in any way currently guess the biochemical content of a given cannabis plant based on its height, branching, or leaf morphology. The degree of interbreeding and hybridization is such that only a biochemical assay tells a potential consumer or scientist what is really in the plant.
>
> ETHAN RUSSO, MD

Growing Your Own

You might also consider growing your own cannabis. In Canada, where I practice, every household is allowed to grow four plants per year. That may not sound like a lot, but when you consider that a good grower can expect yields of 3–5 pounds per plant, it is actually plenty for the year and then some. There are plenty of videos online explaining how to grow, harvest, and process excellent-quality medicine. It may not be as potent as some of the hydroponic, forced, and chemical-laced commercial cannabis products, but it will be pure and effective.

DOSING

Judging your dose requires some trial and error, and not everyone can tolerate this plant medicine. The CBD-rich strains may not get you high, but evidence suggests that all compounds, including the psychoactive THC, have an entourage effect to augment each other, and isolating one compound in excess of the others may disrupt this and diminish the medicinal effects. In other words, you may need to get a bit high to get the best effects; clearly, this is not suitable for everyone and needs to be managed carefully.

For my patients wishing to use medical cannabis, I recommend purchasing high-quality, organically grown bud, activating it in the oven at 240°F (116°C) for 40 minutes, grinding it in a coffee grinder, and putting it into capsules. A capsule-filling device, such as Cap M Quik, can hold "0" (small) or "00" (medium) sized capsules and allows you to fill 50 capsules in just a few minutes.

Initial doses should be taken in a controlled situation, when you do not need to drive, operate machinery, or be out in public, and with someone nearby, in case you feel afraid or get nauseous. The general recommendation is to start low and go slow.

Doses of up to 20–30 mg THC/day are usually safe. Remember that psychoactivity is not the same as clinical or medical effectiveness. The correct dose is the lowest that produces therapeutic benefit without associated adverse effects. First-time users may want to start at 2.5–5 mg of THC and work up from there. To calculate how much herb is required to achieve this dose, you ideally need to know the THC content by percent. For example, a THC content of 20% would yield 200 mg of THC per 1 g of cannabis leaf. Most strains today, bred for high THC yield in the recreational market, are 21–25%. If you grow your own, this information is not available, so some degree of trial and error is necessary.

How cannabis is consumed also makes a difference in how effective it is. When cannabis is smoked, only 60–65% of the THC is bioavailable. When it is cooked and eaten, the effects can be three to five times greater than smoking or vaping the same amount. The effects of inhaled cannabis come on rapidly but also pass more rapidly, and this is a big difference from ingesting it (where the effects come on slowly but stick around for much longer). Some people in severe pain may do best to use both inhaled medicine for rapid effects and oral medicine to avoid peaks and troughs of plasma levels.

OVERDOSING

Overdosing on cannabis is common, especially after eating it, where the dose may be harder to control. Dizziness, disequilibrium, spatial misjudgment, delayed reflex responses, and disordered thinking are subjective states along a continuum from "slightly stoned" to "absolutely zonked." More severe symptoms of high dose, beyond an enjoyable high, may include sedation, lack of muscle control, low blood pressure, mood instability, short-term memory impairment, and, in very high doses, possibility of a dissociative (disconnected) mental state. Individual tolerance may be affected by the strain or strength of the herb, but also by whether you have recently eaten or had any alcohol, coffee, or other mood-altering drugs. Whether you are overtired or stressed also makes a difference.

If you do take too much and feel unwell, simply lying down and waiting it out is probably sufficient. In rare cases an excess dose, or heavy daily use over a long time, will trigger a state of hyperemesis (persistent cycles of vomiting and deep nausea that does not respond to conventional antinausea drugs). This hyperemesis can last several hours in an acute overdose, or days to weeks in chronic overuse, and can be quite debilitating. In patients on other pharmaceutical drugs, vomiting may create a short-term risk of undermedicating.

A person with cannabis-induced hyperemesis is usually deeply cold and shivering and often will urgently seek a hot bath or bundle up in blankets, both of which are useful. If they end up in the emergency room, a common treatment is a generous application of a capsaicin (cayenne) ointment over the abdomen and upper back; this is something that can be done at home as well.

Jamaican Dogwood (*Piscidia piscipula*)

This remedy is made from the bark of a small Central American tree in the pea family. The wood has been known by Indigenous people for generations to stun fish in ponds for an easier harvest. Neurotoxins (called rotenoids) in the wood immobilize the fish and make them float to the surface for capture. (Residual amounts of the neurotoxins in the fish are very small, so the fish are not considered harmful to eat.) For many years Jamaican dogwood was approved in organic agriculture as an insecticide, but it has been phased out and largely removed from sale because of the potential for harm to fish stocks if allowed to leach into creeks. All that is to say, in therapeutic doses the medicine is safe, but if you take too much you will feel dizzy and sick and have a bad headache. The bark extract has a range of other compounds, notably several isoflavones that allow the synergy of constituents to act as a deep central nervous system relaxant and mild narcotic.

This herb is a strong relaxant and can shorten sleep latency (help you fall asleep quicker) and is best combined with other herbs to allow for lower doses without losing overall effectiveness. For skeletal muscle pain, it can be combined with muscle relaxants and pain relievers such as black cohosh, willow, meadowsweet, and kava. For insomnia, combine it with herbs such as skullcap, California poppy, valerian, wild lettuce, and hops. For severe pain, combine it with corydalis, valerian, and kava.

Note that this tree is restricted in habitat and is under threat of overharvesting. As far as possible, try to buy only from sustainable sources.

Dosing. Dried root bark: 1–2 g three times daily. Tincture (1:2 strength made with 60% ethyl alcohol): 3–6 mL daily.

Wild Lettuce (*Lactuca virosa*)

This lettuce relative has traditionally been used as an anti-inflammatory and sedative, with pain-relieving and antianxiety properties. The plant exudes a bitter, white latex (much like what you'd see if you cut the stem of cultivated lettuces), and this is the source of its medicinal power. In times past the thick, 3-foot-tall stalks of wild lettuce were tapped or cut (a bit like a maple tree) and the oozing latex was collected on cotton fabric tied over the cut. This fabric could then be soaked in alcohol to extract the latex and the alkaloids in it. The alcohol was then evaporated off over very low heat, leaving behind a black, tarry substance called "lettuce opium." It is not an opioid at all—rather, it is a sesquiterpene-rich resin substrate—but after processing it *looks* like opium. It also has sedative and pain-killing properties like opium but is milder, nonconstipating, and non-habit-forming.

Modern studies are scant, but in the Perso-Arabic Unani system of traditional medicine the seed of *Lactuca scariola* (prickly lettuce) is an important drug for the treatment of headache, insomnia, nervousness, hypertension, palpitation, and fever. The seed extract is listed in a 2013 review article published in the *Global Journal of Research in Medicinal Plants and Indigenous Medicine* as a "sedative and hypnotic, a diuretic, deobstruent, antipyretic, anti-inflammatory, blood purifier, demulcent, refrigerant, anesthetic and antispasmodic, anticancer, antibacterial, bronchodilator and vasorelaxant."

Lactuca virosa is a variety closely related to *L. scariola,* while *L. sativa* is the nonmedicinal garden variety cultivated worldwide as a vegetable.

Dosing. No standardized dose has been established for wild lettuce. Tea of the leaves and stems is likely to be the mildest form, as the sesquiterpenes are not very water soluble. It will also be quite bitter and unpleasant. Tincture of the leaves and stems, using around 45% alcohol as a solvent, will be stronger, and the concentrated latex "opium" will be the strongest form and can be rolled into a small ball about the size of a pea and taken like a pill.

- Tea: 1–2 teaspoons of dried leaves and stems in 1 cup of water up to three times a day.
- Resin (lettuce opium): 1.5 g as often as needed.
- Tincture (1:5 strength made with 45–65% ethyl alcohol): 0.5–1 mL in water several times daily, as needed. Higher doses may be taken, but sleepiness may result.

There is only one report of acute human poisoning with this herb when a simple water extract was injected intravenously by three individuals, one of whom also injected an alcohol extract of valerian root. Effects included fevers, chills, abdominal pain, flank and back pain, neck stiffness, headache, elevated white cell count, and elevated liver enzymes. All three individuals recovered over the next few days.

Another report described eight individuals in Iran who were mildly sickened by eating excessive quantities of wild lettuce, with symptoms including pupil dilation, anxiety, dizziness, decreased bowel motility, and urinary retention, suggesting an anticholinergic (nervous-stimulating) effect at high doses. This is exactly what we do not want from a supposedly relaxing herb, so wild lettuce appears to have a dose-dependent effect.

Palmitoylethanolamide (PEA)

Palmitoylethanolamide (PEA) is a fatty acid made in the cell wall and is a type of endocannabinoid, closely related to anandamide (AEA), the first endocannabinoid identified. It is available in capsule form as a supplement for self-medication (no prescription required).

PEA binds to receptors in brain cells and exerts a variety of biological functions related to chronic pain and inflammation. PEA does not bind directly to cannabinoid receptors; however, in the presence of PEA and related compounds, anandamide activity is enhanced by an entourage effect. It is used for neuropathic pain, fibromyalgia, MS, carpal tunnel syndrome, and pain from other neuromuscular inflammatory states. PEA induces a feeling of euphoria, energy, stimulation, and overall well-being. It can also promote heightened focus, attention, goal-directed behavior, and task completion, all of which can be helpful if there is postchemotherapy or postsurgical cognitive impairment.

Dosing. The ultramicronized form is preferred as it tends to be more bioavailable, up to 600 mg twice daily, taken with food. PEA has no drug interactions because it's broken down by the body through the cytoplasm, instead of in the liver or kidneys. It also has no side effects and is not addictive. It's safe for use in the elderly and can be used in opioid withdrawal.

Herbs for Topical Use in Pain

Some herbs may be very effective for managing pain but are too toxic for internal use. They are best used as part of a liniment (blended alcohol and oil extract), a salve (herb-infused base oil set firm with beeswax), or an ointment (blended water or hydrosol creamed or emulsified with herb-infused oils). Everything that is put on the skin can be absorbed to some degree (or else the herbs wouldn't work at all), so even with topical applications there may be some restrictions or cautions. They should not be used over broken skin, including on open incisions or ulcerated skin, or on mucous membranes (inside the mouth, on the genitals), and should be used with extra care if you have impaired liver function, to avoid risk of toxic accumulation. Do not ingest these herbs, and be sure to wash your hands well after applying them.

Monkshood (*Aconitum napellus*)

The root of monkshood contains alkaloids that act to reduce the permeability of nerve cells to sodium, thus inhibiting the ability to transmit a nerve impulse. It is used as a strong topical painkiller. Application of aconite produces an initial irritation of nerve endings, with a sensation of heat, then numbing of nerve endings and a sensation of coolness. It is an effective topical treatment for nerve pain such as toothache, sciatica, trigeminal neuralgia (inflammation of the fifth cranial nerve), and rheumatic pains.

This herb should not be ingested. If taken orally it causes central nervous system paralysis with slow heart rate, low blood pressure, irregular heartbeat, respiratory weakness, and heart failure. Death can occur after ingestion of only 5 milliliters of the 1:10 tincture.

It is important to point out here that in Traditional Chinese Medicine *Aconitum carmichaeli* is used. The roots are cooked and processed to reduce any toxicity, and it is frequently prescribed as a very warming herb and as a painkiller, anti-inflammatory, antirheumatic, heart tonic, heart stimulant, and vasodilator (widens blood vessels, to reduce blood pressure). Do not confuse the processed Chinese monkshood with the crude European monkshood.

Topical application dosing. According to the *British Herbal Pharmacopoeia,* the tincture is made to 1:10 strength in 60–65% ethyl alcohol and is incorporated into liniments or lotions at not more than 1.3% in a formula. It can also be diluted to 1:9 with distilled witch hazel and applied directly on the skin. The witch hazel tightens pores in the skin, thus delaying absorption. Monkshood is used over areas of shooting, stabbing, lancing, or searing pain and can be reapplied frequently.

Arnica (*Arnica montana*)

The bright yellow, daisylike flowers of *Arnica montana* and related species are where this traditional medicine is found. The volatile oil is rich in sesquiterpene lactones, including helanin and dihydrohelenalin, which reduce inflammation and act as microvascular tonics. This is why the oil is effective for reducing bruising. It is a frequent ingredient in topical recovery formulas where there has been active soft tissue damage—in addition to treating bruising, it is a specific remedy for sprains and strains, torn or sore muscles, pulled ligaments, arthritis, lower back pain, and other types of musculoskeletal pain, and for recovery and repair of these tissues, including after injury or surgery. The flowers also contain sugars, and a polysaccharide fraction of arnica flowers may have significant immunostimulating properties and increase the rate of phagocytosis by granulocytes, which allows cleanup at sites of inflammation.

The seeds are rich in phenolic acids (chlorogenic acid, caffeic acid, quercetin, and kaempferol) and flavonoids (luteolin and apigenin), and in cell studies they induced cell death in two types of brain cancer cells (anaplastic astrocytoma and glioblastoma multiforme). The essential oil from the roots inhibited the nuclear transcription factor NF-κB, which controls many procancer oncogenes. Overall this suggests some anticancer potential. This potential has not been researched in animals or humans and is not a traditional use of the plant, so safety data is absent and doses are unspecified. Certainly, soaking seeds or roots into base oil for use in a cancer salve is safe, but I am not recommending you take arnica internally in any form except in homeopathic remedies until more research has been done. Homeopathic arnica is made with flowers in a tincture, ultradiluted and potentized. This is exceptionally safe and is given in case of shock, sprain, bruise, strains, blows, or falls. It is especially useful in the immediate recovery phase after surgery.

Arnica for topical use is usually prepared as an infused or macerated oil, made by soaking fresh flowers in a base oil or carrier oil like grapeseed or almond oil for 2 weeks, then straining it off. Alternatively, a tincture can be made with fresh flowers in 65% alcohol at 1:5 strength. The finished tincture is then incorporated into salves or liniments. It is approved by German drug regulation authorities (Commission E) for topical treatment of skin inflammation and is a frequent ingredient in products for seborrheic dermatitis and psoriasis, insect bites, boils, acne eruptions, and hemorrhoids.

Topical application dosing. Do not ingest this remedy except as a homeopathic dilution. When used as a compress, 1 tablespoon (15 mL) of tincture (1:5 strength made with 45–65% ethyl alcohol) is mixed with 0.5 L of water and a cloth is soaked in the fluid and applied. For an infusion, pour 1 L boiling water over 25 g dried arnica flowers, cover, and steep until cool enough to use in a basin or bucket as a soak for the affected part. Cream or ointment preparations should contain a maximum of 15% infused arnica oil or 20–25% tincture.

There are rare reports of contact dermatitis caused by arnica. There are also several reports of irritation when arnica is used at stronger concentrations or for longer periods than are recommended. It is not recommended for use on open wounds or broken skin.

There is some concern about overharvesting and habitat loss for this herb in Europe, and many suppliers now are using the more abundant North American *Arnica cordifolia.*

Cayenne (*Capsicum minimum* and other species)

The fruits and seeds of cayenne contain capsaicin, a compound that binds to vanillinoid receptors under the skin and strongly promotes the release of substance P from peripheral nerve fibers. Initially this induces sensations of heat and itching or prickling; there will also be a rubefacient (reddening) action on the skin. Quickly, however, the substance P is depleted, and a numbing or pain-relieving effect occurs.

Capsaicin ointments and creams are readily available and moderately effective for nerve pain (sciatica, trigeminal neuralgia), a pinched nerve or slipped disc, spasms and crampy types of muscle pain, diabetic neuropathy, post-herpes pain and itching, migraines, cluster headaches, postsurgical pain, and post-amputation pain.

Creams and lotions usually are between 0.025% and 0.075% capsaicin. Several applications daily are necessary to maintain effects. Avoid touching eyes or mucous membranes when applying a cayenne product, and wash hands very well with soap afterward.

For the Practitioner

Herbs for Moderate to Severe Pain

These herbs are toxic. They are only available to qualified herbalists from professional suppliers and not available for the general public or for self-care. Do not pick or purchase these plants and try to make your own medicine; the uncertainty of product potency would preclude safe dose calibration. Doses need to be made from validated plant material in a controlled process yielding a known potency of finished product. When storing them in the dispensary, they should be in a locked cabinet, labeled as poisons, and signed out by the dispenser. Dispensing should be done in a 5-milliliter glass column because most of the 100-milliliter dispensing columns have a 2 percent margin of error and that is too much for these herbs. Both maximum single and maximum daily dose should be written in red pen. I affix stickers to the bottle, one with a skull and crossbones saying "poison," and another suggesting not to drive or operate heavy machinery after use. I also tell the patient what they are getting and how to be safe with them while also getting an effective dose.

USING TOXIC ANALGESICS

Finding the balance between the effective dose and the toxic dose is not a precise science. Factors that influence dose may include many individual metabolic idiosyncrasies (single nucleotide polymorphisms, or SNPs, in the liver that govern detox capacities), age, body mass index, diet, comorbidities, polypharmacy (taking other drugs as well), compliance, and lifestyle. Another important consideration is the quality and potency of the remedy itself. By building doses slowly, by using incremental and carefully calibrated doses, tolerable amounts can be determined in each case.

The reason I am discussing these herbs here, the reason why they would ever be prescribed in clinical practice, is only if the patient is having substantial problems or distress from pharmaceutical pain-management strategies. For example, hydromorphone and morphine, given for severe pain, are notably constipating, and this side effect may end up contributing to even more pain over time. The herbs may possibly be used to reduce drug dosing and make the patient more comfortable.

Actions and Uses

- **Yellow jasmine.** Strong sedative in small amounts, narcotic analgesic in higher dose
- **Belladonna.** Antispasmodic and drying in the gut
- **Henbane.** Antispasmodic and drying in the bladder and urethra
- **Jimson weed.** Antispasmodic and drying in the lungs and airways

YELLOW JASMINE (*GELSEMIUM SEMPERVIRENS*)

This climbing, vining plant with its sweetly scented yellow flowers is not a jasmine at all but was named thus by early white settlers in the southern US who used it as a powerful fever-reducer for the assorted swamp fevers they encountered. Its roots have several alkaloids that make the extract strongly sedative in small amounts and a narcotic painkiller in higher doses. These alkaloids first have a powerful effect on the peripheral nervous system to cause generalized muscle relaxation, drooping or heaviness of eyelids and jaw, a strong sense of ease and relaxation, and reduced sensitivity to pain.

If the dose is just slightly higher, then central nervous system involvement leads to disequilibrium, double vision, pupil enlargement, drooping or heaviness of eyelids and jaw, and feebleness of movement. The pulse may slow to 30–40 beats per minute, and body temperature drops. The respiratory control center of the brain stem is depressed and respiration initially speeds up, then becomes slow and shallow. Still larger doses will cause spinal paralysis, complete loss of muscle power, reduction in sensitivity to pain, coma, and death by heart and respiratory failure.

The Eclectic physicians recommended this herb for hectic or intermittent fevers, especially in the early stages of fever, when there is severe muscle and head pain, and also as a sedative and a painkiller. Specific indications included conditions with bright eyes, contracted pupils, flushed face, great heat and restlessness, mental irritability, insomnia, excitation, hysteria, head pain, nerve pain, chilly sensations upon movement, and convulsions.

Dosing. Tincture is made from fresh root at 1:10 strength in 65% ethyl alcohol. Put 5–15 drops in ½ glass water and take ½ tsp. every 10–15 minutes until physiological effects are noticed. The maximum daily dose is 25 mg of the dried root or rhizome or 0.25 mL (about 6 drops) of 1:10 tincture three times daily. The maximum weekly dose is 5 mL of 1:10 tincture.

BELLADONNA, JIMSON WEED, AND HENBANE (*ATROPA BELLADONNA*, *DATURA STRAMONIUM*, *HYOSCYAMUS NIGER*)

These plants are all in the Solanaceae (tomato and potato) family and contain pyrrolidine and tropane alkaloids—principally atropine (a mix of L- and D-hyoscyamine) and hyoscine (also known as scopolamine), and also apoatropine and belladonnine, among others—that inhibit receptors of the parasympathetic nervous system and hence have a sympathomimetic (sympathetic nervous system) effect that is warming, drying, relaxing to smooth muscle spasms, and overall stimulating.

In very small therapeutic doses there is a sympathomimetic effect that results in midriasis (dilation of pupils); reduction in all bodily secretions (sweat, saliva, tears, and digestive juices); inhibition of the vagus nerve leading to tachycardia, increased cardiac output, and raised blood pressure; and a reduced tension in all smooth muscle, leading to vasodilation, bronchial dilation, and reduced peristalsis. Overall, the effect is to relax the airways, facilitate gaseous exchange, speed up the heart, increase cardiac output, and warm the body, as well as drying secretions and bodily juices and reducing spasms or cramps.

Higher doses are felt more in the central nervous system (brain and spinal cord). There is an initial period of stimulation followed by confusion and hallucinations. If the dose has been large enough, the respiratory rate will increase and the temperature will rise. Ultimately there is central narcotic paralysis with a reduction in all symptoms, followed by coma and death.

Of the three herbs, belladonna is the strongest, followed by Jimson weed, then henbane. These herbs are most often used for their smooth muscle relaxant/antispasmodic effect. Belladonna has some specificity to the gut and is especially indicated for esophageal spasms; colicky bowel cramps; looseness, frequency, and urgency of bowel movement; and biliary (gallbladder) spasms. Jimson weed especially is useful for alleviating the bronchial constriction of asthma or the fruitless, spasmodic coughing of lung cancer and is specific for the tremor of Parkinsonism (corrects the choline/dopamine balance in the brain). The antispasmodic effect of henbane is more pronounced in the urinary system, where it may be useful in the passage of kidney stones, painful spasms in bladder cancer, or the bladder spasms of interstitial cystitis. Henbane may also be used to prevent motion sickness and in the treatment of Ménière's disease, where it helps greatly with nausea and dizziness.

Dosing. The maximum allowable weekly doses according to the UK list of restricted herbs (Schedule 20 list) are:

- Belladonna leaf 1:10 tincture, 10 mL
- Belladonna root 1:10 tincture, 6 mL
- Jimson weed 1:10 tincture, 10 mL
- Henbane 1:10 tincture, 20 mL

One of the first signs of overdosing with belladonna, Jimson weed, or henbane is a dry mouth. The eyes may also become sore and dry. This reduction in secretions can be useful in the treatment of peptic ulceration or hyperacidity but should be employed with mucilaginous herbs to replace the body's own mucus. In the case of coldlike congestion and overproduction of mucus, these alkaloids may act to dry up the excess mucus, but care should be taken not to overdry and thus irritate the delicate and sensitive membranes. Again, soothing herbs may be usefully employed in these cases to promote the production of a healthy quality and quantity of mucus.

Individual sensitivities to these herbs can vary quite extensively, and caution is advised when commencing treatment with these centrally acting pain relievers. Use small doses and slow incremental increases, so that you can calibrate the least dose required for the best effects.

CHAPTER 5

Thriving during Chemotherapy and Radiation

The stronger and healthier the body is at commencement of treatment, the better the outcomes to be expected. If a person is run down, depleted, and nutrient deficient after a long battle with cancer, yet another round of chemotherapy may not be tolerable or effective. But if there has been no previous chemotherapy, if the person is still in reasonably robust health with decent liver function, chemotherapy may be better tolerated. In my clinical experience I have seen a few people go through it with little to no drama, and I have seen others completely prostrated. I recommend preparing the body in advance with a strong prehabilitation plan (page 40) by implementing the Clean and Green Detox Diet, with immune support, liver support, digestive aids, and stress-reducing nerve restoratives (adaptogen nervines), as well as by doing prechemotherapy fasting, then following up with herbal and nutritional strategies to manage side effects and symptoms. With this plan the body will be better able to tolerate and complete a full course of treatment.

CHAPTER 5 CONTENTS

146 Understanding Conventional Cancer Treatment

146 Conventional Cancer Therapies
147 Systemic Drug Therapies
147 Considering Chemotherapy
148 Side Effects of Chemotherapy
149 Tolerating Chemotherapy Better

153 Dosing Models for Chemotherapy

153 Maximum Tolerated Dose
153 Metronomic Dosing
154 Chronotherapy
154 Hypothermic Isolated Limb Perfusion
155 Nanoparticle Drug Delivery
155 Liposomal Drug Delivery
155 Hyperthermic Intraperitoneal Chemotherapy

156 Other Innovative Anticancer Treatments

157 Photodynamic Therapy
157 Hyperthermia

160 Managing Side Effects of Chemotherapy and Radiation

160 Establishing a Healthy Daily Routine
161 Adaptogens for Stress
162 Brain Fog and Chemotherapy Haze
163 Cerebral Circulatory Stimulants
163 Wide Awake Tea

164 Managing Constipation

164 Causes of Constipation
164 Types of Constipation
165 Holistic Treatment of Constipation
166 Herbal Tea for Flaccid or Atonic Constipation
166 Herbal Formula for Tonic Constipation
172 Triphala for Bowel Health

173 Diarrhea Caused by Chemotherapy and Radiation

174 Types of Diarrhea
174 Diarrhea in Cancer Patients
174 Holistic Treatment of Diarrhea
175 Methods for Stopping Diarrhea
176 Carob Drink to Stop Diarrhea
176 Herbal Tea Formula for Loose Stools
177 WHO Rehydration Formula
177 Herbal Tea for Rehydration

176 Cardiac Support

178 Herbs for Cardiac Support
179 Cardiotonic Hawthorn Tea

180 Fatigue and Debility

180 Adaptogens for Rejuvenation
181 Herbs and Nutrition for Building Blood
185 Herbal Formula for Building Blood
185 Dong Quai and Millettia Formula

189 Gastritis and Reflux

189 Mucilaginous Herbs
190 Stomachics
190 Carminative Herbs
191 How You Eat Matters
192 A Powdered Herb Formula to Soothe the Digestive System
192 Herbal Formula to Calm the Nerves and Promote Appetite and Digestion

193 Hand-Foot Syndrome and Skin Rashes

194 Herbs for Soothing and Healing Skin
196 Super Moisturizing Skin Cream

197 Loss of Appetite
197 Holistic Strategies for Treating Appetite Loss
198 Using Herbs to Support Appetite
200 Herbal Bitters Blend
201 Stomach Settler Seed Sprinkle
201 Carminative Chai Tea
202 Cannabis and Appetite Promotion

202 Orthorexia
203 Holistic Strategies for Treating Orthorexia

204 Lymphedema
205 Stages of Lymphedema
205 Moving Lymph Fluid Is Beneficial
206 Herbal Treatments for Lymphedema
207 Herbal Formula for Moving Lymph and Stimulating Lymphocytes
209 Skin Lotion for Lymph Drainage
209 Skin Lotion for Lymph Node Stimulation

210 Mouth Sores
211 Preventing Mouth Sores
212 Conventional Treatment of Mouth Sores
212 Holistic Strategies for Treating Mouth Sores
214 Soothing and Healing Mouthwash
214 Rooty Fruity Herbal Tea Frozen Pops

215 Cracked Lips
215 Holistic Strategies for Treating Chapped Lips
216 Healing Lip Balm

217 Nausea and Vomiting
216 Mineralizing Tea for Replenishing after Vomiting
217 Herbal Formula for Nausea and Vomiting
218 Peppermint-Fennel Essential Oil Emulsion

218 Nephritis and Kidney Damage
219 Herbs for Improved Kidney Function

222 Neuropathy
222 Herbs for Neuropathy
224 Herbal Lotion for Neuropathic Pain
224 Magnesium Lotion
225 Supplements for Neuropathic Pain

226 Special Considerations for Immunotherapies
228 Managing Monoclonal Antibody Therapy and Immunotherapies
229 Diaphoretic Tea

230 Managing Radiation
231 Scans and X-rays
231 Radiotherapy
232 Radio Sensitizing and Radio Protection
234 Consequences of Radiation
234 Topical Herbs for Radiation Burns
235 Herbal Cream for Radiation Burn

Understanding Conventional Cancer Treatment

In choosing the best path through cancer therapies it is helpful to have guidelines for the types of options that may be presented and the decisions that may need to be made. Knowing what may be ahead or what other options could be explored is empowering and useful. The journey begins with a diagnosis (usually through biopsy) followed by commencement of treatment. Treatment may be more or less aggressive according to the type, stage, and grade of the cancer and your overall health status.

Local treatment. Conservative and constrained, this targets the tumor itself and adjacent tissues. This type of treatment is offered only if there is no evidence of distant spread, and it is usually well tolerated and has a reasonable chance of success. Examples of local treatment include surgery, cryotherapy (use of extreme cold), and sometimes targeted radiation therapy.

Systemic treatment. This will affect cells throughout the body and is offered when cancer has already spread or is imminently likely to spread from the primary tissue to metastatic sites. There is a higher risk of side effects from systemic treatment, and overall outcomes are highly variable among cancers and among different population groups. Examples of systemic treatment include chemotherapy, hormonal therapy, immunotherapy, and targeted therapy.

Conventional Cancer Therapies

Neoadjuvant therapy. This refers to the first steps taken to shrink a tumor before surgery to remove it and may include chemotherapy, radiation therapy, or hormone therapy.

Surgery. This is still the first line of defense against cancer that is localized and has not spread. Improved techniques of laparoscopy (minimally invasive surgery) have reduced some of the more extensive open abdominal surgeries, which has led to better outcomes. Sentinel node assessment has replaced the extensive lymph bed dissections that used to be done, with consequent lessening of the incidence of lymphedema (buildup of lymph fluids) in patients today.

Adjuvant therapies. These are additional treatments given after surgery to ensure all malignant cells were removed. They may include chemotherapy, biological drugs (immunotherapies) for systemic effects, or radiation for a local effect.

Palliative therapies. These are used to manage symptoms and are intended to give higher quality of life without necessarily addressing the cancer itself. Palliative therapies may focus on relief of pain, improved appetite, and better sleep.

Supportive therapies. These may be used to relieve or suppress severe side effects from chemotherapy and radiotherapy. They can include treatments such as the prescription of laxatives to avoid constipation from opioids or healing creams to alleviate radiation burns.

Systemic Drug Therapies

Cytotoxic agents. Conventional chemotherapy involves cytotoxic agents (those that are toxic to cells) that mostly target DNA as it unwinds and copies. It is not very specific and carries a high risk of long-term side effects. Effects can be partially predicted through some tissue tests and through sensitivity and resistance testing.

Targeted therapies. These are the biologicals, immunotherapies, or monoclonal antibodies that target specific receptor sites or other tumor-causing molecules on or in the cell and stimulate immune responses. They carry a high risk of short-term side effects and are effective only if the correct drug is given for a specific mutation, which requires careful tissue testing.

Endocrine/hormonal. These types of treatment address estrogen, androgen, and insulin balance. There may be significant risks (for example, tamoxifen for breast cancer may cause endometrial cancer and blood clots) and they are not always very specific (e.g., aromatase inhibitors for breast cancer may also down-regulate, or suppress, cytochrome detox enzyme pathways in the liver).

> The biggest thing I suggest for chemo is doing some form of trauma therapy; get help with mindfulness and letting go. Also develop a solid daily health routine before the treatment starts.
>
> 9+-YEAR CANCER SURVIVOR

Considering Chemotherapy

Chemotherapy is the major treatment strategy for almost all cancers, with just a few treated effectively by surgery alone when caught early, such as cervical dysplasia or squamous cell carcinoma on the skin, and with radiotherapy used largely as a palliative measure or for some extra layer of protection against later recurrence in a primary site.

For anyone undergoing chemotherapy, it is critically important to consider how to get the best results and manage side effects. Timing or frequency as well as dose of drugs can make all the difference to tolerance and effectiveness. Metronomic (timing) and chronotherapy (frequency) dose schedules are worth considering, in collaboration with the oncologist. Fasting before chemotherapy, taking redox regulators (antioxidants) with chemotherapy, using herbs to support the liver, and so on can offer substantive help; patients are encouraged to gather information about these choices and discuss them with their practitioners before making decisions.

Side effects of associated drugs (opioids, steroids, antibiotics) that are routinely prescribed during chemotherapy can be quite significant, including opioid tolerance, immunosuppression, constipation, diarrhea, and dysbiosis (imbalanced gut microbiome). Any herbal or nutritional program that you are reasonably able to implement might help reduce the need for some of these other pharmaceuticals and lessen the risk of side effects, and that is quite aside from addressing the cancer itself with herbs.

There is also the added complication of using cytotoxic drugs in combination to greater effect. This is routinely done by oncologists today, but there is often very poor evidence or data to support any particular choice. Perhaps a study showed that combination A provided 1 or 2 months of increased longevity compared to combination B in mice, or in human cell lines, or even in a human trial, but that does not prove that combination A is actually the best one for you. This is where sensitivity and resistance tissue testing becomes important (see page 357); it helps the decision-making process by providing evidence that a specific drug cocktail is active against your cells.

Side Effects of Chemotherapy

Before pursuing chemotherapy, it's important to understand some of the potential side effects. No one sails through chemotherapy without some disruption to their daily routine or well-being. The toxic nature of chemotherapy is a dose-limiting factor in how much chemotherapy a patient can actually tolerate. Chemotherapy patients may even be told that their bodily wastes are a hazardous material and they should burn bedding, towels, and cloths used in their personal care. It is not unusual to delay the last treatments in a series in order to allow the patient some recovery and some repair of their immune system in between.

ACUTE TOXICITY

Fatigue and malaise, nausea and vomiting, oral mucositis (inflammation in the mouth), hair loss, and myelosuppression (bone marrow suppression) are the most common symptoms, indicative of profound cellular toxicity from conventional chemotherapy drugs. Some symptoms may be more prevalent than others, usually commencing within 1–2 days of receiving the drugs, and they may be cumulative, with reactions to treatments getting progressively worse with each treatment cycle. Certain drugs may cause specific side effects, such as hepatotoxicity (liver poisoning) from methotrexate, chronic cystitis from cyclophosphamide, or renal and neurotoxicity (kidney and nerve poisoning) from platinum drugs.

CHRONIC TOXICITY

Long after the drug treatments have finished, their toxic consequences may linger, including nerve pain from platinum drugs, taxanes, and vinca alkaloids up to 2 years later; cardiac damage from the anthracyclines 5 years or more later; lung compromise and leukemias from cyclophosphamide 8 or even 10 years later; and functional sterility from many of these drugs. In cancer care, the indiscriminate use of toxic drugs often becomes a part of the problem. This is particularly unfortunate when we know that chemotherapy, including the classical or conventional drugs, can work well if it is applied with care and consideration for the individual patient and their capacity to resist or succumb to specific drugs (as determined by resistance and sensitivity testing).

In a study assessing patient satisfaction with drug therapies, most drugs were around 50–75% effective as determined by patient responses. The lowest success as rated by patients was seen with conventional cancer chemotherapy (25%), and the best results were with COX-2-inhibitors given for arthritis inflammation (80%). That means only one-quarter of recipients were satisfied with their chemotherapy, and a shocking 75% of patients were unable to complete the course due to side effects, were left with significant long-term consequences, or ended up having recurrences that indicate drug failure. Those patients were left at higher risk of health breakdown as a consequence of treatment, and the medical and social costs are staggering.

Tolerating Chemotherapy Better

Most conventional chemotherapy drugs, by their very nature, are more effective in the cells that are actively reproducing. Most of the older drugs, those discovered and developed before around the year 2000, target cells while DNA is unwinding or copying, which is indicated by elevated S (synthesis) phase and elevated Ki67 in the mitotic index of the pathology report. This is why the drugs also affect skin, hair, and gut-lining cells that reproduce quickly as well. Examples of the drugs that specifically target DNA unwinding and copying include platinum drugs (cisplatin, oxaliplatin, and carboplatin), alkylating agents (melphalan, bendamustine, doxorubicin, epirubicin, and idarubicin), cyclophosphamide, chlorambucil, etoposide, 5-fluorouracil, gemcitabine, methotrexate, and temozolomide. Assessing cells for Ki67 and for the percent of cells in active synthesis phase is a quick assessment of likely benefit from some chemotherapy drugs. The higher the levels, the better chance chemotherapy has of working.

"STARVING" THE CANCER BEFORE CHEMOTHERAPY

Healthy body cells are naturally evolved to manage the feast-or-famine phenomenon familiar to our ancestors. Healthy cells can slow down their metabolic activities in the absence of freely available sugars or can quite readily use fats and proteins to turn the Krebs cycle and make energy. Cancer cells, in contrast, use a lot of glucose to make energy, struggle to use fats and proteins efficiently, and are quite compromised by lack of sugar. Unfortunately, though, you can't *literally* starve cancer cells, because the liver will release glycogen to keep up blood-sugar levels for as long as possible. And, like all cells, cancer cells can make energy from alternate sources if glucose is restricted.

However, fasting followed by a dose of sugar can make chemotherapy drugs more effective. Fasting for 24–48 hours prior to receiving chemotherapy, taking only water or an electrolyte drink without sugar, causes the healthy cells to slow down their metabolism and hence their energy demand, while cancer cells become metabolically stressed due to lack of sugar. About 30 minutes before receiving chemotherapy, take a small dose of easily digested sugar—eat a ripe banana or drink 6 ounces of fresh orange juice. This small sugar load will be readily taken up by cancer cells and can facilitate uptake of the chemotherapy drug with it. This delivers the drug to the target cells more effectively and reduces collateral damage in other tissues. In many hospitals, before chemotherapy, patients get an infusion of glucose, in which case the other sweet treat before chemotherapy is not needed. Ask your oncologist about this in advance. Some research hospitals are investigating a process called insulin potentiation therapy, in which a sugar dose is given with an insulin dose, which allows for even quicker uptake and for reduced doses of chemotherapy to gain clinical effects.

Patients who underwent chemotherapy with fasting in a clinical trial reported a reduction in fatigue, weakness, and gastrointestinal side effects. Fasting did not prevent the chemotherapy from reducing tumor volume or tumor markers, and the researchers suggested that fasting in combination with chemotherapy is feasible and safe and has the potential to reduce side effects caused by chemotherapies. They were careful to add that more studies are needed, but there is nothing to stop patients from following this suggestion for themselves. In my own practice I can confirm that fasting before chemotherapy has generally reduced the severity of side effects and allowed better chemotherapy adherence.

If actual fasting is too hard, then the following can be consumed.

- Steamed greens with lemon juice
- Green juices or raw green vegetables
- Broth (strained to remove meat and vegetables)

INTRAVENOUS VITAMIN C

This adjunctive treatment is popular with naturopaths and functional medicine doctors. Flooding the body with high doses of vitamin C and naturally associated bioflavonoids 2–4 hours prior to receiving chemotherapy is useful to offer maximum protection to healthy cells. In my clinical practice I may refer a patient to another practitioner to receive these injections because I am not licensed for giving them.

If intravenous vitamin C is not available, it can be taken orally as a supplement, at 1–5 grams daily. It tends to become a laxative in higher quantities, so this limits the daily dose.

A History of Modern Chemotherapy

Chemotherapy today is in a state of flux and transition. For the first half of the twentieth century, cancer care was focused on improving diagnostic and surgical practices and some very primitive radiotherapy that was so spectacularly ineffective and dangerous it is a wonder they continued trying to make it work at all. In the second half of the century, the science of chemical pharmacology progressed rapidly, and drug therapies became a major medical focus for cancer research.

Twentieth-Century Treatments

In the 1940s research was focused on derivatives of mustard gas first used in World War I, known to inhibit bone marrow activity, and this led to the discovery of the first true chemotherapy drugs, the alkylating agents. These drugs work by causing DNA damage sufficient to prevent the cell from replicating. They are effective in all stages of the cell cycle, not just during the active replication phase as many other chemotherapy drugs are. This action may make them more potent drugs for cancer treatment, but it also leads to widespread and profound cell damage in the rest of the body. They are widely used, including for lung, breast, and ovarian cancer, as well as leukemia, lymphoma, multiple myeloma, and sarcoma. The biggest risk from their use is seen up to 10 years later, when they can cause leukemia.

Not long after the discovery of the anthracyclines came folic acid antagonist drugs (such as methotrexate, aminopterin, pyrimethamine, trimethoprim, and triamterene). These can inhibit cell replication but are toxic for the liver. Huge research efforts in the 1950s and 1960s yielded other drugs, such as the plant-derived compounds taxol, podophyllotoxin, camptothecin, and vinca alkaloids, as well as platinum-based drugs.

In the mid-1960s a combination of these drugs was given for the first time, each drug with a different action, to reduce the opportunities for cancer to develop resistance. Using methotrexate (an antifolate), vincristine (an alkaloid from the Madagascar periwinkle plant), 6-mercaptopurine (an antimetabolite that prevents DNA synthesis by inhibiting the production of the purine-containing nucleotides, adenine and guanine), and prednisone (an anti-inflammatory), researchers were able to induce long-term remissions in children with acute lymphoblastic leukemia. This diagnosis had been rapidly fatal until this drug cocktail was developed, and ever since then it has been a survivable diagnosis. There were, and are, considerable adverse effects for children taking these drugs—the drugs can stop other organs growing and maturing as they should, and puberty and maturation can be delayed and disrupted, but the implications of these adverse effects are rarely noted in the celebration of increased longevity. This is a trade-off that cancer patients have been making for decades: a possibility of immediate survival against the risk of catastrophic toxicity or possible long-term health deterioration.

Although calculating the odds is basically impossible—there are so many variables and unknowns in each case—oncologists have to attempt this calculation in order to give their best advice for treatment options. One of the key goals of the holistic treatment approach is to improve the risk-to-benefit calculation for each person by strengthening and reinforcing the terrain in which the cancer is trying to get a foothold, and by increasing the resilience of the body to withstand conventional treatments that may also be required.

Twenty-First-Century Advancements

In the twenty-first century, since the breaking of the genome in 1995, it has become possible to measure molecular signaling networks for proliferation and survival in specific cancer cells. This detailed information has allowed for new targeted therapies that inhibit specific metabolic pathways that underlie each specific type of cancer's behaviors. These are the so-called immunotherapies, and they have been a game changer in many types of cancer.

Some of these drugs are well established now—Herceptin (trastuzumab) for breast cancer (targets the HER2/neu receptor), Gleevec (imatinib) for chronic myelogenous leukemia (targets specific tyrosine kinase proteins that control cell growth and inhibition of apoptosis in cancer cells), and Rituxan (rituximab) for lymphoma (targets CD20 antigen expressed on the surface of B lymphocytes). These were all pioneers in the field, but the past 10 years have seen a multitude of new drugs come to market, all aimed at specific receptor proteins.

Cancer cells are capable of immune evasion, avoiding detection and resisting immune destruction. Monoclonal antibodies (immunotherapies) are engineered to bind to specific antigen proteins that are overexpressed on a cancer cell surface and mark it as "flawed," which then induces and allows cell destruction by the immune system. This is in direct contrast to the old-style chemotherapy that is really just educated guesswork for the right cocktail and the right dosage schedule.

Monoclonal antibody (mAb) drugs may also work as antagonists to receptor sites for various growth factors cancer uses to promote replication, as antiangiogenics to reduce new blood vessel growth to cancer, as immune checkpoint antagonists to prevent the cancer from turning down the immune system, and even as specific inducers of apoptosis (cell death) in cancer cells.

Some targeted therapies can carry toxins to the cancer cells to kill them, while protecting and preserving normal cells. These are the so-called conjugated mAbs, which comprise a mAb plus chemotherapy or a radioactive particle, used as a kind of homing device to deliver treatment directly to the cancer cells. The mAb hooks onto the target antigen (cell-surface protein) and delivers the toxic substance where it is needed most and with less collateral damage to other cells. Conjugated mAbs are also sometimes referred to as "tagged," "labeled," or "loaded" antibodies.

Dosing Models for Chemotherapy

Patients would like to believe that there is some precise mathematical formula that determines the dose and frequency of their drug cocktail. Unfortunately, it is not that simple, and different oncologists in different hospitals might in fact give quite different drugs or different drug schedules for ostensibly the same cancer. While this may be disconcerting in some ways, it is also reassuring: If you want to get a second opinion or seek further advice, there indeed may be good reason to seek out different opinions within the medical profession. This is quite important to understand. As a patient you may find that any questioning of a medical treatment plan and the perceived wisdom of an oncologist may be treated as heretical and challenged vehemently by that oncologist, such that you may need to be strong to hold your ground in choosing how to navigate your cancer journey. It is helpful in this case to know that the doctors and scientists don't always agree, and you may find other treatment options that suit you better.

Maximum Tolerated Dose

Current dosing models for conventional chemotherapy recommend calculating metabolic capacities to assess the maximum tolerated dose (MTD), then giving that amount in specified frequencies based on clearance rates (half-life) and side effects. Following this model will destroy a lot of vulnerable cancer cells fast. The problem is that not all cells will die with each dose, and those that don't die may grow back stronger. The drugs are so toxic that they usually cannot be taken frequently or continuously. While you take a break, the stronger cancer cells may be regrouping and reproducing. Although there may be short-term responsiveness from the MTD, there are also often severe, even life-threatening side effects, and there is high likelihood of recurrent growth.

Metronomic Dosing

There is a growing trend toward using what is called pulsed or metronomic dosing, rather than MTD. In this system, one-tenth to one-third of the MTD of a chemotherapy agent is given, which is often much better tolerated than the full MTD. This method also allows for more frequent dosing, thus reducing the time between treatments and the chance for cells to grown back. Cell cycle–specific agents (those that target the S or M phase of cell reproduction) are especially active when given frequently or continuously in this way. At this lower dose, the drugs primarily act on the tumor microenvironment, including the tumor endothelial cells and immune cells, rather than being catastrophically and systemically toxic. Metronomic chemotherapy has demonstrated some advantages over MTD—in particular, lower complication rates and lower hospital care requirements—but more and larger clinical trials are necessary to determine if it is truly more effective.

Chronotherapy

Multiple aspects of the immune system are under circadian control, ebbing and flowing over 24 hours. Each organ may be more or less metabolically active (for example, the brain and heart are more active during the day, and the gut is more active at night) and specific control hormones should switch on and off accordingly. The immune system is similarly influenced by diurnal (day/night) signals, and interferon gamma, natural killer cells, and regulatory T cells are all disrupted by lack of sleep.

Chronotherapy refers to a way of scheduling chemotherapy doses so that they are synchronous with the patient's biorhythms (sleep–wake cycles and consequent diurnal organ activities). It has demonstrated its effectiveness in several randomized multicenter trials. Both the toxicity and effectiveness of more than 30 anticancer agents may vary by more than 50 percent depending on what time of day the dose is given.

For example, chronotherapy schedules have been applied in studies of oxaliplatin, 5-FU, and leucovorin against metastatic colorectal cancer and have achieved unprecedented long-term survival rates. Clinical trials showed a fivefold improvement in patient tolerability and near doubling of antitumor activity through the chrono-modulated delivery of oxaliplatin, 5-FU, and leucovorin combinations.

In animal studies researchers found that epidermal growth factor receptor (EGFr) signals were suppressed by high glucocorticoids when the animals were active (sympathetic dominance), and that EGFr signals were enhanced during the resting phase (parasympathetic dominance). Thus, they suggested giving targeted EGFr drugs during the resting phase of normal circadian rhythms for quicker access and uptake by receptors and more targeted effects.

Neither metronomic dosing nor chronotherapy is yet routinely or readily obtained outside of large research hospitals. However, I predict that in the next few years these will both become more mainstream and standard of care. Just as it used to be a battle to get HER2/neu testing and Herceptin (trastuzumab) prescribed for patients 20 years ago and now it is routine and expected, so currently novel ways of administering drugs will come to be normal too.

Hypothermic Isolated Limb Perfusion

This is an innovative way of delivering a very high dose of chemotherapy without systemic toxicity. It is currently used only to treat localized melanoma of the arm or leg but may be considered in the future for other cancers that are isolated to a single limb. The technique involves isolating the main artery and vein serving the limb, then redirecting the blood flow from the limb into a bypass machine, similar to the ones used in open heart surgery. This allows delivery of a high doses of chemotherapy that is not recirculated to the heart and the rest of the body but goes back to the machine for reoxygenation and recirculation to the isolated limb. The dose that can be delivered may be up to 10 times higher than what could be tolerated if given systemically to the whole body. Hypothermic isolated limb perfusion works only with drugs that do not need to pass through the liver to be activated, and when delivery is complete and the blood supply of the leg or arm is reattached to the systemic circulation, the drug-infused blood is held back from the body, leaving the patient with a blood deficiency state that may be quite debilitating. However, blood can be rebuilt and restored, and the overall tolerance of treatment is generally very good.

Nanoparticle Drug Delivery

Another innovative means of targeting chemotherapy to cancer cells and reducing collateral damage of healthy cells is seen with nanotechnology. In recent research from Washington State University, tiny proteins called nanotubes, 100,000 times thinner than a human hair, were successfully used as ferries to transport doxorubicin directly into rapidly dividing lung cancer cells. This was further augmented by using the nanotubes to also deliver a photodynamic agent that, when exposed to light, releases reactive oxygen species (ROS) to induce cell death and kill cancer cells. This dual-drug approach allowed for the use of a lower dose of chemotherapy and effective killing of cancer cells with low systemic toxicity.

Nanoparticle drug delivery is still in a research stage and has not yet proven its safety or effectiveness in general practice. Possible limitations include poor bioavailability, instability in the circulation, poor biodegradation, inadequate tissue distribution, and potential toxicity in the liver or kidneys, especially for long-term administration.

Liposomal Drug Delivery

Liposomes are tiny spheres of fat sandwiched between protein layers (a lipid bilayer), and they can carry hydrophilic (water-soluble) drugs in their inner aqueous core and lipophilic (fat-soluble) drugs within the bilayer. Liposomes are the first nanoparticle drug delivery systems successfully applied in clinical applications. Many chemotherapy drugs today are wrapped up this way; it allows better delivery into cells, and perhaps most importantly, the drugs can cross the blood-brain barrier and allow delivery of chemotherapy to brain lesions, which are otherwise hard to access.

Hyperthermic Intraperitoneal Chemotherapy

Ovarian cancer is the eighth most common cause of death for women worldwide and rising, despite aggressive interventions. Research into using heated chemotherapy (cisplatin or carboplatin) to treat ovarian cancer is currently underway at the Mayo Clinic. The heated chemotherapy agents are pumped directly into the peritoneal cavity, immediately after laparoscopic surgery is performed to remove all visible lesions, while the patient is still on the operating table and under anesthesia. This chemotherapy delivery method is poorly tolerated by many patients, and a course of treatment is not always completed because of this, but some patients have shown good results from this procedure.

All of these novel ways of delivering chemotherapy are promising, but few are well developed yet or in wide clinical application, and it is likely that drug treatments for cancer will continue to be refined and improved over time. However, it is still the case today that most cancer patients receive conventional chemotherapy, without specific targeting, delivered intravenously to the maximum tolerated dose, and these patients suffer all the consequences we have come to expect of modern medicalized cancer treatment.

Other Innovative Anticancer Treatments

It can take years if not decades for a new treatment strategy to become widely accepted and used. Sometimes an entirely new treatment approach is developed (for example, photodynamic therapy, discussed on page 157), but sometimes existing drugs are repurposed for specific anticancer actions. In clinical practice, doctors have realized that several pharmaceuticals have wider applications and uses than are generally indicated or licensed, and this situation has led to substantial off-label prescribing for managing aspects of cancer care. Some of these off-label uses are now well researched and well established; others are perhaps less so. The table on pages 158–59 outlines some of the better-known pharmaceutical options that are currently used by functional medicine doctors. They may not be sufficiently powerful to actually replace chemotherapy, but they will be better tolerated for people who are unable to complete conventional treatment protocols, and they may have particular value in the 12–24 months after completing chemotherapy. On page 476, you will find the case history of a patient of mine who had lung cancer and has been on low-dose naltrexone for about 3 years now without recurrence.

These are prescription drugs, so cancer patients will need to discuss these possibilities with their physicians. They are not suitable for everybody but are promising nonetheless. Some of them may have an effect on conventional chemotherapy. For example, metformin tends to lower Ki67 levels in cancer cells, indicating a slowing of cell cycling, and this may lessen the effects of chemotherapy drugs targeting cell replication (such as alkylating agents like busulfan, chlorambucil, cyclophosphamide, and thiotepa) or antimetabolites such as methotrexate. In these cases, using metformin after conventional chemotherapy instead of with it is advised.

Photodynamic Therapy

This is a novel treatment using photosensitive molecules, such as hypericin, delivered into a tumor and then activated using a directed laser beam. Photodynamic therapy (PDT) is usually an outpatient procedure (no overnight stay in hospital) and may be combined with surgery, chemotherapy, or other anticancer drugs.

PDT is very well tolerated with minimal residual effects after completion of treatment. It is not invasive and can be targeted very precisely. However, it is only suitable for smaller cancers without metastases, and the skin over the area can be very sensitive to light for some time afterward. Cancers for which it has been successfully employed include skin cancers of various types and grades, as well as bladder, esophageal, and brain cancers.

Hyperthermia

Hyperthermia uses various forms of heat to treat cancer, either through local or regional application or by heating the whole body. This method has been approved by the US Food and Drug Administration (FDA) for progressive or recurrent solid tumors, when given with radiation therapy. High heat is expected to induce immune responses, including interferon release, and to activate control systems in the body. It requires specialized training and education as well as specialized equipment and is not yet widely available.

OFF-LABEL USES FOR PHARMACEUTICALS IN CANCER CARE

Drug	Approved Conventional Uses
Antabuse (disulfiram)	Alcohol addiction 40+-year history of safe use as an aversion therapy to reduce alcohol craving. Inhibits the enzyme acetaldehyde dehydrogenase that detoxifies alcohol. The drug induces acute sensitivity to alcohol and rapid onset of hangover symptoms.
Celebrex (celecoxib)	Arthritis, autoimmune inflammation
Low molecular weight heparin	Blood clots
Glucophage (metformin)	Diabetes, hyperglycemia
Low-dose naltrexone (4.5 mg)	Opioid and alcohol addiction, at doses > 50 mg Blocks opioid receptors for up to 4 hours; avoid using with opioid agonists (such as narcotic pain medications). Use caution for people taking thyroid hormone, as this drug can suppress autoimmune thyroiditis and reactivate the gland (useful in Hashimoto's thyroiditis and low thyroid function).
Rapamycin (sirolimus)—a soil-derived antibiotic	Autoimmune inflammation
Tagamet (cimetidine)—note that other H2 blockers are not as effective	Antacid; used for acid reflux, gastritis
Tetrathiomolybdate (high-potency molybdenum)	Wilson's disease (copper accumulation)
Valproic acid	Anticonvulsant used for epilepsy and other seizure disorders

Anticancer Actions	Anticancer Mechanisms
Antiangiogenic (inhibits new blood vessel growth) Antitumor, antimetastatic	Copper chelation Is chemosensitizing and overcomes multidrug resistance partly by shutting down the glycoprotein dump. Inhibits NF-κB—downregulates inflammatory chemicals that drive cancer.
Anti-inflammatory	COX-2 inhibition
Antiangiogenic (inhibits new blood vessel growth)	Inhibits blood clots, resists tumor growth and metastases.
Inhibits hepatic (liver) gluconeogenesis and improves peripheral metabolism of glucose. Lowers blood sugar and fasting insulin.	Reduces plasma levels of insulin-like growth factor 1 and leptin, downregulates inflammatory pathways, and makes adiponectin more effective. Inhibits glycolytic shift. Inhibits mTOR activity by stimulating adenosine monophosphate-activated kinase (AMPK), which ultimately inhibits protein synthesis and cell growth. Activates p53; this inhibits the cell cycle. Reduces incidence and mortality from many cancers. Increases cellular response to radiotherapy and chemotherapy. Reduces incidence of relapse.
Immunomodulator, antidepressant, mood elevating	Opioid receptor antagonist. Taken at night to increase endorphin production, induces and activates stem cells and immune cells. Inhibits cancer growth or spread. Improves long-term survival.
Immunomodulator	Inhibits mTOR receptors—controls cell growth, spread, and survival. Downregulates signal transduction and inhibits oncogenes.
May provide survival benefits in surgery. May synergize with chemotherapy. Inhibits multiple CYP450 pathways; delays metabolism of a wide range of drugs; allows lower doses. Strongest research so far is for colon cancer.	Regulates cell adhesion molecules and cell-to-cell communication. Increases tumor infiltrating lymphocytes—increased immunosurveillance. Increases production of antitumor signaling proteins (cytokines). Cancer cells initiate metastasis by binding to receptor sites in blood vessels using sugars called Lewis antigens. The receptor sites can be inhibited by cimetidine. Lewis antigens can be tested in blood to assess likely benefit from cimetidine treatment.
Antiangiogenic (inhibits new blood vessel growth)	Copper chelation Most effective when there is active tumor growth.
Histone deacetylase inhibition	Upregulation of hundreds of genes controlling multiple control pathways, including ATP generation, MAPK signaling, cell cycling, cell death, growth factor signaling, and others.

Managing Side Effects of Chemotherapy and Radiation

Once the decision is made to take chemotherapy drugs or to undergo radiotherapy, it is important to support the body to help it tolerate the treatments as well as possible and to mitigate damage. Side effects of treatment can be quite severe and even dose limiting; in some chemotherapy regimens, as many as 20–30 percent of patients cannot complete the course of treatment. Different drugs may cause different sets of symptoms, and each patient is unique with their specific cancer diagnosis, as well as with other comorbidities and drug tolerances or intolerances. Navigating the best path through this process includes managing the symptoms and making conventional treatment more tolerable, as well as addressing the cancer itself.

The formulas and recipes below are drawn from more than 35 years of clinical prescribing, the last 20 years with a focus on cancer. They are what I have found effective in my clinical practice, with cancer patients and others, and they use ingredients with strong research and good reason for the purpose. Sometimes I may list an herb or ingredient that is difficult to come by but could possibly be exchanged for another herb with equivalent actions (such as licorice if you can't get ashwagandha, or chamomile if you can't get passionflower). These alternatives are intended to give you ideas and the basic proportions so that you can make something customized for your situation.

> The patient . . . sometimes gets well in spite of the medicine.
>
> THOMAS EDISON

Establishing a Healthy Daily Routine

Everything about being diagnosed with cancer and navigating treatment, no matter which choices you make, will take you out of your daily routines and past experience and into previously uncharted territory. It may seem like an insurmountable task to even get out of bed sometimes, never mind making green smoothies, taking supplements, doing yoga, or going for a walk in the woods. It is important to work out what is realistic and practical and essential, to learn to pace yourself, to ask for help, to be okay with saying no, and to make looking after yourself your daily priority. There will be better days and worse days, times when you are able to do more than others. Do not beat yourself up about any of this, but celebrate what you are able to do, and know that every little step is helpful and that it's never too late to start.

Example of a Daily Self-Care Routine during Chemotherapy

This routine was created by E. B., a patient with ovarian cancer.

- Dry skin brushing to promote lymph flow
- Juice of ½ lemon or 1 tablespoon raw apple cider vinegar in a cup of hot water, sweetened with honey to taste (a traditional folk remedy to promote detoxification)
- Stretching or yoga, qi gong, or tai chi, as able
- Coffee/herb enema if needed
- Fresh green juice
- Rest/meditation
- Bitter herbs to promote appetite
- Food (easy to digest, light, and nourishing): eggs, oatmeal, avocado, poached fish, steamed greens
- Herb teas
- Rest/meditation
- Bone broth
- Rest/meditation
- Walk
- Smoothie: frozen or fresh berries and plain goat or sheep yogurt, plus tahini or nut butter for protein and fat if needed
- Rest/meditation
- Food: fish, casserole, or stew; slow-cooked or poached vegetables
- Movie/reading
- Bed: Don't stress if you are not sleeping. Go with it. Make your bed your comfy zone. Don't put the light back on after you go to bed. Plan things you can listen to in the night if you're not sleeping. Have sedative herbal drinks ready by your bed.

Adaptogens for Stress

Adaptogenic herbs support adrenal functions and build resilience and resistance in the immune system. They also support energy systems and anabolic (constructive) pathways and are considered tonics and restoratives.

Adaptogens are absolutely fundamental to treating cancer. They are the foundation and the backbone of all long-term treatment planning, although they are not in and of themselves necessarily directly anticancer. They are especially indicated during and after chemotherapy or radiotherapy because they can support resistance and resilience in the immune system, build endurance and stamina, and build blood and bone. There is almost never a time when adaptogens would not or could not be used, although the individual herbs may rotate in and out of formulas over time to suit the changing needs of the patient.

For brain fog, choose adaptogens that are slightly stimulating (Korean ginseng, rhodiola) in a daytime formula, and consider switching to other adaptogenic herbs in the evening (ashwagandha, for example, will support sleep). Lion's mane mushroom is a strongly restorative adaptogen for the brain. Numerous studies have shown it to be a powerful brain tonic with rejuvenating properties that improve memory, cognitive functions, and mood. For more information on adaptogens, see page 66.

Brain Fog and Chemotherapy Haze

One of the most distressing aspects of undergoing chemotherapy is the impact on clear thinking and memory. The drugs used are often neurotoxins (nerve poisons) in and of themselves, and most of them are also hard on the liver, which has to remove them from the body. This impact may be aggravated by other commonly used drugs, such as hormones or opioids that may be used concurrently. Just when you need your faculties and wits about you to make life-and-death decisions about treatments, your brain is full of cotton wool and your memory is shot. While much of this brain fog may diminish once chemotherapy is over, it is not unusual to still be struggling with these issues a year or more posttreatment. Cognitive deficit after surgery may be a contributing factor, as may fatigue, stress and distress, increasing age, infections, nutritional deficiencies, and alcohol or marijuana use.

These mental changes can make it hard to carry out your normal daily routine including school, work, and social activities, which might require an exhausting amount of mental effort. People often don't tell their care providers about this problem, as it is not something life threatening. As a result, the impact is often downplayed until it is adversely affecting the patient's everyday life.

American Cancer Society Recommendations to Manage "Chemo Brain"

- Use a detailed daily planner, notebooks, reminder notes, or your smartphone. Keeping everything in one place makes it easier to find the reminders you may need. You might want to keep track of appointments and schedules, to-do lists, important dates, websites, phone numbers and addresses, meeting notes, and even movies you'd like to see or books you'd like to read.
- Do the most demanding tasks at the time of the day when you feel your energy levels are the highest (midmorning for most people). Exercise your brain. Take a class, do word puzzles, or learn a musical instrument or a new language.
- Get enough rest and sleep.
- Keep moving. Regular physical activity is not only good for your body, it improves your mood, makes you feel more alert, and decreases tiredness (fatigue).
- Eat veggies. Studies have shown that eating more vegetables is linked to keeping brainpower as people age.
- Set up and follow routines. Try to keep the same daily schedule.
- Pick a certain place for commonly lost objects (like keys) and put them there each time.
- Try not to multitask. Focus on one thing at a time.
- Avoid alcohol and other agents that might change your mental state and sleeping patterns.
- Ask for help when you need it. Friends and loved ones can help with daily tasks to cut down on distractions and help you save mental energy.

Brain fog usually diminishes over time, but it can take weeks or months to feel anything like normal again. To encourage brain recovery and promote clear thinking, numerous supplements available from the health food store or from your natural medicine practitioner can be helpful. These are often the same supplements that might be used in supporting patients with Alzheimer's or dementia or even for students looking to enhance their mental sharpness before exams. More detail on these strategies is given in the section on post-operative cognitive impairment (see page 102).

Natural Agents for Daily Use to Support Cognitive Functions

- Essential fatty acids (omega-3 fats from fish oil), 1,200–1,500 mg—myelin support, mood elevation
- B vitamin complex, 100 mg—cofactors in parasympathetic system
- Acetyl-L-carnitine, 1,000 mg—cell energy/fuel for nervous system
- Glycerophosphocholine (from soy lecithin), 2,000 mg—myelin support
- Phosphatidylserine (from sunflower lecithin), 200 mg—neurotransmitter support
- Ginkgo, gotu kola, lesser periwinkle, rosemary, tulsi—brain tonics, stimulants

Cerebral Circulatory Stimulants

These herbs are known to cause opening of blood vessels and promote increased circulation to the head and brain, enhancing oxygenation and delivery of nutrients for optimal brain function. By default, this enhances venous return—that is, drainage and removal of metabolic wastes from brain tissue. Some of these herbs are extremely well researched. For more information, see page 106.

Wide Awake Tea

This tea blend has a bright, fresh flavor, a hint of caffeine from the green tea or the yerba mate, and a general uplifting effect. If you don't want any caffeine, you can leave out the tea or mate or replace it with something like rooibos.

+ 30 g green tea or yerba mate
+ 20 g tulsi
+ 10 g hibiscus flower
+ 10 g lemongrass
+ 10 g peppermint
+ 10 g rosemary
+ 10 g ginger

Mix all herbs. Use 1 heaping teaspoon of the blend per cup of boiling water and sweeten to taste with honey or stevia. Drink this in the morning or whenever you need a mental boost.

Managing Constipation

Constipation is a condition in which bowel movements occur infrequently, or in which the stool is hard and small, or in which the passage of feces causes difficulty or pain. Ideally, the number of bowel movements in a day should be more or less equal to the number of meals eaten the previous day. Young children and animals evacuate little and often, but that is not convenient or culturally acceptable in many places. So as adults, we train our bowels to need to go only once, usually in the morning. Although medical textbooks may suggest that it is normal to go only every 2–3 days, this is not natural and can be corrected with herbs and diet. Ideally, there should be at least one good elimination each day. The stool should be more or less the size of a banana, soft, but formed and not loose or runny, and should break apart a little in the toilet bowl. The color will vary somewhat according to the diet but generally should be a uniform medium brown.

While occasional constipation (a missed day or two) will not be seriously detrimental to health, chronic constipation can have significant implications in the body. The bowels are a major channel of elimination, and if they are not working sufficiently then the other channels (kidney, skin, and lungs) will have a greater workload. Many metabolites cannot be eliminated easily by other channels, so if the bowels are incompetent, then toxins rapidly accumulate in the body. This may manifest as bad breath, body odor, skin eruptions, visual impairment, headaches, muscle and joint pains, and mental confusion.

Causes of Constipation

There are many possible causes and aggravating factors in constipation in cancer patients. These include the following.

- Dietary factors such as low fiber from excess consumption of refined foods or inadequate fluid intake
- Physical inactivity such as prolonged bed rest or general lack of exercise
- Various drugs such as anesthetics, antacids, anticholinergics, anticonvulsants, antihypertensives, antipsychotics, beta-blockers, diuretics, iron, bismuth, muscle relaxants, and opiates
- Psychogenic factors such as stress and nervous tension or emotional disturbances

Types of Constipation

There are two broad categories of constipation, and knowing which you have as a predominant pattern can make a big difference to the treatment plan.

TONIC CONSTIPATION

- Excess muscle tone in the bowel, a result of tension or holding on—used to be called spastic bowel; insufficient or incomplete bowel movements with hard, dry, pelletlike stool, straining, maybe hemorrhoids or tearing
- May be more common in younger people who are in a hurry in the morning, sharing homes with partners and children and not having much time in the bathroom in the morning, or not having an opportunity for bowel movements during the working day
- Holding a lot of tension generally in the body; may have bowel spasms or cramps from peristalsis
- Worse with a fast-food or low-fiber diet and low fluid intake

FLACCID OR ATONIC CONSTIPATION

This is the type most often seen in cancer care where there is opioid use for pain.

- Lack of tone (hypotonicity) in the bowel allows it to dilate a lot before triggering the stretch defecation reflex; used to be called lazy bowel
- Infrequent bowel movements that are large, bulky, and with relatively complete emptying when they do occur, but only once or twice a week
- Slow transit time leads to fermentation of foods in the upper digestive tract, with bloating, belching, and nausea, as well as colicky abdominal pain and flatulence
- Worse with lack of exercise, obesity, prolonged bed rest, or habitual use of laxatives
- Worse with a high-fiber diet; often better with a low FODMAP (restricted carbohydrate) diet

Holistic Treatment of Constipation

Constipation is a feature of insufficient or inadequate peristalsis. As such, it is a symptom—a result of certain specific circumstances—that needs to be identified and addressed in order to achieve resolution. It is easy to take laxatives, but they do not address the cause and may not help much in the long term.

DIET

Dietary fiber holds water in the colon, which makes the stools softer and bulkier. This stimulates the defecation reflex and makes the stools easier to pass. Fiber also tends to hold toxins in the stool and minimize their reabsorption, as well as making the transit time faster. Because fiber is found exclusively in plant foods (fruits, vegetables, pulses, and grains) and not in animal products, your diet should include lots of vegetables. Oat bran appears to be the gentlest and most effective form of added fiber to use. Add ¼–½ cup of oat bran per day to soups, stews, baked goods, and cooked cereals. Raw foods tend to be more stimulating to the colon and so should be increased to form at least half of your daily intake of food.

Herbal Tea for Flaccid or Atonic Constipation

This tea has a stimulating action and is slightly irritating to the bowel wall, promoting peristalsis to remove waste material. The dandelion leaf promotes the flow of bile, a natural laxative, and the fennel, ginger, and peppermint are carminatives to reduce gas. Ginger also increases blood flow in the pelvis, which thus delivers more oxygen and allows for lessening of tension. The cascara is a stronger laxative, so dosing should start low and build up; it can take 6–8 hours to be effective.

+ 20 g dandelion root
+ 20 g burdock
+ 20 g cascara
+ 10 g fennel seed
+ 10 g ginger
+ 10 g dandelion leaf
+ 10 g peppermint

Mix all herbs. Add 1 teaspoon to 1 tablespoon of the herb mix per cup of cold water to a pan and simmer with the lid on for 10 minutes.

Herbal Formula for Tonic Constipation

This is a sweet and soothing formula that provides healthy fibers to feed the gut flora and coats and protects the gut lining throughout its length. All ingredients are powdered.

+ 30 g marshmallow root
+ 30 g slippery elm
+ 30 g oat bran
+ 10 g ginger

Mix all ingredients. Take 1–2 teaspoons of the powder stirred into water first thing upon rising or last thing before bed.

Chase it down with another glass of water and don't eat for at least 1 hour afterward. Consider also using relaxing and calming herbs for the nervous system and encouraging lifestyle changes to support bowel health (diet, allowing time in the morning, keeping well hydrated).

Muscle-relaxing herbs like ginger, wild yam, and cramp bark may be helpful to ease spasms, as well as using carminatives to reduce gas.

Note that slippery elm is a species suffering habitat loss and endangerment and should only be purchased from certifiably sustainable sources. It can be reduced or omitted in this recipe if preferred, but there is nothing quite like it for mucilage to soothe the bowel, complex sugars to feed the microbiome, and vitamins, minerals, and phytonutrients that nourish the body.

Include high-fiber foods, such as whole-grain breads and cereals, well-cooked or sprouted legumes, and raw fruits and vegetables. Add oat bran or wheat germ to foods such as casseroles, cereals, or homemade breads. Leave the skin on vegetables and fruits.

An additional benefit of eating a high-fiber diet rich in vegetables is that you are providing excellent complex sugars and feeding the microbiome. Beneficial bacteria are supported by leafy greens and other plant materials, and this has wide implications to overall well-being.

Simple Ways to Reduce Constipation

- Soak 4–6 dried prunes in a cup of water overnight, then eat them all in the morning.
- Drink plenty of fluids—at least 8 ounces per 20 pounds of body weight daily—always warm, not cold. Water or herb teas are best. Black tea can be constipating and should be avoided.
- If you have tonic constipation, avoid very bitter herbs (which are drying), and take lots of carminatives and antispasmodics (moistening and relaxing agents). Use psyllium or another bulk laxative as needed. Try 1 heaping teaspoon and increase to 2 tablespoons, if necessary. Stir into a glass of water and take before bed on an empty stomach. Follow with another glass of water. Do not do this if you have flaccid constipation. Consider a warm-water enema for tonic constipation.
- Take a high-potency probiotic supplement that contains 50 billion bacteria, daily. Make sure it contains a good range of bacteria; it should have at least six to eight strains. Fermented foods are also excellent for repopulating the microbiome, as long as they are live and fizzing, not pasteurized and dead.
- Use Triphala powder or capsules to retrain the bowel to be more responsive.
- Magnesium oxide at 200 milligrams and magnesium citrate at 200 grams, taken in water at bedtime, will relax the bowel in the night and allow onward movement of stool.

LIFESTYLE

Adequate exercise is very important to ensure good circulation and muscle tone in the pelvic area. Any exercise that gets the legs and pelvis moving will be good: yoga, rebounding, walking, running, or dancing. The exercise should be reasonably vigorous, should last at least 20 minutes, and should happen three or four times per week. The urge to defecate should never be suppressed. If you need to go, then go! To train the bowel to function optimally, it is recommended to develop the habit of going to the bathroom every morning at a regular time regardless of whether the defecation urge occurs. Over time, the body will learn that this is the time for elimination (though there is nothing wrong with having a bowel movement several times in a day). Evacuation is easiest in a squatting position, which relaxes the pelvic floor muscles. Some countries have toilets designed for this. Where squatting is not possible, it's helpful to raise the feet on a small stool.

LAXATIVES

It is important to determine whether there are tonic (tight) or atonic (flaccid) muscles in the colon. Either situation may lead to constipation, but they will require different treatment approaches. In the hypotonic state (flaccid or atonic constipation, such as seen with use of morphine for pain), stimulating laxatives and liver and gallbladder remedies may be the most appropriate. Loading up on fiber may actually cause more bloating and discomfort. In the hypertonic situation (tight muscles, spastic bowel), however, you should avoid stimulating the bowel and instead use muscle relaxants or antispasmodics, nervines, and maybe the osmotic bulking agents.

Sometimes dietary and lifestyle changes are insufficient to reverse old patterns of constipation, and in those cases a stimulating herbal laxative may be necessary. If you have constipation that does not improve with fiber and water intake or the various measures recommended here, then don't keep adding more fiber. You may have tonic constipation and need to take carminative or spasmolytic herbs (those that relieve smooth-muscle spasms) to relieve the excess tension in the colon. Bowel-moving herbs derive their effects in several ways.

Activate the liver and gallbladder. Hepatics, cholagogues, and choleretics are herbs that improve bowel function by activating the liver and gallbladder, increasing bile production and promoting bile flow. This creates a reflex activation of the bowel and also tends to improve the tension of the colon muscles. These herbs include dandelion, burdock, and greater celandine. They are usually quite gentle in action and may be used on a daily basis to support normal functions, alongside stronger herbs used intermittently as needed.

Draw water to the colon. Hydrophilic and osmotic laxatives are large, complex polysaccharides that draw water to themselves and hold it in the colon. This serves to soften the stool and give it bulk or volume. Osmotic laxatives, such as psyllium or flax, are also called bulking agents or stool softeners and are suitable for tonic/tense constipation. They hold water, filling the bowel and triggering peristalsis, as well as soothing the membranes. They are also high in fructo-oligosaccharides, which are a good prebiotic for the gut flora.

Stimulate the bowel. Bowel wall stimulants promote regular and strong contractions of the colon muscles. Herbal remedies in this category commonly contain related chemicals, the anthraquinone glycosides (found in aloe, yellow dock, cascara, and senna) or resins (found in bryony and pokeroot). These are suitable for the flaccid or atonic type of constipation. Stimulating the bowel can resensitize it to the stretch reflex and trigger a bowel movement. Herbs such as cascara and Cape aloe should be used as little as possible and for as short a time as possible.

Contact stimulants irritate the colon wall and cause it to attempt to evacuate the offending substance. Mineral oil and castor oil are the most common of this type of laxative. However, use of contact stimulants is not a recommended clinical strategy, as it is unnecessarily harsh.

Herbal laxatives of all classes are usually prescribed with an aromatic herb rich in volatile oils. These oils provide a carminative action that serves to promote contractions of smooth muscle around the gut, the circular and longitudinal muscles that control peristalsis and minimize spasms or cramping. These aromatic herbs include spearmint, lemon balm, ginger, chamomile, and peppermint.

Four Types of Herbal Laxative

There are four classes of herbal laxative, each stronger than the last. Only the first two categories are normally used in clinical practice, as the others are too strong for routine use.

Stimulant laxative herbs are often quite bitter. They can be taken in a tea but it is usually unpleasant and so compliance may be poor; a tincture is usually preferred. I will often provide a laxative tincture formula with the aromatic carminative herbs in it as well, and this formula is usually reasonably well tolerated.

Always start by using the gentlest approach first—diet and lifestyle, water and exercise—then the mild laxatives before stepping up to the more aggressive actions.

Aperients

Most bitters have an aperient effect up to a point—stimulating bile production in the liver, as all bitters do, will have a stimulating effect on the bowel. These are the so-called hepatics, cholagogues, and choleretics. Generally gentle and safe, they are mild bowel stimulants and rarely cause spasming or cramping. They include the following.

- Dandelion
- Burdock
- Yellow dock
- Greater celandine

Laxatives

These are effective but still relatively mild bowel stimulants.

GENTLE, BULKING TYPE

These laxatives contain soluble fiber and mucilage and are especially indicated for tonic (tense muscle) or spastic constipation. Use sparingly in cases of iron deficiency anemia, osteoporosis, or cachexia and wasting, as they can bind minerals and impair absorption.

- Flaxseed
- Psyllium seeds
- Aloe gel (mucilage)

STRONGER, IRRITATING TYPE

These laxatives contain anthraquinones that ferment with gut flora and irritate the bowel wall. They may cause cramping; use with carminatives.

- Rhubarb root
- Sheep sorrel
- Cascara sagrada
- Buckthorn

Purgatives (used only short term)

These are notably irritants in the bowel. The body will attempt to flush them away, which causes acute diarrhea. Pokeroot and bryony are used in clinical practice in very small doses and with great care; Cape aloe is no longer a popular remedy. Note that Cape aloe is different from aloe vera, from which we use the mucilaginous gel from the center of the leaf, which acts as a bulk laxative that is very soothing and healing to the entire digestive tract. The medicine in Cape aloe is in the anthraquinones harvested from just beneath the leaf epidermis. The purgative and cathartic effects are dose dependent, so these are not hard-and-fast categories; there will be gradations of action based on individual tolerances.

- Cape aloe
- Senna
- Pokeroot
- Bryony

Cathartics (very rarely necessary)

These herbs are too aggressive to be useful except in extreme situations, and they are indicated only for very short-term use after opioids have stopped the system moving or in declining doses to wean off opioid drugs.

- Black alder/alder
- Cape aloe in higher doses

PROCEDURE FOR REDUCING LAXATIVE USE

This protocol can be used to assist people who are habitually using commercial laxatives as well as those who wish to wean themselves off stronger herbal laxative agents. People who have been taking drugstore laxatives should halve the drug dose and add a stimulating herbal formula for 1 month; the dose will depend on their individual requirement to ensure one bowel movement each day. After this first month the drug dosage should be reduced by one-quarter each week thereafter, until the amount is so small that they can stop altogether. Increase the herbal dose as needed throughout this time and then work on reducing it in similar fashion to establish the lowest dose while still having regular movements. If constipation recurs at any point, repeat the previous week's dose for another week, then try to reduce again.

ENEMAS FOR CONSTIPATION AND PAIN

Enemas are an age-old traditional method for giving herbs to treat the bowel directly, for people who can't take herbs easily by mouth, and for addressing severe spasmodic abdominal pain. An herbal enema using a marshmallow root cold infusion can be soothing, tonifying, and gently laxative. If there is a lot of bowel inflammation, consider a cooled tea of flowers of lavender, chamomile, calendula, or rose petal. If there is bleeding add geranium, shepherd's purse, or plantain. Enemas are not recommended for use on a regular basis, as they can disrupt the microbiome over time, but they are perfectly safe for occasional use.

An enema of strong coffee is specifically effective for pelvic pain and constipation and is often indicated for pelvic or abdominal tumors. The coffee should be organic and freshly ground to preserve its constituents. It contains the alkaloids caffeine, theophylline, and theobromine, which cause relaxation of smooth muscles and expansion of blood vessels and bile ducts. Because the veins of the rectum are very close to the surface of the tissue, the caffeine is absorbed very quickly and in high concentration. Bitter receptors in the colon respond to coffee, which may be able to both relax smooth muscle in the gut and trigger bile production and peristaltic activity. The balance of these actions may allow the bowel to relax and contract more uniformly and ease peristalsis and evacuation. Thus, when the colon is evacuated, the toxins and bile are carried out of the body and this relieves pain.

Preparing a Coffee or Herbal Enema

Bring 8 cups of filtered or distilled water to a boil. Grind enough beans to make 8 teaspoons of organic coffee (any roasting level) and put it in a French press pot. The French press allows for stronger coffee than a percolator will make and can also be used for making a strong herbal tea for enemas. Pour the water over the coffee grounds and let it steep for 1 hour; cool to room temperature. Press the coffee grounds to the bottom of the pot, then pour the coffee liquid through a paper or cloth coffee filter into the bag of an enema kit (which allows more volume of fluid) or a rectal syringe (which is more convenient and easier to use); both are available at pharmacies. Allow at least 20–30 minutes when you can be uninterrupted for the treatment.

An enema should be done after a bowel movement if possible, not more than once per day and not more than four times per week.

Triphala for Bowel Health

No discussion of bowel health would be complete without mention of the traditional Ayurvedic formula called Triphala. Consisting of three herbs—amalaki, bibhitaki, and haritaki—the name means three fruits (Sanskrit; *tri* = three and *phala* = fruits). Triphala is considered a tridoshic rasayana in Ayurvedic medicine, meaning it balances the three *doshas* or constitutional types in the body. It has a written history of more than 1,000 years of use in India, where it is used to promote longevity and rejuvenation.

Triphala is considered a mild, stimulating laxative; it improves the appetite and reduces gastric hyperacidity. Research has suggested numerous other actions that can benefit a person with cancer, including antioxidant, anti-inflammatory, and immunomodulating effects, as well as promising antimutagenic, antineoplastic (inhibiting the growth of malignant cells), chemoprotective, and radioprotective effects. Triphala may increase T lymphocytes and natural killer cells, inhibit cancer growth, suppress oncogenes (genes with the potential for promoting cancerous cell behaviors), reduce cell proliferation, and promote cell death.

The major active constituents appear to be water-soluble polyphenols, including tannins and derivatives. Studies on these constituents suggest they may modulate gut bacteria to promote the growth of beneficial bacteria while inhibiting the growth of pathogenic bacteria. Chebulagic acid is a particular phenolic in the Triphala blend that has been shown to inhibit COX and 5-LOX and to demonstrate immunosuppressive and liver-protective properties.

Both in vitro and in vivo studies have suggested that Triphala may inhibit growth of several malignancies, including breast cancer, prostate, and pancreatic tumors. There is some preliminary evidence that this may be in part due to inhibition of vascular endothelial growth factor and prevention of new blood vessel growth.

Dose makes a big difference in the actions, with bowel toning effects at low doses, mild laxative effects at moderate doses, and a strong laxative action at high doses. Triphala is widely used in Ayurvedic medicine to lower gastric acid levels, reduce constipation and flatulence, and improve volume, frequency, and ease of passing a stool.

Other suggested benefits of Triphala include lowering blood sugar, protecting the oral mucosa and the gut lining from inflammatory effects of chemotherapy or radiation, and inhibiting lipid peroxidation.

Because the active constituents of Triphala are mostly water soluble, teas will work fine, or the powder can be stirred into water or taken in capsules. Triphala should be taken between meals on an empty stomach for maximum absorption. The recommended dose ranges from 500 mg to 1 g daily at bedtime, though larger amounts may be used to treat severe constipation. A study from Thailand established a no-observed-adverse-effect level of 2,400 mg/kg/day. A study of Triphala in HIV-positive patients using just over 1 g daily found no adverse effects demonstrated in liver function or kidney function tests, fasting blood sugar, lipid profiles, or complete blood count compared to the control group over 4 weeks of use and a 2-week follow-up period.

Diarrhea Caused by Chemotherapy and Radiation

Diarrhea refers to unusually frequent bowel movements or the passage of abnormally soft or liquid stools. It is often associated with nausea or vomiting and colicky pain. Cancer patients may be particularly afflicted by diarrhea as a result of chemotherapy drugs and radiation. Both chemotherapy and radiation can cause massive systemic toxicity that the body attempts to eliminate rapidly. Furthermore, surgery may remove sections of the bowel, which reduces surface area for absorption of fluids from feces. Radiation to the bowel can cause nerve damage, which may have a significant adverse effect on bowel control. Chemotherapy can also cause death and sloughing of gut-lining cells, and this contributes to diarrhea too.

Although most cases of diarrhea are self-limiting, acute diarrhea can lead to serious complications. Dehydration, electrolyte imbalance (loss of sodium, potassium, and magnesium), and kidney failure (insufficient renal blood supply) are possible.

Types of Diarrhea

Diarrhea can be exhausting and debilitating and can lead to nutritional deficiencies if there is insufficient time for proper nutrient absorption. There are several possible types and causes of diarrhea, each with different treatment strategies, although symptomatic management may be similar.

Osmotic diarrhea. This occurs when there is an excess of hydrophilic water-soluble substances present in the bowel and they are not absorbed, leading to retention of water in the stool. Possible causes include lactose intolerance, ingestion of large amounts of sugars, excessive intake of vitamin C, overuse of saline laxatives or magnesium oxide ("milk of magnesia"), general nutrient malabsorption, and the use of certain antacids containing magnesium. In this type of diarrhea, the more of the offending substance you take, the worse your symptoms will be. Avoiding the substance will alleviate symptoms.

Secretory diarrhea. This occurs when the large intestine secretes rather than absorbs electrolytes and water (due to the disruption of epithelial electrolyte transport). This type of diarrhea may be due to the presence of bacterial toxins (such as from food poisoning or drinking polluted water), where secretions of fluid are required to wash them away; unabsorbed bile acids after bowel surgery; certain enteropathogenic viruses; unabsorbed dietary fats in liver or gallbladder disease; excessive use of anthraquinone herbal cathartics or other irritating laxatives; certain hormonal imbalances such as secretin or calcitonin; or prostaglandin imbalances.

Exudative diarrhea. This occurs when there is acute or chronic inflammation in the gastrointestinal tract leading to copious production of inflammatory exudate, for example in Crohn's disease or ulcerative colitis.

Diarrhea in Cancer Patients

In cancer, diarrhea may be osmotic due to drugs or exudative due to inflammation (especially in gastrointestinal cancer) or due to surgery to remove portions of the bowel, which will shorten transit time. However, most diarrhea in cancer patients is chemotherapy induced and is secretory in nature, due to the extreme toxicity of the drugs and the attempts by the body to flush them away. Gut-lining cells naturally replicate quickly, as they are constantly being abraded by the passage of food; this high metabolic rate makes them vulnerable to taking up chemotherapy drugs. As they die and slough off, they contribute to diarrhea as well.

Holistic Treatment of Diarrhea

Like constipation, diarrhea is a symptom, not a disease in itself. You must always look for the underlying pathology before attempting to treat the diarrhea. Fortunately, in the case of chemotherapy-induced diarrhea, it usually diminishes or ends after the chemotherapy has ended and the drugs have been cleared from the system. During an acute attack of diarrhea you can implement a symptom management plan, ensuring a high fluid intake, along with astringent and carminative herbal teas.

The best foods to eat during an acute episode is the BRAT diet—banana, rice, applesauce, toast. In this case taking white rice and white toast will be easier on the gut than whole grains. If you are gluten sensitive, or just need a change, try steamed white potatoes instead of toast. You can also try diluted vegetable juices and broth.

When other food is reintroduced, it should be low-allergen and easily digested (such as vegetable soup, yogurt, cooked fruits, grated apple). Take high doses of probiotics to recolonize the bowel flora, which become imbalanced during diarrhea.

Reduce or avoid caffeine, which is a bowel stimulant. This means coffee, sodas, black/green tea, yerba mate tea, and even chocolate. Avoid foods and drinks that cause gas, including beans, cabbage, Brussels sprouts, beer, and carbonated beverages.

Methods for Stopping Diarrhea

If acute or debilitating diarrhea persists longer than 2–3 days, then it may become necessary to stop the diarrhea itself, and astringent (drying/tightening) herbs such as geum, geranium, oak bark, and shepherd's purse may be employed in the form of teas or enemas. Psyllium seeds may also be used to absorb excess water in the colon and thus give form to overly loose stools.

Tannins and fiber should be taken 8–12 hours apart, and both are best away from foods. This means dosing tannins in the morning, preferably at least an hour before food, and dosing fiber at bedtime, at least 2 hours after eating.

In bacterial infections, goldenseal, barberry, or Oregon grape may be useful because of their strong antibacterial properties. Goldenseal also has astringent, vulnerary, and tissue-strengthening effects on mucous membrane, making it especially effective if there is ulceration or incisions in the gut lining. In very severe diarrhea a qualified herbalist might also choose to use belladonna to stop secretions and peristalsis, but this is a short-term solution and is not available without a prescription. Weeding, seeding, and feeding the gut microbiome (see page 55) is required in both constipation and diarrhea, as there is dysbiosis (imbalance) in both states.

After a bout of diarrhea, you're likely to be dehydrated. Possibly the best way to rehydrate is to consume young, green coconut—both the liquid and the jellied flesh inside. This colloid solution of fat in water helps the cell walls hold on to intracellular fluids, keeping the tissues juicy. Other recipes for rehydration after diarrhea are included on page 177.

Carob Drink to Stop Diarrhea

This is a quick and effective remedy to stop acute diarrhea.

+ 1 tablespoon unsweetened carob powder
+ ½–1 cup room-temperature water

Stir the carob powder into the water and take every 15–30 minutes or hourly, as needed.

Herbal Tea Formula for Loose Stools

Raspberry, strawberry, and blackberry leaves are all astringent (cause tightening of tissues). If you cannot get one, then increase the others proportionally. Fennel is a carminative (relieves gas), and valerian is a warming relaxant to ease peristalsis (elimination). All herbs listed below are dried, except for the gingerroot.

+ 60 g blackberry leaf or root
+ 20 g fennel seed
+ 20 g valerian root
+ 60 g raspberry leaf
+ 40 g strawberry leaf
+ 1 inch fresh gingerroot, roughly chopped

Mix the dried roots and seeds in one jar, and the leaves in another. Simmer the chopped gingerroot with 1 tablespoon of the roots and seeds mix in 4 cups of water for 10 minutes with the lid on. Turn off the heat and add 4 tablespoons of the leaf mix. Cover and steep for at least 10 minutes. Add a pinch of salt and honey to taste. Drink 2–4 cups daily, away from meals.

The fennel, ginger, and valerian are all carminative to reduce any cramping or griping. Stronger astringents may be required for short-term use (3–6 days) including geum, geranium, oak bark, and shepherd's purse. These should not be taken for more than a week at a time without a week break, as they can reduce nutrient absorption as well.

Cardiac Support

Many chemotherapy drugs cause significant cardiovascular damage and disease, including arterial high blood pressure, heart failure, and clots. Anthracyclines are of particular concern and can cause considerable heart muscle damage (cardiomyopathy) even 5–10 years after completing treatment. Other chemotherapy drugs that may cause heart damage include cyclophosphamide, ifosfamide, platinum agents (such as cisplatin and oxaloplatin), antimetabolites (such as 5-fluorouracil and capecitabine), antibiotics (such as

WHO Rehydration Formula

The World Health Organization provides the following rehydration formula for use in cases of dehydration.

+ 3.5 g sodium chloride
+ 2.5 g sodium bicarbonate
+ 1.5 g potassium chloride
+ 20 g glucose

Dissolve all the ingredients in 4 cups of boiled water. Drink 1 liter of the formula every hour (proportionately less for children based on weight and age).

Herbal Tea for Rehydration

This is a refreshing tea blend that can be taken hot or iced. If the mouth is very sore, freeze the tea into ice cubes, then chip it and fold into a piece of cheesecloth for sucking on to cool inflamed tissue. It can also be used as the fluid part of the WHO Rehydration Formula.

+ 50 g rooibos
+ 10 g lemongrass
+ 10 g lemon peel
+ 10 g hibiscus flower
+ 10 g plantain
+ 10 g spearmint

Mix all herbs. Steep 1 teaspoon of the dried herb blend in 1 cup of boiled water. The tea can be taken hot or cold, or can be frozen into ice cubes for chipping.

mitoxantrone, mitomycin, and bleomycin), and antimicrotubule agents (such as taxanes). The newer biological or immunotherapies may also cause adverse heart effects.

Before prescribing these drugs, doctors will assess the ejection fraction (amount of blood that leaves the heart in each beat as a percentage of all blood in the heart); it should be over 70 percent. Anything below that may preclude the patient from certain cardiotoxic chemotherapy drugs or from left chest radiation that can further damage the heart. If cardiotoxic drugs are used, or if there is left chest radiation, then it is important to be proactive in protecting the heart. Supplements and herbs can be used in advance of treatment, in even higher doses during treatment, and in lower doses as background support long term.

Herbs for Cardiac Support

Herbal medicine and targeted nutritional supplements may be helpful in supporting and optimizing heart health through strengthening the heart muscle and regulating the force of the beat and the rhythmicity of the heart, through strengthening the vascular tissue (veins and arteries) and controlling vasodilation, and by regulating the blood pressure.

HAWTHORN (*CRATAEGUS* SPP.)

Hawthorn fruit provides traces of vitamin C, flavonoids, tannins, proanthocyanidins, and cofactors that may help build connective tissue and provide structural support of cardiovascular tissue (strengthening the heart muscle, valves, walls of arteries, and veins). Hawthorn flower buds and the young spring leaves are considered to address the functions of the heart, regulating the force of the beat (inotropic action) and the rate and rhythm of the beat (chronotropic action).

A meta-analysis of multiple trials in people with congestive heart failure (but not specifically chemotherapy-induced heart problems) has verified that hawthorn leaf and flower can increase maximal workload tolerance, increase exercise tolerance, decrease cardiac oxygen consumption, and improve symptoms of fatigue and shortness of breath.

Each part of this plant is important medicine for the cardiovascular system, and they are quite different but also quite complementary. Together these parts have synergy and offer a safe, broadly therapeutic and cardiotonic effect, giving strength and resilience to the physical tissue, the valves and vessels, as well as regulating the rate or rhythm and the force of the beat. This is a foundational herb for all seniors in my clinical practice, part of a daily routine of self-care that is easy, palatable, and affordable.

Dosing. Hawthorn extracts and teas have consistently proven to be well tolerated by patients, with low or negligible side effects. Hawthorn is considered safe for seniors and safe in conjunction with cardiac or other prescription drugs.

Hawthorn used in medical studies is usually standardized to its content of flavonoids (around 2 percent) or the even more active proanthocyanidins (just under 20 percent). Clinical trials have dosed between 800 and 1,800 mg of standardized dried herb extract daily, with no significant adverse effects reported.

Desirable constituents are largely water soluble, so tea is an effective way to take hawthorn but may require several cups daily.

Cardiotonic Hawthorn Tea

+ 2 tablespoons hawthorn berries
+ 2 tablespoons hawthorn flower buds and leaves
+ 3 tablespoons linden flowering tips (flowers and bracts)

Soak the berries for 15 minutes in a pan filled with 4 cups of cold water to soften. Cover, bring to a boil, and simmer very low for 10 minutes. Remove from the heat and add the flower buds and leaves. Cover again and infuse (steep) for 10 minutes. Strain off and sweeten to taste. Drink 3–4 cups daily.

ARJUNA (*TERMINALIA ARJUNA*)

The arjuna tree is from India and the bark from at least 15 different varieties may be used. Arjuna was introduced into Ayurveda as a treatment for heart disease by the seventh century CE, traditionally prepared as a milk decoction. Powdered arjuna was also used topically for the treatment of wounds, hemorrhages, and ulcers. Constituents found in the bark of arjuna include triterpene saponin glycosides, a cardenolide (cardioactive glycoside), antioxidant flavones, tannins and proanthocyanidins, and anti-inflammatory beta-sitosterol.

The bark of arjuna raises the levels of cardiac intracellular antioxidants and protects the heart against oxidative stress. Arjuna is indicated for chronic cardiovascular diseases, including chronic, stable angina; mild congestive heart failure; cardiomyopathy; hypertension; hypercholesterolemia; and metabolic syndrome. Arjuna may improve symptoms and signs of heart failure, including a decreased cardiac output. Clinical trials explicitly looking at the protective effects of arjuna in humans with chemotherapy have not yet been done, but, based on many hundreds of years of historic use for strengthening, nourishing, and supporting the heart, it is reasonable to expect that there will be beneficial effects in the case of cardiotoxic chemotherapy as well.

Dosing. 1–2 g daily of dried bark or 1.5–4 mL daily of a 1:2 tincture made with 45% ethyl alcohol.

Arjuna is well tolerated and produces only minor adverse reactions, such as mild gastritis, headache, and constipation. No metabolic or blood-, kidney-, or liver-related toxicity has been reported even for long-term administration of 24 months.

Supplements for Cardiac Protection

- L-carnitine: 1,000 mg twice daily
- CoQ10: 100–200 mg twice daily
- Magnesium glycinate: 500 mg twice daily
- Taurine: 1,000 mg twice daily
- Omega-3 fats: 1,200–1,500 mg daily
- Vitamin E: 400–800 IU daily
- Arginine: 1,000 mg twice daily

Fatigue and Debility

Disabling fatigue can be a very challenging consequence of advanced cancer and of some conventional treatments. Chemotherapy and radiation will profoundly impact bone marrow; not only will white blood cell count drop, leaving the body vulnerable to infections, but red blood cell count may also go down, making the body functionally anemic. This is not an iron-deficiency state but rather an inability of the bone marrow to make sufficient stem cells for red or white blood cells. Because of that, the hemoglobin count is often low as well, and iron and ferritin (stored iron) may be low or normal, or even in the upper range of normal, as iron is not being used up in making hemoglobin.

Taking an iron supplement is not the answer in this case; it won't help restore the bone marrow to replenish stem cells. There are drugs that may occasionally be helpful in this situation—granulocyte colony-stimulating factor (G-CSF) and granulocyte-macrophage colony-stimulating factor (GM-CSF) have been in use for more than 30 years and have generally countered some of the damage to bone marrow functions that is routinely seen with chemotherapy, thereby decreasing infections and bleeding and shortening hospitalizations. However, the immune responses may not be as robust, and the supply of newly formed neutrophils can become depleted over time.

There are many well-designed clinical trials that demonstrate the benefits of individual herbs in mitigating and managing cancer-related fatigue. However, similar trials on herbal formulas and blends for cancer-related fatigue are few and far between. The recommendations given below are based on my own clinical experience and the evidence-based practice of traditional herbal medicine.

Adaptogens for Rejuvenation

A tonic, restorative, and rejuvenative program will help boost energy and reduce fatigue. This may include adaptogens (stress reducers), but only the gentler types, such as ashwagandha, American ginseng, licorice, or eleuthero; reserve the more stimulating Korean ginseng or rhodiola for intermittent or occasional use when an extra energy boost is needed. Use leuzea as an anabolic adaptogen, and pulse dose it, 2 weeks on and 1 week off. Consider, rather, the deeply nourishing and restorative herbs, including rehmannia (prepared or cooked as it is used in Traditional Chinese Medicine) or codonopsis, and the nutritive herbs such as medicinal mushrooms, yellow dock, nettles, alfalfa, and kelp.

GINSENG AND CANCER-RELATED FATIGUE

Dozens of studies over several decades generally support the use of ginseng in cancer-related fatigue, showing that it improves quality of life and supports mood. A 2020 randomized, double-blind, placebo-controlled phase III trial into the use of Korean red ginseng for cancer-related fatigue in colorectal cancer patients taking a chemotherapy cocktail (FOLFOX-6) showed that the herbal medicine improved cancer-related fatigue compared with placebo. A 2021 study into the different types of ginseng in treating cancer-related fatigue showed that American ginseng (> 5% ginsenosides, dosed at 2 grams daily for up to 8 weeks) and Asian or Korean ginseng (≥ 7% ginsenosides, dosed at 400 milligrams daily, or with ginsenoside content not specified, dosed at 3 grams daily for 12 weeks) were all successful in reducing and relieving symptoms of cancer-related fatigue.

There is still some debate about the best species of ginseng to use and the best dose and duration. A 2021 study reviewing past research suggested that American ginseng demonstrates benefits in treating cancer-related fatigue, but Asian ginseng may be less effective. Clearly there is a beneficial effect from ginseng in general, but the preferred species and optimal doses may need to be determined on a case-by-case basis.

Herbs and Nutrition for Building Blood

During and immediately after completing chemotherapy or radiation, digestive symptoms may make it hard to eat well and maintain good nourishment. If there has been radiotherapy to the mouth and throat or to the central chest, or if chemotherapy has caused vomiting and esophagitis, then any hard, hot, spicy, or crunchy foods may be uncomfortable to eat, and the digestive and absorptive capacities may also be compromised by chemotherapy, radiotherapy, and drugs that damage the gut lining. It is important to choose foods that are nutritious but easy to digest and probably relatively bland because the taste buds may also be ultrasensitive. Soups, stews, casseroles, slow-cooked poached and braised foods, mashed root vegetables and squash or pumpkin, soft-boiled eggs, smoothies, oatmeal porridge, and congee (rice porridge) are all suggested.

Add nourishing, mineral-rich herbs such as alfalfa, kelp, and stinging nettle to the diet, as well as deep immune tonic herbs like astragalus and the medicinal mushrooms. These are all easy to take in soups—either as a vegetable for leafy herbs or simmered into the stock if they are woody.

Alfalfa (*Medicago sativa*). Alfalfa can send its thin taproot down 10–15 feet deep into the subsoil, so it pulls up minerals and nutrients from way down. It is for this reason that alfalfa hay is the highest quality and highest price for farmers. Dried alfalfa can be used in teas and soup stocks. If you can get fresh plant material, then it can be juiced and frozen in ice cubes or soaked in apple cider vinegar to extract minerals.

Stinging nettle (*Urtica dioica*). This has been enjoyed as a spring green vegetable by country folk wherever it grows since time immemorial. Like alfalfa, it has a deep root and draws up many minerals into the leaves. The leaves can be harvested when the plant is 6–8 inches high in spring and then steamed, sautéed, or juiced very much as you would spinach. Nettles do have a sting when fresh—wear gloves to pick them! Any processing will remove the sting: drying, blanching, juicing, cooking. You can easily dry stinging nettle in a food dehydrator. It will take 24–36 hours with the setting at 95°F (35°C) and you need to rotate the racks to dry everything evenly. A lower temperature, under 90°F (30°C), is actually better, but most domestic dehydrators don't go that low. I like to keep a big bag of dried stinging nettle in the kitchen and crumble a handful or two into a soup, a curry, a gravy, or even an omelet. You can also powder it and add it to smoothies, gravies, or sauces, or take it in capsules.

Seaweed. Kelp is just one of the many seaweeds you can eat. I like to buy three or four different ones and grind them coarsely, then add them as a condiment at the dining table. Sometimes I mix them with the Stomach Settler Seed Sprinkle (page 201) for a salty, aromatic, mineral booster. Be careful where you source your seaweeds from, as the oceans may not be clean in some locations. Seaweeds can concentrate heavy metals and possibly other toxins, so purity is paramount. A good supplier can provide tests showing levels of pollutants and proof of safety.

Bone broth. Bone marrow and bone broths are useful to provide dense nutrients and good fats. I will admit that this is still something I personally struggle with as a committed vegetarian for more than 40 years. However, there is no gainsaying the fact that our traditional or ancestral diets included significant amounts of fish, lean game, and organ meats from wild animals and that there are core nutrients available in these meats that are critically important for optimal health. When we are weak, depleted, debilitated, or run down, in a convalescent state after chemotherapy, or weak after surgery, then these nutrient-dense, slow-cooked, easy-to-swallow soups can be wonderfully restorative. Bone broths have been a traditional folk healing remedy across many cultures of the world. They provide healthy fats as well as collagen, which is restorative and tonic. People who choose no animal products at all will need to actively seek out good protein sources and to find supplements of vegan omega-3 fats (make sure there are 2 parts EPA to DHA), vitamin B12, and iron.

Mushrooms. Whether in the form of capsules, extracts, or food, mushrooms should be consumed regularly. The sugars and complex sterols in mushrooms (even just the kind found at the grocery store) are all beneficial. Mushroom and yeast extracts, rich in beta-glucans, are some of the most researched agents in integrative cancer therapies.

Beta-glucans are long-chain sugar molecules that are a natural part of the mushroom cell wall. They bind to specific receptors on neutrophils and macrophages and induce the production of various cytokines, which then activate other immune cells such as T cells and B cells. Mushrooms need to be cooked to extract the beneficial compounds properly; the sugars extract in water, and the sterols extract best in a fat or alcohol as a solvent. For this reason, it is ideal to add mushrooms to soups; if you fry onions and garlic in oil to start off with, followed by simmering in stock, you're essentially creating a dual extract into fat and water. Some mushrooms are not palatable; reishi and turkey tail, for example, are woody and tough. These can be tied off in a muslin bag or a clean cotton cloth and cooked down just the same with the onions and the oil as a solvent and then simmered in the broth for the watery extraction phase, but lift out the bag in its entirety before serving the soup.

Whey protein. Whey is a by-product of cheese production; it needs to be handled and processed carefully, as there are immune-supporting proteins in it that are fragile and easily damaged in manufacture. It is sold commercially as a powdered supplement called whey protein concentrate, and it provides a balanced source of essential amino acids and peptides, sulfur amino acids (methionine and cysteine), and the muscle-building branched-chain amino acids (leucine, isoleucine, and valine). It needs to be cold processed and microfiltered with a measured amount of immunoglobulins (lactoferrin, lactalbumin, lactoglobulins). Don't buy the cheap whey supplements used for bodybuilding; they lack these fragile proteins.

Whey has shown benefits in many conditions as part of a nutrient-dense treatment plan. It builds muscles and bones, is immunomodulating, regulates insulin and glucose, and helps regulate cholesterol and blood fat. In particular, whey is notably high in sulfur-containing amino acids (cysteine and methionine), which serve to boost levels of glutathione in the body, providing an antioxidant effect and optimizing various aspects of the immune system.

Maca (*Lepidium meyenii*). This is a root vegetable from the cabbage family, native to the highlands of Bolivia and Peru, that is traditionally eaten to support endurance and stamina at high altitudes. It is considered useful in reducing fatigue, as an antioxidant, for protection of nerves and the liver, to modulate the immune system, for memory enhancement, to address sexual dysfunction, as an antidepressant and antimicrobial, and for its anticancer actions. These combine to make it one of the preeminent food adaptogens.

Three different varieties of maca have different root colors and are traditionally used for different purposes. Yellow maca is the most widely used and researched; it is used for increasing physical and mental energy and stamina, enhancing concentration and learning capacity, and balancing sexual hormones. Red maca is the sweetest; it is thought to be the most effective for balancing hormones in women and for enhancing bone strength. Black maca is traditionally used for men's hormone balancing as well as for enhanced muscle gain and libido.

Chlorophyll. This is the green pigment in plants that reacts to sunlight and conducts photosynthesis. It is chemically and structurally very closely related to hemoglobin, with the exception that there are different side chains and chlorophyll has magnesium at its center while hemoglobin has iron. Numerous studies going back almost 100 years have verified that chlorophyll can act as a substrate for making new hemoglobin. Chlorophyll can literally help replenish hemoglobin and support formation of new red blood cells. Because chlorophyll has magnesium in its core, which needs to be replaced with iron, a practitioner might order blood work to assess iron in the system and determine if supplements are necessary. Iron supplements can be quite constipating, so if supplementation is needed it is helpful instead to seek out iron-rich foods and to cook in cast iron, which will provide a microdose of the mineral. Iron is best absorbed from the digestive tract when there is slight acidity, so adding vitamin C (ascorbic acid) is useful, and vitamin C happens to be an effective natural laxative at the same time, to offset any constipation from the iron.

Additional anticancer actions from chlorophyll include antioxidant and antimutagenic activity, modulation of detoxification pathways, and induction of apoptosis (cell death). There is also preliminary research suggesting a role for chlorophyll in inhibiting multidrug resistance, suggesting a positive benefit from combining chemotherapy with chlorophyll extracts and eating lots of dark green leafy vegetables.

Foods Rich in Chlorophyll

- Alfalfa
- Asparagus
- Broccoli
- Chlorella
- Collard greens
- Green beans and peas
- Green cabbage
- Matcha green tea
- Mustard greens
- Parsley
- Spinach
- Spirulina

Herbal Formula for Building Blood

This is a blend of herbs known for their adaptogenic, restorative, and rejuvenating properties, used to build and nourish the blood both literally and in a more energetic sense of building vitality, inner warmth or life force, and resilience. Some of them are from Traditional Chinese Medicine and some are more Western in origin. This formula has an appreciable amount of licorice in it, which could possibly raise blood pressure in some individuals. Blood pressure should be checked before commencing use and monitored every week or two while using it.

DECOCTION BLEND (20 GRAMS OF EACH HERB)

+ Astragalus root
+ Schisandra berry
+ Burdock root
+ Cat's claw bark
+ Chaga
+ Licorice root
+ Taheebo bark
+ Dandelion root
+ Goji berry
+ Orange peel
+ Reishi mushroom

INFUSION BLEND (10 GRAMS OF EACH HERB)

+ Lemongrass
+ Red clover
+ Hibiscus
+ Nettle leaf

Combine 20 grams of the decoction blend with 3 cups cold water. Put on the lid, bring to a boil, and simmer very low for 15 minutes. Remove from the heat and add 10 grams of the infusion blend. Put on the lid and steep for 15 minutes. Drink this amount daily.

Dong Quai and Millettia Formula

This Traditional Chinese Medicine formula is used to nourish blood and aid circulation; it is indicated for advanced stages of bone marrow disease or when there are deficient white blood cells or platelets during chemotherapy or during radiation. These herbs are nutritive, tonic, restorative, and rejuvenating.

+ 15 g dong quai root
+ 15 g millettia stems
+ 15 g rehmannia (prepared)
+ 9 g dan shen (red sage)
+ 9 g white peony root
+ 9 g longan fruit

This formula is available from TCM providers, usually as a tea to boil up and drink one cup twice daily.

Recipe continues on next page

Dong Quai and Millettia Formula, *continued*

Dong quai (*Angelica sinensis*). This is a well-known herb in TCM, highly regarded for building and nourishing blood, moving blood, and reducing stagnation and congestion in the tissues, especially abdominal organs (viscera) and reproductive organs. It is warming, moistening, and relaxing. It is prescribed for states of depletion, exhaustion, and debility.

Interestingly, traditional use attributes different actions to different parts of the root. The upper portion is considered more tonifying and less blood moving, while the deeper part or tail of the root is thought of as blood moving and less tonic. In practice, the whole root is usually prescribed to give the fullest possible range of effects. Because of its ability to relieve congestive pain in the pelvis, dong quai is especially useful to ease menstrual cramps, pain from ovarian cysts, and colic or spasms with tensive constipation. It has some emmenagogue effects, freeing the menstrual flow and promoting pelvic circulation, hence it is not recommended for anyone with heavy menses or during pregnancy. It is not an anticoagulant and should not be of particular concern in people taking blood thinners or facing surgery.

A note about dong quai and breast cancer. There is some controversy over the possible estrogen-like influence of this herb in breast cancer. However, research also has shown interesting anticancer effects in several other types of cancer.

In a study of invasive ductal breast carcinoma cells, a water extract of *Angelica sinensis* root increased proliferation of MCF-7 cells (estrogen and progesterone receptor positive) while inhibiting the growth of MDA-MB-231 cells (triple negative for estrogen, progesterone, and HER2/neu receptors). This suggests caution when using dong quai in estrogen receptor–positive breast cancers.

In contrast, another 2021 study found that complex polysaccharides from dong quai root reduced cell proliferation (growth/spread), induced apoptosis (cell death), and downregulated (suppressed) the activity of the JAK/STAT signal transduction pathway. The effects were dose dependent, and the researchers concluded that dong quai may be a useful agent for treating breast cancer.

A large-scale epidemiological study in Taiwan in 2020 documented a weak but still significant protective effect on breast cancer, especially in women who first used dong quai when they were 47–55 years old. There was some statistical suggestion that in younger women and with more prolonged use there may be more risk of cancer cell proliferation, but the authors of this study still suggested an overall beneficial effect.

In my clinical practice, I am likely to avoid using dong quai in a patient with a cancer known to overexpress estrogen receptor sites, but in cancers that are not hormone related, especially where there is debility and depletion, dong quai can be a key part of a restorative program.

White peony root (*Paeonia lactiflora*). This is a member of the buttercup family, now widely cultivated in gardens and bred to give many colors and multiple petals. The flower in the wild is creamy white (hence the species name) and the medicine is found in the root. It contains monoterpene glycosides and derivatives, mostly made bioavailable by fermentation with gut flora, another example of the importance of addressing bowel health and microbiome balance in everyone. Paeoniflorin and related monoterpenes inhibit COX-1 and COX-2 enzymes, which reduces inflammation.

Paeoniflorin binds to estrogen and androgen receptors and exerts a modulating agonist/antagonist action. It also activates aromatase enzymes that convert testosterone to estrogen. This may mildly increase estrogen production and reduce testosterone levels accordingly. Paeoniflorin has demonstrated antagonist interactions with alpha- and beta-adrenergic receptors, leading to parasympathetic dominance and enhanced learning capacity, cognition, and memory functions. This action suggests that peony root may be useful as part of a protocol for cognitive impairment.

Paeonia has a strong antispasmodic effect in the intestines, lower back, and uterus and also lowers blood pressure, relieves gas, increases urination, and promotes menstruation. It is traditionally used to treat menstrual disorders and premenstrual tension. The root also exhibits marked antibacterial effects as well as increased macrophage activity and increased numbers and activity of T lymphocytes. It can also reduce body temperature caused by fever.

Peony root is often combined with codonopsis and dong quai for weakness, debility, dizziness, and palpitations from blood deficiency.

Rehmannia (*Rehmannia glutinosa*). Known as Chinese foxglove and with a recorded history of use over 2,000 years, this root is considered one of the most important herbs in Traditional Chinese Medicine. It is especially recommended for disorders of the kidneys and adrenal glands causing weakness and deficiency of function. It is a cooling and anti-inflammatory herb that promotes recovery and longevity.

Rehmannia is traditionally used as a restorative and building agent to treat osteoporosis and adrenal fatigue and as a tonic to treat anemia, palpitations, and arrhythmias. It nourishes the blood and supports the adrenals. It is an adaptogen that modulates stress hormones, mostly due to phytochemicals known as "iridoid glycosides," notably catalpol, which stimulate the production of adrenal cortical hormones and exert an anti-inflammatory effect. Rehmannia is considered a "trophorestorative" for the adrenals, supporting structure and function of the gland and especially indicated for chronic degenerative disease.

Rehmannia increases kidney blood flow and promotes elimination of urine with dissolved wastes and toxins, and it supports kidney production of the hormone erythropoietin, which promotes proliferation of bone marrow stem cells and progression into erythrocytes (red blood cells). In animal studies rehmannia prevented osteoporotic bone loss and increased the bone matrix and thickness of bones. Rehmannia regulates blood glucose and insulin levels and stabilizes blood sugar.

Rehmannia root was traditionally prepared by steaming it repeatedly and sun-drying in between. The root may also be steamed in wine until it turns black and moist (called "prepared" rehmannia, which is energetically warmer and more restorative and tonic). The unprocessed root may be slightly toxic and should be avoided.

Recipe continues on next page

Millettia (*Millettia* spp.). Also known as jixueteng, this is a Traditional Chinese Medicine from the stems of several *Millettia* species. The most common is *M. spatholobus*. Traditionally used to enrich the blood and promote blood circulation, relax tendons, and activate meridians (energy channels in Traditional Chinese Medicine), it is also indicated for blood deficiency and blood stasis syndrome manifesting as anemia, menstrual pain, and heavy bleeding (dysmenorrhea and menorrhagia) or for soreness, numbness, and stiffness of limbs. It's used for joint pains due to wind and dampness (exacerbated when the weather changes and the barometer moves), aching pain in the waist and knees, numbness of the extremities, weakness of the muscles and tendons, and irregular menstruation and low or no flow due to deficiency of the blood.

Millettia contains a range of flavonoids and sterols that contribute to its immunomodulatory action.

- Isoflavones similar to genistein: formononetin, ononin, afrormosin, daidzein
- Chalcones (flavonoids): isoliquiritigenin, tetrahydroxychalcone, licochalcone
- Coumestans (flavones): medicagol
- Condensed flavonoids (tannins): epicatechin

Other flavonoids: pruetin, cajinin, methoxyhydroflavonol

- Triterpenes: friedelan, taraxerone
- Sterols: beta-sitosterol, daucosterol, methoxycoumesterol, camphesterol, stigmasterol
- Phenolic organic acids: protocatechuic acid

Millettia is usually dosed at 15–30 grams per day of dried herb and is often combined with other blood-nourishing herbs such as dong quai, peony, and prepared rehmannia, as well as blood-vitalizing herbs such as dan shen.

Longan (*Dimocarpus longan*). The fruit and seeds contain phenolic compounds with antioxidant activity, as well as antimicrobial and anticancer actions.

Gastritis and Reflux

Gastritis is an uncomfortable and distressing condition that is highly likely in people with cancer who are receiving chemotherapy that makes them vomit and have acid reflux. It's caused by stomach acid coming back up into the esophagus. The esophagus, which leads from the back of the throat down into the stomach, is lined with tissue that is quite resilient. It can withstand the scraping and heat of food passing down but is not designed for exposure to stomach acid. At the bottom is the esophageal sphincter, a valve that should be closed as a default position and open only when the swallowing reflex occurs. However, if that valve does not close tightly or if there is any back pressure from below, then acid from the stomach can leach up into the lower level of the esophagus and act as an irritant and a chronic inflammatory trigger.

Symptoms of gastritis and gastroesophageal reflux disease may be quite marked and unmistakable (acid in the back of the mouth or a bad taste coming up from the stomach, retro sternal pain and discomfort, sensitivity to acid or hot spicy foods, waking at night with central abdominal pain). In some people, however, the reflux is more challenging to identify, diagnose, and treat. In these cases, a chronic cough is often a sign, as is irritation or clearing of the throat, which may be worse at night as the person lies down and gravity no longer helps keep the acid down.

Taking antacids and proton pump inhibitor drugs does not really help, particularly because the problem is not too much acid but, rather, a lax or loose valve. Antacids adjust the pH of the stomach upward, which may cause further acid production in response to rising pH, thus creating a self-perpetuating problem. Furthermore, pH disturbance can disrupt gastrin and pepsin production, which have downstream consequences of poor digestion, malabsorption, and gut microbiome imbalance. In particular, long-term antacid users may run the risk of insufficient calcium absorption and possible bone thinning.

Mucilaginous Herbs

Wherever there are inflamed, irritated, or raw membranes, mucilaginous herbs are indicated. These herbs are rich in complex sugars that hold water. To get a sense of what mucilage does, think of the gel that drips if you cut an aloe leaf or the thickening action of chia or flax in your smoothie. This slippery, slimy action creates a moist, soothing, and healing barrier over mucous membranes to protect them.

In the case of gastritis and reflux, hydrochloric acid from the stomach irritates the esophageal valve and lower esophageal lining when it ascends from the stomach through an incompetent (leaky) esophageal sphincter that allows backwash. This may be compounded by low mucus production from mucous glands in the stomach lining. Mucilaginous herbs that could be indicated here include slippery elm bark; aloe gel; marshmallow flower, leaf, and root; fenugreek seeds; licorice rhizome; and plantain leaf. To avoid gumminess they may be best taken as a cold infusion or cold gruel with powdered herb.

Stomachics

Stomachics are herbs that act as gastric tonics, supporting correct opening of the esophageal (entrance) and pyloric (exit) sphincters; stomach acid, mucus, and gastrin hormone production; and peristalsis. They are used in mild to moderate gastritis and dyspepsia or indigestion.

MEADOWSWEET (*FILIPENDULA ULMARIA*)

This is possibly one of the best stomachics and the most useful herb for treating gastritis. It is a tall and beautiful marsh-dwelling member of the family Rosaceae with a sweet-scented flower. Herbalists in Europe have known it for hundreds of years as an upper digestive tonic, as well as an herb for arthritis and joint pain. It turns out that meadowsweet is rich in salicylates, the same that are found in willow and poplar and that impart anti-inflammatory and pain-relieving effects. Actually, meadowsweet used to be called *Spiraea ulmaris* and gave its name to aspirin when salicylates were first researched and defined. Willow may have been a good source, but the name came from meadowsweet.

Herbalists use it as a tea. It is pleasantly scented and slightly astringent (drying), has the ability to soothe and calm inflammation in the stomach lining, and normalizes acid production to reduce irritation. When taken with demulcent (soothing), mucilaginous herbs like slippery elm and marshmallow, the astringent (drying, tightening, and toning) properties of meadowsweet are tempered and the combination becomes both astringent and demulcent, as well as toning and nutritive. This defines the complex stomachic concept.

Interestingly, synthetic aspirin (acetylsalicylic acid) is a strong gastric irritant and may predispose to ulcers, as well as cause gastric bleeding, none of which the plant compounds do because they are not acetylated.

Carminative Herbs

One of the key therapeutic strategies herbalists would consider for gastritis is the use of carminative herbs. These herbs are rich in volatile oils and hence are aromatic and often quite tasty. The action of carminatives is to relax longitudinal and circular muscle contractions throughout the gut and ensure easy onward movement of foods, and then feces, in a timely manner. They are useful for treating gas accumulation, colicky abdominal pain, tonic or tension constipation, and any derangement of peristalsis. The carminatives open the pyloric and the ileocecal sphincters as waves of peristalsis go through. However, most carminatives (such as lemon balm, chamomile, and lavender) will not markedly affect the esophageal sphincter and can be safely taken for reflux and gastritis. Peppermint, on the other hand, is not recommended with any reflux (although it can be helpful to allay vomiting). Peppermint can open the esophageal valve at the top of the stomach, which allows acid reflux. Sucking on a peppermint candy may not be a problem, because there may be little to no real peppermint in it. Taking an herbal tea or tincture, though, with a noticeable amount of peppermint herb in it might aggravate symptoms.

Holistic Strategies for Gastritis and Reflux

- Put a 4- to 6-inch-thick plank of wood under the head of the bed to raise it slightly so that simple gravity can help direct the flow of acid.
- Don't eat after 6 pm, so that you don't go to bed with food in the stomach. This happens to support the idea of intermittent fasting or the 16/8 method as well (see page 53), but here it is more about the need to lie down with an empty stomach.
- When antacid drugs are used, consider adding digestive enzymes with meals (amylase for starch, lipase for fats, and proteolytic enzymes for protein) as the low acid will diminish all other digestive juices as well. Bitter herbs may be indicated, although that can seem counterintuitive as they promote digestive juices and functions. In small doses, though, and in combination with mucilage, tannins to tighten and astringe tissues, and resins to reduce inflammation, bitters can be helpful to support the whole digestive process. Some herbs even do double duty, such as calendula, which is bitter, anti-inflammatory, and vulnerary, or meadowsweet, which is bitter, carminative, and astringent.

How You Eat Matters

It is very important that you pay attention not only to what you eat but also to *how* you eat. In order to optimize the release of bile and consequent fat digestion at the time it is needed (that is, 1–2 hours after eating), and then pancreatic juices a little later, it is necessary to be in the right frame of mind. Literally that means being in parasympathetic-dominant or relaxation mode. The nervous system is wired to switch off digestion when there is any stress or need for activity. I suggest always making a point of sitting down to eat and not ever eating while doing other things—driving, working, or even watching television (watching the news or a horror movie is definitely not recommended!). Take 5 minutes of quiet time before diving into your food. Eat mindfully and slowly, chew carefully, pay attention to what you're eating, and don't rush.

Additional Herbal Suggestions

- Aloe gel can be taken by the tablespoon. Easy to purchase in any natural health store, it soothes and protects the inflamed mucosa.
- Chamomile tea is anti-inflammatory, carminative, and relaxant.

A Powdered Herb Formula to Soothe the Digestive System

In this formula, the slippery elm provides fructo-oligosaccharides for microbiome support; the slippery elm, marshmallow, and fenugreek all supply mucilage for coating and soothing the gut lining; the psyllium bulks and softens the stool; and the cinnamon is a carminative to relieve any gas, bloating, or cramping. Glutamine is an amino acid that protects against gut mucosal injury or atrophy, promotes mucosal repair and resistance, and may have a nutritive and cytoprotective effect in small bowel and colonic mucosal cells. The ingredients listed below are powdered herbs. The amounts indicated will result in 100 grams, supplying 20 doses at 5 grams per dose (approximately 1 rounded teaspoon of powder).

+ 45 g slippery elm
+ 13 g marshmallow root
+ 15 g meadowsweet
+ 10 g glutamine
+ 10 g licorice
+ 5 g psyllium seed
+ 1 g cinnamon
+ 1 g fenugreek seed

Make a strong chamomile tea, using one small handful of herb per cup of boiling water, and allow to cool. Mix all powdered herbs. Mix ½–1 cup of the cooled tea with 1–3 teaspoons of the herb powder mix and blend into a paste or a gruel. Take 3–4 tablespoons two or three times daily.

Herbal Formula to Calm the Nerves and Promote Appetite and Digestion

This tasty tea blend combines the gentle bitters chamomile, blue vervain, and lavender with the carminatives spearmint and lemon balm. These are all relaxing nervines to calm the nervous system. The linden tastes sweet and has a relaxant and blood-pressure-lowering effect. The damiana and the blue vervain are both thymoleptics, which act as gentle mood elevators. Milky oats are restorative to and feed the nervous system. The amounts listed below will make about 20 cups of tea.

+ 15 g lemon balm
+ 15 g milky oats (young tops, harvested green)
+ 15 g chamomile
+ 10 g linden
+ 10 g damiana
+ 10 g blue vervain
+ 10 g lavender
+ 10 g spearmint
+ 5 g wood betony

Mix all herbs. Use 1 heaping teaspoon of the herb blend per cup of boiling water. Pour the hot water over the herbs, cover, and steep for at least 15 minutes. Use as needed.

- DGL (deglycyrrhizinated) licorice lozenges can be taken for their mucilaginous and soothing qualities, and they won't raise blood pressure, which can happen with higher doses of unprocessed licorice.
- Calendula is bitter, anti-inflammatory, and vulnerary.

Hand-Foot Syndrome and Skin Rashes

A form of dermatitis called palmar-plantar erythrodysesthesia (PPE), or hand-foot syndrome, is a common consequence of chemotherapy drugs—especially doxorubicin, cytarabine, docetaxel, capecitabine, and fluorouracil, as well as some of the newer immunotherapies that target epidermal growth factor receptors that are found in skin and overactive in some cancers.

Though rarely life threatening, the rash is significant because it impairs a person's quality of life. Not only can the rash cause discomfort, but it can bleed or become infected, and in the worst cases can cause deadly sepsis.

Allopathic recommendations for dealing with PPE include high-SPF sunscreen, rich moisturizer, barrier creams, hydrocortisone 1 percent cream, and antibiotics if needed.

Ways to Minimize Skin Irritation

- Use very mild soaps, body washes, and shampoos that do not contain alcohol, perfume, or dye. Unscented products for babies are usually okay.
- Soothe your skin with oatmeal bath products.
- Avoid saunas, steam rooms, and hot tubs.
- Bathe with cool or lukewarm water, take tepid baths instead of showers, and avoid hot, humid places.
- Moisturize your skin at least twice a day with a thick, emollient cream that has no alcohol, perfumes, or dyes. The best time to do this is right after you bathe, while your skin is still damp.
- Wear loose, soft clothing made from natural fabrics—silk or bamboo are ideal next to the skin.
- Use liquid laundry detergents that rinse out easily and avoid fabric softeners and anything that contains strong perfumes. Consider a second rinse cycle in the washing machine. Use 10 drops of lavender essential oil on a cotton cloth in the clothes dryer instead of dryer sheets.
- Stay out of the sun as much as possible; sunlight seems to trigger and/or worsen rashes in some people. If you'll be outside during the day, wear a hat with a wide brim and clothes with long sleeves. Use a broad-spectrum sunscreen with an SPF of at least 30 and zinc oxide or titanium dioxide if you do need to be outside in the sun.

- Do not use acne medicines. Though the rash may look like acne, acne medicines don't work. They can dry out the skin and make the irritation worse.
- Try gel shoe inserts if the soles of your feet are tender. Wear shoes that fit well and aren't tight.

Grading Scale for Hand-Foot Syndrome

- **Grade 1 (mild):** Minimal skin changes or dermatitis (e.g., little redness and inflammation, buildup of fluids, or thickening) and no pain
- **Grade 2 (moderate):** Skin changes (such as peeling, blisters, bleeding, buildup of fluids, or thickening) with pain; limiting functional activities of daily living (work, education, recreation)
- **Grade 3 (severe):** Severe skin changes (such as peeling, blisters, bleeding, buildup of fluids, or thickening) with pain; limiting self-care activities of daily living (bathing, clothing, feeding)
- **Grade 4 (life or limb threatening):** Loss of fluids can contribute to local tissue atrophy and systemic dehydration, risk of infection, and unmanageable pain

Herbs for Soothing and Healing Skin

Herbs can be used topically for cooling, softening, and moistening actions. Oatmeal soaks, plantain or chickweed poultices, chilled aloe gel, and a peppermint lotion (20 drops of pure essential oil in 100 milliliters of base lotion) can all be effective at cooling mild to moderate PPE.

CHICKWEED AND PLANTAIN (*STELLARIA MEDIA* AND *PLANTAGO* SPP.)

Both of these are very common weeds that can easily be picked and processed fresh into a green slurry diluted with water. The slurry can be chilled in the fridge and used as a hand soak that is cooling, anti-itching, and healing. Between them, these two herbs provide mucilage, allantoin, vitamin E, chlorophyll, tannins, and other healing agents to reduce burning and inflammation and promote healing and tissue repair. If they are not in season, then make a tea from the dried herbs, cool it in the fridge, and use it as a soak. Infused oils of these herbs are also helpful as the base of a healing oil blend.

ALOE (*ALOE VERA*)

Aloe gel is a thick mucilage from the center of the leaf; it is hygroscopic (holds water), emollient, and anti-inflammatory. One way to use it is to keep a few aloes as houseplants and break off a leaf or leaf tip as needed. Peel it carefully to remove the outer layers where the laxative constituents are found, and you are left with the inner gel that you can apply to the hands liberally or use in a recipe like the Super Moisturizing Skin Cream (page 196). The gel can be purchased in health food stores as well. Keep it in the fridge for an extra cooling effect.

OATS (*AVENA SATIVA*)

Oats were one of the first cultivated grains in northern Europe. The grains have long been known as an anti-itching, anti-inflammatory, skin-softening, skin-soothing, and tissue-repairing agent. It is important to note that the humble oats actually offer three different medicines: oatmeal (from the mature seed head), green milky oats (harvested when the seed is immature), and oat straw (taken while still fresh and green, shortly after the milky oat tops have been removed).

Colloidal oatmeal. The use of colloidal oatmeal—finely ground oats (the mature oat seeds) stirred into and partly dissolved into water—as a skin protectant was regulated by the US FDA in 2003 for use in skin rashes, erythema, burns, itchiness, and eczema, and its commercial preparation for retail sale is standardized by the US Pharmacopeia.

Oatmeal (mature seed) derives its beneficial effects by several means.

- Starches and beta-glucans. These are hygroscopic (hold water), protective, and emollient.
- Phenols. These are antioxidant and anti-inflammatory, as well as protective against sun damage.
- Saponins. Detergent and cleansing, these are also anti-inflammatory.
- Soluble proteins (globulins and prolamines). These are pH buffering, and research suggests they may be able to activate genes for improved integrity of the skin barrier (for example, tighter junctions between cells, better lipid balance).

The total effect of these different constituents reduces the expression of pro-inflammatory cytokine mediators in keratinocytes (skin cells) and decreases activation of the NF-κB pathway, which could contribute to the anti-inflammatory activity.

Other Uses for Oats

Green milky oats. The immature grain from which a milky fluid can be expressed when fresh, this is considered one of the preeminent nourishing, restorative foods for the nervous system. It lifts the mood and gives energy when you are down, calms and soothes frayed nerves if you are anxious or wrung out, and creates balance between the sympathetic and parasympathetic functions in the central nervous system. An entirely safe and nutritive tea can be made from dried milky oats, or a tincture can be made using fresh green heads.

Oat straw. This is not the dried straw that is left over after the matured and dried grain head is harvested and is typically used for animal bedding. Rather, oat straw comprises the stems and leaves picked fresh and green with the milky oats. The younger, green oat stems and leaves are rich in soluble and bioavailable minerals and are used as a tea, tincture, or capsule to give tensile strength and resilience to connective tissues.

Making an Oatmeal Bath

First of all, here's what *not* to do: Do *not* pour oatmeal directly into a hot bath! Your skin will feel lovely, but you will have a hard time explaining to the plumber why your drains are plugged with porridge (yes, some of us learn the hard way).

Instead, put 1–2 cups of finely ground oatmeal (better than oat flakes) into a cotton bag, a thin sock, or the foot cut off a pair of nylons, and tie the neck tightly. Drop this into a warm bath and squeeze it in your hands a few times to get the bath water to look milky. Add 10 drops of lavender essential oil, lie back, and relax. Your skin will feel soft and silky afterward, and the water will be deeply soothing and nourishing to cells. Be careful, though—the saponins can make the bathtub slippery.

Super Moisturizing Skin Cream

+ 15 mL aloe gel
+ 12.5 mL calendula-infused oil
+ 12.5 mL gotu kola–infused oil
+ 10 mL sea buckthorn oil
+ 10 mL jojoba oil
+ 10 mL propolis tincture (or pine resin for vegans)
+ 10 mL licorice tincture
+ 5 mL squalane oil (derived from olive oil)
+ 5 mL vitamin E oil
+ 1 mL liquid vitamin A
+ 10 g lanolin (or avocado butter for vegans)
+ 10 g cocoa butter
+ 10 g shea butter
+ 20 drops lavender essential oil
+ 10 drops each essential oils of benzoin, blue chamomile, and Peru balsam

Mix all the liquid ingredients except the essential oils, and gently warm them in a double boiler. Do not overheat—the oil should not cook. Add the lanolin, cocoa butter, and shea butter and melt slowly. Remove from the heat and add the essential oils. Pour into a clean glass jar and allow to cool before putting the lid on. Store in the fridge so it feels cool when it goes on the skin. This will last 2–3 months in the fridge.

Loss of Appetite

One of the distressing and debilitating symptoms of chemotherapy and radiotherapy may be loss of appetite. Just when you need to eat to keep your strength up, just when you are trying to improve your diet, you suddenly have no interest in food at all and you struggle to eat well. This is definitely one of those times when being well prepared pays off. If you are able to make soups, broths, and other healthy foods in advance of starting treatment, and freeze them in small portions, then you may be able to eat smaller amounts more often and with little effort required.

Many factors may contribute to loss of appetite (technically called anorexia), including the following.

- Nausea and vomiting from chemotherapy
- Changes in taste buds and bad taste or metallic taste in the mouth—foods don't taste the same
- Mouth sores and esophageal sores that cause pain when eating
- Anxiety, stress, and distress, which stimulate the sympathetic nervous system (driven by adrenaline, the hormone of fight or flight)—this down-regulates digestion so that food is not processed as well or moved down properly through the gut for elimination
- Fatigue and enervation—being too tired to cook or enjoy food
- Fear of eating the "wrong" foods, demonizing certain foods, or rigidly adhering to restrictive diets (technically called orthorexia)
- Unappetizing, stale, or poorly prepared food
- Pain and the opioids or other drugs used to manage pain

Holistic Strategies for Treating Appetite Loss

It is often helpful to have smaller, more frequent meals and snacks. That way you don't need to feel that you have to be hungry; just be sure to be taking something nutritious and balanced at least every 2 hours. If tastes are deranged or swallowing is difficult, then consider using smoothies, broths, and liquids or juices that can be sipped through the day and don't hurt to swallow or make you feel full. Be sure to get the maximum nutrition from everything you eat—add nut butter or an avocado to a smoothie, use high-quality whey protein with immunoglobulins intact, use bee pollen if you need a sweetener, add mushroom powders, turmeric, cinnamon, and other warming spices where you can.

SMALL, NUTRIENT-PACKED MEALS AND SNACKS

Sometimes just figuring out what to eat is the hardest part of making dinner for yourself. When you are tired and weak, when you need to eat but don't have a big appetite, then having just the right food readily at hand can make all the difference. It helps to make meal plans and menus and shopping lists so that your support team can better meet your needs.

Stock your freezer with soups and casseroles in single-serving containers, buy fillets of fish or portions of meat in single servings, and thaw just what you need for a day or two at a time. Buy some of your vegetables prewashed or precut, subscribe to one of the food box delivery programs that brings you meals ready to go, or form a friends cooking club to make it a fun and sociable event.

Use the Immune Boot Camp Nutritional Breakfast Smoothie from Chapter 2 (page 60) as a base and build drinkable meals with concentrated nutrient additives such as whey protein, nut butters, and easily digested puréed vegetables.

Using Herbs to Support Appetite

Herbal medicines can be used in several different ways to support appetite. Teas will usually be the most effective, taken warm and naturally sweetened with stevia, maple syrup, or honey. Warming, aromatic bitters such as angelica, calamus, burdock root, cinnamon sticks, valerian, and fresh gingerroot will relax tension in the gut and promote flow of juices. Taking bitter herbs—especially those with a tendency to stimulate upper digestive functions, including wormwood, centaury, and andrographis—are another option.

BITTER HERBS

The bitter taste is one of the five primary tastes (sweet, salty, sour, bitter, and umami) and serves some very specific physiological roles. Bitter compounds in plants are often alkaloids, which tend to be the more potent and physiologically active "effector" compounds.

Improve appetite and digestion. Bitters are considered to be digestive tonics and stomachics, which are normalizers of gastric activity and will improve the appetite and all digestive functions when taken in moderation. Bitter herbs stimulate the flow of digestive juices (saliva, hydrochloric acid, mucus, pancreatic enzymes, bile) and cause the release of hormones into the bloodstream, including gastrin from the stomach, which regulates and sets the tone for downstream digestive controls, and hormones that govern satiety, hunger, and sugar management and stimulate peristalsis.

Reduce stress responses. When you are digesting properly, you are functioning in parasympathetic dominance—the so-called "rest and digest" state of nervous activity. When bitters promote digestive functions, they are therefore also reducing stress responses and symptoms of anxiety, which are derived from the sympathetic nervous system fueled by adrenaline. It is no surprise that we feel anxiety as "butterflies in the tummy" or that acute stress can cause diarrhea (like right before an exam); chronic stress can cause tonic or tense constipation. Herbalists may even use bitter herbs such as yellow gentian as antidepressants, and now, with the dawning understanding of the impact of gut flora and the microbiome on mental health, it is becoming apparent that

Using Yellow Gentian to Improve Digestion

Yellow gentian (*Gentiana lutea*) is a classic bitter herb with a long history of use for digestive insufficiency or a weak digestive system with symptoms of low appetite, rapid satiety, food sitting heavy in the stomach after meals, belching and acid reflux, low-grade nausea, and upper abdominal bloating. Studies of isolated stomach cells exposed to different levels of gentian root extract increased production of gastric acid in a dose-dependent manner. Gentian extract was effective at concentrations of 10–100 mcg/mL, a range that can be readily achieved. Human trials suggest an effective dose is up to four or five capsules of gentian extract per day, each containing 120 mg of a 5:1 dry extract of gentian root. This achieves rapid and dramatic relief of symptoms, including constipation, flatulence, appetite loss, vomiting, heartburn, abdominal pain, and nausea. Because of habitat loss and overharvesting, this herb is at risk in the wild, and some practitioners recommend dandelion leaf, wormwood, yarrow leaf, or other bitter herbs instead.

alluding to "gut feelings" is not just a turn of speech but actually means something in medicine.

Bitter taste receptors are not restricted to the oral cavity. They are expressed in the gut, including the stomach. Bitter receptors have been found on enteroendocrine (hormone-releasing) cells in the gut lining, and their activation promotes the release of gut peptides, in particular cholecystokinin (CCK), which triggers the secretion of pancreatic enzymes and bile and regulates stomach function, appetite, and acid production. Activation of bitter receptors is also thought to indirectly improve the elimination of absorbed toxins from the gut epithelium. Lower down in the gut, bitter receptors induce fluid secretion, suggesting a mild laxative effect.

Take bitters early. The best time to take bitter herbs is early in the morning or an hour before meals. You should take tincture diluted with water or a tea made from dried or fresh herbs. If you take capsules, you will stimulate the receptors in the stomach and intestines but will miss the whole-mouth experience and the initiation of the effects from sublingual absorption (under the tongue) and from the oral mucosa. This is a rapid and direct route from the mouth to the brain, bypassing the liver, where blood from all the rest of the digestive system ends up prior to entering systemic circulation. The oral route allows delivery to the brain to be fast and direct.

Some Key Bitter Compounds from Plants

Mildest

- Green tea catechins (from green tea leaves)
- Arbutin (from bearberry leaves)
- Lavandin (from lavender)

Stronger

- Arctigenin (from burdock root)
- Berberine (from Oregon grape root, goldenseal root)
- Cynaropicrin (from globe artichoke leaf)
- Humulone (from hops strobiles)
- Marrubiin (from horehound leaves)
- Sinigrin (from horseradish root)

Strongest

- Absinthin (from wormwood)
- Amarogentin (from gentian root)
- Andrographolide (from andrographis bark)
- Parthenolide (from feverfew leaves)

Secondary Actions of Bitter Herbs

Bitter herbs often have secondary actions, which may help determine the exact bitter to choose for an individual.

- Bitter relaxing nervines—hops, motherwort, blue vervain, chamomile, damiana, lavender, wood betony
- Bitter antimicrobials—goldenseal, Oregon grape, andrographis
- Bitter mood elevators—damiana, gentian
- Bitter stimulants—coffee, yerba mate, guarana, kola
- Warming bitters—angelica, sweet flag, calendula
- Cooling bitters—wormwood, feverfew
- Bitter anti-inflammatories—yarrow flower, chamomile, calendula
- Bitter carminatives—angelica, chamomile, lavender, hops

Herbal Bitters Blend

This is a very bitter combination, best taken as a tincture, but the cinnamon, angelica, and peppermint relieve gas and provide a strong flavor that will make it more palatable. The tinctures listed below are all 1:2 strength—1 part dried herb (in grams) to 2 parts alcohol (in milliliters).

+ 15 mL angelica root
+ 15 mL artichoke leaf
+ 10 mL burdock root
+ 10 mL Oregon grape
+ 10 mL bitter melon
+ 10 mL cinnamon
+ 5 mL andrographis
+ 5 mL condor vine
+ 5 mL goldenseal
+ 5 mL bitter orange
+ 5 mL wormwood
+ 5 mL peppermint

Take ½ teaspoon of the tincture blend in ¼ cup water before meals, two or three times daily.

Stomach Settler Seed Sprinkle

This is a delicious blend of flavors to use as a condiment on food; it is easily made by combining aromatic seeds with roughly ground seaweed and grinding it in a pepper grinder. Use any combination of ajwan, anise, black pepper, caraway, celery, coriander, cumin, dill, fennel, fenugreek, mustard, and nigella. Do not grind in advance, as the volatile oils evaporate quickly and the medicine is dissipated. Coarse sea salt or dulse (seaweed) can also be added, especially if you are thirsty or dehydrated, as it will help you hold water in the body. Toasted sesame seeds make a tasty addition to this as well, for a variation on gomasio.

Carminative Chai Tea

This is a rich and delicious tea that we enjoy in our household often. You can make a large pan of it and cool it off without adding the milk, then keep it in the fridge to add milk as desired for a cold drink, or even take the concentrated herbal decoction with or without the tea added, cool it off, and dilute it with sparkling mineral water for a refreshing summer drink.

+ 2- to 3-inch piece fresh gingerroot
+ 1 tablespoon cardamom seed
+ 1 teaspoon fennel seed
+ 1 teaspoon orange peel
+ 1 teaspoon clove bud
+ ½ teaspoon black peppercorns
+ 2 star anise pods
+ 1 stick cinnamon
+ ¼ teaspoon powdered nutmeg
+ 1–2 tablespoons black tea or rooibos leaves
+ 3 cups hot milk (animal or plant based)

1. Chop the ginger into small pieces (no need to peel it). Transfer to a heavy-bottomed pan and add 1 quart water. Cover with a lid and bring to a low boil.
2. Simmer for 5–10 minutes while you grind the cardamom seed, fennel seed, orange peel, clove bud, black peppercorns, star anise pods, and cinnamon stick with a heavy mortar and pestle or an electric coffee grinder.
3. Add the ground spices, including the nutmeg, to the ginger decoction, put the lid back on, and simmer for another 5 minutes.
4. Turn the heat off and add the black tea or rooibos.
5. Cover again and steep for 5 minutes more.
6. Add the hot milk and bring back to a light simmer before serving, strained well and sweetened to taste.

Cannabis and Appetite Promotion

Medical cannabis may be useful in enhancing appetite. Endocannabinoids are neuromodulators made by the nervous system that, among many other positive and beneficial effects, act to enhance appetite in animals and humans. We make cannabinoids in our cells (*endo* means "within"), and we have receptor sites that respond to cannabinoids, whether our own or from plants. Ghrelin is an appetite-promoting peptide that is secreted from the stomach, and THC, the psychotropic compound found in cannabis, is known to promote this secretion.

Dosing. The dose should be the lowest that produces therapeutic benefit without associated adverse effects. Start low and go slow. Doses of up to 20–30 mg THC daily are usually safe, but the upper dose range will produce notable psychoactivity and risk of adverse effects. Do not confuse psychoactivity with effectiveness; just because you are feeling "high" does not mean you have a good-quality medicine. See page 134 for specific information on dosage.

Note that this herb is not legal for use in all parts of the US and not at all in some countries. You should know the legal status of your jurisdiction before using this herb. In Canada, where I practice, it is entirely legal and it is very helpful to a lot of people.

Orthorexia

The term *orthorexia* comes from the Greek word *orthos* (straight, proper) and *orexia* (appetite). It was coined for the first time in 1997 by Dr. Steve Bratman and refers to the pathological obsession for biologically or ideologically pure food, which leads to significant dietary restrictions. Orthorexic patients exclude from their diets any foods that they consider to be impure. Strict maintenance of a diet having these restrictions may cause nutritional deficits and weight loss.

Cancer patients may be particularly vulnerable to slipping into orthorexic behaviors when they implement stringent detoxification diets, undertake extensive juicing or fasting programs, and feel guilty or inadequate when they are unable to meet their own high standards.

Doctors, nutritionists, and psychologists have collaborated to design the Eating Habits Questionnaire (EHQ) to identify individuals with behaviors, thoughts, and feelings that may indicate a problematic fixation on healthy eating. The EHQ is a 21-item reference range that contains three subscales measuring knowledge of healthy eating, problems associated with healthy eating, and feeling positively about healthy eating. Practitioners can use this to help establish boundaries around food choices.

Current best practices suggest that orthorexia can successfully be treated with a combination of cognitive-behavioral therapy, education, and management of weight loss. Medications such as antidepressants, especially serotonin reuptake inhibitors, antipsychotics such as olanzapine to decrease the obsessive nature of food-related thinking, or even occasionally steroids may be used, but these merely suppress the symptoms and do not help the patient build a healthy eating plan or a healthy relationship to food in general.

Holistic Strategies for Treating Orthorexia

Cognitive-behavioral therapy, nutritional counseling, meditation and other stress-release practices, exercise, and psychotherapy may all be useful techniques to manage obsessive healthy eating. The patient may also be encouraged to enroll in whole-food cooking classes to improve their kitchen skills and kitchen confidence.

I am not a big fan of long-term specialized or restrictive diets even when the science is solid and the principles and ideas have merit. It is important to be able to have a treat or a celebration meal sometimes, as long as the daily diet principles are sound. I don't think it is terribly healthy to go through life "on a diet," but it is better, rather, to find a way of eating that is sound in principle, is tailored to your personal preferences and needs, and still gives you pleasure and companionship at the table. That may sound like a tall order, but in fact it boils down to common sense. Not all of the below is possible for everyone, but every little bit helps. A more plant-based diet is quite a lot cheaper than an animal-based one; the cost savings may allow you to purchase more organic and whole foods.

Some Ground Rules for Healthy Eating

- Eat only whole foods—(almost) nothing from a package, can, or box.
- Buy organic—it is worth paying extra to avoid the toxic residues of agrochemicals.
- Eat lots and lots of vegetables. Aim for seven or eight servings daily, including at least two or three green leafy vegetables, plus a couple of servings of fruit daily.
- Eat the rainbow—aim for five colors on the plate.
- Eat only high-quality, grass-fed, or wild meats, and no more than once or twice a week.
- Eat wild-caught fish once or twice a week.
- Eat very few carbohydrates and get your energy from high-quality protein, fats, and small amounts of whole grains or starchy vegetables (two or three servings daily of starch or carbohydrates is plenty for most people).
- Eat protein and vegetables in the daytime, and save the carbohydrates or starch till later in the day; they tend to spike and drop the blood sugar, making you drowsy.

RECONSIDER INTERMITTENT FASTING

Although the practice of intermittent fasting has gained a lot of popularity in the cancer field, and with good reason, if you are depleted, debilitated, or orthorexic, then fasting is possibly not the best plan. You may need to be built up, nourished, and restored, and this may mean small and frequent meals, although a 10- to 12-hour (overnight) fast is achievable for most people anyway.

Lymphedema

Lymphedema is an abnormal buildup of fluid in soft tissues due to a blockage in the lymphatic system, a network of vessels that run parallel to veins. Like veins, the lymphatic vessels drain fluids from the tissues and carry them back to the heart. Lymphedema is usually considered a chronic and incurable condition that requires lifelong management. Lymph fluid is basically serum—blood without cells—and as it passes through nodes (intersections where numerous vessels come together), the lymphocytes (white blood cells in the nodes) are exposed to pathogens and will mount an immune response in defense.

Because cancer can spread via lymph vessels, the nodes adjacent to a tumor may be surgically removed and assessed for the presence of cancer cells to determine the stage of the tumor. However, when the lymph nodes are removed, lymphatic fluid collects in the surrounding tissues and swelling occurs. Lymphedema may develop promptly after surgery or radiation therapy, but more commonly it takes 2–5 years or more to become apparent. Because it is common to remove lymph nodes in the armpit and groin, lymphedema most often affects the arms and legs, but it can also occur in the neck, face, mouth, abdomen, or other parts of the body. The cancers most commonly associated with subsequent lymphedema are breast, gynecologic, prostate, and head and neck cancers as well as melanoma, and other skin cancers.

Lymphedema is seen less today than it used to be due to improved surgical procedures. In the past, anywhere from 20–30 or more lymph nodes could be removed, sometimes only to discover that none carried cancer cells. Modern techniques include sentinel node biopsy whereby a dye is injected into the lymphatic system, and only those nodes that take up the most dye are removed and screened. If they prove negative for cancer cells, then it is highly likely that other adjacent nodes will also be negative and no more need to be removed. If the sentinel nodes are positive, then further lymph bed dissection may be done.

Symptoms of Lymphedema

- Swelling, loss of mobility
- Throbbing pain
- Tight, shiny, warm, or red skin
- Hardened skin, or skin that does not indent when pressed
- Thickening skin

- Skin that may look like an orange peel (swollen with small indentations)
- Small blisters that leak clear fluid

Stages of Lymphedema

Early identification of lymphedema is key to successful treatment. Lymphedema is usually classified from stages 0 to 3, with increasing symptoms and severity. Stage 0 may not display overt swelling, although there may be heaviness or aching in the affected body part, which can last for months or years. In stage 1, swelling becomes visible but can be reduced by elevating the limb and with lymph drainage massage and compression bandaging. There may be visible indentation in the skin when it is pressed upon, but there are few visible signs of skin thickening and scarring. By the time there is progression to stage 2, elevation will no longer drain fluid from the limb, the skin may or may not indent when it is pressed, and there is moderate to severe skin thickening. In stage 3, the skin becomes notably thickened and hardened, there is pronounced swelling and disablement, and there may be pain from the swelling. Stage 0 or 1 lymphedema can realistically be treated with an expectation of good and durable results. Stage 2 may not achieve resolution but is manageable with ongoing care. Full recovery from stage 3 lymphedema is not expected but symptomatic improvement may be achieved.

Moving Lymph Fluid Is Beneficial

Because cancer can spread through the lymph system, there is an erroneous belief that moving lymph fluid with herbs, lymphatic drainage massage, sauna, and so on may be a risk for metastases. In fact, this is not true. If lymphocytes are going to generate effective immune responses, then they need to be exposed to the trigger proteins that activate them, and this will only happen when lymph is flowing through nodes. This also means lymph node removal compromises lymphocyte activation and immune surveillance.

Lymph, like all other fluids in the body, is intended to flow and move. It is sometimes called the "internal ocean" because it has the same electrolytes and water ratio as the sea, and it flushes and detoxifies the tissues. Blockages of lymph flow, such as happen in cancer, can be considered a condition of stagnation or congestion in the tissues. Flushing them, stimulating the lymph flow, is a great way to remove toxicity, draining fluids back to the systemic circulation for filtering through the liver.

Physical Treatments for Lymphedema

- Manual lymphatic drainage is a specialized massage technique that gently encourages lymphatic flow and reduces swelling.
- Aerobic exercise will get the blood flowing and will, by default, support lymph flow.

- Compression sleeves, socks, and bandages may be helpful to prevent tissues refilling too quickly after a drainage treatment.
- Complete decongestive therapy is a protocol that combines skin care, manual lymphatic drainage, exercise, and compression.
- Elevation: Keeping your affected limb raised helps reduce swelling and encourages fluid drainage through the lymphatic system. It may be easy enough to put your foot up, but arms can be more difficult.
- Dry skin brushing with a natural bristle brush can help move lymph. Use long, sweeping strokes up the legs and arms and abdomen, always moving toward the heart. Do this daily before a shower and finish with a seaweed-based lotion to continue the effect.
- Infrared sauna and the rebounder trampoline are other ways of enhancing lymph flow.
- Low-beam laser treatments and cold laser treatments are showing promise but are not routinely used yet.

Herbal Treatments for Lymphedema

Herbal diuretics will help remove fluids from the body. They may function as kidney-secretory stimulants, such as horseradish root or juniper berry, which slightly irritate the kidney membranes and encourage secretions to flush it away. Others exert their diuretic qualities through the large sugars such as are found in marshmallow root, which are excreted into urine, where they exert an osmotic pull upon water and have a demulcent diuretic property as a result.

The purpose of using diuretic herbs in managing lymphedema is to encourage fluid elimination though the kidneys; in the process, excess fluid from the tissues will be drawn through lymph back into the bloodstream, to the kidneys, and hence out of the body. Clinical studies into the efficacy of herbal diuretics for managing lymphedema are not available, although coumarin and flavonoids have been shown to reduce swelling in all types of lymphedema; traditional uses of diuretic herbs support the idea that they can be gently encouraging to lymph flow and promote drainage. In European health spas, specialized massage techniques are combined with herbal infused oils and essential oils to promote lymphatic drainage and encourage proper lymph flow.

Prescription diuretics are not usually recommended, because as they strongly remove excess water from tissues, they may leave proteins behind, which then draw water back to the affected area and contribute to increased lymphedema volume, increased fibrosis, and local inflammation. This is not likely to be a concern with the herbs, which have a much gentler action, especially in the case of cleavers, which actively removes the proteins from the tissues as well. Prescription diuretic use is usually reserved for specific cases where comorbidities may make them more valuable, such as with congestive heart failure.

Herbal Formula for Moving Lymph and Stimulating Lymphocytes

This formula is a mix of tinctures. The ingredients listed below are tinctures prepared from dried herbs extracted at a 1:2 ratio in alcohol and water (except as noted). As an alternative, you can create a tea mix with the dried herbs. Use the same proportions of herbs listed here; simply measure in grams rather than milliliters. Prepare the tea with 1 heaping teaspoon of the herb mixture per cup of boiling water, two or three times daily.

+ 20 mL cleavers
+ 20 mL calendula
+ 10 mL butcher's broom
+ 10 mL red root
+ 10 mL violet
+ 10 mL wild pansy
+ 10 mL blue flag
+ 10 mL pokeroot (1:10 extract from fresh root; use caution with dosing, as this is a toxic herb)

Take 1 teaspoon of the tincture mix in water between meals, two or three times daily. If there is any bowel disturbance, reduce the amount of pokeroot by half.

CLEAVERS (*GALIUM APARINE*)

Cleavers is a diuretic herb that functions to increase lymphatic fluid return into systemic circulation, a feature that raises blood pressure, a result of which is increased glomerular filtration in the kidney and increased urine production to remove fluids and lower the blood pressure again. Cleavers is the archetypal lymph-moving herb. Its constituents are largely water soluble and include iridoids, hydroxycinnamic acid derivatives, caffeic acid derivatives, tannins, flavonoids, and sugars. Cleavers has traditionally been used as a relaxing diuretic that is soothing for the urinary tract, indicated in cystitis, urethritis, prostatitis, kidney infections, and kidney deficiency. It's also specifically used to clear away stagnation and congestion in the lymphatic system, eliminate stasis, and detoxify the body. It's used to increase lymphatic drainage and reduce lymphatic congestion (enlarged lymph nodes), especially in the pelvis and urinary tract.

Cleavers stimulates the activation of white blood cells and supports lymphocyte functions. It promotes macrophages in interstitial fluids to take up albumin that has leached out of blood vessels and is exerting osmotic pull in the tissues. Removing the albumin frees fluids to enter the lymphatic vessels and be transported away back to systemic circulation.

Preliminary studies have also demonstrated some anticancer effects of cleavers, possibly attributed to their flavonoids. One study suggested anticancer effects against breast cancer cells without impairing normal breast epithelial cells, as well as the ability to induce nonapoptotic cell death, which may enable the killing of apoptosis-resistant breast cancer cells.

Cleavers tends to grow freely and abundantly in many parts of the world, and aerial parts can be readily harvested in early spring before it blossoms. It can be chopped up and dried for later use, but it is also an excellent herb to juice and freeze in ice cube trays, which can be stored and taken out for use as needed. One or two ice cubes per day melted into your smoothie or added to a bowl of soup is an easy prescription.

BUTCHER'S BROOM (*RUSCUS ACULEATUS*)

Butcher's broom is a small evergreen shrub that has traditionally been recommended for chronic venous insufficiency, varicose veins, varicose ulcers, lymphedema, hemorrhoids, and the congestive (fluid-retention) symptoms of premenstrual syndrome. The root contains steroidal compounds comprising the aglycones ruscogenin and neoruscogenin and their glycosides, as well as triterpene steroids. It increases tensile strength of veins and strengthens capillary integrity. Butcher's broom improves several markers of venous health and function, including a decrease in plasma viscosity and reduction in red cell damage and in red cell aggregation.

CALENDULA (*CALENDULA OFFICINALIS*)

The bright orange flowers comprise the medicine; they hold a range of water-soluble and non-water-soluble constituents, including flavonoids, carotenoids, terpene resins, coumarins, volatile oils, amino acids, and lipids. This flower is used as an anti-inflammatory, antiviral, and antifungal; in the treatment of poorly healing wounds, minor burns, bruises, and rashes; and also in the treatment of inflammation of the oral and pharyngeal mucosa, gastritis, and colitis.

In cancer care, extensive preclinical research supports using this herb to normalize and stabilize cancer-control pathways. For example, the triterpene glycosides induce cell cycle arrest (inhibit cell replication) and apoptosis (cell death) and have antimetastatic effects in animals.

In one study where calendula lotion was compared to trolamine (Biafine), a standard pharmaceutical cream for radiation burns, acute dermatitis was significantly lower in the patients using calendula than in those using trolamine. Moreover, patients applying calendula had less-frequent interruption of radiotherapy and significantly less radiation-induced pain. Calendula was considered to be more difficult to apply, but self-assessed satisfaction was greater. The authors noted that increasing body mass index and prior use of chemotherapy before radiotherapy were both significant prognostic factors for acute dermatitis. In such patients, overweight and pretreated with chemotherapy, it is probably worth using calendula preemptively over a radiation site to reduce risk.

Skin Lotion for Lymph Drainage

This formula combines the cooling, soothing, and healing properties of aloe with the blood-cleansing and drainage properties of cleavers and pokeroot. Cleavers is traditionally used as a cool compress over lymph swelling, and pokeroot assists with penetration of the lotion through the skin. The essential oils chosen for this lotion are traditionally used for lymphatic drainage in European spas, where they are incorporated into cellulite treatments.

+ 75 g aloe gel
+ 20 mL cleavers-infused oil
+ 5 mL pokeroot-infused oil
+ 10 drops each essential oils of pink grapefruit, cypress, bay laurel, fennel

Combine all ingredients. Apply this from the extremities toward the trunk with long, sweeping movements to aid lymph flow.

Skin Lotion for Lymph Node Stimulation

This lotion is penetrating and decongesting, stimulating lymph nodes to drain and lymphocytes to activate.

+ 50 g neutral base cream (can be purchased from herbal suppliers, or use a simple calendula cream from a health food store)
+ 10 mL chaparral tincture
+ 10 mL pokeroot tincture
+ 10 mL calendula-infused oil
+ 10 mL nigella-infused oil
+ 10 mL arnica flower–infused oil
+ 10 drops each essential oils of bay laurel, cypress, ginger, grapefruit, rosemary, frankincense

Stir the tinctures and infused oils into the base cream. This will make it runnier—a lotion, not a cream. Apply two or three times daily over congested lymph nodes or over areas of lymphedema.

It is worth noting that another study, a blind, randomized clinical trial of more than 400 people, looked at a popular proprietary commercial calendula cream versus a plain aqueous cream in reducing the risk of severe acute radiation skin reactions after radiotherapy for breast cancer and found no statistical difference. However, the patients reported low levels of skin-related symptoms overall, so it is hard to say if the herb may be more successful in more acute conditions.

RED ROOT (*CEANOTHUS AMERICANUS*)

Red root is a warming lymphagogue (promotes flow of lymph fluid) that is indicated for buildup of fluids, mucus congestion of the upper respiratory tract and lungs, the phlegmatic state in humoral medicine, and what is called damp stagnation in Traditional Chinese Medicine or kapha excess in Ayurvedic medicine, especially when accompanied by sluggishness, melancholy, and apathy (mental/emotional stagnation). Red root has tannins in the root bark that tighten and tone tissues, as well as saponins that are anti-inflammatory, making red root an excellent remedy for congestion and fluid stagnation of all sorts. It is traditionally used for chronic sore throats, tonsillitis and enlarged lymph nodes, lymphedema, and restoring the spleen after the acute phase of mononucleosis. Red root can help resolve depression, lethargy, and lack of drive due to emotional blockage. Key indications for red root are swollen, tender lymph nodes, enlarged tonsils, fluid retention in the limbs or extremities, or an enlarged, swollen tongue with a dirty white or yellow coating.

OTHER HERBS FOR LYMPHEDEMA

Violet, wild pansy, and blue flag are all traditional "alteratives" or depurative (blood-cleansing) herbs with a reputation for moving lymph through the nodes, activating lymphocytes, aiding in toxin removal by the liver, and promoting elimination. They are considered safe but may occasionally drive toxins and stagnation to the surface and bring up boils or pimples as they cleanse the tissues. Other lymphagogue herbs that could be used internally to alleviate congestion include echinacea, burdock root, and ocotillo bark.

Mouth Sores

Patients going through chemotherapy and radiation are particularly susceptible to mouth sores. The surface layer of cells lining the mouth is naturally replaced every 2½ hours or so, and this rapid turnover rate makes the cells especially vulnerable to damage from systemic chemotherapy and from local radiation, which impairs cell turnover. Because conventional chemotherapy and radiation impair immune cells, there is higher risk of local infections in the mouth sores. Vomiting from chemotherapy may also bring acids in contact with the oral mucosa, and some of the new immunotherapy drugs for cancer also induce mouth sores and impair the innate healing ability of the tissues.

Mouth sores may occur on any of the soft tissues of the mouth, including inside the lips and on the gums, tongue, roof, or floor of the mouth. Sores can also extend onto the tonsils and into the esophagus, making swallowing painful. Severity is variable, from a mild discomfort all the way to severe pain that may make a patient unable to continue treatment. Sores typically develop within 2–4 days of commencing treatment and may get worse for up to a week after discontinuation of treatment. Usually within 2–4 weeks after completing treatment, mouth sores from chemotherapy are largely resolved, but tenderness and a bad taste in the mouth may persist for weeks or months. Mouth sores from radiation may last 4–6 weeks after the last radiation treatment. Mouth sores are also common after a bone marrow transplant, as the immune system is intentionally suppressed, and can continue as long as the patient uses immunosuppressant drugs.

Chemotherapies Most Likely to Contribute to Mouth Sores*

- Capecitabine
- Cisplatin
- Cytarabine
- Doxorubicin
- Etoposide
- Fluorouracil
- Methotrexate

*According to the Mayo Clinic

Preventing Mouth Sores

Fortunately, there are a few ways to help prevent mouth sores.

Get a dental checkup. Before commencing chemotherapy or oral radiation treatment, you should have a full dental checkup and deep cleaning. This might also be a good opportunity for a fluoride treatment to resist dental decay. All root canals and crowns should be carefully inspected. If there is chronic inflammation or an infection that can't be fixed, you may want to consider pulling the tooth so it does not get further infected later on during chemotherapy if the immune system is low.

Chew on ice chips. Chewing on ice chips or rinsing repeatedly with iced water for up to an hour after receiving chemotherapy may reduce blood flow to the oral mucosa and reduce delivery of drugs that cause the tissue breakdown.

Increase vitamin B intake. A deficiency of B vitamins can contribute to stomatitis (inflammation and cracking in the corners of the mouth), so a high-potency B-complex supplement may be helpful. The US FDA-recommended intake of B vitamins is the lowest possible amount required for normal healthy body functions, and it does not take into account increased need in specific individual cases. Because these vitamins are all water soluble, and hence inherently safe as they do not accumulate in the body, many practitioners recommend doubling these doses or more in cancer care.

Good Food Sources of B Vitamins

- Dairy products
- Eggs
- Fish and seafood (especially clams)
- Leafy green vegetables
- Legumes (beans, peas)
- Liver and meat (from poultry, beef, lamb, pork)
- Nutritional yeast
- Nuts
- Potatoes
- Whole grains

Conventional Treatment of Mouth Sores

Conventional treatment of mouth sores includes good oral hygiene, saline washes, and alcohol washes. A steroid mouthwash may be recommended in severe cases. For patients with known oral herpes simplex infections, an antiviral may be used.

Palifermin (Kepivance) may also be prescribed. This is given intravenously to stimulate the growth of cells in the mouths of people who receive bone marrow transplants. It acts as a keratinocyte growth factor promoter. Side effects are common and may include red, dry, or itchy skin rash, cracked lips, pancreatitis leading to bloating, indigestion, fatty stools, loss of appetite, sweating, abdominal pain, weight loss, fevers, peripheral edema (swelling of the hands, arms, legs, ankles, and feet), and risk of birth defects in children conceived while either the mother or the father is using this drug.

Holistic Strategies for Treating Mouth Sores

Instead of using saline or steroid mouthwashes, or even stronger drugs, you may be able to achieve good symptom management with natural remedies.

- Apply manuka honey or pure propolis to the sores to speed healing.
- Use slippery elm or licorice lozenges to soothe the throat, or echinacea lozenges for their saliva-inducing effect; if sores become infected, use zinc lozenges.
- Take coenzyme Q10 in doses of 100 milligrams two or three times daily to help reduce bleeding of the gums.
- Use the softest toothbrush you can find, and a natural toothpaste. You may even want to make your own tooth powder with ½ teaspoon baking soda and 1 drop of essential oil of peppermint.
- Brush and floss after every meal, or at least rinse well if you cannot brush. Cut foods into small pieces and choose soft foods that are easy to chew, such as congee (rice porridge), oatmeal, poached eggs, and poached fish.

- Avoid foods that may cause irritation to the mouth, including citrus fruits or juices (such as orange, tangerine, grapefruit); spicy or salty foods; and rough, coarse, or dry foods (such as raw vegetables, corn chips, crackers, toast).
- Choose liquid nutrition, such as soups, green juices, and smoothies. Serve foods cool or at room temperature; hot foods may irritate the mouth and throat. Frozen fruits like blueberries and mango are great.
- Add sauces or gravies to food to make them easier to swallow.
- Drink from a straw to reduce exposure of sore areas to the liquid.

PREVENTIVE MEASURES FOR CARRIERS OF HERPES SIMPLEX

In people who carry the herpes simplex (cold sore) virus, outbreaks are likely while they're undergoing chemotherapy or oral radiation treatment. In fact, treatment with an antiviral drug is usually part of the chemotherapy protocol and antivirals are prescribed routinely. As a preventive, patients should avoid foods rich in the amino acid arginine and emphasize those rich in lysine. Arginine-rich proteins are required for viral replication, and the presence of a high lysine content seems to be antiviral by antagonizing (counteracting) the metabolism of arginine. The two amino acids compete for intestinal absorption.

Boost your lysine intake. Consider supplementing with 500 milligrams of lysine two to four times daily. High doses like this over many months may elevate cholesterol, so monitor cholesterol levels periodically. Choose foods that are high in lysine. This includes fruits and vegetables, such as apricots, avocados, beets, green and red peppers, leeks, mangoes, pears, potatoes, and tomatoes; legumes, such as black beans, edamame, kidney beans, navy beans, soybeans, tempeh, and tofu; and certain nuts and seeds, such as pumpkin seeds, pistachios, cashews, macadamia nuts, quinoa, and amaranth.

Significantly reduce or avoid foods that are high in arginine. This includes most nuts (almonds, Brazil nuts, filberts, peanuts, walnuts), bacon, gelatin, chocolate, sesame seeds, sunflower seeds, yeast extract, bleached flour, refined sugars, and all sugar-rich foods.

Foods that are moderately high in arginine, which can be eaten with discretion, include chicken; shellfish; chickpeas, lentils, and all other legumes/pulses; liver; pork; salmon; sardines; turkey; and oats, corn, rice, and all other grains.

TREATING ORAL THRUSH

Oral thrush or yeast infection can be a complicating factor with mouth sores. Yeast infections are more common when the immune system is depleted and after antibiotics have deranged the microbiome (gut flora). White patches on the oral mucosa and a sour, moldy taste in the mouth are indications to treat it with antifungal tinctures added to the mouthwash, such as goldenseal, oregano, Oregon grape, taheebo, thuja, or thyme.

Soothing and Healing Mouthwash

- 30 mL colloidal silver solution at 10 ppm
- 20 mL aloe gel
- 10 mL calendula juice
- 10 mL gotu kola tincture
- 10 mL licorice tincture
- 5 mL propolis tincture
- 5 mL goldenseal tincture
- 5 mL myrrh tincture
- 5 mL frankincense hydrosol

This formula can be diluted with a marshmallow leaf tea at a 1:2 ratio (10 mL formula to 20 mL tea) and used as a mouthwash for swilling and spitting.

In this formula, the colloidal silver is strongly antimicrobial and included to prevent secondary infections, and it reduces sensations of burning and irritation. Propolis, goldenseal, and myrrh tinctures are likewise antimicrobial. Myrrh is leukocytic, drawing white blood cells to tissues where it is applied. Aloe gel and calendula juice are soothing, promote tissue healing, and relieve burning pain in tissues they come into contact with. Licorice is antimicrobial, soothing, healing, and anti-inflammatory. Licorice is also antiviral and may help reduce outbreaks of herpes simplex. Gotu kola promotes repair of the lining of the mouth and healing of sores. Frankincense has powerful anticancer and anti-inflammatory actions, though it doesn't taste great.

Rooty Fruity Herbal Tea Frozen Pops

An ice pop feels so good in a sore mouth! In this recipe, marshmallow root brings mucilage to soothe and heal the mouth, the berries provide polyphenols and flavonoids, and the licorice is an adaptogen to support the immune system, as well as having mucilage. And it tastes good!

- 35 g chopped, dried marshmallow root
- 40 g any combination of dried blueberries, cherries, cranberries, and blackberries
- 20 g each of dried licorice root, elderberries, and goji berries
- ¾ cup (200 mL) manuka honey
- 20 drops mandarin or tangerine essential oil

1. Steep the chopped, dried marshmallow root overnight in 1 cup (250 mL) of cold water. Press out, keep the liquid, and discard the marshmallow root.
2. Add all the fruit and licorice root to 3⅔ cups of cold water. Bring to a boil, covered, and decoct (simmer very low) until it reduces down to 2 cups (500 mL). Strain and press out the liquid.
3. Add the honey while the decoction is still warm, then add the marshmallow tea.
4. Allow to cool, then add the mandarin or tangerine essential oil and stir well.
5. Pour into ice pop molds and freeze. Suck on the pops as desired.

Other Herbs for Mouth Sores

Some other herbs and constituents showing promise in treating chemotherapy- or radiotherapy-induced mouth sores and mucositis include yarrow, isatis (woad), curcumin (from turmeric), chamomile, psyllium husk gel, and silymarin (from milk thistle). There is even a 1995 study suggesting use of chewed capsaicin taffy to reduce oral pain from mucositis. Honey lozenges or a honey water mouthwash may also be helpful in reducing inflammation and infection.

Cracked Lips

Like the oral mucosa, the lips are particularly vulnerable to damage from chemotherapy. The hard, dry, outer layer of skin (called the stratum corneum) is very thin on the lips (this is why the lips are soft), so they are less protected from sunlight, heat and cold, cracking, or being burned from vomiting. Lips also lack sebaceous glands, so they cannot make their own lubricant as the skin elsewhere on the body does. The lips are reliant on moisture from saliva, and if you have a dry mouth from chemotherapy, this also means dry lips.

The dry air of hospitals and nursing homes can aggravate chapped lips, as can a dry wind or strong sunlight. There are no truly natural sunblocks for lips, or for applying to the skin in general, except zinc oxide or titanium dioxide, and those tend to leave a white chalkiness on the surface. A commercial SPF lip cover is a good idea if your lips are sun sensitive.

Holistic Strategies for Treating Chapped Lips

Keep well hydrated by drinking lots of plain water. Ensure you have a high intake of essential fatty acids (e.g., evening primrose oil and fish oils), as these are incorporated into the cell membrane and are required for the cell to take up and hold water. There are two main types of fish oil—EPA (eicosapentaenoic acid) and DHA (docosahexaenoic acid)—and you need both in your supplement. Aim for at least 750–1,000 milligrams of EPA and 350–500 milligrams of DHA daily. If you are bothered by fishy burps, then keep the supplement in the fridge or even the freezer and always take it with food and followed by food.

Note: Fish oil is not the same as fish liver oil, which is a source of vitamin A and D and not so high in omega-3 fatty acids.

The very best thing to put on cracked or peeling lips is lanolin—the fat from sheep wool. It is sold in pharmacies as a nipple balm for nursing mothers, and people use it on cracked heels and very dry skin. A small amount of lanolin can be incorporated into a lip balm. If you are strictly vegetarian, then shea or cocoa butter is a good substitute.

Healing Lip Balm

This recipe will make around 70 grams (2½ oz.). You can purchase push-up tubes for lip balms and pour carefully with a steady hand, or you can use small glass jars.

- + 15 g coconut oil
- + 10 g beeswax
- + 10 g cocoa butter
- + 10 g shea butter
- + 5 g argan butter
- + 4 g lanolin (or extra shea or cocoa butter, for vegans)
- + 5 mL babassu oil
- + 2 mL sea buckthorn oil

Melt the coconut oil, beeswax, cocoa butter, shea butter, argan butter, and lanolin, then stir in the babassu oil and sea buckthorn oil. Pour into containers and let cool.

Argan seed oil is rich in essential fatty acids and is more resistant to oxidation than olive oil. The butter moisturizes and deeply nourishes the skin and strengthens its elasticity.

Babassu seeds yield an oil that is 40–48 percent lauric acid, making it useful against yeast (candida) infections. It is an effective emollient, soothing, protective, and nongreasy; it melts upon contact with the skin and penetrates quickly.

Sea buckthorn oil is expressed from the fruit pulp or seed and is rich in fatty acids that contribute to faster epithelial cell growth and wound healing. The pressed oil contains anti-inflammatory phytosterols, which promote factors that control and regulate the laying down of connective tissue matrix and control new blood vessel growth at the site of an injury, wound, or lesion. It also possesses antioxidant properties, with studies showing significant increase in bioactive glutathione levels and reduced production of reactive oxygen species in wound granulation tissue. The oil also has antibacterial activity.

Mineralizing Tea for Replenishing after Vomiting

- + 25 g alfalfa
- + 25 g dandelion leaf
- + 25 g horsetail
- + 25 g nettles
- + 25 g oat straw
- + 25 g plantain
- + 25 g red clover
- + 25 g rose hips

Blend the herbs together and store in an airtight container. When needed, steep 2 tablespoons of the herb blend in 2 cups boiling water for at least 15 minutes. Add lemon juice or mint for flavor.

Nausea and Vomiting

For the most part, nausea and vomiting are relatively short-lived concerns, occurring mostly during the immediate aftermath of a chemotherapy or radiation treatment. However, they can be truly miserable while they last and may also contribute to significant loss of appetite and weight loss.

Practical Strategies for Counteracting Nausea

- Try easy-to-digest food such as clear liquids, broths, light egg custards, toast, rice, porridge with steel-cut oats or rice, and crackers.
- Drink smoothies to get some concentrated nutrition with minimal digestive effort.
- Avoid foods that are fried, greasy, very sweet, spicy, hot, or strongly flavored.
- Eat small, frequent meals.
- Take sips of water, smoothies, or herbal teas throughout the day.
- Smell citrus fruit such as tangerine or orange. Even just peeling an orange can help, or use sweet orange essential oil in a diffuser in the room.
- Drink chamomile or mint tea, or ginger if it isn't too spicy for a sensitive stomach.
- Try wearing acupressure wrist bands, sold for motion sickness.

Herbal Formula for Nausea and Vomiting

All ingredients listed below are tinctures made at a 1:2 ratio of herbs to alcohol.

+ 25 mL chamomile
+ 25 mL meadowsweet
+ 15 mL black horehound
+ 15 mL peppermint
+ 15 mL fennel
+ 5 mL ginger

Combine all tinctures. Mix ½ teaspoon of the tincture blend with ½ cup of water or herbal tea and take 1 tablespoon every 15–20 minutes as needed.

Experienced herbalists may incorporate belladonna (1:10 from dried root, 65% ethyl alcohol, using 2 mL belladonna per 100 mL tincture formula) to dry out secretions in the gut and reduce spasms. If belladonna is used, decrease the fennel to 13 mL. Belladonna is toxic and should be used only by practitioners. Reduce the dose volume or frequency if eyes or mouth feel dry.

Peppermint-Fennel Essential Oil Emulsion

This is one of the most powerful antispasmodic and antiemetic formulas I have ever come across; for upper or lower digestive gas and bloating, abdominal cramping, and nausea, this remedy is unparalleled. It features acacia powder as an emulsifying agent, which reduces the surface tension between the water and the oil, allowing them to mix. Using acacia powder is a way to make an essential oil product for internal use. Do not use this formula if you have reflux, as peppermint can open the esophageal sphincter and worsen the symptoms.

*Caution: Professional supervision is recommended for using most essential oils internally. This particular formula is safe at this dilution of 2 percent, but not all volatile oils are.

+ 10 g acacia powder
+ 10 mL peppermint essential oil
+ 10 mL fennel essential oil
+ 20 mL water

The proportions for this emulsion are 1:2:2 (that is, 10 g acacia powder, 20 mL essential oil, and 20 mL water).

1. Place the acacia powder and essential oils in a bone-dry, smooth ceramic mortar and stir with a pestle until they're thoroughly mixed.
2. Add the water and stir in one direction only, until the mixture emulsifies and "clicks"—it will have a sticky consistency and will pull away from the walls of the mortar with an audible "click."
3. Dilute this primary emulsion with 980 milliliters of pure water to yield a total of 1 liter of a 2 percent emulsion (safe for internal use). Take 1 teaspoon as needed in ¼–½ cup of water. Be careful—it is strong and can take your breath away!

Nephritis and Kidney Damage

The incidence of low-grade, chronic, progressive kidney failure in the population at large is surprisingly high, especially in our aging population. A slow decrease in kidney filtering capacity, the so-called glomerular filtration rate (GFR), is often part of the clinical picture of patients. Cancer patients are particularly susceptible to kidney damage. Many chemotherapy drugs, most notably the platinum drugs (carboplatin, cisplatin, oxaliplatin), as well as methotrexate and others, are profoundly damaging to kidney tubule-lining cells and can significantly compromise kidney function.

Herbs for Improved Kidney Function

Herbs that are taken by mouth, whether in tea, tincture, or capsule form, will all be absorbed in the enteric (intestinal) circulation and taken to the liver for filtering and processing. Residues or wastes from this process and from other metabolic functions of the body may then be eliminated into bile and the bowel and leave the body in the stool, or they may be dumped back into the bloodstream for eventual delivery to the kidneys, where a secondary elimination system will take them out in urine. Evidence-based medicine, over hundreds if not thousands of years, has validated and verified some herbs quite specifically to be supportive and healing in the kidneys. These include renal tonics or trophorestoratives, herbs that support tissue repair and are regenerative to kidney structure and function and can restore compromised GFR. Other herbs may be used as vulneraries to repair lining tissues and to heal lesions in the mucous membranes of the kidneys, ureters, bladder, and urethra; as demulcent (soothing) diuretics to support overall flushing of the system; and as cystorestoratives to improve tone and control to the bladder.

Horsetail, plantain, and corn silk (*Equisetum arvense*, *Plantago* spp., and *Zea mays*). This traditional triad of herbs has been used as a restorative and healing mix for kidney disease in folk medicine for hundreds of years. Horsetail is astringent, toning, and strengthening to kidney tissues and to connective tissues such as skin, hair, lungs, and bone. It restores integrity of the bladder outlet valve and improves muscle tone of the trigone (the neuromuscular zone comprising the bladder floor and involved with opening and closing the valve). Plantain is healing, soothing, tightening, toning, and strengthening to the tissues. A cooling herb, gentle and strong, it rebuilds the structure of the kidneys after chemotherapy. Corn silk is vulnerary, demulcent, and a gentle osmotic diuretic (pulls water into the tubules).

Pellitory (*Parietaria* spp.). This is in the nettle family (Urticaceae) and includes several species, of which *Parietaria judaica* and *P. officinalis* are the most common. *Parietaria judaica* grows on the Mediterranean coasts while *P. officinalis* grows farther north into France, Italy, and eastern Europe. They are used interchangeably in medicine. Clinical trials are lacking but evidence-based clinical practice supports pellitory's use.

Pellitory has traditionally been used as an antilithic, meaning it inhibits the formation of kidney stones by improving renal drainage and acts as a kidney trophorestorative (tissue restorative). *Parietaria judaica* has shown potent antimicrobial effects against eight microbial strains, and one extract also showed potent antifungal activity against *Candida albicans*. It has antiobesity and antidiabetic activity due to potential alpha-amylase and lipase enzyme inhibition, comparable to pharmaceuticals aimed at inhibiting fat uptake, such as orlistat.

Stinging nettle (*Urtica dioica*). This is one of the most useful herbal medicines because it is incredibly easy to grow, it can be found growing wild in many parts of the world, and every part of it has something to offer.

Nettle leaf is widely used as a diuretic, a nutritive edible spring green, and a traditional blood purifier. It can be eaten as a dried green added into soups, stews, casseroles, and chilis all winter.

Nettle root is known as a remedy for benign prostate enlargement, where it upregulates the binding capacity of sex hormone binding globulin (SHBG), a protein in blood that binds testosterone and prevents it from stimulating cells. While the hormone is bound to the protein it is inactive, so higher SHBG is a good thing in prostate enlargement or prostate cancer.

Nettle seed has a direct supportive effect on kidney function. Taken over the course of several weeks, nettle seed tincture can notably improve serum measurements like urea, nitrogen, creatinine, and glomerular filtration rate. Clinical studies are lacking, but herbalist Jonathan Treasure suggested in a case report that there are omega-3 unsaturated fatty acids that may contribute to the effect. A lectin isolated from the seeds of Turkish stinging nettle has shown immunomodulating effects, but it is not known if this is found in other species.

Cordyceps (*Cordyceps* spp.). This is one of the most powerful adaptogenic (stress-reducing) medicinal mushrooms. In the wild, this parasitic fungus grows on insects, which the fungus eventually consumes and kills. It's now mostly grown in laboratories, both for hygienic control and to avoid depleting it in the wild. Its natural habitat is high elevations of remote mountain peaks in northern China and Tibet—places where the air is thin. One thing it offers as a medicine is improved oxygenation of the blood by means of enhanced gaseous exchange in the lung. Cordyceps has a particular reputation for nourishing and healing kidney tissue and promoting kidney function. It is anabolic and rejuvenating to the body, has potent anticancer action from the fungal polysaccharides, and has been successful in clinical trials for chronic kidney failure. Doses of up to 5 grams daily of the mushroom and for up to 1 year were shown to be safe and without adverse side effects.

Hydrangea (*Hydrangea* spp.). The root of this wild American flowering shrub has a long folk history as a drainage herb for the kidneys, helping to better clear wastes. In clinical studies, the Chinese *Hydrangea paniculata* has been shown to protect kidney function because of its anti-inflammatory and antioxidant activities, and it has potential in the critical care of acute kidney infection leading to kidney failure.

Crataeva (*Crataeva nurvala*). Also known as varuna, this deciduous tree is found throughout India, especially in semiarid regions, as well as Southeast Asia and China. In Ayurvedic medicine, crataeva is widely used as a blood purifier and to treat heart and lung weakness, arthritis, memory loss, wound healing, and a weak immune system. In folk medicine, the leaves and inner bark were applied to the skin to treat abscesses and swellings, for relief of rheumatic joint pain, and across the abdomen to reduce enlarged spleen.

The root and bark are considered to have a particular affinity to kidney and bladder systems and to regulate endogenous oxalate synthesis. The plant is rich in saponins, triterpenes and phytosterols, tannins and flavonoids, alkaloids, and glucosinolates. Both the root and bark of *Crataeva nurvala* are laxative and help dissolve kidney stones—probably due to the high content of lupeol, a pentacyclic triterpene isolated from the root bark, which significantly minimizes the deposition of stone-forming constituents in kidneys. Crataeva is used for treating and preventing kidney stones or bladder stones and for prostatic enlargement. Crataeva also promotes appetite and increases the secretion of bile.

A 2004 rat study demonstrated that crataeva could significantly reduce symptoms of kidney dysfunction caused by chemotherapy. A crataeva tincture was administered orally for 10 days at either 250 or 500 mg/kg body weight, starting 5 days after administration of a single intraperitoneal dose of cisplatin (5 mg/kg). Kidney dysfunction was measured through assessing blood urea nitrogen, serum creatinine, and lipid peroxidation; oxidative stress was measured by assessing glutathione and catalase activity in the kidney cortex. The results demonstrated that both 250 and 500 mg/kg significantly lowered symptoms of cisplatin-induced dysfunction of kidney proximal tubule cells and increased glutathione and catalase activity, indicative of the antioxidant properties of *C. nurvala* stem bark extract.

Studies have suggested an active anticancer effect as well, possibly explained by the high lupeol content. In human hepatocellular carcinoma cells, lupeol inhibited cell growth and induced the apoptosis (cell death) by downregulation of "death receptor 3" expression. In animal studies, topical applications of lupeol at 40 mg/kg three times per week for 28 weeks significantly decreased tumor burden and slowed tumor growth, in part by targeting NF-κB signaling.

Beta-sitosterol. This is a phytosterol with antioxidant, anticancer, antidiabetic, androgenic (promotes testosterone), anti-HIV, cholesterol- and plaque-reducing, and immunosuppressant effects.

Betulinic acid. This triterpenoid is normally found in birch sap and in chaga mushrooms growing on birch trees. It has antibacterial, anti-inflammatory, cholesterol-normalizing, cytotoxic, antitumor, and antidiabetic effects.

Diosgenin. This has anticancer, antioxidant, anti-inflammatory, hypolipidemic, cardiovascular-protective, and neuroprotective properties. It relaxes muscle spasms in the pelvis and contributes to the passage of urinary stones.

Neuropathy

As many as 30–40 percent of patients treated with conventional chemotherapy will develop some degree of peripheral neuropathy—nerve damage that causes pain, tingling, and numbness, often in the hands and feet. This is a common dose-limiting side effect of treatment. Symptoms may include numbness; prickling, tingling, burning, or cold sensations; hypersensitivity to mechanical and/or cold stimuli in hands and feet; difficulty with fine finger movement, such as buttoning up clothes or tying shoelaces; unsteady gait (due to numbness and loss of joint position sense); pain on walking; and cold weather hypersensitivity.

Some anticancer drugs cause more neuropathy than others; paclitaxel, oxaliplatin, thalidomide, and Velcade (bortezomib) are particularly problematic. Neurotoxicity is usually dependent on cumulative dose; higher, more frequent, or more prolonged doses will result in more nerve damage. Severity of neuropathy increases with duration of treatment and usually diminishes once drug treatment is completed. The platinum-based chemotherapy drugs are an exception, where sensory disturbance may continue for several months after cessation of treatment.

Conventional drug therapies for chemotherapy-induced neuropathic pain include intravenous calcium and magnesium infusions, and glutathione, gabapentin, and even antidepressants may be offered. Topical pain relievers may include baclofen/amitriptyline/ketamine gel. However, none of these drugs are very effective in treating neuropathy. Severe symptoms may require reduction or cessation of cancer treatment, with adverse effects on patient survival.

Practical Strategies for Reducing Neuropathy

- Avoid very hot or very cold water (showers, baths, swimming).
- Avoid saunas, steam rooms, hot tubs, and tanning beds.
- Avoid getting overheated with exercise or sun.
- Wear soft, brushed cotton, hemp, bamboo, or silk next to your skin.

Herbs for Neuropathy

In the case of chemotherapy, neuropathy is caused by a poisoning of the nerve endings, which causes structural damage to the nerve tissue. Detoxification programs may be helpful to remove drug residues; chelation therapy may be considered in really severe cases to chemically draw toxins out of the tissues. Restorative, rebuilding herbs are used to regenerate damaged nerve tissue. A number of herbs may have neuroprotective and neuro-healing qualities. Not all are specific to the brain and nervous system, but they will be helpful nonetheless.

ST. JOHN'S WORT (*HYPERICUM PERFORATUM*)

St. John's wort ointment has traditionally been used on first- and second-degree burns and on wounds and generally results in a good cosmetic appearance of the affected skin areas, with regeneration of the epithelium and the normal arrangements of the collagen fibers, and so less scarring. Ointments containing St. John's wort extract can reduce fluid retention under the skin and support the normal flow of fluids in the skin after a burn. Interestingly, a study of intestinal permeability determined that flavonoids and other compounds, such as phenolic acids or proanthocyanidins, substantially improved the permeation characteristics (absorption rate and uptake into the blood) of hypericin, one of the plant's primary active constituents. It is not known if this is also true of transdermal (skin) absorption.

If St. John's wort is applied to the skin or is ingested in higher doses before sun exposure, pronounced sun sensitivity can occur and photodermatitis, or sun poisoning, will result. This can happen with ingested doses of hypericin over 0.5 mg/kg of body weight. Patients using St. John's wort topically should avoid sun exposure on the affected area.

OTHER HERBS WITH BENEFITS IN NEUROPATHY

Gotu kola and plantain (*Centella asiatica* and *Plantago* spp.). These are classified as tonics or trophorestoratives for connective tissues, including nerve tissues. They can be taken to build and strengthen physical tissue, to assist in repair of nerve damage, and to improve the integrity and strength of the nerves.

Cannabis (*Cannabis* spp.). Patients often self-medicate with various forms of cannabis, and many case reports suggest that cannabis CBD (cannabidiol) has beneficial effects on neuropathic pain. Certainly, it is known that there are cannabinoid receptors in skin, and topical cannabis has a local anti-inflammatory action. However, the extent to which this is effective in neuropathy is still being defined.

A 2018 report published in the medical journal *Current Pain and Headache Report* presented several randomized controlled trials assessing medical cannabis for the treatment of neuropathic pain from diverse causes and including different THC concentrations and routes of administration. The authors stated that multiple randomized controlled clinical trials (the "gold standard" of research models) demonstrated a high level of effectiveness of medical cannabis for treating neuropathic pain.

Conversely, a report from the Cochrane Collaboration, also in 2018, reviewed 16 studies with 1,750 participants. All were randomized, double-blind, controlled trials using medical cannabis or plant-derived and synthetic cannabis-based medicines against placebo or against conventional drug therapies for chronic neuropathic pain in adults, with a treatment duration of at least

Herbal Lotion for Neuropathic Pain

This is a rich and creamy formula that soothes and numbs the skin. St. John's wort and gotu kola both have a nerve-healing, restorative action, while the cayenne and aconite inhibit pain impulse transmission. Magnesium gel is cooling and soothing, vitamin E is anti-inflammatory, and the essential oils are numbing, cooling, and pain relieving.

+ 15 mL St. John's wort–infused oil
+ 10 mL gotu kola–infused oil
+ 5 mL vitamin E oil
+ 10 drops each (2 mL total) essential oils of bay laurel, nutmeg, wintergreen, and peppermint
+ 50 g neutral base cream
+ 5 mL capsicum tincture
+ 2 mL aconite tincture (1:10 tincture made with 60% ethyl alcohol; this is a toxic herb, so use it only topically)
+ 10 mL magnesium gel

Blend the oils into the base cream, then add the tinctures slowly, followed by the magnesium gel, and mix until all is smoothly incorporated. Apply to the affected part as needed. Wash hands after applying.

Magnesium Lotion

This lotion is deeply penetrating and relaxes smooth muscles, widening blood vessels to promote distal blood flow (in the areas farthest from the center of the body) and thus support toxin removal from tissues and nerve repair in neuropathy after chemotherapy.

+ ½–1 cup magnesium chloride flakes
+ 2 tablespoons methylsulfonylmethane (MSM) powder
+ ½ cup coconut oil infused with cannabis
+ ½ cup unrefined shea butter
+ 2–4 tablespoons beeswax
+ 1 teaspoon liquid soy lecithin (can be found at most natural foods stores)

ESSENTIAL OILS

+ 10 drops lavender
+ 5 drops frankincense
+ 5 drops ginger
+ 5 drops blue chamomile

Stir the magnesium chloride flakes into ½ cup water, then add the MSM (a connective tissue restorative).

Using a double boiler, gently melt the infused coconut oil, shea butter, and beeswax. Use more beeswax if you want a firmer product, more like a cream than a lotion.

Add the liquid soy lecithin as an emulsifier (allowing you to blend water into oil). Stir the magnesium solution into the warm oils and allow to cool for 15 minutes. Then stir in the essential oils.

Transfer the mixture to a food processor and whip until light and creamy. Put in a clean jar with a tight-fitting lid and keep in a cool, dark place.

2 weeks and in some trials running up to 26 weeks. Cannabis-based medicines were better than placebo for inducing pain relief and global improvement (pain intensity, sleep problems, and psychological distress), but there were more side effects reported in the cannabis users than in the other groups, and more cannabis users than placebo users dropped out of the studies. The side effects reported were largely the result of getting high on the THC, and the reviewers concluded that the potential benefits of cannabis-based medicine in chronic neuropathic pain might be outweighed by the higher incidence of side effects.

I think the answer to this conundrum probably lies in the fact that not all patients enjoy or want the THC component; those patients may be able to use the herb topically, and they may still get benefits from oral ingestion of CBD alone.

GOSHAJINKIGAN

Goshajinkigan, a traditional Japanese (kampo) medicine, also widely used in Traditional Chinese Medicine, is effective against acute neuropathy, notably from platinum drugs. Extreme sensitivity to cold is a common side effect of platinum drugs, especially in the hands and feet, due to drug-induced damage to thermosensitive receptors in nerves. The herbs in this formula inhibit this sensitivity. The formula also acts as a muscle relaxant and antispasmodic in skeletal muscle. Dosed at ½ teaspoon two or three times daily, it has remarkable effects on neuropathies. I have been supplying it to patients for some years now and have had exceptional feedback. The taste isn't great, but the effects are notable—less neuropathic pain (reduced tingling, burning, itching) and less neuromuscular pain generally.

Ingredients in Goshajinkigan

- Rehmannia (prepared)/shēng dì huáng (*Rehmannia glutinosa*)
- Ox knee/niú xī (*Achyranthis bidentata*)
- Cornelian cherry/shān zhū yú (*Cornus officinalis*)
- Chinese yam/shān yào (*Dioscorea opposita*)
- Hoelen/fú ling (*Poria cocos*)
- Plantain seed/chē qián zǐ (*Plantago asiatica*)
- Water plantain/zé xiè (*Alisma orientale*)
- Tree peony bark/mǔ dān pí (*Paeonia suffruticosa*)
- Cassia bark/guì pí (*Cinnamomum cassia*)
- Aconite root (heat processed)/fù zǐ (*Aconitum lateralis*)

Supplements for Neuropathic Pain

Several types of supplements may offer help in alleviating neuropathic pain. Vitamins B6 and B12 and folic acid are very important for methylation, a detoxification process in the liver, and for proper DNA copying, but in addition these three water-soluble nutrients are critical for helping to rebuild myelin (the covering of a nerve) and for healing neuropathy. Fish oil (omega-3 fats) is anti-inflammatory and can help with nerve healing. Eating cold-water fish (herring, mackerel, wild salmon, sardines) can also be helpful. Acetyl-L-carnitine supports nerve function and is particularly good for neuropathy caused by chemotherapy. Alpha-lipoic acid is a fat- and water-soluble antioxidant specific for neuropathy.

- Methylcobalamin (B12): 1,000 mcg daily
- Folic acid (B9): 1,200 mcg daily
- N-acetylcysteine: 500 mg twice daily
- Magnesium glycinate: 500 mg in afternoon and again at bedtime
- Acetyl-L-carnitine: 500 mg twice daily
- Pyridoxine (B6): 50 mg twice daily
- R+ alpha-lipoic acid: 500 mg twice daily
- Omega-3 fish oil: 1,500 mg EPA and 700 mg DHA daily

Special Considerations for Immunotherapies

In the last 15–20 years an abundance of new drugs designed to approach cancer in a completely new way have come to market. They include a whole new generation of anticancer drugs—the so-called immunotherapies or biological agents. They are also called "targeted therapies" because they interface specifically with cancer cells. They can block or turn off chemical signals that tell the cancer cell to grow and divide, change proteins within the cancer cells so the cells die, prevent the creation of new blood vessels to feed the cancer cells, and trigger the immune system to kill the cancer cells. In the case of conjugated monoclonal antibodies, the therapy carries toxins to the cancer cells to kill them, while protecting and preserving normal cells.

Monoclonal antibodies (mAbs). With names all ending in the suffix "mab," these are given by intravenous infusion, and they either inhibit intracellular transduction pathways or induce immune responses to destroy the cell. Conjugated mAbs comprise a mAb plus chemotherapy or a radioactive particle used as a kind of homing device to deliver treatment directly to the cancer cells. The mAb hooks onto the target antigen (cell-surface protein) and delivers the toxic substance where it is needed most. This can reduce damage to normal cells in other parts of the body. Conjugated mAbs are also sometimes referred to as tagged, labeled, or loaded antibodies.

Small molecules. With names all ending in the suffix "ib," these can cross the cell membrane and bind to intracellular signal transduction targets, disrupt gene expression, and bring about cell death. They are removed by efflux pumps (protein transporters). Resistance to these small molecules develops quickly unless they are taken in combination with other drugs to reduce the pumping, but doing so also has an increased risk of side effects.

Checkpoint inhibitors. These are a particular type of monoclonal antibody that target the so-called checkpoint receptor molecules on immune cells, which regulate and control immune responses. Cancer cells activate these checkpoints to avoid being recognized and attacked by the immune system. Checkpoint inhibitor drugs allow immune cells to recognize cancer cells and flag them for destruction. Common side effects of checkpoint inhibitor drugs include kidney infections, diarrhea, pneumonitis (inflammation in the lungs), skin rashes and itchiness, and inflammation of the pituitary gland (also known as hypophysitis). With some drugs, as many as 20 percent of patients experience disturbances in some hormone levels—notably autoimmune thyroiditis with subsequent thyroid disturbance (hypothyroidism and occasionally hyperthyroidism)—caused by inflammation of the pituitary gland.

Several checkpoint inhibitor drugs, including pembrolizumab (Keytruda), ipilimumab (Yervoy), nivolumab (Opdivo), and atezolizumab (Tecentriq), are now approved by the US FDA for specific cancers, and some more widely for other types of cancer. For example, pembrolizumab is used to treat any metastatic tumor that meets specific criteria of a molecular alteration called microsatellite instability-high (MSI-H) or shows DNA mismatch repair deficiency (dMMR), both of which can be screened for in biopsy material.

An important but often overlooked factor in checkpoint inhibitor therapy success is the condition of the gut microbiome. Although the mechanisms of action are not yet defined, research suggests that a healthy and well-balanced gut flora is critical to the drug action, and if this type of therapy is chosen it would be prudent to go through a 6-week program of "weeding, seeding, and feeding" the gut prior to commencing drug treatment (see page 55).

Cancer virus therapy. This is a biological therapy using a genetically modified virus injected into the tumor. The virus causes the cancer cells to die and release proteins that trigger the immune system to target any cancer cells in the body that have the same proteins as the dead cancer cells. The virus does not enter healthy cells.

The first genetically modified virus drug was approved by the FDA in 2015 to treat late-stage melanoma. Imlygic (talimogene laherparepvec) uses a modified herpes simplex virus as the delivery vector, but other virus-enhanced drug regimens are currently being researched.

Cancer vaccines. These may be preventive (for example, the human papilloma virus vaccine protects against cervical cancer) or may be used as a treatment strategy to induce immune responses against a tumor. To make a vaccine that is active against an existing cancer, pieces of the cancer tissue are cultured in a lab and used to induce or trigger immune responses against the cancer when the manipulated protein is reintroduced to the body. Vaccines are not widely available and not yet well researched, but they hold promise for the future of cancer therapies, especially now that messenger RNA can be used for vaccines, as with the novel COVID-19 vaccines. One cancer vaccine currently in use is Provenge, for prostate cancer.

Chimeric antigen receptor T cell therapy. T cell lymphocytes are specialized white blood cells that fight infection. In T cell therapy, T cells are removed from the blood of a person with cancer and then introduced in the lab to specific proteins that enable the T cells to recognize cancer cells. The trained T cells are replaced into the body, where they find and destroy cancer cells. Chimeric antigen receptor T cell therapy shows promise in treating certain blood cancers and multiple myeloma. Side effects have been severe and dose limiting, including fevers, confusion, low blood pressure, and seizures.

Early in 2022, it was announced that some of the first patients ever to receive this therapy were still cancer-free after 10 years; the treatment is now considered a successful cure. Although this technique is not widely practiced yet, it is promising. In the UK, the therapy is approved for use in children and young adults with B-cell acute lymphoblastic leukemia and in adults with certain types of lymphoma.

Managing Monoclonal Antibody Therapy and Immunotherapies

To date, most of these newer drugs have been approved in the marketplace for use only after conventional chemotherapy has been attempted and found unsuccessful. This is unfortunate, as in many cases these drugs are more targeted, better tolerated, and likely to be at least as successful as most of the conventional chemotherapies. The key to success with the targeted drugs is to have comprehensive testing done in advance of treatment to determine the correct drug for targeting specific proteins found on the cell. This is still not routine practice in many countries, but it is the subject of much excited speculation in the medical literature about the future of cancer care and the customizing and targeting of treatment. This branch of medicine is in active development and will certainly be the future of drug treatment for cancer, with conventional "one size fits all" chemotherapy eventually falling out of favor. Because cancer cells overexpress specific receptor sites, they may be very sensitized to targeted drugs like this, which can have a significantly deleterious effect upon the cancer cell, with somewhat less collateral damage than conventional chemotherapy.

The interferon release caused by the immune stimulation from these drugs is one reason for some of the recognized side effects of treatment with the drugs. These side effects may include fever and chills, weakness and lassitude, headache, nausea and vomiting, diarrhea, and low blood pressure. Interferon is a part of the body's natural defenses. It tells the immune system that pathogens or cancer cells are present, and it triggers immune cells like natural killer cells to fight those invaders. The drugs trigger immune responses that cause the same symptoms as a viral infection—fever, muscle aches, fatigue, and headaches. Another common, and sometimes dose-limiting, side effect is skin rashes. For example, the drug cetuximab (Erbitux) targets specific receptor sites normally found on skin cells as well as some types of cancer cells. This drug can cause serious rashes in some people.

Rare but High-Risk Side Effects Occasionally Seen

- Clotting disorders—for example, bevacizumab (Avastin) targets VEGF (a signal protein), which affects tumor blood vessel growth; it can cause high blood pressure, bleeding, poor wound healing, blood clots, and kidney damage
- Congestive heart failure and heart attacks
- Inflammatory lung disease

Because these are relatively new drugs and are not yet widely used, there is less understanding about how to manage them and mitigate side effects. Specific natural medicine strategies may be employed, much like in conventional chemotherapy, for symptoms such as diarrhea, skin rashes, clotting disorders, and so on. However, there is some evidence that these side effects are actually evidence of the drug working—for example, if you don't get skin rashes from EGFr inhibition, you may not have as good a cancer response as those with more severe rash. There is likely to be a lower risk of herb–drug interactions with these targeted immunotherapy drugs than with conventional chemotherapy, and so far no herbs have been identified as specifically contraindicated.

ENCOURAGING IMMUNE RESPONSE WITH SWEATING AND FEVER

Herbalists are inducing interferon when recommending diaphoretics and fever treatments in influenza or other feverish conditions, and there is some suggestion that it might be helpful to manage immunotherapy drug reactions in a similar way—to encourage the immune responses as we would for a flu. On the day of receiving the drug and for 2–3 days afterward, use a diaphoretic tea plus hot baths to promote a fever and promote natural interferon release.

Diaphoretic Tea

Make a strong tea of herbs that induce sweating. Catnip, yarrow flower, elderflower, ginger, and peppermint are all useful here. Prepare as an infusion, using 1 ounce of dried herbal mix to 1 pint of water (30 g per 500 mL), and drink it very hot over the course of 1 day. To maximize immune responsiveness, add echinacea capsules at 500 mg per capsule, three capsules twice daily.

Fever Treatment

Taking a very hot bath is an old folk technique for increasing the core temperature and promoting interferon release in the early stages of a viral infection. Do not use this treatment if you have skin rashes from immunotherapies or neuropathy, which may be thermosensitive.

Run a hot bath and after getting into it add more hot water—as hot as you can tolerate. Take care not to scald your skin. Drink a large cup of diaphoretic tea while soaking in the tub. Have a bucket or basin of iced water nearby and wring out a washcloth in the ice water to lay on your forehead if you feel dizzy.

You will also need a thermometer; take your temperature every 10 minutes or so. Soak in the tub for 15–20 minutes, then go straight to bed, wrap up well, drink some water or electrolyte solution, and be prepared to sweat some more.

Unless someone is quite weak or debilitated, it is generally safe to increase the temperature up to 101°F (38°C) in children and 103°F (39–40°C) in adults, provided there is active perspiration. Evaporation of sweat is how we cool down, so as long as you are sweating you won't overheat. If you feel dizzy or nauseous and wish to bring your temperature down quickly, place an iced cloth around your neck or wrists.

Fever Treatment Cautions

- Do not use this treatment if you have high or very low blood pressure.
- It's best to do this when there is someone else in the house and not to lock the bathroom door, in case you feel dizzy.
- Do not stand up quickly from the bath. Stand up slowly and keep your head down until any dizziness wears off.
- If you feel nauseated during the treatment, drink a 50-50 mixture of an electrolyte sports drink and water.
- Watch for signs of hyperventilation: numbness and tingling around the mouth or in the hands and feet. If necessary, add cold water to the bath. Breathe from the abdomen, not the chest. Get out of the bath if you feel distressed or unwell.

Managing Radiation

Virtually every person going through cancer treatment will experience a higher-than-usual exposure to ionizing radiation. This may be from treatment but can also be from diagnostic procedures required to achieve a reliable diagnosis or to monitor progression. Added to the routine background levels of radiation that we are all exposed to, radiation exposure may become problematic and detrimental to well-being.

Scans and X-rays

CT scans and x-rays are frequently used to visualize cancer and measure its dimensions for assessing response to chemotherapy or to measure cancer progression and growth. However, these techniques bring their own risk of radiation exposure, which may become a limiting factor over time. Around half the lifetime radiation exposure of the average American comes from medical tests and procedures not associated with cancer, so the additive effect of cancer diagnosis, treatment, and monitoring can rapidly become significant. Cancer patients can quickly surpass the safe lifetime amount, especially if they receive radiotherapy. PET scans use a radioisotope-labeled sugar to track cells that are metabolically active; this can identify very small growths and is useful for seeking out dispersed metastases. A PET scan is more accurate than a CT scan but is almost always combined with CT, which means that patients receive double or triple the ionizing radiation that they do with a simple CT.

Thus, it is desirable to take steps to reduce the radiation load. Diagnostic and monitoring scans can be scheduled further apart if it is deemed safe to do so. Avoid other radiation exposure wherever possible—long flights at high altitude, for example, or occupational exposures (such as those experienced by x-ray technicians or miners). The risk from body scanners at airports, from cell phones and transmission towers, and from radon exposure or other environmental sources is hard to quantify. However, even though each of these may be very low exposures, they are summative, and over time this is not optimal.

Radiotherapy

Although radiotherapy only occasionally offers curative potential in and of itself, somewhere upwards of 50 percent of patients will receive it as part of their treatment. Often it is prescribed for managing symptoms, including pain, bleeding, and nerve compression. It is also used after surgery or chemotherapy to prevent local recurrence, most notably in breast, lung, urological, and lower gastrointestinal cancers. It is important to note that radiotherapy will not prevent distant metastases that have already been seeded from the primary tumor into peripheral tissues and may not lead to better long-term outcomes.

Radiotherapy may comprise external beam therapy (photons, electrons, protons, and other particles), which is the most common approach, and, less commonly, internal treatments (brachytherapy or insertion of radioactive pellets into the tumor, or injected radiopharmaceuticals, for example attached to monoclonal antibodies for targeted delivery). For radiotherapy to work, oxygen is essential. Tumors are generally somewhat low in oxygen, which promotes new blood vessel growth and contributes to radio-resistance. Because of the low sensitivity of most tumors to radiation, a high dose of radiation is often needed, and this leads to severe damage to adjacent tissues.

Modern nanotechnology is now allowing for delivery of radioactive particles to tumors even when they are low in oxygen. Proton beam therapy—a specialized form of external beam therapy—allows more precise targeting and less collateral damage. Stereotactic body radiotherapy and intensity-modulated radiotherapy are other novel delivery models allowing dose reduction and greater precision and thus minimizing toxicity.

Radio Sensitizing and Radio Protection

Resistance to treatment and recurrences after treatment are two major concerns when considering whether to do radiation. A long-term concern is post-radiotherapy incidence of a second tumor, usually at a new location in the body, because radiotherapy does not protect against metastases. A more immediate concern is the risk of developing radio-resistance, where any beneficial value of radiotherapy (even for palliative care) becomes unavailable. This is where herbs—specifically those containing large amounts of polyphenols—can be effective. There are numerous studies that demonstrate how plant polyphenols sensitize tumor cells to chemotherapy agents and radiation therapy by inhibiting pathways that lead to treatment resistance, mostly through regulating and adjusting tightly balanced redox cycling and by inhibiting oxidative stress. These so-called radiosensitizers enhance the radiation-induced cell death inflicted to the tumor and thereby allow lower doses and hence fewer side effects.

Many of these herbs also protect healthy cells from therapy-associated toxicities. Radioprotective activity of these herbs is associated with scavenging of free radicals and depletion of lipid peroxidation with increased glutathione, catalase, and lactate dehydrogenase enzymes—the cleanup crew for intracellular detoxification. These radioprotectors lessen the undesired or collateral damage caused to the normal cells, minimizing the side effects of radiation therapy.

As is so often the case in medical research, most of the reports use animal models and cell cultures, especially when studying radiation, due to ethics constraints in running human trials. However, studies support a long list of radioprotective and radiosensitizing herbs, some of which are not readily available in the marketplace (yet) and others that are routinely and regularly used by herbal oncology prescribers. This research corroborates the clinical experience of herbalists, but human clinical trials are still needed for final confirmation.

Any of these may reasonably be used to support patients through radiotherapy, without concern of negating the effects of radiation. Understanding of the complex redox-regulating and cell-normalizing effects of these compounds creates clinical confidence.

Many members of the mint family can be used effectively, not just for redox- and inflammation-modulating actions but also to stimulate DNA repair mechanisms. Both peppermint and field mint protected mice against radiation-induced sickness and mortality. Aqueous extract (tea) of peppermint leaves protected the organs, including gastrointestinal organs and bone marrow, due to free radical scavenging, antioxidant, metal chelating, anti-inflammatory and antimutagenic actions, and enhancement of the DNA repair processes.

Ginseng confers a radioprotective effect from a water-soluble extract of whole ginseng that appears to give a better protection against radiation-induced DNA damage than do the isolated ginsenoside fractions, implying that a whole-root tea would be effective.

Herbs and Constituents for Radiotherapy

This selection of herbs and constituents has been shown to be beneficial during and immediately after radiation treatment.

- Allicin from garlic
- Betulinic acid from chaga mushroom
- Camptothecin from camptotheca (actually a chemotherapy drug)
- Ellagic acid from pomegranate
- Genistein and daidzein (isoflavones) from soy
- Beta-lapachone from taheebo
- Oleuropein from olive
- Plumbagin from sundew
- Resveratrol
- Alpha-santolol from sandalwood
- Silymarin from milk thistle
- Tangeritin from citrus rinds

Other Herbs Known to Provide Radioprotective Effects

- Green tea
- Gotu kola
- Turmeric
- Echinacea
- Ginger
- Triphala, "three fruits" formula: *Emblica officinalis* (amlaki), *Terminalia bellirica* (bibhitaki), *Terminalia chebula* (haritaki)

Herbal Constituents That Have Demonstrated Radiosensitizing Capacity

- Withaferin A (from ashwagandha)
- Berberine and herbs that contain this substance
- Artemisinin (from annual wormwood, qing hao)
- Honokiol (from magnolia)
- Sulforaphane (from cruciferous vegetables)

Consequences of Radiation

Side effects of radiation will vary according to the site, intensity, and duration but may include dry mouth, burning tongue, mouth sores, and dysphagia from oral treatment and loss of appetite, nausea, vomiting, and diarrhea from abdominal treatment. Fatigue, hair loss, and neutropenia (low white blood cell count) are almost universal symptoms. External beam therapy often causes skin burns, sometimes occurring weeks after completion of treatment, which are very slow to heal.

Natural Agents to Assist in Removal of Radiation from the Body

- Flavonoids—quercetin, genistein, catechins from green tea, epicatechin, apigenin, silibinin (blueberries, mulberries, citrus fruits, green tea, chamomile, propolis)
- Phenylpropanoids—propolis, curcumin, thymol, zingerone, resveratrol (green tea, turmeric, ginger, rosemary, oregano, thyme)
- Vitamin C (naturally sourced acerola cherry extract is best)
- Gallic acid (tannin derivative found in green tea and astringent herbs like raspberry leaf, bearberry, sumac, oak bark)

Seaweed for Removing Radiation

According to Dr. Ryan Drum, a seaweed expert in Washington State, seaweed contains alginic acid, a complex sugar that binds to radioactive isotopes and facilitates their transport out of the body. He suggests that anyone who wants to remove radiation from the body could benefit from eating seaweed. One way to add seaweed to the diet is to keep coarse ground seaweed on the dining table to add as a condiment. I sometimes mix it with toasted sesame seeds to make a tasty gomasio. Aim for 3–10 grams (dry weight) of unrefined seaweed daily.

Topical Herbs for Radiation Burns

Radiotherapy burns the skin. This is often a limitation to the treatment, and many patients do not complete the recommended course of treatment for this reason. There is also a risk of impaired healing of the tissue due to the radiation, and weeks or months later there may still be thin or fragile skin and burning sensations. Scarring can also complicate healing of a radiation burn.

Do not apply anything to the treated area for 24 hours prior to radiotherapy, as any oil on the skin will increase burning. If radiation is being applied daily, then topical help with treatments needs to be delayed until the completion of the treatment; if radiation is intermittent, then herbs can be used in between treatments.

Herbal Cream for Radiation Burn

This cooling, soothing, and healing cream will promote tissue repair, inhibit infection, and minimize scarring.

+ 5 mL sea buckthorn oil
+ 5 mL vitamin E oil
+ 1 mL vitamin A liquid
+ 5 mL propolis tincture
+ 20 drops lavender essential oil
+ 10 drops blue chamomile essential oil
+ 10 drops helichrysum essential oil
+ 5 mL manuka honey (or other raw, unpasteurized honey)
+ 50 g calendula cream
+ 10 mL colloidal silver gel
+ 10 mL aloe gel
+ 5 mL calendula juice (of flowers)
+ 2 g comfrey root powder

Blend the sea buckthorn oil, vitamin E, vitamin A, propolis, essential oils, and honey together. Slowly add this mixture to the calendula cream, stirring well, then set aside. In a separate bowl blend the silver and aloe gels with the calendula juice and add the comfrey powder. Then fold the two mixes together and stir well. Apply over closed skin (not over open wounds, to avoid absorption of comfrey).

Turmeric (*Curcuma longa*). A study of a proprietary cream from India containing turmeric and sandalwood oil on posttreatment radiodermatitis in 50 patients with head and neck cancer showed a significant reduction in all grades of dermatitis in the cohort applying turmeric and sandalwood cream.

Aloe (*Aloe vera*). Another study investigated the effectiveness of an aloe vera–based cream for the prevention of radiation-induced dermatitis in head and neck cancer. It concluded that there was a statistically significant delay in the incidence and severity of dermatitis in the aloe group and indicated that the benefit continued for some weeks after cessation of radiotherapy. There are some contradictory studies involving aloe, and although both traditional use and evidence-based medicine suggest it helps, not all the clinical research supports that.

HONEY

Honey has a long history of use in medicine. In cancer care, it is especially useful as a topical agent.

Skin healing. Honey is used for burns and other skin injuries; it speeds up wound healing, treats postoperative infections, and inhibits bacterial infections. It is used for abscesses, bedsores, fistulas, cracked nipples, diabetic ulcers, and surgical wounds. In the US, medical-grade honey products have been approved by the FDA for use in treating minor wounds and burns. In the UK, the National Health Service wound care protocols include manuka honey–infused bandages over open wounds.

Antibacterial action. Honey has broad-spectrum antibacterial activity against many types of bacteria. This means it is useful in treating surgical incisions or cancers that have breached the surface of the skin. The high sugar content draws moisture out of the bacteria into the honey, and the bacteria die. Honey also destroys biofilms—the communities of bacteria dwelling behind a self-produced protective layer and routinely found adhering to surfaces, including wounds, teeth, mucosal surfaces, and implanted devices. Microbes living in biofilms can't be reached by conventional antibiotics and they can cause persistent, chronic infections. Manuka honey, in particular, has been shown to disrupt and disperse the cellular aggregates and prevent the formation of biofilms by a wide range of problematic pathogens, including *Streptococcus* and *Staphylococcus* species, *Escherichia coli*, *Klebsiella pneumoniae*, and more. Manuka honey is made by bees in New Zealand visiting the manuka tree.

Anticancer activity. In addition to its benefits from topical use, honey contains flavonoids and phenolic acids with known anticancer activity. Honey modulates oxidative stress, inhibits cancer cell growth, supports normal cell death, and has anti-inflammatory, immunomodulatory, tumor necrosis factor–inhibiting, antimetastatic properties and (phyto)estrogenic effects.

One study looked at the effects of honey where bees had visited different plants, including thyme, fir, and pine, on the modulation of estrogenic activity and viability of breast cancer cells in vitro. They found that the honey demonstrated variable and opposing effects depending on the concentrations. Notably, the extracts exhibited antiestrogenic effect at low concentrations and estrogenic activity at high concentrations. After considering different sourced honeys and differing cell line toxicities, the researchers concluded that thyme honey in the diet showed the most anticancer activity in breast, prostate, and endometrial cancer cells.

Natural honey is relatively free of any toxicity. Although being allergic to honey is rare, it can occur, and people allergic to bee stings should exercise caution when using it. Honey can also harbor botulinum bacteria normally found in soil; infants or people of any age taking immunosuppressive drugs may be at risk of infection and should not use honey.

Anticancer Mechanisms of Honey

- Downregulates cell-signaling pathways, mitochondrial activation, and oxidative stress
- Induces cell death and cell cycle arrest; stabilizes p53
- Inhibits new blood vessel growth and cell proliferation
- Immunomodulating and anti-inflammatory through regulating TNF-α, COX-2, lipoxygenases, and prostaglandin E2 inhibition
- Improves both the activity of agents that inhibit cancer cell growth and the quality-of-life parameters in patients undergoing chemotherapy

CHAPTER 6

Materia Medica: A Directory of Herbs for Cancer

From the polyphenols in green tea, the immunomodulating mushroom polysaccharides, and the anti-inflammatory pigments in turmeric to the plant-derived chemotherapy drugs like taxol and etoposide, there is a general agreement in the scientific literature that plant medicines can be profoundly effective in treating cancer. This is borne out in clinical practice as well.

There are many dozens of herbs to choose from. Those discussed in this chapter are some of the key herbs that I regularly use when formulating for cancer care. They are the synergists or supportive herbs in a pyramid prescribing model (see Chapter 7 on herbal formulating). These are the herbs that direct the treatment to target tissues, encourage and support healthy physiology functions, and work in harmony with the more targeted or specific herbs to help them be more effective. Although they may contain constituents that have been shown in empirical use and in research studies to have anticancer activity, the whole herbs and their extracts are not considered to be systemically toxic like the cytotoxic herbs discussed in Chapter 9. The herbs listed here are active against cancer but are largely safe for regular use in most people.

CHAPTER 6 CONTENTS

239 **Dosing Herbs for Cancer Care**
239 Herbal Teas
240 Tinctures
241 **Aloe** (*Aloe vera, A. barbadensis*)
244 **Andrographis** (*Andrographis paniculata*)
245 **Baikal Skullcap** (*Scutellaria baicalensis*)
247 **Bupleurum** (*Bupleurum falcatum*)
249 **Cacao** (*Theobroma cacao*)
251 **Calendula** (*Calendula officinalis*)
253 **Corydalis** (*Corydalis yanhusuo, C. ambigua*)
255 **Dan Shen** (*Salvia miltiorrhiza*)
257 **Echinacea** (*Echinacea purpurea, E. angustifolia, E. pallida*)
259 **Feverfew** (*Tanacetum parthenium*)
261 **Garlic** (*Allium sativum*)
263 **Ginger** (*Zingiber officinale*)
265 **Gotu Kola** (*Centella asiatica*)
268 **Green Tea** (*Camellia sinensis*)
271 **Horse Chestnut** (*Aesculus hippocastanum*)
272 **Indian Frankincense** (*Boswellia serrata*)
273 **Magnolia** (*Magnolia grandiflora, M. virginiana, M. acuminata, M. macrophylla, M. officinalis*)
276 **Nigella** (*Nigella sativa*)
278 **Pomegranate** (*Punica granatum*)
281 **Propolis**
283 **Red Clover** (*Trifolium pratense*)
285 **Sea Buckthorn** (*Hippophae rhamnoides*)
288 **St. John's Wort** (*Hypericum perforatum*)
292 **Taheebo** (*Tabebuia impetiginosa, T. avellanedae, T. rosea,* a.k.a. *Handroanthus impetiginosus*)
294 **Tulsi** (*Ocimum sanctum, O. tenuiflorum*)
298 **Turmeric** (*Curcuma longa*)
303 Golden Milk
303 **Medicinal Mushrooms**

Dosing Herbs for Cancer Care

Depending on the time and energy you have, you can either make your own herbal preparations or purchase them. You can easily make herbal teas at home with simple kitchen equipment. You could also make infused oils, tinctures, lotions, and capsules yourself, but because making them may require some special equipment or expertise, you might be inclined to purchase them from a natural foods store or a practitioner.

Herbal Teas

A tea will extract an herb's water-soluble constituents (such as tannins and bitters) but will not readily extract components like resins, oils, or alkaloids, which are less soluble in water. Alkaloids can be made more soluble in tea by the addition of a splash of vinegar to lower the pH, and the volatile terpenoids and phenylpropanoids can be extracted by inhaling the steam rising from hot tea.

To achieve a therapeutic dose of the herbs from tea, however, it is sometimes necessary to drink either copious amounts or rather strong and often bitter brews. Because of that, patients are less likely to follow through with taking it. It may also be difficult to get a sufficient dose and potency from a tea to rely on it for a primary part of a cancer protocol. More often, teas are used as an adjunct to a tincture and capsule regimen, addressing secondary concerns and symptoms, not directly working on the cancer. In addition to drinking them, you can also use teas as a foot or hand soak, a gargle, an enema or a douche, in a bath, or on a gauze pad as a compress.

Teas are made either by infusion (steeping herbs in water) or by decoction (simmering herbs in water). A medicinal tea would usually be made at a strength of 1–2 tablespoons of dried herb per cup of water. Roots, barks, and seeds tend to be denser and heavier, so lesser amounts may be needed. Leaves and flowers are often light and fluffy, so a larger amount is called for. A typical dose is 2–3 cups daily.

Infusions. These are used to prepare leaves, stems, flowers, and other soft plant tissues. Put the herbs into a teapot or a glass or stainless steel vessel and pour the boiling water over them. Steep the herbs for about 10 minutes and drink the infusion hot or cold, as the condition requires.

Decoctions. These are used to prepare roots, twigs, berries, and other hard plant tissues. Put the herbs into a stainless steel pan. Cover them with water, bring it to a boil, then simmer for 5–15 minutes.

It is important to cover teas with a lid while infusing or simmering to capture any volatile oils that condense on the lid so they fall back into the tea. It is always advisable to use pure spring or filtered water to make your infusion or decoction. If you strain out the spent herbs after steeping them, the resulting tea can be kept for 3 or 4 days in the refrigerator.

Tinctures

Tinctures are made with a solvent to extract all the fat-soluble constituents like resins and alkaloids, as well as the water-soluble ones. The most common solvent is alcohol (usually ethyl alcohol), but vinegar or glycerin is occasionally used. The quantity of alcohol in a tincture is written as a percentage—from 25–60%—with the balance being pure water (or it can be made up with an herbal tea from the same plant for a really full-spectrum extraction). A tincture must always be at least 25% alcohol to ensure shelf stability. Remember that if you use vodka or another commercially available alcohol, you need to account for the water content it has. For example, vodka is a popular choice for home tincture making as it is readily available and has little to no flavor of its own (you can use gin, brandy, or whiskey if you prefer). It is only 45–50% alcohol, though, so it is not suitable for some herbal extracts, such as the resins that need a higher percent of the alcohol as a solvent. The proportion of herb to solvent is always shown as a ratio of weight in volume—for example, 200 grams of herb in 1,000 milliliters of fluid (alcohol plus water) is a 1:5 tincture, while 500 grams of herb in 1,000 milliliters of fluid is a 1:2 tincture.

In the descriptions below, I have generally referenced tinctures at a 1:2 strength and have indicated the preferred alcohol ratio. If the potencies you work with are different than these, the doses can be adjusted up or down as needed. Generally speaking, the daily dose of herbal remedy should be divided into three or four doses taken throughout the day to keep the blood levels as stable as possible, and in a range that is safe and effective.

> Until man duplicates a blade of grass, nature can laugh at his so-called scientific knowledge. Remedies from chemicals will never stand in favor compared with the products of nature, the living cell of the plant, the final result of the rays of the sun, the mother of all life.
>
> THOMAS A. EDISON

A Word about Threatened Species

A few of the herbs listed in this chapter may be threatened or endangered in the wild, and for this reason many practitioners will choose not to use them unless they are very specifically indicated. For example, taheebo, or pau d'arco (*Tabebuia impetiginosa* and *T. avellandae*), is overharvested for timber and lost to forest clearing in Brazil. It exhibits potent anticancer activity, though, and is specific where there is a comorbidity of viral, fungal, or parasitic infection. In these cases, it may be reasonable to substitute with other antiparasitic and anticancer herbs, like black walnut or Chinese wormwood (*Artemisia annua*). Similarly, Indian frankincense (*Boswellia serrata*) is overharvested for perfumery. In this case, you can substitute other anti-inflammatory and anticancer herbs that are cultivated and more abundant, notably turmeric and ginger.

I have included information about these herbs in clinical practice but have also indicated which are notably at risk and to be used with restraint. Similarly, I hesitated over recommending coconut oil or avocados in the diet, despite their manifest benefits, because plantations are replacing tropical rain forest and there are complex questions of carbon footprint and sustainability that may affect our food choices. These are dilemmas of our times that have no easy answers. At the least, we should seek out herbal remedies from organically cultivated sources where possible, not wild harvested, and we should aim to buy as much organic and fairly traded food as possible and to localize our food (and herbal medicine) sources.

Aloe

Aloe vera, A. barbadensis

Plant family: Asphodelaceae
Part used: leaf (inner gel)
Medicinal actions: The inner gel of the leaf is a soothing demulcent and emollient; anthraquinones just below the leaf surface are laxative but also anticancer.

This fleshy-leaved plant is found in kitchens all over the world, where it lives happily neglected on a windowsill and serves as an instant first-aid burn remedy. A slice of the leaf will ooze and drip slippery mucilage, a gel-like substance that cools, soothes, and heals tissue. The gel contains a complex sugar that attracts and holds water (essential for this desert-living plant), and this water-retention action is deeply emollient on the skin; it holds moisture in the surface layer, hydrating and plumping cells and promoting elasticity. When ingested, the gel has a demulcent action that is essentially the same effect—cooling, soothing, and healing mucous membranes with which it comes into contact.

The demulcent action may be useful if there is inflammation, tissue damage, or lesions in the gut after surgery or chemotherapy, if the esophagus and throat are sore and burning from radiotherapy or from vomiting, or if there is rectal or vaginal inflammation or burning after radiotherapy. It can be ingested, but it can also be applied in a douche or an enema. The emollient effect is invaluable when treating radiation burns, hand-foot syndrome, or rashes from chemotherapy.

What Makes It Medicinal

The inner gel from aloe leaves also has direct anticancer activity. A polysaccharide in the gel, called acemannan, stimulates the immune system. Aloe gel is also antioxidant.

A 2009 clinical trial of 240 patients with metastatic solid tumors, randomized to receive standard chemotherapy with or without aloe gel, suggested that aloe can be a synergist, or promotor, of chemotherapy. In this study, patients with lung, colorectal, gastric, or pancreatic cancer received chemotherapy alone or with aloe gel, given orally at 10 milliliters three times daily. Patients receiving aloe with their chemotherapy showed improved tumor regression and higher disease control than patients treated with chemotherapy alone, and 3-year survival was higher too.

ALOE EMODIN

Aloe emodin, aloin, and related compounds are water-soluble polyphenolic (antioxidant) anthraquinone derivatives found just under the outer layer of the leaf. This material is harvested by carefully filleting the leaf to separate the outer layer from the mucilaginous center.

Emodin demonstrates some interesting anticancer activity, specifically when it comes to skin cancer. In vitro studies have indicated that aloe emodin can inhibit proliferation and induce cell death in adult human keratinocytes, suggesting particular value in squamous or basal cell skin cancers. In vitro studies also suggest that emodin inhibits critical cell pathways such as toll-like receptors, MAPK, and NF-κB pathways, which downregulate cancer.

Caveats

Taking aloe internally should be done with some caution. Overconsumption of emodin elevates liver enzyme concentrations. Other adverse effects—such as seizures, nephritis, gastrointestinal hemorrhage, and dyspnea (shortness of breath)—have been seen in animal studies. However, these acute symptoms in response to isolates are highly unlikely to occur in clinical practice using whole herb extract, because no herbal practitioner would be giving a large enough dose to cause these effects. In fact, the dose for herbs high in emodin is to take only as much as is needed to generate a bowel movement 6–8 hours later, and no more. The few case reports in the literature of acute toxic hepatitis induced by aloe in humans also note that patients showed improved conditions after discontinuing aloe medication.

Although the gel of the inner leaf of aloe is nontoxic, as evaluated by the Cosmetic Ingredient Review Expert Panel, the whole-leaf extract (with anthraquinones) is classified by the International Agency for Research on Cancer as a possible human carcinogen (group 2B), when taken internally, due to carcinogenic activity in rats. The National Toxicology Program in the US conducted toxicity studies on rats given oral doses of aloe vera whole-leaf extracts and found a dose-related increase in mucosal hyperplasia in the large intestine as well as nonmalignant lesions in the large intestine and mesenteric lymph nodes. The researchers concluded that the intestinal tumors developed in chronic use or with high doses, due to emodin being transformed into mutagenic components in the intestine.

Aloe as a Laxative

Aloe emodin is an anthroquinone and an irritant to the bowel. It is safe and may be effective for short-term relief of situational constipation, but it is not recommended for longer than 2–4 weeks unless as part of a program to reduce habituation and lower doses over time. This is not because it is inherently risky or toxic, but rather because addressing the cause of the constipation and reducing the need for a laxative should be the goal. Nevertheless, children under 12 years of age and pregnant or lactating women should not use aloe as a laxative. See page 170 for more information on using Cape aloe (*A. barbadensis*) as a laxative.

Chronic users of anthraquinone-based laxatives tend to develop a condition called pseudomelanosis coli, a brown discoloration of the bowel lining cells due to oxidative damage and lipid peroxidation. Although this condition was previously thought to be a risk factor for colorectal cancer, a 2021 review of the literature suggested that human studies do not demonstrate a significant correlation between anthraquinone laxative use, pseudomelanosis coli, and colorectal carcinoma. Interestingly, the authors of this review suggested that the slightly increased incidence of polyps seen in anthraquinone laxative users could be attributed to the pigmentation of the bowel wall, which allowed for better visualization on colonoscopy. As such, it provided a diagnostic benefit rather than a cause of the polyps themselves.

Dosing

There is no risk or dose restriction when using the mucilaginous gel on the skin; if it is properly prepared, without anthraquinones (achieved by separating the outer layer of the leaf from the mucilage), it should be safe for internal use as well. The International Aloe Science Council suggests that the maximum allowable aloin content in aloe-derived material for oral consumption is less than 10 ppm (parts per million).

The vast majority of studies have verified and validated the claims for aloe as a great skin-healing and wound-healing herb, but there is at least one contradictory study. A study of 21 women who had wound complications requiring a second surgery after cesarean delivery or laparotomy for gynecologic surgery demonstrated significant delay in wound healing in the aloe-treated cohort. This was a very small study, but it does serve as a reminder that herbs work in pluripotent ways, and a natural practitioner will need to consider each herb in the context of each patient and their diagnosis and state of well-being.

Andrographis

Andrographis paniculata

Alternate common name: chiretta
Plant family: Acanthaceae
Part used: aerial parts
Medicinal actions: blood-sugar balancing, hepatoprotective, anticoagulant, antiviral, and immunostimulating

Sometimes called the king of bitters, this annual herb from India and southeast Asia is remarkably bitter, largely due to the andrographolides—bitter diterpene lactones that constitute up to 50 percent of the plant material by dry weight. Although the most common traditional use is for bacterial infections, especially with hectic fevers and sweating, where it is considered to clear "toxic heat," this herb is also known for eliminating parasites and for treating viral infections, including herpes, tuberculosis, HIV, influenza, and dysentery. It is indicated for viral infections of the liver, where the cooling, bitter, and bile-promoting (choleretic) properties and the hepatoprotective properties are particularly helpful. Andrographis is indicated where there is loss of appetite and weight loss.

Benefits in Cancer Care

The antiviral, liver-protective, blood-sugar-lowering, and anticoagulant effects of andrographis are generally helpful in cancer care, and its nonspecific immune-stimulating properties are also important. It improves cardiac perfusion, or circulation to the heart muscle, meaning better oxygenation of the heart. It reduces platelet aggregation and functions indirectly as a blood thinner through reducing various cytokines and other inflammatory molecules that tend to stimulate coagulation (thickening).

Andrographis regulates blood sugar and may increase the effectiveness of metformin in type 2 diabetes. This makes it especially helpful in treating cancer, where blood-sugar management is a critical aspect of a holistic treatment plan. It is also an immunostimulant; it helps white cells conduct phagocytosis, which is a direct attack on pathogens, and in studies it shows promise against cancer of the stomach, breast, and prostate, against melanoma, and against lymphocytic leukemias.

In addition, it has demonstrated anticancer effects. In studies, the active constituent in andrographis—called andrographolide—demonstrated cytotoxic and anticancer effects on almost all types of cell lines. This was due to multiple regulatory pathways, including modulation of oxidative stress, induction of cell cycle arrest and cell death, anti-inflammatory and immunomodulating effects, and inhibition of migration, invasion, and development of new blood vessels. Cell line and animal studies have shown combined treatment with the chemotherapy drug 5-FU and andrographis was significantly more effective than either 5-FU or andrographis alone, and that these effects were even more effective when the andrographis was combined with oligomeric proanthocyanidins (OPCs), a group of flavonoids present in grapeseed extract and pine bark extract.

Dosing

Dried herb: 2–6 g daily of dried herb.

Tincture: 3–12 mL daily of a 1:2 tincture made with 45% ethyl alcohol.

Use caution with higher doses, as it can cause gastric distress, loss of appetite, and vomiting. Animal studies have suggested an antiandrogenic and antispermatogenic effect that could affect fertility, so long-term use is not recommended. However, it is commonly used long term in Traditional Chinese Medicine with no evidence in humans of any toxicity like that seen in rodents.

Clinical Pearls

Because it is so cooling to the body, andrographis may be used with warming herbs, such as prickly ash, ginger, or turmeric, for balance. The bitterness of this herb gives it a tropism, or direction of action, toward the liver. It may be especially supportive in viral hepatitis, primary or metastatic liver cancer, gallstones, and cancer of the bile duct. It is also a specific herb in the rare case of hepatic parasite infections (for example, amoebic dysentery can ascend and reside in the liver).

The antiviral properties of andrographis may be helpful in preventing some virally induced cancers. Effects on cancer are uncertain because the viral infection may have been long ago (10–20 years in hepatitis C and liver cancer), but at the least, resisting progression can be expected.

Baikal Skullcap

Scutellaria baicalensis

Alternate common name: Chinese skullcap

Plant family: Lamiaceae

Part used: root

Medicinal actions: bitter, cooling, anti-inflammatory, antimicrobial

Baikal skullcap root contains more than 35 flavonoids, which give it the yellow color that inspires its name *huang qin,* or golden root. In Traditional Chinese Medicine, Baikal skullcap is characterized as bitter and cold and is prescribed for infections, inflammations, and fevers. It is antimicrobial and anti-inflammatory and is used for treating high fevers that are accompanied by irritability, thirst, cough, and productive coughing. The closely related species *Scutellaria barbata* is also used in the same ways.

What Makes It Medicinal

It is likely that there is synergistic action among the many flavonoid compounds in Baikal skullcap. One of them, baicalin, has been especially well researched. It ferments in the gut to produce a flavone called baicalein, which is readily absorbed into the bloodstream and exerts a broad spectrum of important biological activities, including marked anti-inflammatory action and anticancer effects.

Traditional Indications for Baikal Skullcap

- Diarrhea, dysentery, and other bowel infections
- Upper respiratory infections with fever, earaches, and full sinuses
- Thick sputum or mucous discharges
- Urinary tract infections, jaundice, and hepatitis
- Nervous tension, irritability, insomnia, seizures
- Tension or fluid retention–type headache
- Red face or eyes
- Coughing or vomiting blood, nosebleeds, and blood in the stool
- Abdominal pain and vaginal bleeding, threatened miscarriage during pregnancy, and premenstrual stress
- Water retention

Benefits in Cancer Care

Baicalein exhibits antioxidant and anti-inflammatory effects that can inhibit cell cycling by inhibition of telomerase activity. Telomerases are enzymes required to initiate the unwinding of DNA prior to copying and cell replication. If DNA cannot unwind, then the cell cannot replicate, and this can slow cancer. Baicalein regulates fatty acid metabolism and prostaglandin production and shows powerful mediating effects on inflammatory pathways. It also suppresses NF-κB oncogenic transcription factor in the nucleus.

Another flavonoid from Baikal skullcap, called wogonin, sensitizes cells to cisplatin chemotherapy and induces apoptosis or cell death. In a study of cancer cells with resistance to the chemotherapy drug doxorubicin, wogonin reversed the drug resistance by suppressing nuclear factor erythroid 2-related factor 2 (NRF2) transcription factors, which normally act to protect cells from oxidative stress.

Baicalein has other benefits as well. It is neuroprotective and anticonvulsant, which can be helpful if there are metastases in the brain, and it protects the liver and reduces liver stress from chemotherapy. The herbal extract is also beneficial for postoperative cognitive impairment. A human study providing two flavonoids from roots of *Scutellaria baicalensis* and the heartwood of *Acacia catechu* at 300 milligrams twice daily for 30 days demonstrated improvement in speed and accuracy of processing complex information and improved recall and memory.

One study showed that Baikal skullcap extract had a weak blood-building effect in lung cancer patients undergoing chemotherapy and also some immune benefits in the same population.

Dosing

Dried root: 8–15 g daily in a decoction. Capsules are usually sold in 500 mg doses, with a recommendation to take two to four capsules daily. That is a low dose compared to the decocted tea; it is safe to take six to eight capsules daily, if indicated.

Tincture: Up to 40 mL daily of 1:5 tincture made with 45% ethyl alcohol. There is no specified upper limit and no expected risk. The plant flavonoids are activated by fermentation in the gut, indicating that attention to the gut flora and microbiome may be necessary to obtain best effects from the herb. Weeding, seeding, and feeding the gut flora (see page 55) may maximize the herbal effects.

Bupleurum

Bupleurum falcatum

Alternate common name: chai hu or hare's foot

Plant family: Apiaceae

Part used: root

Medicinal actions: immunomodulating, anti-inflammatory, hepatoprotective

The root of this herb from the celery family is widely used in Traditional Chinese Medicine and is recognized for its immunomodulating and inflammation-mediating properties. These have particular value in cancer. The root is considered bitter and cooling to the body; it is used as a diaphoretic, or sweat inducer, at the onset of colds and flus and a cough suppressant for chest infections that are disturbing sleep or becoming debilitating.

What Makes It Medicinal

Bupleurum root contains several triterpene saponins, collectively called the saikosaponins, and these are largely responsible for the anti-inflammatory properties, including increased macrophage (white blood cell) activity, inhibition of the inflammatory prostaglandins, and regulation of tissue granulation in wound repair. The saikosaponins also inhibit platelet aggregation and are thus slightly blood thinning. Saikosaponins have a liver-protective effect after toxin exposures and promote liver repair. They improve the integrity of the gut wall, thus reducing toxin absorption, and they improve kidney function and promote elimination. Complex polysaccharides, the bupleurans, are immunomodulating and support the saponins in normalizing adrenal cortex functions, making this herb an effective adaptogen.

Benefits in Cancer Care

Numerous constituents in bupleurum have been identified in lab research and show promise in the treatment of cancer. The root is used in herbal medicine, but modern research is finding potentially useful constituents in the leaves as well. Harvesting leaves instead of roots allows for a more sustainable harvest cycle; it also means that the medicine is often more affordable to the patient.

In studies involving human colon cancer cell lines, the steroid fraction of bupleurum root induced cell death in a dose-dependent manner, inhibited p-glycoprotein-mediated multidrug resistance, and sensitized cancer cells to chemotherapy and radiotherapy. It protected against inflammatory disorders, such as asthma, arthritis, and sepsis, and it protected the liver against injury and fibrosis by suppressing cytokines, including platelet-derived growth factor and transforming growth factor-β1.

A paper published in 2021 identified a new phenolic glycoside—malconenoside A, from leaves of *Bupleurum malconense*—that inhibited human liver and gastric cancer cells and indicates the potential for antitumor activity. Another study of the aerial parts of *Bupleurum marginatum* identified a new triterpenoid and a new flavonoid; in vitro, they inhibited oncogenic NF-κB induction by 60 and 24 percent, respectively. This is all promising, but caution is suggested as these are not the species or parts traditionally used in herbal medicine, so it is harder to know what to expect from them.

Dosing

This herb rarely causes side effects, but drowsiness may occur at higher doses, and it can occasionally have a laxative effect.

Tincture: 3–12 mL daily of 1:2 tincture made with 60% ethyl alcohol.

Dried root: Up to 6 g daily decocted into tea. Tincture is preferred, to better access the saikosaponins.

Cacao
Theobroma cacao

Plant family: Malvaceae
Part used: seed/bean
Medicinal actions: antioxidant, blood-sugar balancer

It was a good day for patients and practitioners alike when research confirmed that chocolate is good for you! As well as being a sweet treat the world over, cacao is known to have numerous health benefits, including regulation of blood pressure and insulin levels, improved vascular health, inhibition of oxidation processes, increased prebiotic intestinal effects, and more stable blood sugar and better metabolism of fats.

What Makes It Medicinal

Cacao seeds are rich in flavonoids, polyphenols, and procyanidins, which have been shown to inhibit new tumor formation, tumor growth, and new blood vessel growth. With its high levels of antioxidants, cacao may decrease damage caused by carcinogens and inhibit oxidative processes that lead to cancer. Polyphenols contribute to antiulcer, antithrombotic (blood clot–reducing), anti-inflammatory, immunomodulating, antimicrobial, blood pressure–decreasing, and pain-relieving effects. Cacao reduces atheroma (blocking of arteries by cholesterol) through an antioxidant effect on cholesterol. Along with green tea and red wine, dark chocolate is one of the most polyphenol-rich foods consumed regularly by many people. Dark chocolate contains more nonfat cocoa solids (cocoa powder) than milk chocolate, and therefore more flavonoids per gram, although total catechin content may vary.

These polyphenols contribute to the bitter aftertaste of cocoa. To decrease the bitterness and achieve a sweeter taste, processing techniques (such as "dutching") are used. Dutching involves washing the cacao beans in an alkaline solution of potassium carbonate to counteract their acidity, so that the finished cocoa powder won't neutralize baking soda if used in cooking. However, it also decreases the polyphenol content substantially, creating a more palatable but markedly less medicinal product.

This means you should always look for raw, unprocessed cacao. Cacao bean is the richest known source of an alkaloid called theobromine, a xanthine alkaloid related to caffeine and to the asthma drug theophylline. Theobromine is a mood enhancer and antidepressant. Cacao also contains phenethylamine, which triggers the release of endorphins and increases the action of dopamine, a neurotransmitter associated with sexual arousal and pleasure. Another substance found in cacao is a cannabinoid called anandamide, which is normally found in the brain. It binds to the same receptor sites in the brain as cannabis does and produces feelings of happiness and pleasure. Cacao also boosts brain levels of serotonin—maybe one reason why people with depression and women with PMS crave chocolate (because they are deficient in serotonin). Cacao is also high in minerals, notably potassium, phosphorus, copper, iron, zinc, and magnesium.

Cocoa butter, made from roasted cacao beans, has a melting point around body temperature, is very emollient, and prevents rancidity of other fats—all of which make it an excellent addition to herbal skin-care products.

Food of the Gods

The Latin genus name for cacao translates to "food of the gods" (*theo* meaning "god" and *broma* meaning "food"). The words *cacao* and *chocolate* are corruptions of the ancient Indigenous names *kakaw,* for the plant, and *cacahuatl* or *xocolatl,* from the Aztec words *xococ* (bitter) and *atl* (water), for the traditional drink made of the seed.

What we recognize today as chocolate is also made from the seeds. When the seeds are harvested, they are first fermented, then dried and roasted to make "nibs" that contain more than 50 percent cocoa butter. These are crushed in heated rollers to yield cocoa liquor, which is combined with varying amounts of milk and sugar to make chocolate. The chocolate nibs are unsweetened, as is cocoa powder, and this is what you should purchase if you want to eat chocolate, or very dark (> 85% cacao) chocolate bars.

Benefits in Cancer Care

Cacao polyphenols reduce vascular endothelial growth factor (VEGF) activity and inhibit new blood vessel growth. In vitro studies of catechins, flavonoids, and procyanidins from cacao have shown that these compounds downregulate (suppress) the nuclear transcription factors NF-κB and AP-1 in cancer cell lines. Many of the same redox-regulating and free radical–quenching effects of catechins that are seen with green tea are mirrored with the catechins of chocolate. These effects provide a broad antiproliferative influence that is a strong preventive of cancer.

BLOOD-SUGAR REGULATION

The various flavanols in cacao slow carbohydrate digestion and absorption in the gut. Cacao flavanols improve insulin sensitivity by regulating glucose transport and insulin-signaling proteins in insulin-sensitive tissues (liver, fat tissue, and skeletal muscle). This has anticancer effects by reducing readily available sugars for a tumor.

IMMUNOMODULATION

Dark chocolate (low sugar) has anti-inflammatory effects after 4 weeks of use, with measurable reduction in postchallenge responses of cytokines, vascular markers, white blood cells, and leukocyte-activation markers as well as lower serum concentrations of immunoglobulins. Reducing these inflammatory pathways has an anticancer effect.

HEART HEALTH

Cacao lowers blood pressure, inhibits insulin resistance, improves vascular functions, and helps regulate several of the detrimental blood fats, including total cholesterol, low-density lipoprotein (LDL) cholesterol, and apolipoprotein B concentrations. It increases production of nitric oxide (NO) in blood vessels, causing vasodilation and reducing blood pressure, and it inhibits oxidation of LDL cholesterol and prevents atherosclerosis (thickening and hardening of the blood vessel walls). The nitric oxide also activates the prostacyclin synthesis pathway, which has the effect of acting as an anti-inflammatory and widening and protecting the blood vessels by inhibiting plasma leukotrienes.

Cocoa butter is approximately 33% oleic acid, 25% palmitic acid, and 33% stearic acid. Rather than raising plasma cholesterol levels, these acids act in the body much like the monounsaturated fat in olive oil to help keep cholesterol liquid and flowing in vessels, instead of forming atheroma plaques.

Dosing

Dark chocolate (84% cacao or higher): Not more than 1 oz. (30 g) daily, preferably sweetened with stevia or xylitol to avoid sugar.

The *American Journal of Clinical Nutrition* suggests that consuming just ½ ounce (15 g) of dark chocolate daily will be sufficient to reduce damaging oxidation of LDL cholesterol. Even in healthy younger adults a daily intake of 20 g of very dark chocolate (90% cacao) for 30 days can improve vascular function by reducing central brachial artery pressures and promoting vascular relaxation.

Raw cacao nibs: A particular favorite sweet treat in my household is 1 tablespoon each of raw cacao nibs and bee pollen combined. We sometimes eat it right off the spoon, or if we are being really decadent, we sprinkle it over French toast or stir it into thick Greek yogurt.

Calendula

Calendula officinalis

Alternate common name: pot marigold
Plant family: Asteraceae
Part used: flowers
Medicinal actions: anticancer, redox regulator, bitter, vulnerary, antimicrobial

Calendula is one of the most useful herbs in the dispensary. It is a redox regulator that reduces oxidative stress in tissues without compromising conventional cancer treatments. It is a bitter digestive aid, a skin and mucous membrane restorative, and a vulnerary herb that promotes wound healing both internally and topically after surgery. Furthermore, it has antifungal and antiviral effects.

What Makes It Medicinal

The flowers are rich in carotenoids and xanthophyll pigments with strong redox-regulating properties, as well as polysaccharides, triterpenes, and saponins that are immunomodulating and a bitter resin that is antimicrobial.

Calendula has a long history of traditional use for any inflammations or ulcerations of the digestive system. It inhibits the enzymes responsible for making inflammatory leukotrienes or prostaglandins, and it stimulates phagocytosis by white blood cells, which cleans up the cellular debris at the site of an inflammation.

Calendula promotes lymphatic drainage and supports tissue detoxification, especially in lymphatic or breast cancers and as a uterine and endometrial anti-inflammatory tonic agent. Topically, it is well known to treat fungal infections of the skin, as well as burns, wounds, varicose eczema, chilblains, skin infections, and skin cancers. It can be included in a bloodroot salve for skin cancer and will ameliorate some of the burning symptoms.

Benefits in Cancer Care

The antioxidant, immunostimulating, antiviral, and vulnerary actions of calendula make it valuable as an adjunct in most cancer treatments. However, it has active anticancer effects as well. The cytotoxic effects of calendula extract on tumor cell lines were first identified more than 25 years ago, and research has confirmed several active constituents.

Cytotoxic activity. Lutein, a flavonoid found in *Calendula officinalis* flowers, possesses selective cytotoxic activity toward breast cancer cell lines in vitro, in particular triple-negative breast cancer cells. Studies have shown that several proteins that drive cell death, including p53, Bax, and caspase-3, are increased in lutein-treated cancer cells, while expression of Bcl-2, a protein that inhibits cell death, is decreased after exposure to lutein.

Two triterpene glycosides from calendula flowers were tested in vitro for their cytotoxic activity in 60 cell lines derived from leukemia, non–small cell lung cancer, colon cancer, central nervous system cancer, melanoma, ovarian cancer, renal cancer, prostate cancer, and breast cancer and were found to exert wide inhibition.

Reducing skin damage from radiation. In a placebo-controlled clinical trial of 40 patients, calendula flower extract proved to be helpful as a mouthwash to significantly decrease the severity of radiation-induced oral inflammation after local radiotherapy. Topical use of calendula flowers has also shown benefits in reducing dermatitis and radiation damage to skin.

Dosing

Several methods of extraction have been studied, including various solvents such as methanol and hexane, and even a water infusion potentized with laser beams. None of these is practical for the prescribing herbalist, and the studies have tended to show a need for higher doses than is easily achievable through simple teas, so tinctures or concentrated extracts are recommended.

No acute toxicity was recorded after oral administration of calendula flower tincture in doses of up to 5 g/kg of body weight. There is no upper limit on the dose of this herb, and the flower petals can be added to food quite safely—they look lovely sprinkled over a salad or a dessert or frozen into decorative ice cubes.

Tincture: 1.5–3.5 mL daily of a 1:2 tincture comprising equal amounts of 25% extract and 95% extract. Because it has water-soluble and non-water-soluble active constituents, the tincture of calendula is best made in two separate vessels, at 25% alcohol and at 95% alcohol respectively, then the two extracts can be combined.

Growing Calendula

Calendula is so easy and satisfying to grow that it lends itself to a simple horticulture-therapy project everyone can engage in. Simply get some seeds, sow them according to the directions, plant the seedlings out into flowerpots or window boxes, and keep them watered. It won't be long before you can have the immense pleasure of seeing your flowers pushing on up and bursting out in bright orange blossoms. Don't be shy to pick them—the more you pick, the more the flowers keep growing. Toward the end of the season you can let some of them mature through to seeds that are dry and browning on the plant and ready to harvest, store, and plant again the next year.

Corydalis

Corydalis yanhusuo, C. ambigua

Plant family: Papaveraceae

Part used: root

Medicinal actions: antispasmodic, analgesic, blood moving and decongesting, anticancer

Corydalis is a type of poppy with a number of traditional uses: as a blood-moving herb, for clearing stagnation in tissues, and as an anticonvulsant for seizures, an antiarrhythmic, an antiviral, and a sleep aid. Perhaps its most helpful role in a cancer scenario, though, is to relieve pain with fewer side effects, such as constipation, than pharmaceutical opioids. Importantly, corydalis is not habit-forming and may in fact help decrease the opioid cravings in patients who have become habituated.

What Makes It Medicinal

Opioids work through binding with three types of opioid receptors (mu, delta, or kappa receptors) in nervous tissue, all of which suppress conduction of calcium and inhibit neurotransmitter release. Corydalis root has isoquinoline alkaloids that can act selectively on kappa opioid receptors; these receptors are especially active in mediating abdominal pain perception, as well as regulating mood and the craving/reward systems that control addiction. Kappa opioid receptor agonists have potent pain-relieving effects and elicit fewer side effects than agonists of the other opioid receptor subtypes. They are not habit-forming and do not cause constipation and respiratory depression like morphine does. Indeed, several human studies have demonstrated that corydalis may be helpful in reducing morphine cravings.

The alkaloids corydine and corydaline are also mu opioid receptor agonists and contribute to pain-relieving effects that way as well, but the addictive properties are tempered by the kappa agonist effects. Numerous other isoquinoline and protoberberine alkaloids may also inhibit the enzyme cholinesterase, which breaks down the acetylcholine that runs the parasympathetic nervous system and thus promotes rest and relaxation.

Corydalis is also a mediator of inflammation, inhibiting the enzymes responsible for production of inflammatory prostaglandin E2, leukotrienes, and thromboxanes. In practice corydalis is often combined with anti-inflammatory herbs, antispasmodics, and anxiolytics or other sedatives for its sleep-inducing or pain-relieving effects, and with blood-moving herbs like dong quai and ginger for decongesting and anticoagulant (blood-thinning) effects.

Benefits in Cancer Care

Corydalis is primarily used for pain relief, but it does have direct anticancer activity as well. Specifically, it is a blood-moving and blood-vitalizing agent, which is useful as a restorative agent in myelosuppression (bone marrow depletion) from chemotherapy or radiotherapy. It is also helpful for pain and sleep disturbance.

Corydalis can also play an important role in managing opioid addiction. Morphine is widely prescribed for cancer pain, but brings with it the risk of increasing drug tolerance and decreasing effects over time; patients require more and more of it, but experience diminishing benefits. There is also the concern of opioid-induced hyperalgesia (a paradoxical increase in pain sensitivity).

Tetrahydropalmatine, one of the key alkaloids in corydalis, binds to dopamine receptors and acts as an antagonist at D1 and D2 and as an agonist for D3, α-adrenergic, and serotonin receptors. This has a balancing and regulating effect on sympathetic/parasympathetic balance.

Dosing

Dried herb: 5–10 g per day of the dried rhizome.

Tincture: Take 2–4 mL daily of a 1:2 tincture made with 45% ethyl alcohol.

The American Herbal Products Association has assigned corydalis a class 2B rating, meaning that it should not be taken if pregnant or breastfeeding.

Clinical Pearls

Use corydalis in small or moderate doses (3–6 g daily) for deep restorative action and blood-building effect and to induce deeper sleep. Use in higher doses (6–10 g daily) for severe pain, especially crampy abdominal pain with blood stasis (feeling of fullness in lower abdomen, bearing-down sensation, throbbing in thighs). Higher doses can lead to morning grogginess and headaches. This herb is quite powerful, so dosing should start low and increase as needed.

Dan Shen

Salvia miltiorrhiza

Alternate common name: Chinese red sage

Plant family: Lamiaceae

Part used: root

Medicinal actions: bitter, cooling, blood moving

Dan shen is an herb with a long history of use in Traditional Chinese Medicine, in which it is considered to have bitter and slightly cooling properties. As long ago as the 1500s, Chinese medicine practitioners recognized that dan shen could improve blood circulation into microvasculature and alleviate blood stasis. Traditionally it is used for angina, palpitations, menstrual problems, insomnia, liver diseases, and cancer.

The main compounds of dan shen root have beneficial cardiovascular and cerebrovascular effects and are antioxidant, neuroprotective, antifibrotic, and anti-inflammatory, and they also inhibit the growth of malignant cells. Caffeic acid derivatives found in dan shen contribute to antioxidant, antithrombotic (prevention of blood clots), antihypertensive (prevention of high blood pressure), antiviral, and antitumor properties. It improves peripheral blood flow. Other recognized actions and uses of dan shen include increased bone-building activity and enhanced bone healing after fractures, after immobilization, or from osteopenia (age-related bone thinning), as well as reducing both the number and activity of osteoclasts that break down bone. Dan shen root is protective and anti-inflammatory in the liver, and it increases macrophage synthesis and immune activation. It is also a mild sedative and relaxant.

What Makes It Medicinal

More than 200 compounds have been identified from dan shen, classified into two major groups: water-soluble (hydrophilic) phenolic compounds (such as salvianolic acids and flavonoids) and nonpolar (lipid-soluble) essential oils and diterpene ketones collectively called the tanshinones. The most abundant of this last group is tanshinone IIA.

Benefits in Cancer Care

The tanshinones have several important therapeutic effects, including antioxidant effects, protection from/prevention of angina and heart attacks, and anticancer properties. They also induce cell death in liver cancer cells.

The blood-moving or decongestant properties of dan shen are of particular relevance in cancer treatment because cancer can be considered, energetically, as a condition of stasis and congestion in the tissues. Similarly, the recognized bone-building properties of the root are especially indicated in cancer as part of a protocol to build bone, strengthen resilience of bone, and resist bony metastasis. Liver-protection and kidney-repair actions as well as neuroprotective actions may also be directly useful to cancer patients.

BLOOD-MOVING ACTION

Dan shen root is used by herbalists today to increase coronary blood flow, improve cardiac oxygenation, reduce angina, and increase cardiac energy production and cardiac output. The tanshinones found in dan shen are actually a type of phytoestrogen molecule that docks into estrogen receptors in the cardiovascular tissues and causes opening of the blood vessels to enable blood flow. Dan shen is not used as a phytoestrogen to regulate reproductive cycles, treat fertility, or alleviate hot flashes of menopause, but it is used to target the cardiovascular tissues specifically and reduces tension, pressure, and congestion in the system. This action promotes overall circulation through the system. The herb also inhibits platelet aggregation and has an antithrombotic effect. It is used to treat cardiac insufficiency, palpitations, hypertension, bruising, and blood clots.

BRAIN-REPAIR EFFECTS

A frequent consequence of chemotherapy and radiotherapy is varying degrees of cognitive impairment, usually worst during and in the immediate aftermath of treatment, and typically improving with time after completion of treatment. This symptom of "brain fog" is one of the key indicators for choosing to use this herb in a formula.

A polyphenolic compound from dan shen root called salvianolic acid B is a powerful antioxidant that activates NRF2 in cell nuclei, thus regulating immune functions, and possesses neuroprotective properties that are beneficial for diseases of cerebral vasculature and cognitive function. Salvianolic acid B also activates sirtuin 1 (SIRT1), a protein that regulates cellular response to inflammation and to metabolic and oxidative stressors. SIRT1 is a key participant in neuronal plasticity, whereby nerve tissue can redirect impulses and form new neural pathways, which allows for improved cognitive function.

KIDNEY-REPAIR EFFECTS

Low-grade or subclinical chronic kidney deficiency is a very common finding in the general population, especially in seniors. This may be particularly aggravated after chemotherapy drugs, especially those of the platinum family, many of which are toxic and can cause some considerable inflammation or tissue damage in the kidney. Renal fibrosis is the final stage of chronic kidney disease, and this stage can be delayed or slowed by using dan shen as an antifibrotic agent.

Dosing

Dried root: 2–6 g daily (according to how it's used in Traditional Chinese Medicine).

Tincture: 4–12 mL daily of 1:2 tincture made with 50–60% ethyl alcohol.

Use caution if you're taking anticoagulant drugs, as dan shen and these drugs together may thin the blood more than is required. This can be an opportunity for a practitioner to carefully and slowly reduce the drug dose, replacing it with the herb, and hence reducing risk of drug side effects. It is also, for the same reasons, an herb to discontinue in the week before and the week after surgery. There are clinical trials showing that giving dan shen before surgery actually lowers surgical complications without causing excess bleeding, but I recommend avoiding it out of an abundance of caution, not because of strong evidence of harm.

Echinacea

Echinacea purpurea, E. angustifolia, E. pallida

Plant family: Asteraceae
Parts used: root, stem, leaves, flowers, seeds
Medicinal actions: immune tonic and normalizing, inhibits hyaluronidase

All parts of this beautiful flowering plant are medicinal. It was well known to Indigenous peoples in what is now North America for treating infections. They chewed the root for toothaches, sore throats, mouth sores, coughing, and tonsillitis. It was also highly regarded as a treatment for snake and spider bites, scorpion stings, and bee stings; in these cases, it was applied as a poultice over the injury, as well as taken orally.

Early European settlers quickly recognized it as an excellent alterative and blood cleanser and used it for boils, abscesses, chronic infections, ulcerating wounds, and lymphatic swellings. It was one of the most rapidly adopted and successful native plant medicines to be commercialized, and it remains one of the world's best-selling herbs today.

Echinacea extract has immunostimulating, antioxidant, anti-inflammatory, antiviral, antifungal, and antitumor activity. *Echinacea purpurea* is a large, bulky plant that is easy to grow and is often the predominant species in the market. However, the research suggests that although *E. purpurea* is especially useful as an immunomodulator (regulating and promoting the numbers and ratios of white cells), *E. pallida* and *E. angustifolia* are more clearly immunostimulants (promoting neutrophil and macrophage functions).

Indigenous peoples of North America mostly utilized the roots (of *Echinacea pallida*), but research into constituents and pharmacology in the twentieth century was largely done on fresh juice of the aerial parts. Some herbalists today will use all parts of the plant—root, stem, leaves, flowers, and seeds—and all three species.

What Makes It Medicinal

Active constituents include echinacein, an alkylamide that causes almost immediate numbness and tingling in the mucous membranes of the mouth, along with salivation, if any part of the plant is chewed—in fact the presence of alkylamides is a test of having the correct plant. Alkylamides stimulate macrophages (white blood cells) to remove inflammatory debris.

Echinacea also contains polysaccharides, especially in the root, which stimulate phagocytosis of pathogens by macrophages and increase T lymphocyte counts. It also has polyacetylenes, which inhibit bacterial and fungal infections, and multiple flavonoids that inhibit the activity of metalloproteinases, a family of enzymes in the body that degrade the extracellular matrix to facilitate the growth of new blood vessels in tumors. Polyphenolic caffeic acid derivatives also provide a redox-regulating effect and may block VEGF binding to its receptor.

Benefits in Cancer Care

In cancer treatment, echinacea plays a number of roles. Flavonoids in echinacea extract inhibit the growth of new blood vessels in tumors. In studies, an echinacea constituent called cichoric acid downregulated new blood vessel growth and induced cell death in colon cancer cells. Cichoric acid is a caffeic acid derivative that also has antiviral action against the herpes family. In studies using gastric cancer cell lines, *Echinacea purpurea* extract inhibited proliferation and migration of cancer cells; it also inhibited colony formation and induced cell death.

Interestingly, the same constituents that make echinacea effective for snakebites also work to resist tumor expansion and the creation of new blood vessels in cancer. In a snakebite, these constituents act by inhibiting the active enzyme (hyaluronidase) that breaks down connective tissue to facilitate spreading the venom. Cancer also promotes hyaluronidase to facilitate spread, so echinacea may inhibit infiltration and metastases.

An interesting human clinical trial showed that echinacea can prevent relapse of genital warts, which provides some of the better evidence to suggest that echinacea might help prevent cervical (and anal) cancer.

One more promising use of echinacea in cancer is as a synergist with chemotherapy. A study using ethyl acetate extract of echinacea root and paclitaxel showed that echinacea alone exerted a cytotoxic activity toward breast cancer, inhibiting both MDA-MB-231 (triple negative) cells and MCF-7 (estrogen, progesterone, and glucocorticoid receptor positive) cells, with no effect observed in normal breast cells. The echinacea extract induced cell cycle arrest in the G1 phase and caspase-mediated cell death. In vitro, a combination of echinacea extract and paclitaxel showed a synergistic effect on both cancer cell lines.

Dosing

With immune-stimulating and selective cytotoxic properties, anti-metastatic action, and a very high safety profile, there is a strong case for using this herb in cancer care. Because echinacea has some immune-stimulating properties, it may be advisable to consider pulse dosing it, 1 month on and 1 month off, possibly alternating with deep immune tonic and modulating herbs such as astragalus and the medicinal mushrooms.

Dried root: 2–4 g daily of dried root is a safe and effective dose.

Tincture: 4–8 mL daily of a 1:2 tincture made with 40% ethyl alcohol.

Higher doses can be used for a few days in acute infections, and lower doses if the infection continues longer term.

A 2019 study of echinacea extract found no toxicity in vitro or in vivo and no signs of toxicity or death at 2,000 mg/kg in rodents.

People with autoimmune disease can safely use echinacea for an acute infection (1–2 weeks), but there is no longitudinal study to show safety with longer-term use in this population. Therefore, patients with autoimmune conditions should discontinue use after the acute infection has passed. People on immunosuppressive drugs should not use this herb.

Feverfew

Tanacetum parthenium

Plant family: Asteraceae

Part used: flowering tops

Medicinal actions: cooling, bitter, anti-inflammatory, antiarthritic, antimigraine, anticancer

Feverfew is easy to grow and popular in cottage gardens. The bright green foliage and the flowers are harvested for medicine. Feverfew is used as an anti-inflammatory and pain reliever in arthritis, with a long folk tradition upheld by modern research. It is widely used to prevent migraine headaches, reducing the frequency and severity of migraines by keeping the blood vessels toned but not spasmed. These effects are achieved through interfering with the actions of arachidonic acid and histamine and by the release of serotonin from white blood cells. Feverfew inhibits prostaglandin synthesis, decreases vascular smooth muscle spasm, and inhibits platelet granule secretion. Feverfew extract has a blood-thinning action that contributes to its benefits for migraines and arthritis. It should be used with caution in people taking anticoagulants and should be discontinued before surgery.

What Makes It Medicinal

Like so many members of the daisy family, feverfew is rich in volatile oils, including an appreciable amount of a sesquiterpene lactone called parthenolide, as well as flavonoids that are pharmacologically active. A distinctive feature of parthenolide is its ability to induce cell death in cancer cells through inhibition of NF-κB and other prosurvival signaling pathways while sparing normal cells.

Parthenolide also inhibits acquired resistance to chemotherapy. It works in synergy with various chemotherapy agents to increase their anticancer effects, resist metastases, and impair new blood vessel growth. Acquired resistance to radiotherapy involves activation of NF-κB. Treatment with parthenolide may inhibit this, leading to lesser doses of radiation required and reduced radiation toxicity to surrounding cells.

Several studies in different cancers and with different delivery mechanisms have demonstrated that parthenolide may be useful in combination with taxanes (paclitaxel and docetaxol) as well as with vinorelbine (a semisynthetic vinca alkaloid) to enhance the anticancer effects of the drugs. Effectiveness of doxorubicin may also be increased when it is combined with parthenolide. Other drugs with strong in vitro and in vivo evidence of benefits with parthenolide include temozolomide, cisplatin, 5-fluorouracil (5-FU), gemcitabine, temsirolimus, and retinoids.

Parthenolide shows promise as a cofactor to enhance the benefits of hyperthermia (heat) in an exciting novel cancer treatment currently under investigation. Hyperthermia, either organ-specific or body-wide temperature elevation, activates many tissue-healing pathways, and parthenolide augments this.

Dosing

Freeze-dried fresh herb: Capsules of freeze-dried fresh herb are the best option; freeze-drying preserves the volatile oils. Doses of 500–1,000 mg (one or two capsules) daily are recommended.

Fresh herb: Some folk literature suggests eating two or three leaves from the plant daily. This is quite feasible in a mild climate where it may grow for 8–9 months a year. To prevent the volatile oils from irritating the oral mucosa over time, roll up the fresh leaf tightly into a little ball and swallow it like a pill, without chewing. Alternatively, you can fold it into a corner of soft white bread to make a bolus.

Tincture: Tinctures of feverfew are sometimes standardized for parthenolide content at not less than 0.4 mg/mL. Research suggests an effective dose to be 0.25–0.50 mg parthenolide daily, so a tincture dose of 0.5–1.5 mL daily of 1:2 tincture will usually be sufficient. Tinctures should be made from fresh herb and with 45% ethyl alcohol.

Many herbalists report mixed results with this herb, which possibly reflects a variability in quality from one product to the next. Due to the high content of volatile compounds, it is subject to rapid aging and degrading on contact with air or heat. Fresh or freshly dried herb is considered the best; it should be replaced seasonally and not kept for more than a year.

Garlic

Allium sativum

Plant family: Amaryllidaceae

Part used: bulb

Medicinal actions: antibacterial, antiviral, antifungal, regulates and normalizes cholesterol (lowers LDL while raising HDL), anticancer, antiparasitic

The "stinking rose," as it is sometimes called, is the perfect example of a food/medicine. The same chemical compounds that make it so tasty are also those that give it the medicinal effects. It can be eaten liberally and can be taken in capsule form. Onion, shallot, leek, and chive are all related to garlic, as are wild onion, ramps, and nodding onion. None are likely to be as potent, but all can be useful in similar, if milder, ways to garlic.

What Makes It Medicinal

The high content of sulfur-containing compounds in garlic gives it potent antibacterial, antiviral, and antifungal actions, as well as making it effective against intestinal protozoans, worms, and parasites. This may be useful for preventing and treating viral infections and for opportunistic infections during chemotherapy or postsurgical sepsis. Garlic is also recognized as a hypolipidemic that lowers triglycerides, LDL, and total cholesterol while raising HDL.

The most researched and studied active compound, found mostly in the bulb, is alliin, a sulfur-rich volatile compound. An unstable compound, it readily degrades into several derivatives, all of which may be medicinal.

Indeed, whole garlic and whole garlic extract are what I recommend, not purified isolates. Fresh garlic contains up to 15 milligrams of alliin per gram and dried garlic contains 45 milligrams per gram. Alliin is held in an inactive form in whole garlic cells, hence the absence of significant odor from a whole bulb of garlic. But as soon as cell walls are breached (by cutting or crushing), oxidation occurs, an enzyme in the plant cell converts the alliin to allicin, and the distinctive odor occurs. Commercial odorless garlic products are an option for people who experience bowel cramps and excessive flatulence after eating fresh garlic. Odorless garlic is processed at very low heat to preserve the alliin, which will then activate after ingestion and deliver the medicine into the gut, not allowing it to dissipate into the air during processing. Odorless garlic is better tolerated by some people with sensitive digestive systems.

Benefits in Cancer Care

Actions of garlic that contribute to overall anticancer effect include enhanced detoxification of carcinogens, inhibition of cell replication/cell cycling, induction of cell death, suppression of metastasis, and induction of immune responses in cancer cells. Studies on long-term garlic supplementation even show that it reduces the risk of gastric cancer, possibly through prevention of infection by *Helicobacter pylori*, the bacteria associated with stomach ulcers and risk of gastric cancer.

Human studies have shown that garlic also reduces platelet aggregation and increases fibrinolytic activity, which can be useful in cancer, as clotting is a real risk. But this is a mild effect; two clinical trials with patients taking warfarin, and one with patients taking garlic, aspirin, and clopidogrel (a pharmaceutical blood thinner), did not show any interaction and, in particular, no increase in bleeding episodes. Moderate amounts of garlic in the diet, or small amounts of concentrated extract as a medicine, will not cause bleeding episodes.

People taking blood thinners, however, may want to monitor clotting factors and look for unexplained bruising if they are also taking high doses of garlic. As an extra precaution, you may wish to stop using garlic supplements for 1 week before surgery, but there's no need to modify the diet.

Dosing

Powdered garlic: Research has suggested 600–900 mg daily of powdered garlic is effective, which is not a very high dose. This is roughly equivalent to eating one large fresh clove of garlic daily.

CAVEATS

High doses of garlic may interact with warfarin, antiplatelets, antihypertensives, calcium channel blockers, quinolone antibiotics such as ciprofloxacin, and hypoglycemic drugs, but in all cases this is a positive interaction and may allow for lowering of drug dose. This needs to be supervised by a practitioner with weekly or twice-monthly blood tests to check clotting factors.

How to Take Garlic (and Keep Your Friends)

Some people don't want to take garlic because they don't want garlic breath. This is how to prepare and take it without that happening. Peel and finely chop one or two cloves of fresh garlic, then set it aside for 10 minutes to allow the enzymes to convert the alliin to allicin. While you're waiting, eat something starchy—a couple of bites of toast or spoonfuls of cereal—so that you have something in your stomach for the garlic to land on. Otherwise, it can be an irritant or even an emetic (induce vomiting).

Scoop up the chopped garlic with a spoon, put it to the back of your throat, and swallow it without chewing. This keeps the oils out of the mouth and avoids the lingering taste. Follow this with a slightly thick drink, such as milk, nut milk, or a mouthful of smoothie, rather than plain water. Do this twice a day during an infection.

Roasting Garlic the Quick-and-Easy Way

Some fancy restaurants roast garlic bulbs whole and unpeeled; it looks lovely on the plate but you then have to squeeze individual cloves to get to the garlic flesh, making a big mess and wasting a lot. In our house we simply peel as much garlic as we want, toss the cloves very lightly in olive oil, and put them in a baking dish. Spread them out, so they're one clove deep, cover the dish with a lid or aluminum foil, and bake at 375°F (190°C) for 30 minutes. Turn them with a spatula and continue to bake without the lid for a further 10–15 minutes to caramelize to taste. Note that this is a relatively hot oven, and you may want to cook them a little lower if they start to scorch.

Ginger

Zingiber officinale

Plant family: Zingiberaceae

Part used: rhizome

Medicinal actions: anti-inflammatory, warming, carminative, antiemetic

Ginger is widely used as a kitchen spice, for which purpose it is usually sold dried and powdered. The drying and powdering process causes many of the valuable volatile oils to be lost; the fresh root of ginger is readily available in the grocery store and is much better to use in the kitchen. Fresh ginger has a very pungent flavor and leaves a hot sensation in the mouth, reflecting its warming and stimulating properties. Drying of ginger forms the cardiotonic shogaols, so there is value in both fresh and dried plant material for different purposes. Interestingly, the genus *Zingiber* includes at least 85 species of aromatic herbs—including galangal, turmeric, and cardamom—and the ginger we use (*Z. officinale*) is just one of many that may be medicinally helpful. In

Traditional Chinese Medicine, ginger is used to expel cold, wind, and dampness as a warming, invigorating tonic.

What Makes It Medicinal

Ginger rhizome contains up to 7.5 percent oleoresin, which is rich in volatile oils and pungent constituents called gingerols. These gingerols are a series of phenolic compounds. They inhibit synthesis of pro-inflammatory prostaglandins and have a marked anti-inflammatory action. Drying converts the gingerols to shogaols, which makes them two to three times spicier, but they all still exhibit a host of biological activities, ranging from anticancer to antioxidant, circulatory tonic, antimicrobial, anti-inflammatory, and anti-allergic. The volatile oil of ginger also includes many terpenes, which are anti-inflammatory.

Benefits in Cancer Care

Ginger extract and gingerol exert anticancer action through numerous mediators and cell-signaling pathways to exert antiproliferative, anti-invasive, and anti-inflammatory activities. Ginger inhibits NF-κB activation and suppresses gene expression induced by carcinogens. Gingerols induce cell death and inhibit cell cycle progression by reducing cyclin D1 expression, inhibiting secretion of angiogenic factors such as VEGF and IL-8, damaging microtubules required by replicating cells, and inducing mitotic arrest. Ginger exerts a significant preventive effect on many types of cancer by reducing oxidative and inflammatory damage, inhibiting the growth of cells, and inducing cell death.

In cancer therapy, ginger is useful in peripheral neuropathy and in hand-foot syndrome, where both the anti-inflammatory effects and the warming, circulation-stimulating properties are beneficial. The use of ginger in cancer treatment is particularly indicated when there is nausea, gastric spasming or cramping, or poor circulation and cold hands or feet, and it can be used as a synergist to improve the uptake and distribution of other herbs in a formula. The warming, carminative properties make this a useful addition to other herbal formulas used during chemotherapy or after surgery. Numerous clinical trials support ginger's value for this purpose, and a recent meta-analysis confirmed this.

OTHER ACTIONS OF GINGER

The shogaols formed during the drying process exert a calming influence on the heart, slowing the rate and regulating the rhythm. They also slow the breathing rate, reduce blood pressure, and have heart-supportive properties.

The oleoresin reduces blood cholesterol levels, and it exerts a cholagogue (bile-releasing) and gallbladder-supporting action. It is thus indicated for the spasming and cramping of gallbladder disease and gallstones.

Ginger especially stimulates the blood supply to the hands and feet and is therefore useful in conditions involving poor circulation to these areas. Chilblains, cramps, pins and needles, and cold hands and feet can all be helped by drinking ginger tea. Ginger rhizome is also useful for cramps of the digestive system, such as painful menstruation, or for cramps of the large intestine, especially where there is associated flatulence.

Dosing

Tincture: 2–4 mL daily (in divided doses) of 1:2 tincture made with 90% ethyl alcohol.

Dried root: 1–3 g daily of dried root, or two to six capsules of 500 mg each.

Ginger is on the FDA's "generally regarded as safe (GRAS)" list and is considered safe at dosages of up to 4 grams daily. The doses given here are quite high and may cause upper digestive burning in a few people, in which case the dose can be reduced by half.

Ginger is warming and tonifying. It can be easily added to any herbal tea or tincture to improve peripheral and abdominal circulation and reduce queasiness, nausea, gas, or cramps. It acts as an adjuvant to other herbs, improving their absorption and assimilation. I use ginger for patients that feel chilly, have digestive cramps and gas, and have poor peripheral circulation, or simply those in need of a warming, stimulating tonic and digestive aid. In Traditional Chinese Medicine, dried ginger is believed to act more deeply in the body than fresh ginger does.

Caution is recommended for patients taking blood-thinner medications. Dietary use of ginger is considered safe, but doses over 4–5 grams daily may theoretically contribute to blood thinning.

Gotu Kola

Centella asiatica

Plant family: Apiaceae

Parts used: leaves and other aerial parts

Medicinal actions: anticancer, cerebral circulatory stimulant, anxiolytic, connective tissue tonic

This is a creeping groundcover plant that grows throughout the tropics. It's probably native to southern India, where it is cooked as a green vegetable and treated much like spinach. It has been recognized for more than 2,000 years in Ayurvedic medicine as a brain tonic to enhance concentration, mental focus, and memory, while also calming the mind and reducing anxiety. It is sometimes called brahmi, but this is also a name given to *Bacopa monnieri*, so "gotu kola" is preferred to avoid confusion.

What Makes It Medicinal

Gotu kola contains a series of triterpene saponins that work synergistically, including asiatic acid, madecassic acid, and asiaticoside; these are responsible for many of its medicinal effects. In the raw fresh plant, these saponins can occasionally irritate the hands, mouth, and throat in some sensitive people. This does not happen with dried plant material or extracts. Other active constituents include flavonoids, volatile oils, and immunomodulating phytosterols. It also contains a range of antiproliferative polyphenols including rosmarinic acid.

BRAIN TONIC

In traditional Ayurvedic medicine this herb is considered to be a brain tonic, to improve memory, and to nourish and strengthen the central nervous system. Research has shown that the asiatic acids from the leaves are agonists for gamma-aminobutyric acid (GABA) receptors, bringing a calming and relaxing effect to the mind. Gotu kola also enhances cerebral circulation, so it is simultaneously invigorating and enlivening to the mind. It was traditionally prescribed for enhancing meditation, to help keep sustained focus on one thing, while also encouraging meditators to be completely calm and relaxed. Today we can see this being valuable to students or anyone struggling or stressed by trying to learn something new or think in new ways. Anxiety impairs short-term memory, and gotu kola inhibits this stress response, thus aiding learning and recall. Gotu kola is used to revitalize the brain and nervous system, to increase attention span and concentration, and to combat age-related cognitive decline or postoperative cognitive impairment.

CONNECTIVE TISSUE TONIC

Gotu kola is a notable connective tissue tonic, helping to lay down proper amounts of collagen and elastic fibers and in the proper alignments, as well as to nourish the interstitial gel or ground substance. It is used as a primary, leading herb to treat many connective tissue diseases, including lupus, scleroderma, sarcoidosis, myasthenia gravis, and multiple sclerosis.

This effect also supports its well-known wound-healing properties. Gotu kola has a long tradition of use in India for healing leprosy, burns, eczema, psoriasis, pressure sores, and diabetic ulcers. One of the main bioactive compounds (called madecassoside) reduces infiltration of inflammatory cells into a wound and promotes enhanced skin repair, antioxidant activity, collagen synthesis, and blood vessel repair. Note that controlled new blood vessel growth is required for wound healing, and gotu kola controls the rate and extent of this growth.

Benefits in Cancer Care

Postoperative cognitive impairment, chemo-induced brain fog, stress, and (understandably) fear-based thinking are all hallmarks of people with cancer, and all of these can be an obstruction to the kind of clear thinking that is needed to properly manage the decision-making related to treatment and postoperative support. Gotu kola's ability to stimulate cerebral circulation can be helpful in mitigating this cloudy thinking, while the antianxiety aspects help with stress and anxiety. Gotu kola may also help with memory loss, cognitive impairment, dizziness, and tinnitus (ringing in the ears).

The wound-healing effects of the herb can be helpful after surgery, both internally for systemic delivery and also topically to speed healing and reduce scarring. An ointment or cream using a gotu kola extract or a gotu kola–infused oil, when applied to open wounds, increases cellular proliferation and collagen synthesis at the wound site and enhances tensile strength. Significantly, cell proliferation is not induced in cancer cells.

CYTOTOXIC EFFECTS

The anticancer actions of gotu kola include inhibiting multiple transduction pathways and transcription factors to induce cell death. Asiatic acid interacts with molecular targets like NRF2, NF-κB, and protein kinase C (PKC), and it has a chemosensitizing effect. In a study with licorice and olive leaf, gotu kola protected human bronchial cells from oxidative and inflammatory injury through enhancing mitochondrial stability, decreasing oxidative stress and inflammation, and promoting the regulatory proteins in the cells.

In studies of kidney and bladder cells exposed to gotu kola alongside chemotherapy, asiaticoside showed synergy with the drug vincristine, inducing cell cycle arrest and cell death and enhancing the antitumor activity of the drug. In animal studies of Adriamycin (doxorubicin), a chemotherapy drug widely used in breast cancer, pretreatment with gotu kola extract at 200 milligrams per kilogram, given orally, significantly prevented the heart muscle damage that would normally occur.

GOTU KOLA AND RADIATION

In cell studies, asiatic acid, madecassic acid, and asiaticoside inhibited radiation-induced migration and invasion of human lung cancer cells at noncytotoxic concentrations, suggesting that they may be useful to enhance the effect of radiotherapy in patients with non–small cell lung cancer. Asiatic acid can act as a natural chemoprotective agent against UVB-mediated injury in human skin cells.

Dosing

Tincture: 3–6 mL daily of a 1:2 tincture made with 45–65% ethyl alcohol for best extraction of triterpenes.

Powdered extract: 150–300 mg daily of 10% triterpene-rich powdered extract.

Clinical Pearls

Gotu kola is the herb I prescribe most frequently in my cancer practice. Gotu kola extract used internally before and after surgery promotes tissue repair and reduces cognitive compromise. I also make an infused (macerated) oil using dried gotu kola leaves and grapeseed oil for topical use over incision sites.

Green Tea

Camellia sinensis

Plant family: Theaceae

Parts used: leaf, twig

Medicinal actions: anticancer, redox regulator, stimulant, metabolic activator

Tea is one of the most widely consumed beverages in the world, second only to water. Green and black teas, as well as oolong, white, bancha, and kukicha, all come from the same plant but are processed differently. Black and oolong tea require partial oxidation of the leaves (the process is frequently called "fermentation," but no microbes are used so "oxidation" is technically incorrect). Green tea is produced by steaming fresh leaves, which inactivates enzymes in the leaves to inhibit oxidation and preserve the polyphenol content; hence green tea has more flavonoids and black tea has more tannins (which form as the flavonoids oxidize). White tea is made from the immature leaf buds; it's low in tannin and has a very mild flavor. Bancha is from the second flush of leaves after the first annual harvest, and kukicha is made from the twigs and stems that can be green or oxidized. All have redox-regulating polyphenols, but green tea contains the most. The polyphenols (flavonols or catechins) in tea comprise 30–40 percent of the extractable solids of dried green tea leaves. An infusion of dried green tea leaves has numerous anticancer activities, including antimutagenic, antioxidant, antitumor, and cancer-preventive actions.

What Makes It Medicinal

Of course, as with all herbs, there are numerous and abundant constituents in green tea with layers of mutual influences, and only a few have been isolated and studied. The most abundant phenolic in green tea, and the most researched, is epigallocatechin gallate or EGCG. This polyphenolic catechin is antiviral, antibacterial, and redox regulating and has strong anticancer effects across numerous cell pathways. It is not directly cytotoxic—in fact it is very safe—but the overall effect is to disable cancer cells and inhibit cancer initiation and progression, achieved through diverse mechanisms including antioxidant activity, cell cycle regulation, tyrosine kinase receptor inhibition (downregulating of VEGF, EGF, and IGF-1), immunomodulation, inhibition of NF-κB and AP-1 transcription factors, and epigenetic control.

A green tea catechin extract applied to the site of genital warts after laser ablation reduced the recurrence rate from up to 77 percent to below 6.5 percent at 3 months after completion of the therapy. This strong antiviral effect is expected to contribute to inhibition of cervical cancer.

Some of the Anticancer Effects of Catechins and Green Tea

Note that most of these effects were seen in preclinical research and not human trials.

- Anti-inflammatory
- Antioxidant (redox regulating)
- Suppress tumor initiation and growth; inhibit topoisomerase I enzyme, which is required for DNA copying before a cell can replicate, thereby blocking tumor cell replication
- Inhibit NF-κB, an oncogenic transcription factor in the nucleus
- Induce or switch on cancer-suppressor genes
- Inhibit genetic mutations
- Inhibit VEGF and protein kinase C, which downregulates new blood vessel growth
- Inactivate matrix metalloproteinase (MMP) enzymes, which break down connective tissue to help cancer spread
- Inhibit aromatase activity to downregulate estrogen influence
- Inhibit multidrug resistance to make chemotherapy more targeted and effective
- Prevent cardiac toxicity in chemotherapy
- Promote liver detoxification pathways
- Reduce serum lipids and lipoproteins; protective effect on lipid peroxidation
- Protect skin from UV radiation
- Thermogenic effect—turn up the body's thermostat so it burns more calories (only from higher doses)
- Decrease muscle loss in cancer
- Enhance fat metabolism

Modern research has revealed a unique amino acid in tea, N-ethyl-L-glutamine, otherwise known as L-theanine. L-theanine increases brain levels of serotonin, dopamine, and GABA, the mood-elevating and relaxing neurotransmitters, and animal studies suggest it improves learning and memory. It is recognized for its neuroprotective and relaxant effects, which can calm the mind and ease anxiety without creating drowsiness. This is somewhat uncommon in herbs, where most antianxiety agents are also sedatives, and capsules of a standardized extract of theanine have become popular as a nervine and antianxiety aid, and, with other more sedating herbs, it is used as a sleep support.

The Question of Caffeine

Caffeine has been shown to activate tea polyphenols, such as EGCG, so it is preferable not to decaffeinate the tea. If this is a problem for somebody very sensitive to stimulants, then taking it in the morning, taking it with food, and possibly taking it with a nervine like chamomile might be helpful. Calming theanine capsules can also be taken alongside green tea if desired.

Dosing

Extract: An appropriate dose for cancer inhibition would be 3–4 g daily of standardized green tea extract (95% polyphenols/60% catechins). This would normally be taken in capsules, equivalent to four to six capsules daily.

Matcha: This is a super-concentrated green tea powder from Japan. A daily dose of 1–2 tsp. is great. It is bitter, so consider adding cardamom, vanilla, coconut sugar, or stevia. It can be made latte-style in a milk or nut milk base, a little bit like making golden milk with turmeric.

CAVEAT

Do not use green tea or green tea products if you are undergoing treatment with the anticancer drug Velcade (bortezomib). EGCG binds with Velcade, which may significantly reduce its bioavailability and make it less effective. This drug is mostly used for multiple myeloma and mantle cell lymphoma, but sometimes for other cancers as well.

It is also worth noting that a review of the literature on green tea and cancer published in 2020 by the *Cochrane Database of Systematic Reviews* was inconclusive, citing poorly designed studies and difficulty of controlling intake of polyphenols in study groups as reasons. This does not negate the value of the compelling in vitro and preclinical research, but it does raise questions about effective doses and delivery methods.

Clinical Pearls

Green tea is another plant that functions as both food and medicine. It is widely drunk across all of Asia on a daily basis by millions of people, which may have some preventive, antioxidant effects that are generally useful, but it is hard to drink enough green tea to have a marked effect on cancer. For patients who want to avoid yet more capsules, a concentrated matcha powder may be more effective.

Horse Chestnut

Aesculus hippocastanum

Plant family: Sapindaceae

Part used: whole, hulled fresh nut (not the spiny green outer casing)

Medicinal actions: inhibits tumor growth and metastases, reduces swelling, strengthens and repairs blood vessels

The horse chestnut is a large and stately tree with beautiful flowers and big leaves. It is a prominent tree in British forests and widely planted as an ornamental. Unlike the sweet chestnut, the Spanish chestnut, and the Chinese chestnut—all of which are in the beech family and are quite edible—horse chestnuts are in the Sapindaceae (soapberry) family. Most parts of the tree are mildly poisonous and the nuts should not be consumed as a food.

What Makes It Medicinal

The brown skin of the nut is rich in astringent tannins, and the nut meat (which is not edible) has several triterpene saponins collectively called aescin (also sometimes spelled *escin*). These tannins and the aescin saponins combine to give a strong anti-inflammatory and astringent property with a tropism, or attraction, to veins. Horse chestnut is recommended for toning and tightening the walls of veins that may be stretched or flaccid in varicose veins, as an anti-inflammatory, and for its free radical–scavenging effects that protect endothelial vein linings from oxidative damage.

Benefits in Cancer Care

In cancer care, horse chestnuts may help resist brain tumor growth and metastases, as well as reduce brain swelling. The aescin found in horse chestnut inhibits cancer's ability to break down hyaluronic acid (the main component of connective tissue), which inhibits cancer growth through tissues and organs. Horse chestnut also strengthens and repairs vascular tissue and increases the integrity of the capillary lining, which reduces fluid leakage into tissues and improves fluid uptake into lymph vessels, with a net effect of reducing swelling.

Horse chestnut contains a coumarin glycoside called aesculin that is activated by fermentation with gut flora to release the pharmacologically active aglycone called aesculetin. Aesculetin is a mild blood thinner that may be especially indicated in cancer, which tends toward stickier blood. Aesculetin may also help resist bone metastases by inhibiting bone breakdown.

Dosing

Tincture: 1–3 mL daily of 1:2 tincture made with 45% ethyl alcohol.

Commercial products: Commercial seed extracts are usually standardized to around 20% aescin. Up to 100–300 mg of aescin daily is considered effective and safe to help reduce symptoms of poor blood circulation, such as varicose veins, leg aching and pain, leg tiredness, swelling in the legs, itching, and water retention. These symptoms may be caused by cancer if there is notable impairment of blood return from the legs—for example, after inguinal lymph node removal—but can also occur independent of cancer.

Topical use: Horse chestnut can be safely used as a topical application for varicose veins or hemorrhoids. A cold compress made by soaking a cloth in cooled tea is effective for toning and tightening tissue, and creams or ointments are often made for treating hemorrhoids.

Clinical Pearls

Some of the tannins may break down in the gut to yield compounds that are potentially toxic to the liver, and aesculitin, the coumarin aglycone, is neurotoxic in higher doses. High doses of horse chestnut will cause dizziness, headache, nausea, stomach upset, and diarrhea.

This herb should be pulse dosed, 1 month on and 1 month off, and liver enzymes should be monitored every 2–3 months. It is safe for longer-term topical use over varicose veins, hemorrhoids, and bruising.

Due to its blood-thinning qualities horse chestnut might increase the risk of bleeding if used before surgery. Stop using it 1–2 weeks before surgery.

Indian Frankincense

Boswellia serrata

Alternate common name: boswellia

Plant family: Burseraceae

Part used: resin (often standardized to boswellic acids content)

Medicinal actions: anti-inflammatory, antiviral, anticancer

This is a small tree from India, Arabia, and North Africa. The medicinal part is the oleo gum resin, which oozes out from cut or broken branches and contains a high amount of terpenoids, oils, and gums; up to 16 percent of the resin may be composed of essential oils. Frankincense extract has shown great promise for treating chronic inflammatory conditions, including osteoarthritis, rheumatoid arthritis, asthma, and inflammatory bowel disease.

Unfortunately, this slow-growing desert shrub is under threat from habitat loss and climate change. Because of that, sustainable sourcing is very important.

What Makes It Medicinal

The resin contains a number of triterpene acids collectively called the boswellic acids. The best-researched one is acetyl-11-keto-beta-boswellic acid (AKBA), which is a potent inhibitor of the inflammatory enzymes 5-, 10-, and 15-lipoxygenase and regulates prostaglandin production.

Benefits in Cancer Care

Research suggests that AKBA inhibits T lymphocyte immune responses, including inflammation; inhibits enzymes required for cell division; reduces Ki67 (indicating slower cell cycling); normalizes blood markers, including those of proliferation, invasion, and angiogenesis; and inhibits metastases.

Recent research using Indian frankincense extracts has confirmed antiproliferative activity of cinnamaldehyde, an organic compound also found in cinnamon. Research showed that it caused cell death in liver tumor cancer cell lines and blocked cell proliferation in several cancer cell lines, suggesting benefits in breast, colon, and prostate cancer. Cinnamaldehyde also decreases blood sugar, widens blood vessels, and is an antifungal agent, a flavoring agent, and a skin sensitizer for some people. Indian frankincense combines well with turmeric, bromelain, and quercetin as a potent mediator of inflammation.

Dosing

This herb doesn't taste great and requires a high percentage of alcohol as a solvent in a tincture, which usually translates to a higher cost, so it is often recommended in a capsule format for convenience.

Dried herb: A typical dose would be 300–500 mg of a product standardized to 60% boswellic acids, taken two or three times a day.

Tincture: 1–2 mL daily of a 1:2 tincture made with 90% ethyl alcohol.

Magnolia

Magnolia grandiflora, M. virginiana, M. acuminata, M. macrophylla, M. officinalis

Plant family: Magnoliaceae

Part used: bark

Medicinal actions: anti-inflammatory, antioxidant, cooling, aromatic tonic bitter, antianxiety

Magnolia bark is traditionally used in folk medicine in the southern US for intermittent or hectic fevers. It is considered mildly diaphoretic, laxative, and an invigorating tonic. In Traditional Chinese Medicine, the bark is used for treating "qi stagnation" (low energy, low vital force) as well as digestive disturbances, especially those brought on by emotional distress. The bark is also reported to have antianxiety action and to support the cortisol balance of the adrenal cortex, to have antifungal and antibacterial properties, to reduce inflammation and pain, and to protect against seizures. Magnolia bark is used to treat menstrual cramps, abdominal pain, abdominal bloating and gas, nausea and indigestion, coughing, and asthma. The anxiolytic, neuroprotective, and relaxant/sedative effects make magnolia especially indicated during chemotherapy or after surgery.

What Makes It Medicinal

Clinical studies of magnolia's medicinal properties have focused on two key lignan constituents: honokiol and magnolol. Laboratory studies have demonstrated that honokiol protects the liver from oxidative stress and protects the brain from inflammation after an ischemic stroke by inhibiting white blood cell overactivity and oxidative damage. It is an antidepressant, and it may delay onset or slow progression of Alzheimer's disease. Preclinical research supports its use for anxiolytic, analgesic, antidepressant, antithrombotic, antimicrobial, antispasmodic, antitumorigenic, and neuroprotective properties.

Honokiol in particular exhibits anticancer and anti-inflammatory effects by inhibition of cyclooxygenase-2, an enzyme that makes inflammatory prostaglandins. Studies suggest it may specifically target cancer cells in the brain while preserving and protecting healthy neurons and preventing deleterious results from ischemia, seizures, and pain.

Magnolia extract interacts in complex ways with the endocannabinoid receptor sites in the brain and body. Magnolol is a partial or mild agonist at endocannabinoid receptor subtype CB1 and has a stronger agonist effect at CB2; honokiol shows strong agonist properties at CB1 receptors, while acting as an antagonist at the CB2 receptor. This agonist/antagonist effect allows modulation of magnolia effects on mood, brain activity, and parasympathetic/sympathetic balance and promotes alertness without anxiety.

Magnolia compounds are also agonists for the inhibitory neurotransmitter gamma-aminobutyric acid A (GABA-A) and for muscarinic receptors in the central nervous system, both of which contribute to the marked antianxiety and relaxant effects. These complex and layered effects are a good example of the importance of using whole herb extract wherever possible, because constituent interactions and synergies are usually a key part of the therapeutic effect.

Benefits in Cancer Care

Both magnolol and honokiol have been reported to inhibit the growth of several tumor cell lines in laboratory and animal studies. Magnolol downregulates inducible nitric oxide synthase (iNOS), the inflammatory cytokines interleukin-8 and TNF-α, and prostaglandin E2, all of which serve to reduce inflammation.

Honokiol blocks intracellular Ras proteins involved in signal transduction that would otherwise switch on oncogenes, and it inhibits some of the pathways driving multidrug resistance pumping. Furthermore, it modulates the transcription factor NF-κB, which controls a large number of genes involved in new blood vessel growth, metastasis, and cell survival, as well as epidermal growth factor receptor (EGFr) and mammalian target of rapamycin (mTOR).

Honokiol is synergistic with the immunotherapy drugs lapatinib and imatinib in breast cancer cells. Use of honokiol with lapatinib or imatinib resulted in synergistic inhibition of cell proliferation and induction of cell death in HER2-positive breast cancer cell lines, and this may represent an opportunity to prevent or delay drug resistance in breast cancer patients.

Honokiol induces cell death and inhibits tumor growth. The antitumor effect of chemotherapy may be increased by combining honokiol with another agent that suppresses the production of new blood vessels. For example, in one study honokiol alone resulted in effective suppression of the tumor growth, and the combined treatment with honokiol plus platinum chemotherapy markedly inhibited tumor growth and resulted in increased life span. In another study, honokiol enhanced the anticancer effects of doxorubicin chemotherapy.

Dosing

Traditional Chinese Medicine suggests doses of 3–10 g per day of crude magnolia bark in decoctions, taken in divided doses for all-day effects or at bedtime for sleep support. This would be equivalent to 1.5–5 mL daily of a tincture made at 1:2 strength. *Magnolia officinalis* extract found in supplement capsules is typically standardized to 90% honokiol and magnolol and dosed at around 30 mg daily.

CAVEATS

Dietary administration in rats at doses of up to 480 mg/kg in a 21-day study and 240 mg/kg in a 90-day study resulted in no toxicity, although some sources suggest a correlation between progressive interstitial kidney fibrosis and long-term use of magnolia. To put this in context, a 480 mg/kg dose is equivalent to a whopping 26.4 g dose for a 55 kg (121-pound) adult, something that is basically impossible to achieve with ingested supplements. In Traditional Chinese Medicine, doses of 3–10 g per day of crude magnolia bark have been used in decoctions over weeks or months with no indication of risk or harm.

Magnolia may have some mild antiplatelet effect due to inhibition of thromboxane formation as well as inhibition of intracellular calcium mobilization. Some in vitro studies suggest that it might be a blood thinner, but this has not been shown in humans. However, caution is advised in patients with increased bleeding potential or on blood-thinning medication.

Magnolia officinalis is endangered in the wild. Even though almost all of the medicinal supply now comes from cultivated trees, the wild populations are still declining.

Nigella
Nigella sativa

Alternate common name: black seed
Plant family: Ranunculaceae
Part used: seed
Medicinal actions: antidiabetic, anticancer, immunomodulating, analgesic, antimicrobial, anti-inflammatory, spasmolytic, bronchodilator, hepatoprotective, renal protective, gastroprotective, antioxidant

Nigella has a pretty blue annual flower and is native to the Mediterranean and North Africa but widely grown in cottage gardens. Traditional uses of nigella seed in Persian medicine include treatment of asthma, hypertension, diabetes, inflammation, cough, bronchitis, headache, eczema, fever, dizziness, influenza, protozoal and parasitic infections, skin infestations (scabies, lice), and fungal infections.

What Makes It Medicinal
Thymoquinone is a monoterpene molecule that is abundant in the volatile oil of nigella (and found in lesser amounts in a few other herbs), and it is one of the key active ingredients of nigella oil. It is an antioxidant, anti-inflammatory, antiviral, antimicrobial, immunomodulatory, and anticoagulant. Thymoquinone also increases the activity and number of lymphocytes, NK cells, and macrophages in the immune system, and it has demonstrated antiviral potential against a number of viruses.

Benefits in Cancer Care
There are several ways nigella seed can be helpful in cancer treatment, including decreased production of fibroblastic growth factor (FGF), an angiogenic protein made by tumor cells, and inhibition of collagenase and other matrix metalloproteinases, enzymes that break down extracellular matrix and permit new blood vessel growth and metastases.

In vitro laboratory studies show thymoquinone to be a synergist for the chemotherapy drug doxorubicin, in part through improvements in drug effectiveness and selectivity, and in part through inhibition of multidrug resistance. In pancreatic cancer, thymoquinone can increase the sensitivity of pancreatic tumors to chemotherapy drugs by preventing gemcitabine- or oxaliplatin-induced activation of NF-κB.

Laboratory studies have shown that pretreatment of gastric cancer cells with thymoquinone significantly increased the cell-death effects of the chemotherapy drug 5-FU and enhanced the toxicity of 5-FU to gastric cancer cells.

Nigella seed oil can be helpful during radiation treatment as well. Thymoquinone protects brain tissue from radiation-induced oxidative stress. It also shows promise in synergizing with radiotherapy to allow lower doses of radiation with maximal effect.

In studies, both whole nigella seed and isolated thymoquinone have been shown to be effective in protecting the liver against a range of toxins. They reduced levels of serum markers of liver stress or liver damage, including ALT, total bilirubin, alkaline phosphatase (ALP), and gamma-glutamyl transferase (gamma-GT) enzymes and ameliorated the reduced levels of glutathione S-transferase (GST) and other intracellular redox regulators seen after toxin exposure. Thymoquinone also induces programmed death in cancer cells by activation of caspases and modulation of the Bax/Bcl-2 ratio (upregulation of pro-apoptotic Bax and downregulation of antiapoptotic Bcl-2 proteins).

The seeds also contain isoquinoline alkaloids (e.g., nigellicimine and nigellicimine-N-oxide) and pyrazole alkaloids, including nigellidine and nigellicine, as well as triterpenes and saponins, which are all promising potential anticancer agents. It is highly probable that synergy between these complex constituents enhances and promotes the anticancer activities.

BLOOD-SUGAR BALANCING AND METABOLIC SYNDROME

Nigella seeds are traditionally used to treat metabolic syndrome in patients with poor glycemic control. A study in human subjects reported a significant decrease in blood glucose level after 1 week of oral ingestion of nigella seed powder at a dose of 2 grams daily.

Both *Nigella sativa* and thymoquinone offer significant support in cardiotoxicity, hypertension, hyperlipidemia, and atherosclerosis, probably due to the antioxidant and anti-inflammatory properties.

A literature review published in 2014 reported that different preparations of nigella, including seed powder (100 mg–20 g daily), seed oil (20–800 mg daily), thymoquinone (3.5–20 mg daily), and seed extract (methanolic extract, especially), had demonstrated reduced plasma levels of total cholesterol, LDL cholesterol, and triglycerides, but there was little effect on HDL cholesterol. Another human trial did suggest that increased HDL may only be associated with nigella seed powder (in other words, ground whole seed).

ALLEVIATING GASTRIC ULCERS

Nigella seeds possess clinically effective antiulcer activity, through an inhibition of the bacteria *Helicobacter pylori,* comparable to that of conventional drug therapies.

Dosing

Dried seed: 2–4 g daily is a safe and effective dose.

Tincture: 2–10 mL daily of a 1:2 tincture made with 65% ethyl alcohol.

The seed can also be cracked or crushed and macerated into oil for topical use. This is a traditional Middle Eastern treatment for skin lesions, including infections, ulcers, and skin cancers. It can also be poulticed over an area for even stronger effect. In addition, it can be taken internally; try it in salad dressings and sauces.

SAFETY OF NIGELLA

Nigella seed oil has low toxicity and a wide margin of safety for therapeutic doses. In a rat study using a daily oral dose of 2 mL/kg of body weight, no changes were observed in liver enzyme levels, nor were there any histopathological modifications (heart, liver, kidneys, and pancreas), but white blood cells and platelets dropped considerably with higher doses, so this may be an herb for short-term use internally but is entirely safe for topical use.

Pomegranate

Punica granatum

Plant family: Punicaceae or Lythraceae

Parts used: fruit and seed

Medicinal actions: antioxidant, anticancer, antidiabetic, and hypolipidemic

This small, long-lived tree is from the Mediterranean region, where it has been known as a food and a medicine since pre-biblical times. The Babylonians considered pomegranate seeds an agent of resurrection, the Persians believed the seeds conferred invincibility on the battlefields, and the seeds symbolized longevity and immortality for the ancient Chinese. The eastern European wedding ritual of breaking a pomegranate on the steps of the church was said to bring fertility to a marriage.

What Makes It Medicinal

Pomegranate juice has a higher antioxidant rating (as measured by its oxygen radical absorbance capacity, or ORAC) than most other juices, including apple, acai, black cherry, blueberry, cranberry, grape, and orange juice; it also has a higher antioxidant rating than red wine. The chemical composition of the fruit differs according to cultivar, growing region and climate, maturity at harvest and maturity of the tree, cultivation practices, and storage conditions, but the active constituents are predominantly polyphenols.

Numerous cell line, animal, and human studies have demonstrated how this fruit acts as an antioxidant, antidiabetic, and hypolipidemic and shows antibacterial, anti-inflammatory, antiviral, and anticarcinogenic activities. It downregulates antibiotic resistance and lessens ultraviolet radiation–induced skin damage. The fruit also improves cardiovascular and oral health.

The peel of pomegranate has the highest concentration of the medicinal properties. The peel can weigh as much as 50 percent of the total fruit weight and is an important source of phenolics, flavonoids, ellagitannins, and proanthocyanidin compounds, as well as a concentrated source of nutrition with complex polysaccharides and minerals, mainly potassium, nitrogen, calcium, phosphorus, and magnesium.

The flesh of the fruit contains mostly water, with fructose and glucose, pectin, ascorbic acid, citric acid, malic acid, phenolics, and some antioxidant flavonoids. The seeds can weigh up to 20 percent of the total weight of the fruit. They have polyunsaturated omega-3 and omega-6 fatty acids, as well as polyphenols, phytoestrogens—mostly coumestrol and the isoflavone genistein—and traces of estrone (a type of estrogen).

As with so many herbs and foods, the synergistic action of the pomegranate constituents are more effective than the single constituents. Do not throw away the skin. Many of the phenolic constituents are at least partially water soluble, and if nothing else, you can dry it and make teas out of it.

Benefits in Cancer Care

The whole pomegranate fruit has anti-inflammatory, antiangiogenic (inhibiting new blood vessel growth), and antimetastatic properties, and it induces cell death. It is antiproliferative and antitumorigenic by modulating multiple signaling pathways. Pomegranate fruit has strong antioxidant activity from the anthocyanins, ellagitannins, and hydrolysable tannins.

Pomegranate seed oil and polyphenols in the fermented juice inhibit oxidation and synthesis of inflammatory prostaglandins, inhibit breast cancer cell proliferation and invasion, and promote breast cancer cell death. They arrest proliferation and stimulate death in prostate cancer cells, induce death in colon cancer cells, inhibit cell growth and cell viability, and induce death in several other types of cancer cells. Pomegranate further inhibits cancer by downregulating signaling molecules such as NF-κB and mTOR, and downregulating the expression of genes that are responsible in cancer development, such as antiapoptotic genes, MMPs, VEGF, cyclins, cyclin-dependent kinases, and pro-inflammatory cytokines.

Fermenting pomegranate juice with *Lactobacillus plantarum* is reported to increase the concentration of ellagic acid and enhance the antimicrobial activity of the juice. Polyphenols from fermented pomegranate juice showed greater antiproliferative effect than did polyphenols from fresh pomegranate juice. Fermented juice also has an overall estrogen-inhibiting effect; it inhibits the activity of aromatase enzymes that make estrogen and inhibits the enzyme

17-beta-hydroxysteroid dehydrogenase type 1, which turns weakly proliferative estrone into the more potent estradiol.

Pomegranate fruit extract enhances the action of tamoxifen in both tamoxifen-sensitive and tamoxifen-resistant breast cancer cells, making it a food medicine of particular interest in treating breast cancer. It also inhibits the expression of genes for key androgen-synthesizing enzymes and androgen receptors, which adds to the anticancer effects. There are preliminary trials of pomegranate in prostate cancer patients showing overall benefits.

ANTIMICROBIAL

In laboratory studies, extracts from pomegranate fruit show strong antibacterial activity against many bacterial strains, including *Escherichia coli, Staphylococcus aureus, Enterobacter* spp., *Bacillus* spp., and *Micrococcus* spp. Pomegranate fruit rind is active against *S. aureus, Proteus vulgaris, E. coli, Klebsiella pneumoniae, Bacillus subtilis, Salmonella typhi, Listeria monocytogenes*, and *Yersinia enterocolitica.*

BALANCING BLOOD SUGAR AND FAT

Pomegranate leaf extract given to mice inhibited pancreatic lipase activity and caused a decrease in feeding and loss of body weight. The main compounds that present antidiabetic properties are polyphenols, which may affect glycemia through different mechanisms, including inhibiting glucose absorption in the gut or inhibiting its uptake by peripheral tissues. The seed extract (300 and 600 mg/kg, orally) caused a significant reduction of blood glucose levels in induced diabetic rats (47 and 52 percent, respectively) after 12 hours. Although these are not human studies, they may be relevant when considering cancer care given the correlation between high blood sugar, high blood fats, metabolic syndrome, and cancer.

Dosing

Juice: 100–300 mL daily. The higher dose is for active treatment and the lower dose is for longer-term maintenance.

Pomegranate extract is available in capsules from health food stores and from practitioners, but I hesitate to recommend it that way because it seems like such an easy medicine to take as a food; save the pills and capsules for things that can't be eaten.

SAFETY OF POMEGRANATE

In animal studies, there were no toxic effects from large doses of pomegranate extract, up to 5 g/kg body weight. In a human study, 64 overweight people took up to three 710 mg capsules of pomegranate extract (435 mg of gallic acid each) daily for 28 days, and no serious adverse effects were seen on complete blood count, blood chemistry, and urinalysis. As a fruit, it is not expected to be toxic to humans at any normal physiological amounts.

I recommend eating/juicing one to two whole fruits weekly at least, and unsweetened, commercial fruit juices are also available for easy dosing.

Propolis

Propolis (also known as bee resin) is a compound made by bees from collected plant resins and waxes. It serves as a glue or cement in the hive and provides powerful antimicrobial action to keep the hive healthy. The name derives from the Greek words *pro*, meaning "for" or "in defense of," and *polis*, meaning "city" (in this case, the hive). Propolis has been used in folk medicine since at least the time of the ancient Egyptians, when it was combined with myrrh and frankincense resins to embalm the dead. It has long been known as a topical agent for burns, bites, infections, ulcers, pressure sores, and wounds. It is a cicatrant, an elegant term meaning to bind the lips of a wound together. Propolis will form a seal over a lesion to protect it from airborne infection, while healing the tissues below. It was used in times past on the umbilical stump of newborns and on amputations.

What Makes It Medicinal

Propolis comprises a complex mix of terpenes; caffeic, cinnamic, and phenolic acids; and more than 500 bioactive flavonoids, which vary regionally and seasonally according to the plants the bees are visiting. Overall, it is considered to have antioxidant, anti-inflammatory, cytotoxic, antiviral, antifungal, antiprotozoal, liver-protective, and anticancer properties in human applications.

Propolis increases natural killer cell activity against tumor cells and shows strong antibacterial effect against *Streptococcus mutans* and several other streptococcus species that cause strep throat and dental decay and against *Staphylococcus aureus* that causes skin infections and cellulitis. It has a synergistic effect on the antibiotic drugs streptomycin and cloxacillin and is strongly indicated in treating methicillin-resistant *Staphylococcus aureus* (MRSA) infections.

Benefits in Cancer Care

Propolis has cytotoxic, immunomodulatory, and antitumor activity. Multiple effects are brought about by molecular mechanisms directed toward cell-death-signaling pathways in cancer cells. Propolis shows cytotoxicity against cancer cells in numerous studies, including against cancer of the tongue, breast, pancreas, and bone. Two phenolics in propolis with notable anticancer activity are caffeic acid phenethyl ester (CAPE) and apigenin. Both of these polyphenols are powerful redox-regulating agents with multiple overlapping effects that normalize cell behaviors. They inhibit the cell cycle, diminish oxidative stress, improve detoxification enzymes, induce cell death, and stimulate the immune system.

APIGENIN

Apigenin is a flavone widely distributed in the plant kingdom, present in significant amounts in vegetables (parsley, celery, onions), fruits (oranges), herbs (chamomile, thyme, oregano, basil and tulsi, feverfew, annual wormwood, yarrow), and plant-based beverages (tea, beer, and wine).

In addition to its marked redox-regulating properties, apigenin shows hypoglycemic, anti-inflammatory, and cytotoxic activities in cancer cell studies. It inhibits hyaluronidase, the enzyme cancer makes that breaks down the extracellular matrix. Furthermore, it protects against hypertension, enlarged heart, and autoimmune heart inflammation.

CAFFEIC ACID PHENETHYL ESTER (CAPE)

Caffeic acid phenethyl ester (CAPE) is a derivative of caffeic acid, and both occur naturally in high amounts in propolis. In a study of motility and migration of breast cancer cells, both CAPE and caffeic acid were cytotoxic, with greater effects at higher doses and over longer periods of time. CAPE was nearly twice as potent as caffeic acid. CAPE has been extensively studied in both laboratory and animal tests and has been shown to be effective in treating infections, oxidative stress, inflammation, cancer, diabetes, neurodegeneration, and anxiety. CAPE also offers neuroprotective activity; it can reduce inflammatory damage from brain or spinal cord injuries or from toxin-induced neurotoxicity. CAPE is also an effective adjuvant of chemotherapy for enhancing the effectiveness of chemotherapy drugs and diminishing chemotherapy-induced toxicities by suppressing free radical formation.

Dosing

Propolis itself is a thick, sticky, tarry substance that is difficult to work with. It's usually tinctured into alcohol or macerated into a fixed oil. In the dispensary, it is worth having a measuring column just for propolis, or be prepared to use rubbing alcohol to clean up after use.

Alcohol of 70–75% is preferred—the percentage needs to be high enough to extract the resin but not so high that water-soluble constituents are lost. A macerated oil will yield the same range of compounds but may need longer to steep and may not be as complete an extraction (in other words, it won't be as strong as a tincture at the same weight in volume). An oil extract is useful for topical applications—it can be incorporated into salves and liniments.

Tincture: 5–10 mL twice daily of a 1:10 tincture made with 75% ethyl alcohol. Note that with this remedy a tincture that is more concentrated than 1:10 is too sticky to work with easily.

SAFETY OF PROPOLIS

People who are allergic to bee stings should not be concerned about using propolis. There is no evidence of risk of anaphylaxis from the resin. However, occasional hypersensitive reactions can be induced by propolis on the skin, probably due to cinnamic acids. Propolis is used in the polishing and finishing of violins, and edema and rashes from contact dermatitis have been reported in the craftspeople making them. Propolis has low acute oral toxicity.

Sustainability of Propolis

Harvesting and removal of propolis from the hive can be harmful to the bees. Herbalists still use it, but only in small amounts and with due appreciation for its rarity. As a more sustainable alternative, a resinous compound with more or less equivalent constituents and uses can be extracted from the buds of cottonwoods or balsam poplars of the Pacific Northwest (*Populus candicans* and *Populus balsamifera*), also known as balm of Gilead.

Red Clover

Trifolium pratense

Plant family: Fabaceae
Part used: flowering tops
Medicinal actions: alterative for the skin, mild phytoestrogen, fertility aid, menstrual balancer; a depurative or alterative especially indicated for teenage acne in girls, for eczema, and for acne rosacea

The flowers of red clover have long been used in European folk medicine as an alterative or blood cleanser. More recent research has revealed that isoflavones in the leaves and flowering tops have mild phytoestrogen actions (agonist/antagonist balancing action), which may support its other traditional use as a women's fertility aid and menstrual normalizer. Red clover is widely recommended by herbalists for the treatment of menopausal hot flushes, osteoporosis, and cardiovascular disease as well as for treating hormonally driven cancers.

Benefits in Cancer Care

Numerous in vitro studies suggest that isolated red clover isoflavones have antiangiogenic and antioxidant effects and phytoestrogenic properties that enhance the anticancer effects.

Effects on estrogen signaling. The phytoestrogenic effects vary depending on the natural estrogen level of the patient. Isoflavones from red clover extract have weak estrogenic action (estrogen agonist) when administered alone.

However, when provided with estradiol, they act as an estrogen antagonist, thus making it a natural selective estrogen receptor modulator (SERM) in the presence of normal physiological amounts of estrogens. In clinical practice this suggests that red clover extract can be used in a low-estrogen state, such as menopause, where the agonist effect will support symptom management, but it can also be used to inhibit estrogen signaling in a situation where it is upregulated, such as estrogen-dependent breast cancer in a younger (menstruating) woman.

As is true for many herbs, robust clinical studies of the whole herb are lacking; evidence of isoflavones binding androgen or progesterone receptors is also weak. A review in 2018 concluded that the mechanism by which isoflavones exert their influence on androgen receptors is poorly understood. This study was on soy, but similar claims are made for red clover, and with possibly even less certainty about the effects.

Increased apoptosis in prostate cancer cells. In a small human trial of men undergoing prostatectomy, patients were randomly assigned to be given either 160 mg daily of red clover isoflavones or a placebo. There was no change in serum testosterone levels or PSA in the treatment group compared to the placebo, but histological analysis showed a higher rate of cell death in the prostate cells of the treated group, indicating a beneficial effect.

Synergy with chemotherapy. In a study of mice bred to get breast cancer, concurrent treatment with doxorubicin and red clover extract (100–400 mg/kg) inhibited the proliferation of tumor cells in dose- and time-dependent manners, which indicates beneficial effects in cancer. The drug/herb combination resulted in decreased serum levels of estradiol (E2), a type of estrogen that stimulates breast cancer cells, encouraging them to proliferate. It also resulted in increased serum levels of anti-inflammatory and immune-stimulating interleukin 12 (IL-12) and interferon gamma (IFN-y) and significant increases in antioxidant serum glutathione peroxidase (GPx). When doxorubicin was given concurrently with red clover, there was lower expression of Ki67 proliferation marker and increased cell death, and the researchers concluded that the herb/drug combination had beneficial synergistic effects.

OTHER BENEFITS OF RED CLOVER

Red clover isoflavones are effective in reducing bone loss in rats with ovaries removed by increasing bone mineral content, providing for enhanced mechanical strength of the tibia, femoral weight, and femoral density, and significantly reducing the number of osteoclasts (cells that break down bone) and the rate of the bone turnover.

Red clover extract reduces total cholesterol in peri- and postmenopausal women and improves arterial compliance, an index of large artery elasticity, which is an important cardiovascular risk factor.

Dosing

Tincture: Up to 6 mL daily of 1:2 tincture made with 45% ethyl alcohol.

Traditional Eastern European Red Clover Salve

This is an old folk remedy that has stood the test of time. It is anti-inflammatory and soothing and healing to the skin, and it has been used to treat skin and breast cancers (although, again, no clinical trials have been done). Making this salve requires a good supply of fresh red clover blossoms, so not everybody will be able to do it, but I believe that picking the flowers is also part of the medicine. It is applied over skin cancer or another cancer that has breached the skin surface. Apply it liberally, cover with clean gauze, and bandage lightly. Replace daily. No irritation should occur with this product. It is not intended to replace surgery or other treatments for cancer.

1. Fill a slow cooker or a Dutch oven with fresh red clover flowers and add enough water to just cover them.
2. Set on the "keep warm" level and simmer, covered, for 12 hours.
3. Remove the spent flowers, replace with fresh flowers, and simmer for another 12 hours. Repeat this five to seven times.
4. Remove the last batch of flowers and simmer the liquid very low, uncovered, until it reduces to half the original volume. It should be dark and tarry.

SAFETY OF RED CLOVER

Red clover has a long history in folk traditions of many countries in the temperate northern regions, and the ethnobotany and traditions are remarkably similar wherever it is used, with no reliable reports of significant adverse effects or risks.

Sea Buckthorn

Hippophae rhamnoides

Plant family: Elaeagnaceae
Parts used: leaf, fruit, and seed
Medicinal actions: antioxidant (redox regulator)

Many parts of this large shrub with a bright orange fruit and wicked thorns are medicinal. This is one of those medicines that is also a food. The leaves make a pleasant refreshing tea. The berry was known in ancient Greece for use in horse feed to increase the shine of the coat. The Latin name is derived from the Greek words for horse (*hippos*) and shiny (*phaos*). The berries can be pressed to collect the juice, which is rich in vitamins A, B1, B2, C, E, and K, carotenoids, and flavonoids. The seeds can be crushed to release the essential fats.

The oil from the seed is especially rich in omega-3 and omega-6 fatty acids, while the fruit pulp oil is notably high in omega-7 fatty acids. A detailed review of this plant published in 2017 suggests that these omega-7 fatty acids protect, regenerate, and soften the skin surface (the stratum corneum), relieve inflammation, and promote stability and integrity in the extracellular matrix, as well as in the diffuse connective tissues of the skin.

To get a full-spectrum extract of all the desirable constituents into a form that can be manufactured into capsules and marketed, both the pressed fruit juice and crushed berry oil are used. As a food, it isn't quite as palatable as the bright orange color might suggest; it is quite sour with a thick skin.

In my garden, I'm lucky enough to have two large bushes of a thornless hybrid, which is much easier to pick from. We have discovered that the best way to handle the crop when it all comes in at the same time from the garden is to put it through the dehydrator and make a sort of raisin.

What Makes It Medicinal

Both the seed oil and the fruit pulp or juice have a high content of essential fatty acids, carotenoids (alpha- and beta-carotenes, lycopene, cryptoxanthin, zeaxanthin), tocopherols, and phytosterols including beta-sitosterol. All these complex phytonutrients combine to give strong antioxidant and anti-inflammatory effects, which are useful in preventing and treating cancer. The fruit pulp and skin of sea buckthorn is especially high in an omega-7 fatty acid called palmitoleic acid, which is responsible for many of the therapeutic effects. This fatty acid is almost absent in the seed. It is a component of the lipids found in skin and stimulates regenerative processes in skin damage and wound healing. It may be useful in providing heart disease–fighting benefits as well as reducing microvascular problems from type 2 diabetes.

Daily doses of 3–5 grams of sea buckthorn oil with a high palmitoleic acid level, taken by mouth, have shown promising results in vaginal atrophy (a common consequence of pelvic radiation), in significantly decreasing LDL cholesterol and increasing HDL cholesterol in people with high cholesterol, in controlling insulin resistance, and in reducing the fatty deposits in the liver.

Clinically validated actions of sea buckthorn fruit and seed extract include:

- Prevents or treats coronary heart disease and other circulatory disorders
- Reduces inflammation
- Increases the regeneration of epithelial (lining and skin) cells
- Offers protective effect against exposure to radiation
- Increases the detoxifying functions of the liver (stimulates bile secretion)
- Relaxes the smooth muscles of the stomach and intestines
- Adaptogenic (stress reducing)

The peel of the stem and the skin of the fruit contain traces of 5-hydroxy-tryptophan (5-HTP), a precursor for serotonin and melatonin pathways that helps regulate emotion, blood pressure, body temperature, and stress hormone levels. The amount in sea buckthorn may not be sufficient to exert a clinical effect, but it can be part of setting the "background tone" of the physiology and metabolism and biorhythms.

Benefits in Cancer Care

The triterpene ursolic acid is found in the fruit pulp and has many anticancer actions. It suppresses NF-κB signaling in the cancer cell nucleus and thus downregulates oncogenes. It improves insulin signaling in fat cells, reduces markers of cardiac damage in the heart, decreases inflammation and increases antioxidants in the brain, is antioxidant to liver cells specifically, reduces programmed cell death signaling in healthy cells, and reduces skeletal muscle atrophy.

Sea buckthorn oil, pressed from the fruit pulp, skin, and seed, has a number of anticancer uses and actions, including:

- Antioxidant and free radical scavenging
- Reduces inflammation
- Increases the regeneration of epithelial cells and skin repair (topical and internal)
- Builds blood after chemotherapy—increases red cell count and inhibits myelosuppression
- Protective effect against exposure to radiation
- Immunosupportive—induces phagocytic functions of the macrophage and strengthens nonspecific immune functions
- Increases the detoxifying functions of the liver (stimulates bile secretion)

Carotenoids and xanthophylls from the fruit pulp also have specific anticancer actions, including:

- Scavenging oxidative damage; lessening of oxidative damage to lipids, proteins, and DNA
- Enhancing cell-to-cell communication for better collective control of cell behaviors
- Inhibition of the insulin-like growth factor 1 (IGF-1), a protein that works with sugar to promote cancer
- Inhibition of the key enzyme (HMGR) in fat metabolism that makes Ras proteins used for signal transduction, which has the effect of reducing oncogenic (cancer-promoting) signals traveling to the cell nucleus

Dosing

Fresh fruit juice: 2–4 tbsp. twice daily.

Pressed oil: 1–2 tsp. daily.

Supplement: Capsules of the pressed oil are typically made at 500–750 mg per cap and a daily dose would be two to four capsules of pure sea buckthorn oil twice daily.

St. John's Wort

Hypericum perforatum

Plant family: Hypericaceae

Part used: flowering tops

Medicinal actions: hepatic, antidepressant, relaxing and restorative tonic nervine, antiviral, anti-inflammatory, vulnerary

The Latin name derives from the Greek *hyper* (over) and *eikon* (image or apparition), referring to the plant's supposed ability to ward off evil spirits and to the practice of suspending a stem of St. John's wort over an icon or an altar as a good luck charm. As long ago as 1525, Paracelsus recommended it for treating depression, melancholy, and overexcitation. These nervine actions are supported by extensive clinical and analytical research, but St. John's wort is also active in many other useful ways.

As well as exerting these effects upon functions of the nervous system, it has particular benefits in restoring and repairing the structure of the nervous system and is valuable in treating nerve inflammation and nerve damage, including chemotherapy-induced neuropathy as well as sciatica and trigeminal neuralgia. Spinal cord injuries, severed or crushed nerves, and autoimmune inflammatory nerve diseases are all situations when high doses of St. John's wort may be used.

What Makes It Medicinal?

Key active constituents of St. John's wort include several phenolic compounds with an extensive range of actions in the body. Hypericin and several of its derivatives have antiviral and anticancer properties. Hyperforin is a red-pigmented compound that has antibacterial, nerve restorative, and antidepressant properties. The flavones and flavonoids in St. John's wort are antioxidant and anti-inflammatory, and quercetin and kaempferol support energy production in nerve cells.

HYPERICIN

This light-sensitive compound is responsible for the red color when St. John's wort flowers are infused in carrier oils and is found particularly in the black oil glands that dot the outer edge of the petals and leaves. It is highly lipophilic and poorly soluble in aqueous solutions, so a tea does not work well to extract the medicine; a tincture, infused oil, or capsules are required.

A unique feature of hypericin is that it requires photoactivation for maximum effects. Due to its chemical structure, it is highly photoreactive. It has a unique capacity to bounce electrons between two adjacent oxygen atoms when exposed to certain light frequencies, thus generating superoxide radicals that can kill tumor cells through oxidative stress. In this way, hypericin can be used as a component of photodynamic therapy (PDT), where a measured dose of hypericin is introduced into a tumor and then a targeted laser beam is used to activate the oxidative reaction right inside the target tissue.

PDT is an established treatment option in a variety of skin diseases, including acne and psoriasis, as well as other conditions such as age-related macular degeneration, and is an emerging treatment for several cancers, including skin, lung, brain, bladder, pancreas, bile duct, esophagus, and head and neck. PDT may also help treat bacterial, fungal, and viral infections and can trigger the body's immune response to help destroy cancerous and precancerous cells.

In vitro studies have suggested that hypericin inhibits the growth of glioma, neuroblastoma, adenoma, mesothelioma, melanoma, carcinoma, sarcoma, and leukemia cells. An additional benefit of hypericin is its notable antiviral properties, including against herpes simplex virus types 1 and 2 and human immunodeficiency virus (HIV). Given that viral infections including herpes and HIV are associated with certain cancers, this is a good example of the overlapping and complementary action of herbs and herbal constituents.

HYPERFORIN

This is a type of molecule called a phloroglucinol (technically a trihydroxybenzene phenolic) that is relatively soluble in water and with an antispasmodic effect, especially in the urinary tract, where it may reduce the urge to void. This may go some way toward explaining why St. John's wort is used for treating incontinence and bed-wetting.

Phloroglucinol itself is a drug prescribed for gallstones and spasmodic upper digestive pain, which may explain in some part how St. John's wort functions as a bitter digestive aid and, by that action, also supports parasympathetic dominance and a restful state of mind that may allow the mood to rise (thymoleptic action). This may be a link between traditional humoral indications for using St. John's wort for balancing and clearing excess earth energy, "morbid black bile," and melancholia that resided in the liver and the modern use for mild to moderate depression.

Hyperforin inhibits the reuptake of serotonin, norepinephrine, and dopamine in the nervous system, thus extending the active life of these neurotransmitters. Hyperforin also inhibits the uptake of GABA and L-glutamate. The end result of this is a marked antidepressant action, equivalent to that of some of the milder prescription drugs and with particular value in treating mild to moderate depression.

Other mild but effective actions of St. John's wort in the nervous system are to promote mental relaxation and aid sleep. The flowering tops contain traces of melatonin, which may be partially responsible for this effect.

AN ANTI-INFLAMMATORY

St. John's wort shows great promise as an anti-inflammatory agent. Extracts of the flowering tops inhibit the expression of pro-inflammatory genes like cyclooxygenase-2, interleukin-6, and inducible nitric oxide synthase (iNOS). Hyperforin plays an important role in inhibiting lymphocyte reaction around epidermal cells and in regulating T lymphocyte proliferation. Hyperforin regulates (promotes and inhibits) key enzymes required for prostaglandin E2 (PGE2) biosynthesis, which play key roles in inflammation and tumor promotion.

Benefits in Cancer Care

Hypericin has demonstrated significant antitumor activity in vitro against several cancer lines. However, it is likely that there is a synergy of at least several of the other known constituents and that the inflammation-modulating, liver enzyme–stimulating, and mood-elevating effects also contribute to resisting the onset or progression of cancer.

As a vulnerary or skin repair herb that can be applied topically over a lesion of any sort, St. John's wort excels in healing burns after completion of radiation, in reducing scarring over surgical incisions, and in healing hand-foot syndrome, where the skin breaks down with tingling and tenderness, swelling, and pain in the palm of the hands and soles of the feet. An oil extract works best, as a foot and hand rub, or incorporated into lotions or ointments.

Making St. John's Wort–Infused Oil

Flower buds are picked just as they start to show yellow but before they open. This is traditionally Saint John's day (June 24) because, in the northern hemisphere at least, that is when they are said to be at the peak of perfection.

Place the buds in a clean glass jar, mark their height, and cover with six times that amount of a neutral carrier oil, such as grapeseed oil. Cover with cheesecloth secured with a rubber band, which will allow any natural moisture evaporating from the plant to escape the jar. (With a nonporous lid, rising moisture condenses and drips back into the oil, which can cause mold to grow.)

Keep the jar in a cool place but by a window where it can get some sun, as this activates the hypericin and turns the oil a dark wine red. Stir daily with a clean chopstick.

Strain off after 2 weeks, pour the oil into a clean glass bottle, label and date it, and keep in a cool, dark place.

Dosing

Dried herb: ½–1 tsp. of dried herb in a tea blend.

Tincture: 2–6 mL of a 1:2 tincture made with 45–55% ethyl alcohol.

CONTRAINDICATIONS

Avoid using the following drugs while taking St. John's wort: antipsychotics (risperidone and 9-hydroxyrisperidone), cyclosporine, digoxin, HIV drugs, SSRI antidepressants (could lead to increased serotonin levels, causing serotonin syndrome), and estrogen-containing oral contraceptives (can lead to decreased effectiveness of the contraceptive and, potentially, unplanned pregnancies). Use of St. John's wort is discouraged for those with bipolar disorder, schizophrenia, or dementia and for people using blood thinners or birth control pills.

Because of how it interacts with certain metabolic enzymes, it is wise to avoid drinking grapefruit juice or eating grapefruit while taking St. John's wort. (For more information, see St. John's Wort and Drug Interactions, below.)

CLINICAL PEARL

Tincture potency can be calibrated to hypericin content, with 0.2 mg/mL as a minimum desirable range. High doses of hypericin (over 0.5 mg/kg) may result in skin sensitivity in sunlight, risk of sunburn, and photodermatitis. People taking St. John's wort internally should limit sunlight exposure to early morning and late afternoon, and if you use St. John's wort oil topically, the area of use should not be exposed to direct sunlight for at least 1 week after application.

Do not ingest St. John's wort or apply it to the skin during active radiotherapy treatment.

For the Practitioner: St. John's Wort and Drug Interactions

Much has been made in the medical press about the risk of herb–drug interactions with this herb—and it is a genuine concern. St. John's wort can significantly reduce effects of a wide range of pharmaceuticals (by inducing intestinal and hepatic CYP3A4/5/7 and P-glycoprotein). This will not make most drugs more dangerous, but it may make them less effective if they clear too quickly, with wide variations in how much of an effect it has between different people. Conversely, some drugs require activation by going through phase 1 enzymes in the liver. For example, taking drugs such as clopidogrel (an anticoagulant platelet inhibitor) with St. John's wort may lead to increased drug doses and higher risk of side effects. Given that around 60 percent of prescribed drugs go through this pathway, it is easy to see that some drugs may be of concern.

The cytochrome enzymes are protein complexes involved in electron transport, the pumping of protons to create the gradient that generates ATP. These complexes play a vital role in cellular energy production. They are also key enzymes in phase I detoxification pathways in the liver and catalyze thousands of endogenous and exogenous chemicals, including most drugs, hormones, metabolic wastes, and toxins. Most drugs undergo deactivation by CYPs and many inactive substances are metabolized by CYPs to form their active compounds. Although there are dozens of CYP series in the human body, just five of them are involved in the metabolism of around 90 percent of pharmaceutical drugs. These enzyme series are CYP1A2, CYP2C9, CYP2D6, CYP3A4, and CYP3A5, with the most active and significant being CYP3A4 and CYP2D6.

As well as providing the phase I detox series in the liver, CYP enzymes are also found in other tissues, such as in the kidneys, lungs, adrenals, ovaries, testes, and brain. For example, the aromatase enzyme in abdominal fat that converts testosterone to estrogen (also called estrogen synthetase or estrogen synthase) is CYP 19A1. Some CYPs metabolize only one (or a very few) substrates, while others may metabolize multiple substrates. Furthermore, many drugs metabolize through several pathways, so inducing or inhibiting one may not affect all substrates equally.

Many drugs may induce or inhibit the activity of various CYP isozymes, as can many natural compounds and otherwise innocuous foods, including St. John's wort, which increases clearance rates. In contrast, bergamottin and dihydroxybergamottin—found in the pulp of grapefruit and some other citrus fruits, including pomelos, and in the peel and pulp of the bergamot orange, used to flavor Earl Grey tea—are natural furanocoumarins that actively inhibit CYP3A4-mediated metabolism of several pharmaceutical drugs, leading to increased bioavailability and the possibility of overdosing of the drugs. One whole grapefruit, or a small glass (200 mL) of grapefruit juice, can cause some drugs to overload in the blood, and this overdose reaction can last for 1–3 days.

Taheebo

Tabebuia impetiginosa, T. avellanedae, T. rosea, a.k.a. *Handroanthus impetiginosus*

Alternate common names: pau d'arco, lapacho
Plant family: Bignoniaceae
Part used: inner bark of branches
Medicinal actions: anti-inflammatory, antiallergic, immune-stimulating, antiviral, antiparasitic

This is a large tree from the Amazon rain forest. The timber is dense, durable, and rot resistant—very useful for building houses and boats. Because of that, the tree is endangered; only purchase this herb from a sustainable source. Research shows that the leaves have antioxidant activity; harvesting the leaves is obviously much more sustainable than harvesting the branches. Taheebo should be used in cancer care only in specific cases where there are known comorbidities, such as viral or fungal infection, or bloodborne parasites.

The inner bark of the branches was traditionally used by Indigenous people of rain forests and jungles from southern Mexico to Argentina for treating fever, malaria, bacterial and fungal infections, and skin diseases. It is used today with good results to treat malaria, tropical fluke, candida, ringworm, herpes virus, HIV, polio, influenza, and Epstein Barr virus. Current research confirms it as having anti-inflammatory, antiallergic, immunostimulating, antibacterial, antioxidant, antifungal, antidiabetic, anti-edema, cytotoxic, antiproliferative, and anticancer properties.

What Makes It Medicinal

While human clinical trials of taheebo use for cancer treatment are lacking, taheebo contains numerous compounds with known anticancer activity, notably a group of phenolics called naphthoquinones. There are more than 1,200 different quinones and derivatives known in plants; many act as pigments, giving yellow, orange, red, purple, or black coloration. As such, many dye plants—including henna, coffee, madder, and alkanet—are rich in quinones. Quinones in wood such as teak and ebony confer dark color and rot resistance to the wood, but they also contribute to allergic reactions among mill workers and woodworkers. Quinone-containing anticancer drugs include Adriamycin (doxorubicin), daunorubicin, and mitomycin C, to name just a few.

There are three main groupings of quinones: benzoquinones (simple quinones as are found in bearberry and buchu [*Barosma betulina*]), anthraquinones (laxatives such as senna and cascara), and naphthoquinones. Naphthoquinones have particular uses in herbal medicine, mostly as antimicrobials, antiprotozoals, anthelmintics (deworming), and anticancer agents. Juglone is the naphthoquinone found in the foliage, wood, and green hulls of black walnut trees that inhibits the growth of adjacent plants. It's also an effective antifungal, anthelmintic, and antiviral agent in humans. Plumbagin, the particular naphthoquinone found in sundew (*Drosera rotundifolia* and related species), is immunostimulating at low doses and cytotoxic in higher doses. It modulates cellular proliferation, carcinogenesis, and radioresistance and increases the tumor cell death effects of chemotherapy.

Benefits in Cancer Care

The principal active constituents of taheebo are a series of naphthoquinones and derivatives, most notably lapachol and beta-lapachone. Lapachol inhibits proliferation of tumor cells, and beta-lapachone exhibits strong toxicity in human cancer cells such as breast, lung, cervical, and hepatocellular carcinoma. It also suppresses growth of the human keratinocyte cell line and has been suggested as a promising antipsoriatic agent.

Lapachol is selectively cytotoxic to rapidly metabolizing cells. This is achieved by disruption to the end stage of energy production in the Krebs cycle, which starves the cell of energy and triggers cell death. It has demonstrated activity against carcinomas, sarcomas, melanoma, and leukemia cell lines. Beta-lapachone resensitizes radiation-resistant human melanoma cells to radiotherapy.

Suggested mechanisms of action of taheebo against cancer include mitochondrial disturbance, inhibition of pro-inflammatory immune fractions, inhibition of cell surface receptors that promote cancer cell activities, reduced lipid peroxidation, downregulation of genes driving cell replication and of proliferative genes that respond to estrogen, and upregulation of genes driving cell death. This makes it particularly indicated for estrogen-sensitive cancers. Due to the suppression of keratinocytes, taheebo is especially indicated where there is dermatitis from chemotherapy, especially the extreme sloughing rashes of the hands and feet seen with immunotherapies.

Which Species Should Be Used?

Most of what is sold in North America and the UK is *Tahebuia avellanedae* or *T. impetiginosa*. Certainly other species are interesting and research is ongoing as to what benefits they offer. It may well be that all of the genus is useful, but other species are not routinely used yet.

Dosing

Dried bark: 1.5–3 g per day of dried bark.

Tincture: 3–7 mL of 1:2 tincture made with 45% ethyl alcohol.

Because this is a shredded bark, it lends itself to decoctions. I often prescribe it in equal parts with mushrooms and astragalus as part of a soup blend, with a bone marrow broth to build blood.

Tulsi

Ocimum sanctum, O. tenuiflorum

Alternate common name: holy basil

Plant family: Lamiaceae

Parts used: leaf and aerial parts

Medicinal actions: anti-inflammatory, analgesic, lowers fevers, normalizes blood sugar, adaptogen, immunomodulator, protects the liver, reduces cholesterol, mood elevating

The genus *Ocimum* comprises more than 60 species, including the classic sweet basil (*Ocimum basilicum)* used in Italian cooking, Thai basil (*O. basilicum* var. *thyrsiflora)* with its anise flavor, and more than 40 other subspecies and cultivars, each with slightly different flavor profiles. *Ocimum sanctum* (synonym *Ocimum tenuiflorum*) is the species properly called tulsi or holy basil. It is native to the Indian subcontinent, where it has been a revered medicine in Ayurveda for thousands of years.

What Makes It Medicinal

Like many members of the mint family, tulsi is rich in volatile oils, which confer most of the plant's flavor as well as its medicinal effects. These include the triterpenoid ursolic acid and eugenol, both of which exert anticancer effects.

Eugenol. The predominant volatile molecule in many medicinal cultivars of tulsi is eugenol, which has antibacterial, pain-relieving, and antioxidant properties. It inhibits the growth of malignant cells, induces cell death, numbs tissues, and is an anti-inflammatory. The essential oil with the highest content of eugenol is actually clove, which is well known for its pain-relieving and antimicrobial properties in tooth infections. Tulsi and clove produce very different essential oils with very different applications, but the eugenol is a predominant feature of both, and their differences come from their medley of other constituents. This is yet another example of the intricacy of constituent interaction and synergy within an herb and another strong indicator for using whole-plant medicine rather than isolated and purified or semisynthetic compounds.

MEDICINAL ACTIONS

The list of medicinal actions and benefits of this herb is so long that it's no surprise to find that in India it is worshipped as a goddess and given names like "Queen of All Herbs" and "The Incomparable One." In Ayurvedic medicine, every part of the plant is revered: the leaves, stem, flower, root, seeds, and oil. Even the soil around the plant is considered sacred. Modern research has documented the presence of a very specific symbiotic fungus in the soil adjacent to the plant and penetrating the roots that augments the essential oil composition and antioxidant properties of the plant. In addition, a range of fungi found in the aerial parts of the plant contribute to the specific range of constituents in the crop. It is suggested that different colonies of fungi may be responsible, at least in part, for the different chemotypes of tulsi that are identified.

Different varieties of tulsi include:

- 'Krishna'—purple-hued leaves and stems; has the highest phenolic content and antioxidant capacity
- 'Rama'—has a sweeter, more clove-like flavor
- 'Vana'—(*Ocimum gratissimum*) or "wild tulsi," which has a mild licorice flavor

According to Eric Yarnell of Heron Botanicals in Washington State, African basil (*Ocimum* × *africanum*) appears to have comparable clinical efficacy to *O. sanctum* and is more suitable for growing in temperate climates.

Overall, tulsi can be considered a mild but effective adaptogen. It can modulate and mitigate responses to physical, chemical, metabolic, and psychological stress. It can counter metabolic stress through normalizing blood glucose, blood pressure, and lipid levels, and it can reduce reactions to psychological stress through positive effects on memory and cognitive function and through its anxiety-reducing and antidepressant properties.

Benefits in Cancer Care

The volatile oil content of tulsi, combined with its polyphenolics and ursolic acid, give it potent anti-inflammatory and anticancer actions through multiple metabolic pathways. In studies, eugenol, rosmarinic acid, apigenin, myretenal, luteolin, beta-sitosterol, and carnosic acid have been shown to prevent chemical-induced skin, liver, oral, and lung cancers by increasing antioxidant activity, altering oncogenic and tumor-suppressive gene expressions, inducing cell death, and inhibiting new blood vessel growth and metastasis. Extracts of tulsi have been shown in cell line studies (in vitro) to inhibit the proliferation, migration, and invasion of prostate cancer cells and induce their apoptosis (cell death). A study in 2013 reported that in mice given tulsi, "genes that inhibit metastasis and induce apoptosis were significantly upregulated and genes that promote survival of the cancer cells and chemo/radiation resistance were downregulated." Cancers for which tulsi shows promise in preclinical research include lung, pancreatic, cervical, skin (basal cell type and melanoma), prostate, gastric, breast, and oral cancers. Clinical trials are needed to verify the good clinical results seen in practice.

Tulsi may protect against toxin-induced cancer by promoting the biochemical transformation and elimination of ingested or inhaled environmental toxins through redox regulation in organs and by inducing phase I liver detoxification enzymes. This is a nonspecific action and assists in removal of industrial pollutants, pesticides, pharmaceuticals, heavy metals, and radiation. This action has not yet been studied in humans, but in studies with mice, tulsi showed notable antioxidant action and liver protection by modulating glutathione, the major antioxidant made by the liver, and by increasing phase II detox enzymes.

Tulsi scavenges free radicals and reduces the oxidative cellular and chromosomal damage induced by radiation. A water extract of tulsi with an appreciable amount of the flavonoids orientin and vicenin protected mice against radiation-induced sickness and mortality and may selectively protect normal tissues against the tissue damaging and carcinogenic effects of radiation.

METABOLIC SYNDROME

Metabolic syndrome is characterized by abdominal weight gain, high cholesterol, high blood insulin, and high blood pressure and is the predominant condition of middle-aged and older adults in the developed world. It is a significant contributor to a procancer terrain through perpetuating a chronic, low-grade inflammatory state. Studies in animals have confirmed that tulsi can reduce blood glucose, correct abnormal lipid profiles, prevent weight gain, reduce blood levels of insulin, and lessen insulin resistance. It protects the liver and kidneys from the metabolic damage caused by high glucose levels. In human trials, tulsi decreased glucose levels, improved blood pressure and lipid profiles, and reduced many symptoms of type 2 diabetes. Furthermore, tulsi may be active in enhancing bile acid synthesis in the liver, thus assisting in detoxification of the body as well as lowering blood fats, while also reducing hepatic lipid synthesis.

OTHER USES OF TULSI

Anti-inflammatory. The eugenol and linoleic acid content of tulsi were responsible for reducing both acute and chronic inflammation and lowering cortisol levels in animal studies (by inhibition of both the COX-2 and LOX enzymes, thus inhibiting arachidonic acid metabolism and production of inflammatory prostaglandins). The anti-inflammatory effects have been found comparable to those of nonsteroidal anti-inflammatory drugs such as phenylbutazone, ibuprofen, naproxen, aspirin, and indomethacin.

Wound care. The volatile oil content of tulsi provides potent antibacterial activity against a range of bacterial pathogens that can enter wounds and cause infection. The antioxidant and anti-inflammatory activities contribute to its traditional topical use in wound healing.

Mood and cognitive support. Tulsi has antianxiety and antidepressant properties, with mood-elevating qualities comparable or superior to mild prescription antianxiety drugs and antidepressants, in my clinical experience. It has a relaxing and calming effect on the mind, supports memory and cognitive function, and protects against age-induced memory deficits.

Dosing

Tulsi has a distinctive flavor that is intensely aromatic, sweet, floral, fresh, and almost minty. It is quite strong; a leaf or two finely minced on a salad might taste quite nice but you are unlikely to want to make pesto with it. Tulsi makes a delightful, delicious tea and is often drunk as part of a tea blend, usually with some kind of tonic nervines or other antidepressant herbs. It combines well with wood betony, skullcap, and lavender as a relaxing and calming, mind-clearing, and uplifting tea, or with green tea, damiana, and blue vervain for a mood-elevating and invigorating tea.

Dried herb: Doses in capsule form of 500 mg of tulsi leaf extract up to four times (2 g total) daily is safe and effective.

Tincture: 2–4 mL daily of 1:2 tincture made with 45% ethyl alcohol.

CAVEATS

As with all herbal remedies, proper botanical identification is important. Purchase from a reputable supplier, preferably one who is collecting and replanting their own seeds, to ensure authentication. Tulsi also has an ability to concentrate environmental toxins in the leaves, which is promising in remediation of industrial sites (hundreds of thousands of tulsi plants have been planted around the Taj Mahal in India to help protect the fragile marble building from damage due to environmental pollution), but it also means that you must choose a supplier carefully; tulsi grown in contaminated soil will increase your toxin exposure.

Turmeric

Curcuma longa

Plant family: Zingiberaceae

Part used: rhizome

Medicinal actions: inflammation modulating, anticancer, antioxidant (redox regulating), antilipidemic, cholagogue (promotes bile flow)

There is so much research available today about the health benefits of turmeric that it is hard to know where to start. Much of this research looks only at a very few constituents in the rhizome (a mixture known as curcumin) and not the whole plant. The aromatic rhizome is a warming stimulant, alterative, stomachic, carminative, cholagogue, choleretic, anti-inflammatory, and detoxifier and regenerator of liver tissue, and, not least of which, a potent anticarcinogenic. It also exhibits strong antimicrobial properties, especially against gram-positive bacteria (e.g., streptococcus, staphylococcus, and salmonella infections).

Turmeric has traditionally been used as a remedy for biliousness, gallstones, liver disease, and jaundice, among many other conditions. Modern research has shown it to be a powerful antioxidant in the liver cell membranes and to be liver protective and a liver rejuvenator, akin to milk thistle or artichoke. It stabilizes lysozymes responsible for removing metabolic wastes in liver cells and raises hepatic glutathione-S-transferase (a detoxifying enzyme).

Interestingly, turmeric can bind iron in the gut and thus indirectly inhibit both inflammation and cancer, which use high levels of iron to fuel metabolic processes. Turmeric is also used to lower cholesterol. This is achieved by inhibiting intestinal absorption and by inducing the enzymes that convert cholesterol to bile acids for excretion, as well as lowering the LDL and triglycerides and raising HDL levels. It also inhibits lipid peroxidation, which lowers the risks from hypercholesterolemia. High cholesterol itself is not directly a cause of cancer, but is a metabolic syndrome of the common health profile of high blood fats, high blood pressure, high blood sugar, and abdominal weight gain, which all contribute to the background, baseline pro-inflammatory state that so many people in the developed world experience and is hospitable terrain for cancer to occur.

In my practice, I use turmeric extensively as an alterative that promotes detoxification while also protecting the liver from oxidative stress. As a warming herb, it may counteract the cooling effect of bitters traditionally used for liver stimulation and detoxification (such as yellow dock or barberry) that may be too cooling if used alone.

What Makes It Medicinal

The volatile oil fraction and the curcumin pigment in it have demonstrated powerful anti-inflammatory effects, comparable to hydrocortisone and phenylbutazone in treating acute inflammation, but without the significant side effects of these prescription drugs. Turmeric inhibits the formation of pain-mediating prostaglandins by regulating the cyclooxygenase-2 (COX-2) cascade. Curcumin has been shown to be more effective in animals in which the adrenal glands are intact and functioning normally, indicating that it may work in part by increasing the sensitivity of receptor sites to adrenal hormones.

Benefits in Cancer Care

One of the most-studied constituents of turmeric is curcumin, a resin pigment comprising several curcuminoids. In cancer care, curcumin acts as a mediator of inflammation and an antioxidant (redox regulator). Some of the specific anti-cancer effects of curcumin include regulation of cell-survival and cell-signaling pathways and inhibition of platelet aggregation, new blood vessel growth, and metastasis. It inhibits cell division (is antimitotic) and induces cell death (is pro-apoptotic).

TURMERIC AND CHEMOTHERAPY

Curcumin may slow the activity of certain enzymes that are required for the metabolism and excretion of drugs (including cytochrome P450 enzymes in phase I liver detox and glutathione-S-transferase and glucuronosyltransferase in phase II). Because of this, curcumin may extend the half-life of chemotherapy drugs in the body, thus possibly enabling a lower overall dose of chemotherapy to still be effective. Preliminary clinical trials have shown curcumin is safe with, and may increase effectiveness of, docetaxel, 5-fluorouracil/oxaliplatin, and gemcitabine chemotherapies in particular, though the exact mechanisms of interaction were not determined.

Curcumin has also been shown to augment the cytotoxic effects of numerous chemotherapy drugs, including doxorubicin, tamoxifen, cisplatin, camptothecin, gemcitabine, daunorubicin, vincristine, and melphalan in preclinical studies. Curcumin crosses the blood-brain barrier and has potentially therapeutic redox-regulating and anticancer effects on brain tissue.

APPLICATIONS FOR ORAL CARE

Several preclinical and clinical trials have now confirmed the usefulness of topical applications (mouthwash or gel) of turmeric in oral inflammation from chemotherapy. There are also promising early studies on various turmeric products for treating precancerous conditions of the mouth as a way to prevent oral cancers.

One study found that gargling with turmeric can delay and reduce the severity of oral mucositis for patients with head and neck cancer who are undergoing radiation therapy. In the single-blind, randomized study, patients were assigned to receive either a turmeric gargle made with whole-plant material, not isolated curcumin, or an iodine-based mouthwash during the treatment period. Assessment included the frequency of mucositis during the 7-week period and the effect of turmeric gargle on the incidence of treatment breaks, loss of scheduled treatment days, and decrease in body weight at the end of the treatment (an indirect sign of difficulty eating due to oral inflammation). At the end of the study the results showed unequivocally that the turmeric-treated patients had less frequent and less severe oral mucositis than the iodine-treated group, as well as less incidence of treatment breaks and less weight loss.

Dosing

As with other food medicines, there is no explicit dosing for this herb. Research has shown doses of up to 12 g per day of turmeric root powder for 3 months to be safe.

Curcumin and the curcuminoids are present in turmeric at around 22–40 mg/g in the rhizomes. Curcumin undergoes extensive metabolism in the intestine and liver, and it is actually quite hard to get a substantial amount of curcumin into the blood.

Turmeric should be taken with black pepper and some kind of oil or oily food to improve absorption. The bioavailability of standardized curcumin is enhanced when you take whole powdered root alongside it.

In my clinical practice I use capsules and whole-root powder together. Capsules are usually up to 500 mg two to four times daily and standardized at 94% curcuminoids. Bromelain, black pepper (specifically the alkaloid extract called piperine), and quercetin will help absorption and are usually included in the capsule. Additionally, take 1–2 tsp. (5–10 g) of powdered turmeric 5 days per week in the form of golden milk (see page 303).

CAVEATS

There is some concern that curcumin can induce DNA damage and chromosomal alterations both in vitro and in vivo at concentrations similar to those reported to exert beneficial effects. This gives reason not to stop using the herb, but rather to note the complexity of herbal medicine and human health.

Curcumin can act as an antioxidant or pro-oxidant, depending on dose. However, these adverse effects may be mediated by redox-regulating mechanisms, and controlled oxidative stress induced by the herb is often what's

Is Curcumin Actually Absorbed?

A lot of research has investigated whether curcumin compounds are absorbed, and many products are touted based on whether they are absorbed or not. Ultimately, the goal of treatment is not absorption; the goal is patients actually getting and staying better. Since studies consistently show people who take turmeric and curcumin have beneficial clinical results, one can surmise that absorption, or at least how we are measuring it, doesn't matter. This is plausible in light of the many effects curcumin has in the gut and on the bacteria that live there, which may cause systemic changes without the curcumin ever being directly absorbed. It is also possible we just don't understand the complex metabolism of the compounds from turmeric, and thus absorption studies may not even be looking for the right molecules. There is some research suggesting that the breakdown products of curcumin—its many and varied derivatives—may be even more therapeutically active, so measuring curcumin in the blood as a gauge of effectiveness may not be useful at all.

inhibiting the cancer, with collateral damage also managed by curcumin-driven redox regulation. This is a classic example of the "amphoteric" effect in herbal medicine—balancing, stabilizing, and normalizing a pathway. In chemistry, an amphoteric substance can act as either an acid or a base, and in herbal medicine it indicates an herb with apparently paradoxical actions that work together to generate the benefits. An analogy might be in managing forest fire risk—better a controlled burn than a conflagration. Similarly with turmeric—better some pro-oxidative stress that weakens cancer, as well as redox-regulating action to protect healthy cells, than allowing an inflammation to become acute or a cancer to grow.

There is some evidence that taking curcumin in higher doses over the long term may cause anemia. Curcumin is an active iron chelator, and animals fed iron-deficient diets in clinical studies became anemic more quickly when given curcumin than animals on the same diet that were not given the herb. This may actually be beneficial in cancer, which requires a high iron load for optimal metabolism. Practitioners often aim to keep the iron load of cancer patients at 20–40 percent of normal range, and blood iron load should be monitored regularly in cancer patients. It may be advisable to avoid using turmeric/curcumin supplements concurrently with annual wormwood (*Artemisia annua*), which functions most effectively when iron is slightly higher than median, so these two herbs could contradict each other. Prudence suggests pulse-dosed curcumin delivery may be helpful to avoid suppressing beneficial acute inflammatory and immune responses needed for healing and tissue maintenance, while also minimizing exposure to continuous high dosages.

One of the biggest drawbacks in all of the impressive modern research around this herb is that it is mostly conducted on the isolated curcuminoids, which comprise only 3–5 percent of the whole herb. When these are purified and isolated in research, the herbalist is left wondering what has been thrown away. All of the traditional uses are predicated on using the whole herb in dietary doses and including all cofactors or synergistic compounds naturally occurring in the root. This is also true of the piperine extracted from black pepper that is often included in curcumin supplements—it is far removed from the whole fresh black pepper used in traditional dietary or medicinal contexts.

The number of studies showing positive effects of curcumin is much higher than those showing negative effects. The preponderance of evidence is that the herb is largely safe. However, it is worth noting that historic dietary use was substantially lower than therapeutic doses being recommended in popular literature today, so historic evidence of safe use cannot necessarily be relied upon for evidence of safety today.

Clinical Pearls

Turmeric helps set circadian rhythms in the body; curcumin delivery at night may promote the ability of melatonin to prevent oncogene activation and cancer cell migration, especially for cancer patients at risk of metastasis or infiltration of tumor into adjacent tissues. Conversely, morning curcumin delivery might complement melatonin effects by suppressing cancer stem cells after melatonin levels have declined. To take advantage of these diurnal changes, twice-daily dosing is recommended.

The underground stem or rhizome of turmeric is comprised by up to 5 percent of essential oils in which the pigmented resin curcuminoids, collectively called curcumin, are found. These compounds require a strong solvent, and water-based decoctions will not be sufficient for good extraction. It is hard to take enough in the diet (although Golden Milk—see facing page—can achieve quite a decent dose and is reasonably well absorbed), so capsule supplements are often recommended. These are not just ground-up turmeric powder; rather, they are dried and powdered super-concentrated extracts. The curcuminoids are usually standardized to around 90–95 percent in the capsule. Because of this, capsules are inevitably missing other key constituents, so ideally the whole root should be taken in addition to capsules.

Golden Milk

Turmeric is best absorbed with black pepper and some dietary fat, and this tasty, warming drink makes it quick, easy, and affordable to take daily.

+ 12 ounces coconut milk*
+ 1 teaspoon–1 tablespoon powdered turmeric (start with a small amount and work up to full dose)
+ Pinch of freshly ground black pepper
+ Cardamom, cinnamon, cloves, fennel, as desired
+ Honey to taste

Warm the milk and stir in the powders and honey to taste. I like to use my latte whisk to froth it a bit, but this isn't essential.

*May be from a fresh green coconut or packaged. If using canned coconut milk, make sure it is full fat. If using fresh or Tetra Pak coconut milk, consider adding 1–2 teaspoons coconut oil.

Other herbs may be added to this blend: eleuthero, maca, and ashwagandha as adaptogens; shatavari as a nutritive, moistening agent; marshmallow as a food for beneficial bowel flora.

Medicinal Mushrooms

There is so much research today on myco-medicinals that whole books have been written just about the use of mushrooms for cancer care.

Although each mushroom species is unique, overall it is safe to say that almost all the 2,000 or so species of mushrooms eaten worldwide are likely to have an overall immunomodulating action—that is, stimulating, tonic, and normalizing immune activities. Constituents of mushrooms include large and complex polysaccharides, triterpenes, sterols, and polyphenols, all of which may provide immunomodulating properties.

BETA-GLUCANS AND IMMUNOMODULATION

The immunomodulating effects of mushrooms appear to be largely the result of beta-glucans—large, complex, branched sugars that make up most of the cell walls of mushrooms. Beta-glucans act on lymphocytes, macrophages, neutrophils, natural killer cells, and dendritic cells and regulate cytokine production and release, such as triggering the release of interferons, which increases immune surveillance against and attack on cancer cells.

Beta-glucans cross the intestinal wall via the M (microfold) cells of the epithelium, which allows the uptake of large glucans into the gut-associated lymphoid tissue (GALT). There, the glucans bind to a range of receptors, including toll-like receptors, and are taken up primarily into the macrophages, where they are broken down and presented to other immune cells in the GALT or transported to the spleen, lymph nodes, and bone marrow to activate immune pathways. Smaller beta-glucan fragments are also taken up by a different process into intestinal epithelial-lining cells.

Beta-glucans from mushrooms, unlike those in oats and other cereals, are quite resistant to solvents and require a slow simmer in water for a couple of hours to extract them well. Although they are sugars, they do not change fasting glucose levels in the blood and are perfectly safe in diabetics. The beta-glucans in mushrooms have a unique triple-helix arrangement; those found in cereals are linear and those in yeast form single-helix chains, so neither of these offer the strong immune activation that the mushroom beta-glucans do.

OTHER KEY ACTIVE CONSTITUENTS OF MEDICINAL MUSHROOMS

Chitin. This is another type of sugar arrangement that makes up the major structural component of fungal cell walls. It comprises a long-chain polymer of N-acetylglucosamine. It is also the main constituent of the exoskeleton of shellfish and insects, making it the second most abundant polysaccharide in nature. Chitin may be partially responsible for promoting the innate immune activation and cytokine production seen with ingesting mushrooms.

Ergothioneine. This is a sulfur-containing amino acid made by some mushrooms—especially oyster, lion's mane, shiitake, maitake, and enoki—as well as by some bacteria and the fungus of tempeh. It is not synthesized by plants or animals, who must acquire it from the soil or the diet. Ergothioneine is readily taken up by human cells, using specific receptor sites, and is strongly retained by cells so it can accumulate to high levels in many human and animal tissues, including red blood cells. It seems that more or less all humans and animals are continually exposed to this molecule throughout their life.

Ergothioneine acts as a powerful antioxidant in the brain, enhancing memory and cognition. Overall, it serves as an antioxidant and cellular protectant against a wide range of stressors. It is a neurotonic brain stress reducer and an anti-aging and rejuvenating medicine. Studies have demonstrated decreased blood and/or plasma levels of ergothioneine in some diseases compared to population average, suggesting that a deficiency could be correlated to disease onset or progression. Some researchers have even begun to call for this amino acid to be classified as essential. It is "generally recognized as safe" by the US FDA, and there are no reports of toxicity or harm.

Lectins. These are sugar/protein complexes that are immunomodulating and antiproliferative (inhibit the growth of malignant cells). They are found especially in button mushrooms, cordyceps, enoki, and oyster mushrooms. More than 100 lectins have been identified in diverse mushroom species. Lectins are critical for regulating various biological processes, including cell signaling, cell differentiation, immune functions, inflammation, and cell death. The antiproliferative activity of mushroom lectins is highest in white button mushrooms, lion's mane mushrooms, straw mushrooms (*Volvariella volvacea*), and maitake mushrooms.

Statins. These are found in some fungi, notably in red yeast (*Monascus purpureus*) but also in reishi mycelium, in oyster mushroom fruiting body, and in sun-dried mushrooms. Just like pharmaceutical statins, these mushroom statins can lower total cholesterol by reversible competitive inhibition of the enzyme HMGR required for cholesterol synthesis, but with less risk of muscle pain (rhabdomyolysis). Because these same pathways also upregulate Ras proteins and laminin, there has been an argument made in favor of using statins for cancer prevention, but side effects of the drugs can be considerable. Mushrooms or red yeast rice supplement may potentially be effective and sufficient to modulate the enzyme without the risk of drug side effects.

Terpenes. Terpenes (including diterpenes and triterpenes) are fat-soluble molecules with potent immunomodulating, anti-inflammatory effects as well as the ability to regulate blood sugar and fasting insulin and reduce blood lipids. It is volatile terpenes in the forest that deliver the Shinrin Yoku effect (see page 74), and these may come from mushrooms and fungal growth on the trees and the forest floor, as well as the emissions from the leaves and needles themselves.

Vitamin D2. A trace of vitamin D2 is made by mushrooms exposed to sunlight. Shiitake mushrooms make the more bioavailable D3 but not sufficient for a daily dose. Vitamin D is a steroidal prohormone that, after being activated by the liver, kidney, and other cells, has immune-stimulating and antidepressant effects and is critical for the absorption of calcium and regulation of bone growth.

MUSHROOMS WITH SPECIFIC ANTICANCER CONSTITUENTS

Numerous animal studies and a few human studies have confirmed that these mushrooms as a whole are immunostimulating, immunomodulating, and antiproliferative (inhibit cancer cell growth) through multiple mechanisms.

Reishi. Ganoderic acids are lanosteroid triterpenes found in the fruiting body of reishi (but not in the subterranean mycelia or "root system"). There are many subtypes, of which ganoderic acid A and ganoderic acid B are the most prevalent. They downregulate growth factors including IGF-1, VEGF, and EGFR receptor sites and inhibit the mTOR pathway of signal transduction, which causes cell death. Ganoderic acids also have a prebiotic action and support a healthy microbiome, and in animal studies they have shown to increase beta cell production in the pancreas, which reduces blood sugar.

Chaga. This is a fungus that grows on the trunks of living birch trees in colder northern climates. Water extracts of chaga have cytotoxic and antimitotic activity and can induce cell death in human colorectal cancer cell lines and liver cancer cells. Several triterpenoids have been identified with anticarcinogenic effects in vivo, and there are unique polyphenolic compounds with marked topoisomerase II–inhibiting activity that prevent DNA copying. These polyphenols also inhibited NF-κB activation of human cancer cell lines, leading to suppressed synthesis of proliferative, antiapoptotic, and pro-metastatic proteins. Polysaccharides from chaga also exert antimetastatic activity and inhibit cancer cell migration by blocking matrix metalloproteinases 2 and 9. It should be noted that this mushroom has the highest-ever reported content of oxalic acid; consuming too much could be damaging to the kidneys as a result. To be safe, limit consumption to 5 grams per day.

Turkey tail. This mushroom has marked cytotoxic, cytostatic, and pro-apoptotic actions on various cancer cell lines. Studies have shown that water-ethanol extracts can inhibit proliferation of human breast cancer cell lines, cervical cancer, B cell lymphoma, promyelocytic leukemia, and liver cancer cell lines. The unique immunomodulating polysaccharides of turkey tail stimulate immune responses by boosting production of cytokines and chemokines such as TNF-α, interleukins, histamine, and prostaglandin E.

Cordyceps. Like many of the Asian mushrooms, cordyceps (also known as caterpillar fungus) has a long and illustrious history of use for improving vitality and energy and for promoting recuperation, recovery, rejuvenation, and longevity. There are more than 900 different species, many of them requiring intricate symbiotic life cycles with various insects, and many found only in very restricted areas of high mountain lands.

To satisfy the high market demand in the West today, most commercially available cordyceps is now cultivated in laboratories on special growth mediums, which may be much more sustainable but inevitably are not identical to the wild-harvested material. It's not clear whether this is detrimental or not, but the truth is that most patients cannot afford the real mushroom even if they can find it to buy. The cultivated form is called CS4 and is widely used and apparently successful. In vitro studies of cultivated cordyceps extract in cancer cells has demonstrated inhibition of mTOR and induction of cell death in gallbladder cells and inhibition of both leukemia and melanoma cell growth.

Clinical trials of cordyceps in cancer patients have demonstrated reduced tumor size, improved tolerance for chemotherapy and radiation, and enhanced immune functions with better outcomes after chemotherapy. Complex sugars from cordyceps can regulate and lower blood sugar levels by improving metabolism of glucose and conserving glycogen in the liver by increasing secretion of glucose-regulating enzymes from the liver. Cordyceps improves kidney functions, mitigating some of the damage induced by certain chemotherapies, and it is antioxidant and anti-inflammatory.

Overall, cordyceps demonstrates many of the same effects as adaptogens, balancing metabolic disturbances and normalizing functions. Studies over several decades have demonstrated mild sedative, anticonvulsant, and cooling effects; it has a broncho-relaxant and broncho-dilating effect, with reduced tracheal spasming; and it has antiasthmatic, expectorant, and antitussive effects. In cancer care, this can be very helpful if there is respiratory compromise.

Dosing

In order for the beta-glucans to be metabolized, they must first be broken down by cooking. Simmer mushrooms in water for around 2 hours before incorporating them into a prepared dish. The boiled mushroom slurry can also be dehydrated and ground to a powder to add to food or to encapsulate. Because the mushrooms represent one of the food medicine herbs, there really is no designated or specified dose. Herbalists generally recommend eating cooked mushrooms freely in the diet, several ounces per meal, several times per week. Capsules and standardized extracts may be used for convenience but are an expensive way to take them, which often means people don't take enough.

Medicinal mushrooms can be prohibitively expensive—especially the highly processed, dual-extract tinctures and capsules and branded products. However, growing or foraging mushrooms can be very inexpensive. Some mushrooms, such as turkey tail and reishi, are prolific and easy to identify. Some are easy to grow even on a balcony or in a small urban yard. Even the edible mushrooms from the grocery store have value. Button mushrooms, cremini, portabello, and shiitake mushrooms are widely available and effective. I encourage my patients to eat a mushroom-based meal at least once or twice a week as an affordable way to get some medicine.

PART 2

For the Practitioner and Herbal Prescriber

CHAPTER 7

Herbal Formulating for Cancer Care

The practice of herbal medicine is both an art and a science. Certainly, knowing the biochemistry and pharmacology of the remedies is interesting and useful and supports safe practice, but there is so much more that goes into creating an effective remedy. In this chapter, we will explore some of the building blocks of successful herbal formulating and discuss the key considerations of safety and efficacy, pharmacy (the form of medicine), and posology (the dose and dosing frequency), and we will apply these principles directly to cancer care.

CHAPTER 7 CONTENTS

311 **The Multifaceted Role of the Holistic Practitioner**

311 Developing the Logic of the Formula

312 **The Causal Chain of Disease**

312 Predisposing Causes

313 Excitatory or Precipitating Causes

313 Sustaining or Perpetuating Causes

313 **The Therapeutic Order**

314 **Creating a Balanced Herbal Formula**

316 Physiological Enhancement

317 Pathological Correction: Strategies and Protocols

318 **The Pyramid Prescribing Protocol**

318 Three Levels of Herbs

319 **Synergy of Constituents in Herbs and Drugs**

320 Clinical Studies on Synergy

322 Formulating for Synergy

323 Key Considerations when Combining Herbs

325 **Formulating for Pathological Correction**

325 Addressing Oxidative Stress

325 Incorporating Targeted Activator and Effector Herbs

327 Taking the Cytotoxics

329 **Timelines for Herbal Treatment**

331 **Safety and Toxicology with Herbs**

331 Isolated Constituents vs. Whole Herbs

332 Variability in Herbal Products

332 Determining Herb Safety

334 Herbal Medicines and Anticoagulants

335 Chemotherapy, Herbal Medicine, and Supplements

337 **Research Showing Positive Benefits from Herbs**

337 Astragalus

338 Redox Regulators

338 Turmeric, Curcumin, and Chemotherapy

340 Ashwagandha and Chemotherapy

340 Green Tea and Chemotherapy

The Multifaceted Role of the Holistic Practitioner

The modern herbal practitioner needs to be adept both in contemporary biomedical thinking and in historical and evidence-based medicine—to be able, for example, to properly assess for herb-drug interactions at the same time as knowing when to warm or cool and dry or moisten a constitutional imbalance. In this maze of options, opportunities, and dangers, there is no single right way or wrong way to prescribe for cancer patients, no "one size fits all" answers, and no single herb that will fix all the problems.

The great strength of phytotherapy lies in its ability to be fitted to the individual, using overlapping herbs, custom blended for the patient, taking account of factors such as age, mental health, and comorbidities, to create a coherent formula that is balanced, with each herb serving a purpose and being in proportion to one another.

Developing the Logic of the Formula

I think of this treatment planning as a process for developing the internal logic of the formula. Does it hang together? Do all the parts fit together and support each other? Creating a coherent formula requires that you know not only the primary actions of the herbs but also the secondary, tertiary, or even more nuanced actions. What is each herb capable of, and is it placed as the lead herb in a formula, as the activator or effector, or as a supportive or a foundation herb that complements another lead herb? By bringing an herb forward in the formula or by reducing it, the balance can be adjusted and the focus repositioned as the case progresses.

This is where the art of phytotherapy takes over from the science. It could be likened to a dance, where there are one or two principal dancers, but the story would be incomplete without the corps de ballet. Or like a piece of music where there are soloists that feature, but without the orchestra in the background the symphony would be rather thin. Each piece and each part of the whole is strengthened and expanded by the presence and interactions of the others. So it is with an herbal formula, where the herbal prescriber is akin to the choreographer or composer, with infinite possibilities to choose from.

With so many herbal options, so many drugs and other therapies in the mix, and so much at stake, in providing cancer care it becomes more relevant than ever to get to know the patient and their particular circumstances and needs. This is important so that we know which herbs will give not only the precision required to treat the cancer but also the breadth required to change the terrain—improving the foundations of health in a person, as well as altering how cancer functions in their body.

> It is more important to know what kind of person has a disease than to know what kind of disease a person has.
>
> ATTRIBUTED TO HIPPOCRATES

The Causal Chain of Disease

All diseases follow a trajectory called the causal chain. Symptoms may present differently in each case, but there are three basic steps or stages in all disease progression: predisposing, excitatory, and sustaining causes. Identifying these and determining a logical sequence for treatment is a key part of the diagnosis and formulating process. Generally speaking, predisposing causes can be managed through a process of physiological enhancement or normalizing of function. Herbs are not expected to undo the damage of a lifetime but to reduce symptoms and slow progression. Excitatory (triggering and precipitating) causes, as well as sustaining or perpetuating causes, may need a more targeted and specific treatment plan through a process of pathological correction (enforced cell or tissue behavior adjustment). This may entail herbal cytotoxics all the way up to targeted chemotherapy, as needed in each case.

The optimal principle in clinical practice is to use as little pathological correction as is required to effect the desired change, and to use physiological enhancement strategies to sustain the changes. This may not be feasible at the outset of a cancer treatment plan, where more aggressive and targeted treatment may be required, but if anticancer strategies are successful, then the restorative and rejuvenating approach will follow. A detailed discussion of physiological enhancement and pathological correction in herbal medicine can be found in the seminal textbook by Mills and Bone, *Principles and Practice of Phytotherapy*, as well as in Bone's book *Functional Herbal Therapy*.

Predisposing Causes

These are the conditions that increase risk before any disease strikes. They are also, therefore, where the greatest opportunity lies for preventing cancer through self-care and lifestyle choices. Some of these predisposing factors cannot be changed but may be managed; for example, genetics are set at conception, but epigenetics (switching genes on and off through environmental influences) can be directed toward good health or ill health by lifestyle choices. To a large extent, these predisposing causes may be addressed through the diet and herbal strategies suggested in Chapters 1 and 2; these are the proactive and preventive strategies recommended by holistic practitioners for warding off cancer and for reducing the risk and severity of most other chronic degenerative diseases.

Predisposing causes of cancer include:

- **Genetics:** inherited or epigenetically acquired defects
- **Mental outlook and stress:** chronic cortisol demand and adrenal dysregulation, impaired healing response
- **Immune dysregulation:** hygiene and infection, chronic inflammation (chronic unresolved infection generates a persistent inflammatory state and prevents resolution)
- **Nutrition:** dietary toxins, nutritional deficiencies, obesity, microbiome dysregulation

- **Physical trauma:** repeated injury, UV (sun) exposure, radiation
- **Environment:** toxins and pollution

Excitatory or Precipitating Causes

These are events or exposures that "flip the switch" and turn a stressed or dysfunctional state into an active pathology, up to and including cancer. They may include:

- **Acute infection:** overwhelming of the immune system and reduced oversight of tumor tissue
- **Acute trauma:** may be physical or emotional/mental
- **Acute exposure or sudden increased load of toxins:** environmental pollution, dietary or occupational exposures
- **Radiation or drugs:** overly frequent use of x-rays or CT scans, immunosuppressive drugs for autoimmune diseases, many chemotherapy drugs

Sustaining or Perpetuating Causes

These are what keep a person sick, delay or inhibit healing, and worsen the prognosis in cancer. They may include:

- **Unresolved excitation:** infection that doesn't heal, repeated trauma or excessive radiation, including CT scans, PET scans, and x-rays
- **Inflammation:** chronic inflammation that doesn't resolve will deplete the immune reserves over time
- **Senescence:** aging of organs with reduced repair and recuperation capacity
- **Drugs:** pharmaceuticals that suppress disease symptoms without addressing the underlying pathology, or that actually contribute to side effects and symptoms themselves

The Therapeutic Order

The therapeutic order is a template or guideline for treatment planning that has its roots in the 1800s, in Eclectic and traditional herbal medicine practice, and was written into modern American naturopathic medicine philosophy of practice by Dr. Jared Zeff and Dr. Pamela Snider. In principle, it suggests working from least to most invasive interventions—from the inside out, from more general strategies to more symptom-specific and targeted therapies. It includes seven steps that should be applied each in turn, the degree of intervention increasing as needed to restore health. This is not a rigid process but a "road map" that can be adapted to each patient as required over time.

1. Remove obstacles to health and establish the conditions for wellness—build the foundation with nutrition and detoxification, stress management, exercise, and sleep. Address all the epigenetic influences you can to reduce risks.

2. Stimulate the healing power of nature and the body's self-healing mechanisms—including bone marrow support, immune normalization, digestive support.

3. Support and balance physiologic and bioenergetic systems—strengthen weakened or damaged systems, restore and regenerate.
4. Correct structural integrity—body work and exercise to improve anatomical functions and tissue repair.
5. Use specific natural therapies to address pathology and symptoms—targeted herbal and nutritional formulas.
6. Use pharmaceutical or synthetic substances and invasive therapies to suppress pathology—chemotherapy and radiation.
7. Use surgery or other invasive procedures to arrest pathology.

Based on this model, it quickly becomes apparent that the holistic practitioner has an opportunity to promote wellness at all of these levels. From the simplest lifestyle and dietary changes (level 1) right up to supporting the patient through chemotherapy or surgery (level 6 or 7), herbs and natural medicines have a significant role to play. If the practitioner needs time to properly assess the case, if some of the conventional allopathic treatments have not yet been decided, or if the patient is too debilitated and weak to take some of the cytotoxic herbs, then addressing the lower levels in the therapeutic order will still be helpful. More specific and targeted treatments can then be added as information becomes available and the patient's condition changes.

In my clinical practice, I usually start a new patient with foundation building first, addressing lifestyle, nutrition, immune tonics, and adaptogens. While they implement as much of this as they feel able into their daily activities, I can then take a bit more time to research their diagnosis and any prescription drugs they take and to come up with a comprehensive and collaborative care plan for each person.

Creating a Balanced Herbal Formula

A properly balanced formula should be a part of a comprehensive protocol that addresses predisposing, excitatory, and sustaining causes. Building a strong foundation, treating and resolving underlying causes and comorbidities, and managing symptoms (physiological enhancement) all need to be balanced and measured so that they aren't overwhelming for the patient to realistically implement, but you'll still need to provide a sufficient dose of each herb or supplement for them to be effective. For the cancer patient, layered on top of that will be the cytotoxic herbs, anti-inflammatories, redox regulators (pathological correction), and herbs for managing acute symptoms from conventional treatments, as well as from the cancer itself.

Questions to Ask before Blending a Formula

- Which actions are most desirable? Which constituents are most desirable?
- What is the pharmacology of these constituents? What is the best way to extract them?

- Does the herb have tissue specificity? What body system or organ is the treatment or herb targeting?
- Does the herb have a traditional use? Is there any current research on it?
- Are there any constituents or herbs to avoid in this particular patient?
- What are the possible signs of toxicity?
- Are there any contraindications or cautions? Are there any anticipated interactions (drug or herbal)?
- What other herbs might it combine well with (for plant synergy)?
- What does the herb taste like?
- What form should be administered (tincture, capsule, infusion, decoction, poultice, lotion, or liniment)?
- How much of each herb is required for a therapeutic dose?
- How often will the herbs be given?
- When or what time of day will the medicine be taken? Will it be taken with or away from food?
- How long will the patient stay on the formula?
- How will you know if the formula is working?

Thanks to Dr. Marisa Marciano, ND, for this list.

Physiological Enhancement: Deep Terrain Support

- Build the foundation through nutrition and diet, lifestyle (exercise, sleep, healthy habits), supporting constitution, and reducing stressors.
- Address the predisposing causes of disease and remove identifiable risks or triggers.

Optimizing Capacity for Wellness

- Optimize the internal chemistry. Detoxification—heal gut lining, support microbiome, and promote hepatic and other metabolic detox pathways—alteratives/blood purifiers, cholagogues, aperients. Exercise and weight management. Avoidance of alcohol, tobacco, environmental toxins.
- Optimize vitality. Sleep, rest, and stress management—adaptogens, nervine tonics, sedatives or relaxants (nighttime), energizers (daytime). Build community—sense of belonging, sense of meaning and purpose.
- Optimize immune function. Build resistance and resilience, enhance white blood cell functions.
- Correct metabolic imbalances. Enhance physiology (e.g., bitters to promote digestive functions, diuretics to promote renal excretion, circulatory stimulants to deliver oxygen and invigorate tissues).

Supportive and Directing Actions

- Promote hepatic and other metabolic detox pathways
- Support bone marrow and immune activity
- Reduce local inflammation
- Strengthen connective tissue, inhibit collagenases and proteases
- Inhibit hypercoagulation
- Normalize angiogenesis

Pathological Correction

- Stronger herbs used to break a vicious cycle; specific pharmacology and targeted actions cause measurable physiological change.

Higher risk of side effects, shorter dose duration. Herbs may include anti-inflammatories, analgesics, antihemorrhagics, cytotoxics.

Addressing Specific Causes of Disease

- Increase mitochondrial energy transfer (promote Krebs cycle)
- Normalize gene expression and gene repair
- Disrupt cancer cell metabolism and normalize growth factors, signal transduction, and signal transcription
- Inhibit mitosis and downregulate cell cycling
- Induce apoptosis

Physiological Enhancement

The concept of building the foundation, strengthening the terrain, and promoting strong inner resources for healing to occur is fundamental to holistic treatment planning and is used to create a strong scaffold for the cytotoxic herbs, chemotherapy, surgery, and radiation to do their work.

Restore vitality. First and foremost, the most important principle of building the foundation is to restore and revitalize the vital force of the patient. Vital force energizes and activates living organisms and governs resistance to disease and healing from disease. Herbal medicine is always aimed at restoring and strengthening the vitality of the patient.

Vitality or vital force is that ineffable feeling of wellness, of physical ease, strength, and stamina, mental balance and tranquility, and spiritual wholeness, that we struggle to articulate but recognize immediately when it presents. It is the joy and motivation that gets us up in the morning and the peace of mind that allows us to rest easy at night. It represents the capacity of the body to repair, restore, and recuperate, or the resilience and adaptation that is possible in an individual. According to English herbalists Priest and Priest (1982) "The manifestations of health and disease are considered as the aggregate expression of this vital force as it endeavors to maintain the functional integrity of the organism."

Vital force functions in a state of dynamic equilibrium. It is not static or stagnant—indeed, that would be associated with a *lack* of vital force, which ultimately means death and decay. Vitality defines aliveness. The effort of healing is to promote this vitality and to resist quenching the spark. Homeostasis—a term that implies a steady state of physiology and an optimal balance point—is an idea that has been supplanted in recent years by the concept of allostasis (from the Greek *allo*, meaning "variable," and *stasis*, meaning "stable"). This is a concept of variable stability that adjusts constantly to best suit the circumstances and environment—an active state of dynamic equilibrium. This balance is best supported with adaptogen herbs that govern stress responses and set the sympathetic/parasympathetic tone.

Because cancer is both caused by and actively contributes to stress in the system, I recommend using tonic herbs, adaptogens, bitters, and nutritives. Consider a morning formula with uplifting and invigorating nervines (ginseng, rhodiola, leuzea—all stimulant adaptogens) and an evening formula with relaxant nervines (damiana, verbena, chamomile, lemon balm, hops—all bitter nervines with relaxing and tonic nervine properties).

Pathological Correction: Strategies and Protocols

Pathological correction strategies achieve known results on a specific condition or symptom.This approach uses herbs that have a specific biochemical impact on a certain aspect of physiology, often directed or targeted by single known constituents, although also influenced and adjusted through other constituents of the whole plant. This quasi-pharmacological understanding of herbs entails a higher level of risk and usually more specific dosing than the nutritive and tonic herbs. They are considered to be activators or effectors in a formula, the potent herbs that effect measurable and tangible change, and in cancer care they include cytotoxics and the narcotic painkillers. These are combined with synergists—supportive or directing herbs, as discussed on page 328.

Pathological correction requires accurate diagnosis and knowledge of correct dosing and safety. The herbs used may require a lower dose than the tonic or normalizing herbs. The cytotoxics and analgesics may even be given in drop doses; the risk of side effects is higher and the duration of use is shorter. These herbs are described in detail, with specific dosing, in Chapter 9.

States of Allostasis

Allostasis is a fundamental biological principle defined as a variable stability or dynamic equilibrium. Disease and health breakdown, as well as healing and recovery from disease, are part of a continuum from negative to positive.

- Negative state = progressive pathology, deterioration and disease; catabolic state
- Positive state = restorative, repairing, healing, may even be a healing crisis; anabolic state
- Tolerant state = state of balance and equilibrium, adaptation has occurred

The Pyramid Prescribing Protocol

Western herbal prescribing is often built upon a pyramid pattern or triangle for layering herbs into formulas. The base of the triangle represents the foundation or the overall state of health, and the two sides of the triangle represent the disease and the terrain, respectively—the immediate or acute disease state and the case-specific background considerations that need addressing. We can expand upon this traditional three-part model to show how the principles of physiological enhancement and pathological correction can be layered into a coherent protocol with an internal logic required to make a nuanced herbal blend that does exactly what is needed.

Many herbalists use variations on this pattern today, including derivations from the work of the late William LeSassier (what he called the "triune" system) and extensive further development of the concept from David Winston, a US herbalist and herbal historian. Dr. Jillian Stansbury illustrates this pyramid prescribing pattern most elegantly in her books in the *Herbal Formularies for Health Professionals* series. She calls the three sides of the pyramid the base, the synergists, and the specifics.

Three Levels of Herbs

There are three fundamental effects to consider: herbs that do something active to exert specific change, herbs that support and promote that change, and herbs that support the body to build stronger terrain.

Base or foundation. This base layer includes herbs that address physiological enhancement at the deepest level; they are normalizing, tonic, and regenerative. They do not address specific diseases but optimize the terrain for attaining and sustaining wellness. They provide

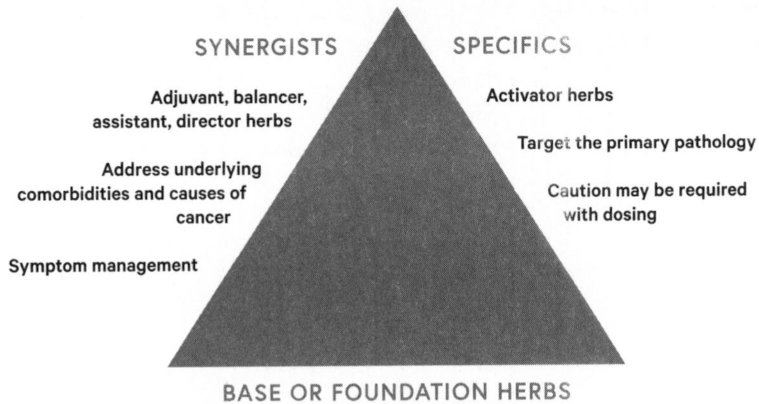
SYNERGISTS
Adjuvant, balancer, assistant, director herbs
Address underlying comorbidities and causes of cancer
Symptom management
SPECIFICS
Activator herbs
Target the primary pathology
Caution may be required with dosing
BASE OR FOUNDATION HERBS
Tonic, nourishing herbs
Generally safe, less specific, more general

physiological normalizing and balancing effects; they support weak organ systems, promoting constitutional balance and maintaining metabolic functions and allostasis. They do not fight cancer directly but promote resilience, resistance, rejuvenation, and repair.

The foundation or base is traditionally focused around three core actions seen as critical to good health and optimal physiological function:

- Supporting anabolic/catabolic balance
- Opening the channels of elimination (the bowels, kidney, skin, mucus, lungs)
- Supporting circulation (meaning to promote heat or life force)

Many herbal recipes for cancer from the Eclectic doctors of the 1800s feature laxatives and warming stimulants as a foundation for this reason, and there is still some value in that. But with modern clinical research and a more exact understanding of the actions of the plants, the herbal practitioner today is able to apply the effector or activator herbs in more specific ways than previously, and to use the supportive, synergistic herbs to augment the efficacy and mitigate risk.

Synergistic or supportive. These are herbs that synergize with or direct other herbs to target organs or that treat comorbidities. They may also change the operating conditions of the body, but in a more symptom-specific way than the foundation herbs do, activating organ systems and promoting tissue functions. They provide directing, regulating, and correcting effects. They harmonize and carry the herbal effects to specific parts of the body—they direct, support, nourish, and tonify.

Specifics or targeted effectors and activators. These are the leading herbs that target the specific tissue derangement or pathology. They are usually given in lower doses or for a shorter duration or may be rotated in and out of protocols to reduce risk of cumulative toxicity. These herbs address pathological correction. They are the main active herbs, targeting the primary pathology and setting the direction of the whole formula.

In further refinements of the pyramid prescribing protocol, it is also possible to consider herbs that are warming and stimulate or induce metabolic changes, herbs that are cooling and sedate or inhibit metabolic changes, herbs that are moistening and relaxing, herbs that are toning, tightening, and drying, and other nuanced constitutional and pharmacological considerations per patient.

Synergy of Constituents in Herbs and Drugs

The word *synergy* comes from the Greek *synergos*, meaning “working together.” In medicine this means combining different drugs or remedies to achieve greater effects and better outcomes. Surprisingly little robust research has been done on synergy in herbal medicine, possibly because conventional medicine hasn’t built capacity in this regard, as synergy in pharmaceutical medicine is largely ignored.

Herbal practitioners use preparations and mixtures that are pluripotent and may target several enzyme or biochemical systems simultaneously, making each one hard to measure in isolation. The challenges of conducting good clinical research on synergies and antagonisms in herbal medicine are described in a 2019 paper by Caesar and Cech (see page 514), but they conclude that, overall, the synergy of constituents in a single herb tends to provide a wider range of benefits than the isolates.

Synergistic interactions between the components of individual herbs or mixtures of herbs are considered a vital part of their therapeutic efficacy, and when herbs are put together in a formula the whole can be greater than the sum of the parts. Similarly, agonist and antagonist interactions between herbs and drugs can augment benefits and ameliorate side effects simultaneously. These synergies are brought about by several mechanisms, which may include protection of active compounds from gastric or hepatic degradation, facilitation of active transport across cell and organelle walls, enhanced hepatic and intestinal metabolism (promoting bioavailability of drugs, speeding a drug's clearance, and shortening half-life), inhibition of multidrug resistance efflux pumping, or eliminating adverse effects and enhancing potency of drugs. In this regard, synergy in clinical practice can often be a positive interaction.

Clinical Studies on Synergy

A number of well-designed human trials, innumerable cell line and animal studies with isolated plant constituents, and some trials with whole herbs or whole herb extracts add up to a strong body of evidence that favors the idea of synergy in formulating and prescribing.

EXAMPLES OF SYNERGY WITHIN ONE PLANT

Isoflavones from crude extract of kudzu (*Pueraria lobata*) achieve greater plasma concentrations than does an equivalent dose of purified isoflavone without naturally occurring cofactors.

Hypericin and pseudohypericin from St. John's wort are coactive constituents that mediate a broad-spectrum inhibition of neurotransmitter reuptake—in particular serotonin, dopamine, noradrenaline, glutamate, and gamma-aminobutyric acid—which leads to a mood-elevating, uplifting, and calming effect. They have considerably less antidepressant activity individually than does whole herb extract with equivalent amounts of these compounds together.

Sennoside A and C, the active constituents of senna, both have similar laxative effects in mice. However, a mixture of the two, administered in a 7:3 ratio (reflecting the proportions found in senna leaf), has nearly double the laxative activity of either constituent alone.

An in vitro study of flavonoids from the leaf of goldenseal synergistically enhanced the antimicrobial activity of the alkaloid berberine from the goldenseal root against *Staphylococcus aureus* by inhibition of the multidrug resistance efflux pump. This suggests it may be helpful to use a combination of both goldenseal roots and leaves for maximum activity against *S. aureus.*

EXAMPLES OF SYNERGY BETWEEN DIFFERENT PLANTS

In a double-blind, crossover, human trial using 20 healthy young adult volunteers, a product containing *Panax ginseng* with ginkgo was more effective in improving cognitive function than either herb taken alone, as measured by the performance in various arithmetic tasks.

A study looking at redox-regulating actions of green tea and ginger confirmed that the combination of both was more effective in quenching free radicals than either herb given alone.

A robust study into the antioxidant and anticancer activities of a diet rich in fruits and vegetables suggests that additive and synergistic effects of phytochemicals are responsible and that no single antioxidant can replace the combination of natural bioactive compounds found in whole foods. This supports the recommendation that people eat 5–10 servings of fruits and vegetables daily.

EXAMPLES OF SYNERGY BETWEEN PLANT COMPOUNDS AND CHEMOTHERAPY

Beet extract enhanced the cytotoxicity of doxorubicin against human pancreatic cancer cells.

Beta-caryophyllene, a sesquiterpene from the essential oil of clove, given with paclitaxel against human breast cells and human colon cells, potentiated the entry of the drug to the cancer cells and enhanced overall anticancer activity of the drug.

Beta-elemene, a sesquiterpene from the essential oil of mint, given with a taxane drug, reduced cell viability and increased cell apoptosis to a greater extent than the drug alone. Beta-elemene also enhanced cisplatin sensitivity and amplified cisplatin cytotoxicity in bladder, brain, cervix, breast, colorectal, ovary, and small cell lung cancer cell lines.

Curcumin sensitized glioma cells to cisplatin, etoposide, camptothecin, and doxorubicin and to radiation, in part by inhibiting AP-1 and NF-κB signaling pathways. In another study, curcumin and 5-FU showed synergistic inhibition of growth against a human colon cancer cell line, with the level of COX-2 protein expression reduced almost sixfold after the combination treatment.

D-limonene, a cyclic terpene from citrus rind, was synergistic in prostate cells with docetaxel, resulting in higher reactive oxygen species (ROS) generation, glutathione depletion, and increased caspase activity.

Geraniol, a monoterpene from the essential oil of geranium, among other flowers, diminished tumor mass volume by acting on cell cycle and apoptosis pathways and enhanced docetaxel chemosensitivity.

Methyleugenol from the essential oil of clove, nutmeg, cinnamon, basil, and bay leaf significantly enhanced the anticancer activity of platinum drugs on apoptosis, cell cycle arrest, and mitochondrial membrane potential loss.

Quercetin significantly reduced the proliferation of cell lines, regulated cell cycling, and induced apoptosis, and the combination of quercetin and cisplatin was found to be more effective than either agent given individually.

Resveratrol (a stilbene from grape skin and seed, peanuts, soy, and Japanese knotweed) resensitized acute myeloid leukemia cells to doxorubicin and induced cell growth arrest and apoptotic death in doxorubicin-resistant cells.

Thymoquinone, from *Nigella sativa* essential oil, improved the antineoplastic properties of doxorubicin by inhibiting cancer cell growth in human leukemia, melanoma, colon, cervix, and breast cells. In a mouse model of triple-negative breast cancer, thymoquinone sensitized cancer cells to paclitaxel through inducing apoptosis, tumor suppressor genes, and p53 signaling.

Formulating for Synergy

Although it may be challenging to find good human clinical research into herbal synergies, it is nonetheless standard practice in most herbal prescribing traditions to use several plants combined to refine the treatment. In TCM and Ayurveda these are formalized into recipes that may be hundreds or even thousands of years old, some of them quite complex. The modern Western herbal practice of formulating and blending may include elements of the traditional energetic principles of prescribing (humoral/constitutional assessment), as well as consideration of the function and actions of individual herbs and herbal constituents.

COMPLEMENTARY HERBS

These are herbs that have different effects but can work together to help each other. Examples include:

Systemic relaxants and circulatory stimulants. Lobelia and cayenne are examples. Cayenne moves blood by cardiac stimulation, and lobelia is a muscle relaxant for peripheral vasodilation, which allows for better distal perfusion.

Antibiotics and immunostimulants. Bearberry and echinacea are examples. Bearberry leaf is an antibiotic active mainly in the urinary tract. It is combined with echinacea in bladder infections for general white blood cell activation and systemic immune upregulation.

Hepatoprotectives and choleretics. Milk thistle and dandelion root are examples. Dandelion root is a bitter hepatic choleretic; it makes bile and promotes detoxification. Milk thistle protects liver cells from the oxidative stress of transiting toxins.

Rubefacients and anti-inflammatories. Mustard plaster and turmeric are examples. A mustard plaster over an arthritic joint will be rubefacient and attract blood, delivering more turmeric to the area.

AMPLIFYING HERBS

These are herbs with comparable effects that augment each other's actions. Examples include:

Cerebral and peripheral circulatory stimulants. Ginkgo and rosemary both increase blood supply to the brain and help memory and cognition.

Anxiolytic and calming herbs. Skullcap and chamomile are both effective relaxants, with skullcap having more antispasmodic or muscle-relaxing actions. Taken together they augment each other to calm the mind and body.

BALANCING HERBS

These are herbs that offset each other and neutralize some traits. Examples include:

Cooling and warming. Perhaps you want the antinausea and anti-inflammatory effects of ginger, but the patient is experiencing hot flashes; gentian can cool them down. Or if you want the sedative and muscle-relaxing effect of valerian, but it can be warming, combining it with hops can be cooling and estrogen balancing for a patient with hot flashes.

Drying and lubricating. Osha is used for deep, sticky lung infections as a stimulating expectorant that tends to be warming and drying. Licorice can be added for its mucilaginous properties to soften and loosen mucus.

DIRECTING HERBS

This refers to the inexplicable phenomenon of tissue specificity, whereby certain herbs have a tropism for certain organs or functions and can be used to "carry" other herbs—to direct their actions to target areas. This is observed but not fully explained in contemporary herbal medicine literature but is often based on traditional indications and historical or empirical uses. It may involve consideration of the energetic principles—the qualities, humors, and temperaments of the herb. It may or may not be readily explicable by modern analytical science. The example given here is from a classic mid-twentieth-century book (now sadly out of print) on the physiomedical prescribing principle, *Herbal Medication* by Priest and Priest.

Valerian is a broadly acting sedative as well as a physical (muscle) and mental relaxant. It can be paired with:

- Passionflower for nervous excitability
- Hops for nervous insomnia
- Lily of the valley for nervous palpitations
- Pasque flower and black cohosh for menopausal anxiety
- Wild yam and ginger for nervous colic
- Prickly ash for restless leg syndrome
- Licorice, milky oat seed, and lobelia for tobacco cravings
- Linden and mistletoe for hypertension
- Datura, ephedra, and lobelia for an acute asthma attack

In these examples the valerian is relaxing and warming to the muscles and tissues (including the heart and smooth muscle), as well as calming and sedating to the mind. It is indicated with the synergist herbs to bring the relaxing and warming effects of the valerian to the target area.

Key Considerations when Combining Herbs

The key questions to consider for each herb in a blend are the actions, the energetics, the synergies and conflicts, any safety concerns or contraindications, availability and sustainability (ecological impact), affordability, and compliance. My teacher, Hein Zeylstra, used to say that the overall aim is to use only as many herbs as are necessary to achieve the clinical goals and to be safe, effective, palatable, and affordable. In principle, "less is more" because using fewer herbs affords greater control and less risk of unexpected interactions, as well as better opportunity to reach therapeutic intake from each herb. If you feel compelled to use isolates and super concentrates because of the urgency of the case and the need for high doses, then I recommend adding the whole herb extract as well, or using it in food, if possible.

Weighting formulas toward a goal. A formula may be weighted more toward physiological enhancement or toward pathological correction and may not necessarily include both approaches in the one product. It is useful to consider prescribing cytotoxic blends or strong formulas separately from the herbs for foundation health or support and synergy. This allows for fine adjustment of dosing of the tertiary herbs in the formula—increasing or decreasing the dose, per individual need—without disturbing the foundation or background herbs.

Person + purpose + potency = proportion. This useful aphorism means the personal parameters of the individual patient and the intention or expectation of treatment tells us how much of each herb to use. In addition, there are several other factors I consider. Liver disease can slow clearance and prolong half-life. Kidney disease may induce rapid clearance of drugs, shortening their half-life, or may slow clearance and lengthen half-life if constituents can't be as efficiently filtered or metabolized by the ailing kidneys. Bowel function should also be considered, as constipation slows clearance, while diarrhea speeds it. Gut flora, height, weight, age, severity/chronicity of the disease, comorbidities, and any other adjunctive treatments are also important. When all of these considerations are accounted for, the protocol can reasonably be expected to be safe and effective.

Therapeutic Intentions in Treating Cancer

Improve quality of life. Of primary importance is reducing stress, building vitality and healing capacity, and nourishing the foundation through physiological enhancement. Address underlying imbalances, including blood stagnation, redox cycling, and mitochondrial efficiency. Enhance potencies and efficacy of conventional treatment; seek beneficial herb-drug interactions, use herbs to maximize efficacy, and mitigate harm. Relieve side effects of conventional treatments, and treat symptoms as required (pain, infection, and wound healing, for example).

Increase longevity. Delay or inhibit the progression of cancer. There are many strategies or ways to achieve this, but fundamentally the intention is to inhibit cell cycling and induce apoptosis. This will require use of cytotoxics in an active cancer case and restorative and rejuvenating herbs for cancer recovery.

Formulating for Pathological Correction

Formulating for pathological correction requires that we target cancer-promoting pathways and cell behaviors specifically, and different herbs or nutritional supplements may be pluripotent or multitargeting through different pathways. Research suggests that maybe only 5–10% of all cancer cases can be attributed directly to genetic defects, whereas perhaps as much as 90–95% are caused by epigenetic defects due to environmental and lifestyle factors.

Addressing Oxidative Stress

After exploring all of the details about how cancer starts, progresses, and proliferates, it becomes apparent that a state of cellular oxidative stress is probably the single most significant process that drives the development of cancer. This means that all the dietary and natural medicine strategies that address redox regulation are acting broadly across myriad metabolic derangements that are creating and perpetuating an optimal environment for cancer to grow. Time and time again, the same herbs and supplements, the same active constituents, are found to be effective in multiple pathways. This creates a broad scope for prescribing, allowing the practitioner to layer and weave herbs and supplements to customize a protocol.

Incorporating Targeted Activator and Effector Herbs

In some ways approaching cancer with herbs and nutrition can feel overwhelming. How can we possibly get enough herbs into someone to make a difference if chemotherapy is not enough? Certainly dose sufficiency matters, and I sometimes tell my patients that "big disease takes big medicine." This misses the critical point, however, that one herb can be effective against multiple pathways, so just a few potent herbs can "punch above their weight" when combined. Individual cytotoxic herbs are the effectors or activators specific to cancer. They are described in detail, along with guidance for their safe and effective use, in Chapter 9.

If the patient is also receiving chemotherapy currently, it is possible to incorporate specific herbs to augment or support drug actions and to reduce side effects as well. For example, alongside taxane drugs, a low dose of Pacific yew extract may enhance the efficacy of the drug while downregulating efflux pumping so that side effects are reduced and cancer response is increased.

As well as addressing the cancer directly, specific herbs are chosen that are secondarily beneficial to the individual patient. For example, in traditional herbal formulas it is very common to see at least one herb that addresses liver function, either as a foundation herb or for a secondary action. A carefully crafted formula may, for example, contain the bitter cytotoxic herb greater celandine, which has direct anticancer action in the upper abdominal organs as well as promoting bile flow and elimination; barberry, which aids in acid waste removal from tissues and inhibits multidrug resistant pumping to enhance chemotherapy effects; and hops, which functions as a phyoestrogenic and a bitter digestive stimulant for low appetite and dyspepsia and also promotes deep and restful sleep. These three bitter herbs are all useful in cancer care, support liver function, and have three unique additional targeted actions. Similarly with supplements, resveratrol, CoQ10, and vitamin E have particular benefits if heart disease is a comorbidity. Diindolylmethane (DIM), indole-3-carbinol (I3C), isoflavones, and coumestans may be specifically indicated if the cancer patient is also menopausal. All of these may have redox-regulating, hormone-balancing, or other anticancer action, but secondary attributes give them specificity in a given patient.

ACTIVATOR OR EFFECTOR CONSTITUENTS IN HERBS

Because plant constituents have been studied in such exacting detail for many years, there is now some fascinating research that goes at least partway toward explaining some of the myriad functions of how plants treat cancer. This is reductionistic and not holistic but still fascinating to consider.

Terpenes. These complex molecules comprising isoprene subunits are broadly active through numerous pathways. They may induce apoptosis through induction of p53, p21, and caspases, as well as inhibition of Bcl-2. They inhibit angiogenesis through downregulating MMPs, HIF-1α, and VEGF, and they can induce cell cycle arrest through inhibition of cyclin-dependent kinases. They can also suppress nuclear transcription factors including nuclear factor-kappa B (NF-κB).

Terpenoid Compounds with Anticancer Activity

- Sterols—beta-sitosterol, stigmasterol, campesterol
- Phytoecdysterones—leuzeasterone, ecdysterone
- Monoterpenes—camphene, carvone, citral, citronellol, eucalyptol, geraniol, limonene, linolool, menthol, myrcene, ocimene, perillic acid, thymol
- Diterpenes—forskolin, taxanes
- Sesquiterpenes—artemisinin, parthenolide, zingiberene, humulone, caryophyllene, azulene, vetivazulene
- Terpenoid quinones—ubiquinone (CoQ10)
- Triterpenes—ginsenosides, withanolides, ursolic acid, glycyrrhizic acid, astragalosides, oleanolic acid, betulinic acid
- Tetraterpenes—carotenoids, lutein, lycopene

Flavonoids. These are polyphenolics found in most plants that have significant redox-regulating capacity. They can donate and regain electrons through a process called resonance stabilization, which allows continual redox control, normalizes multiple oncogenic pathways, and limits proliferation, angiogenesis, and metastasis. Flavonoids may induce cell cycle arrest or apoptosis via modulation of multiple signaling pathways. For example, EGCG from green tea inhibits MAPK, epidermal growth factor (EGF), NF-κB, VEGF, and MMP.

Flavonoids That Downregulate Transduction and Transcription Pathways through Redox Regulation

- Genistein, resveratrol, catechins—block EGFr
- Catechins, silymarin, emodin, resveratrol—inhibit the NF-κB pathway
- Capsaicin, resveratrol, green tea catechins—inhibit AP-1 pathway
- EGCG (green tea)—blocks the MAPK signaling pathway

Flavonoids That Induce Apoptosis

- Hesperidin induced the expression of cytochrome c, caspase-3, and caspase-9 and reduced the Bax:Bcl-2 ratio in gastric cancer cells. It also increased ROS and decreased glutathione concentrations in human esophageal carcinoma cells.
- Naringenin increased p53 expression, PARP cleaving, Bax, and caspase-3 cleaving and decreased expression of Bcl-2 and survivin in human gastric cancer cells.
- Quercetin induced apoptosis via increase of Bax and caspase-3 and decrease of Bcl-2 in breast cancer cells.

Taking the Cytotoxics

Because of the difficulty of obtaining quality and reliable extracts of some of these cytotoxic herbs, it is my usual practice to purchase a proprietary blended formula with several cytotoxic herbs in specified concentrations, which can then be supplemented or augmented with other herbs in a customized blend if necessary. For example, in a case of liver, gallbladder, or pancreatic cancer, you may wish to increase the dose of chelidonium, while in a case with lymphatic nodule involvement, you may wish to have more pokeroot. This illustrates the aspect of tissue specificity that so many herbs demonstrate—including the cytotoxics, which may be able to direct an anticancer treatment to target tissues.

Start herbal cytotoxics before chemotherapy commences, if there is time. Most patients and oncologists will probably choose to stop or reduce herbs and supplements on the days of chemo- or radiotherapy, although herbal practitioners may question the need or benefit of pausing. If the program is paused, recommence 2 weeks after the last chemotherapy session. Some people may not tolerate the cytotoxics during chemotherapy but can start them afterward and continue for 2–4 months.

It is generally recommended that herbs and supplements be rotated in and out of treatment protocols in 6- to 12-week cycles as they may be inadvertently inducing or inhibiting cytochrome enzymes, and that can have secondary effects over time. Some herbs, like *Artemisia annua*, need shorter pulse dosing on alternate weeks due to enzyme induction by

THE PYRAMID PRESCRIBING MODEL IN CANCER

When we put together all of the moving parts, from the simplest to the most complex, from the mildest to the most potent, from the background to the foreground, considering physiological enhancement and pathological corrections, we arrive at a model based on the pyramid pattern of prescribing as described earlier in this chapter. No one model will ever capture the complexities of cancer, never mind those of herbal medicine, but this template or foundation can act as a checklist or guidepost to the principles that the practitioner can then apply to the patient in each case.

Foundation: Restorative/Repairing Herbs

Foundation herbs are tonic, nourishing, less specific, less targeted, and generally safe. They include herbs that are adaptogens, neuroendocrine balancing, relaxants and sedatives, immune tonics, blood building, nutritives, and supportive of the bowel and microbiome.

Synergists: Supportive and Directing Herbs

Also called adjuvant, balancer, assistant, or director herbs, these support the actions of the activator or effector herbs and address comorbidities, symptoms, and side effects of treatment. They may include herbs that are alteratives and hepatics, connective tissue tonics, anti-inflammatories, anti-angiogenics, and symptomatics (to address symptoms like nausea, skin rash, pain, neuropathy, coagulopathies, and others).

In the case of cancer, they:

- Promote hepatic and other metabolic detox pathways
- Reduce local inflammation
- Normalize angiogenesis, strengthen blood vessel walls, and inhibit collagenases and proteases
- Support bone marrow, lymph, and immune activity and build blood
- Inhibit hypercoagulation (blood clots)

Specifics: Cytotoxic and Activator Herbs

These herbs target the primary pathology. Caution may be required with dosing. This category also includes narcotic analgesics.

The cytotoxics:

- Disrupt cancer cell metabolism: reverse glycolytic shift, normalize growth factors, and inhibit signal transduction and transcription
- Inhibit mitosis and slow the rate of cell cycling
- Induce apoptosis

The activator herbs:

- Increase mitochondrial energy transfer
- Stabilize genes and normalize gene expression and gene repair
- Correct for specific genetic defects/epigenetics
- Induce immune response

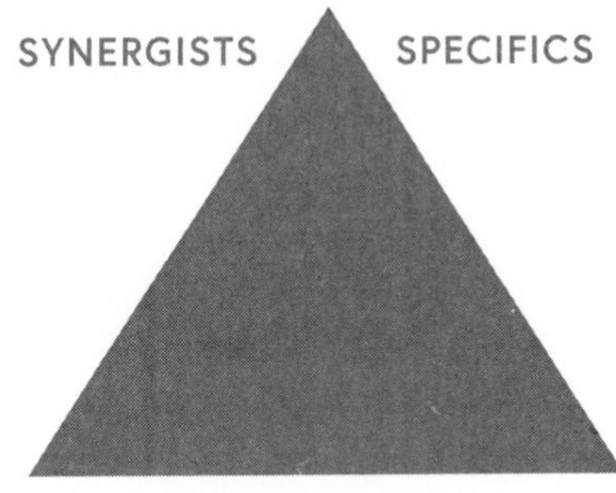

artemisinin. The closer an item is to its natural state—that is, whole herb, not standardized isolates—the safer and less risky it's likely to be. By layering in multiple agents, by including foods in the diet that contain these constituents in natural forms, and by closely monitoring the patient, a very high safety profile is anticipated with most herbs. With the cytotoxics, however, there may be a propensity for side effects. I have certainly seen at least two patients in my clinic with acute liver enzyme (ALT and AST) elevations showing in the blood work shortly after commencing high doses of isolated artemisinin with *Artemisia annua*. For this reason, it is always recommended to start at lower doses and build up and optimally to be testing a range of blood work on a regular basis.

Timelines for Herbal Treatment

Follow an initial protocol for 4–6 weeks, then review all the new test results and make adjustments as required. Develop a monitoring plan for the next 3, 6, and 12 months. Blood work may be more frequent if there are suitable markers. Avoid scans involving ionizing radiation where possible, due to the risk of radiation accumulation; utilize ultrasound or MRI as possible alternatives.

Very common and entirely fair questions from patients are "How long will the process take? How long will I have to take all these pills and potions, and when will I start to feel better?" These are the million-dollar questions with many possible answers, but there are certainly some realistic guidelines. If a patient has an acute symptom and takes an herbal remedy for it—for example, herbs for nausea, headache, or pain—they should reasonably expect to feel relief within 15–30 minutes. If nothing has happened within 30–40 minutes, then either the dose is too low or it's not the right remedy. After consideration of safety factors and dosing guidelines, you may choose to raise the patient's dose at this point.

Other remedies may take weeks or months to be demonstrably effective. Herbs directed to build blood should show response within 1–2 months, but herbs that are directed at normalizing reproductive hormones might take 3–6 months to really make a difference.

Again, we can see this as an opportunity for the herbalist to adjust and revise the protocols over time, in response to the individual needs of the patient. In my original analogy of the composer or the choreographer, this is where the artistry happens. This ability to dance with the herbs, understanding their subtleties, anticipating the nuances that they can bring to the formula, knowing how much to give and when, and when to stop—this is the art of the herbal practitioner at work.

Summary of Treatment Planning

Foundation interventions to change terrain. These address the extracellular area, the tumor microenvironment, and foster ongoing physiological enhancement.

- Assess nutritional status and plan diet; lower the serum glucose and fasting insulin
- Manage inflammation
- Optimize immune functions
- Balance hormones
- Support liver and detox
- Restore the microbiome

Request further testing. If possible, ask for additional blood work, genetic screening, and cancer risk assessment.

Implement strategies for treating cancers. Use these strategies for the first 3 months, continuing for up to 12 months while chemotherapy is ongoing. Adjust according to progress.

- Manage blood clotting with proteolytic enzymes
- Stabilize redox regulation
- Promote immune activation and lymph drainage
- Protect liver, kidneys, heart, and nerves from chemotherapy (reduce toxicity)
- Sensitize cancer cells to drug therapies
- Inhibit multidrug resistance
- Prescribe cytotoxic herbs between chemotherapy cycles or after it is over
- Manage symptoms as needed

Plan a long-term maintenance protocol. This protocol should be followed for up to 3 years after completing conventional care (such as chemotherapy, radiation).

- Support and sustain organ systems (gut health, liver, kidneys, nervous tissue)
- Boost immune system and mediators of inflammation
- Use adaptogens to manage stress and promote tissue healing
- Optimize redox regulation
- Consider personalized off-label drugs like metformin and low-dose naltrexone

Consider other factors when creating a treatment protocol. These might include:

- Specifics of the patient (constitutional weaknesses, psychological and physical environment)
- Specifics of the cancer (growth factors, hormones, gene mutations, angiogenic rate, etc.)
- Symptom-specific herbs, including those for nausea, vomiting, anorexia, cachexia, cardiac support, diarrhea, constipation, fear and depression, pain, neuropathy, hand-foot syndrome, burns, sores, and infection

Take coexisting health conditions into account. Are there herbs or other natural agents that can work broadly across more than one area of concern? For example, hawthorn and CoQ10 can help in cardiovascular disease as well as in cancer, turmeric can help in arthritis, and fish oil in eczema.

Anticipate drug interactions. Are there expected interactions between natural health products and conventional medicine (chemotherapy, radiotherapy, or other medication)? Can it be advantageous or is it a risk factor?

Safety and Toxicology with Herbs

What is there that is not poison? All things are poison and nothing is without poison. Solely the dose determines that a thing is not poison.

PARACELSUS (1493–1541)

Paracelsus may have glossed over the importance of absorption, distribution, metabolism, and excretion of medicines, but there is truth in the old adage that toxicology is simply pharmacology at a higher dose. All drugs are double-edged swords, and few drugs are completely selective at eliciting only the desired effects. Furthermore, in vitro cytotoxicity results often do not translate into in vivo activities, and agents that are effective in animals may not be suitable for human use. Millions of dollars have been spent detecting and isolating in vitro active compounds that are later found to be inactive or even dangerous when tested in vivo.

If we accept that herbs work, then we also have to accept that there may be side effects or unwanted actions as well. Just as with pharmaceutical drug use, the range of people taking herbs, their unique constitutions and wide array of lifestyle practices, makes it next to impossible to completely predict adverse effects in each case, and it takes extensive studies across a broad population to make reasonable pronouncements on toxicity and risks.

Isolated Constituents vs. Whole Herbs

As with the problems of assessing isolated constituents in laboratory settings for beneficial effects, the majority of toxicology research is not very relevant to how practitioners actually use herbs and is hard to extrapolate to clinical practice. Hepatotoxicity is one of the biggest concerns and may take years of use to show up. A meta-analysis of literature concluded that of 15 herbal compounds known to be hepatotoxic in widely used remedies, the anthraquinone emodin was the most toxic. But emodin is present in rhubarb root and sheep sorrel root used in the Essiac traditional cancer formula, and in the laxative part of aloe leaf. Liver cell viability decreased by 30–45 percent when mice were given a very high dose of pure emodin extract by mouth over 24 hours, but this is not whole herb and is not how it is used in clinical practice.

There are some case reports of emodin causing acute toxic hepatitis in humans, but again, doses were not normal. One woman, for example, developed liver inflammation after eating 500 milligrams of aloe vera leaf powder (amount of emodin unspecified) as a laxative every 2–3 days for 5 years, but had she asked an herbal practitioner, they would certainly have told her to change out the herbs periodically, and the fact that she had needed a laxative regularly for 5 years meant she needed professional help. The problem here is not the herb but the way it is used (or abused).

Variability in Herbal Products

Herbal products, being natural botanical extracts, are prone to seasonal as well as year-to-year changes in quality and may be vulnerable to issues of botanical authentication, adulteration, and substitution due to variable factors during growth, harvest, and post-harvest processing and management.

Unfortunately, unsuspecting patients don't know the minefields they are stepping into, and unscrupulous operators sell some very dodgy herbal products and may make a range of unsupportable claims. In one study, less than 8% of retail herbal sales sites provided information regarding potential adverse effects, drug interactions, and other safety information; only 10.5% recommended consultation with a healthcare professional; and less than 3% cited good scientific literature to accompany their claim (which doesn't, of course, mean their products don't work, but only that the data is absent).

Determining Herb Safety

In the textbook *Stockley's Herbal Medicine Interactions*, the authors pose the following questions to ascertain drug safety, and they are equally applicable to herbs.

- Are the drugs and substances in question known to interact in clinical use, or is the interaction only theoretical and speculative?
- If they do interact, how serious is it?
- Has the adverse response been described many times or only once?
- Are all patients affected or only a few?
- Is it best to avoid these two substances altogether, or can the interaction be accommodated in some way?
- What alternative and safer drugs can be used instead?

Dr. Glen Nagel, a naturopath in Portland, Oregon, suggests assessment along a continuum of risk based on several parameters, including:

- Whether the remedy is a simple tea, whole-plant extract (tincture or juice), ground whole herb capsules or powder (very low risk), a standardized extract or concentrate (relatively greater risk), or an isolated concentrate or purified compound (highest risk)
- Low, moderate, or high potency extract (e.g., 1:1 or 1:10)
- Low, moderate, or high dose
- Short or long duration
- Used alone or in combination
- Known interactions with drugs
- Whether the remedy is a known inducer or inhibitor of CYP450 detox pathways

A bit of perspective. It is important to keep a good perspective on real versus potential risks. For example, the annual reports of the American Association of Poison Control Centers (which collects data from poison control centers across the country) indicate that just one or two people die from ingesting poisonous mushrooms in the United State during an average year, and one or two people die from ingesting poisonous plants. Even though not all poisonings are reported and recorded if patients do not end up in a hospital, it is apparent that if herbs were terribly dangerous, we would be hearing about it. Systematic reviews of clinical trials on herbs have also broadly shown safety of herbal medicines when properly prescribed.

Timing of doses. Because we mostly do not know the half-life of herbs, they are usually prescribed to be taken at least twice if not three or even four times daily, in an attempt to sustain effective blood levels of active compounds. This is not a great concern with the herbs of physiological enhancement—the tonic, nutritive, regenerative herbs often have no particular upper limits (except, perhaps, some of the adaptogens, such as ginseng, ashwagandha, or rhodiola, that could be a little stimulating if taken in excess). But this simplistic approach to dosing is not appropriate for the cytotoxic herbs or herbs for pain, where the therapeutic index or window is narrow and toxicity is easily reached. This may be an appropriate place to consider using standardized extracts with known quantities of the active constituents for greater safety in dosing.

If a patient is weak, debilitated, and depleted, they may not be able to tolerate the cytotoxic herbs immediately and may need to build the foundation with tonic, restorative, and adaptogen herbs for several weeks before introducing the stronger herbs. When they are strong enough and have garnered the inner resources for healing, cytotoxic herbs can be used if warranted.

Hepatotoxicity. Some herbs are known to have hepatotoxic compounds, such as the pyrrolizidine alkaloids in comfrey or toxins in some mushrooms, but few herbs in clinical use are outright toxic. The risk is also generally reduced in whole herb and multiherb formulas, in contrast to purified or synthesized isolates.

In Taiwan, where traditional herbal medicine has been included in Taiwan's National Health Insurance system since 1996 and where 90 percent of hospitals have departments of traditional medicine, record keeping is exemplary and it is apparent that the rate and extent of liver injury after using herbal medicine is worse after use of highly concentrated and purified extracts compared to herbal formulas or admixtures. This is in accordance with the traditional practice of combining several whole herbs in moderate doses that enhance safety, in the expectation that some degree of summation or synergy occurs between them, bringing greater efficacy at lower individual doses and hence lower risk as well. As described on page 319, considering herbal synergy is a significant aspect of formulating, both to enhance potency and to mitigate risks.

Herbal Medicines and Anticoagulants

This is perhaps the riskiest herb-drug interaction, because the drugs have such a narrow therapeutic window that any induction or inhibition of the drug can elicit marked effects in the body. Any deviations from the safety range can result in bleeding due to overzealous anticoagulation or a thrombus (clot) because of insufficient anticoagulant action. Vitamin K antagonists (VKAs) such as warfarin are the most commonly prescribed oral anticoagulants worldwide, and they have a high risk threshold. VKAs interact with many foods and herbal supplements. Interactions causing over- or under-anticoagulation significantly increase the risk of major hemorrhagic or thrombotic events. Newer drugs called direct oral anticoagulants (DOACs) may reduce this risk because they have shorter half-lives, demonstrate decreased drug-drug interactions, and do not require frequent blood monitoring. However, they are not in widespread use yet.

A patient taking high-risk anticoagulants should have specific blood work in advance of commencing therapeutic doses of herbs to establish clotting baselines, and then at regular intervals thereafter. This allows close monitoring of changes and gives the ability to adjust doses of herbs or drugs accordingly. If herbs are seen to be antagonistic (inhibiting) to the drugs, then the herbs can be changed or doses adjusted down, but, conversely, if herbs are seen to be agonists—increasing the anticoagulant effects—then it is possible to consider lowering the drug dose. This is considered a positive interaction and can be very useful. In collaborative medicine, frequent blood work to monitor clotting factors allows both the physician and the herbalist to make regular herb or drug dose adjustments. In this way, drug dosing can be slowly decreased, the herbs slowly increased, and safety maintained.

SUPPLEMENTS AND HERBS TO USE WITH CAUTION IF PATIENT IS TAKING ANTICOAGULANTS

Although the risk with herbs in normal dosing is actually very low, and none of these agents is expected to cause notable bleeding in moderate (clinically appropriate) amounts, it is prudent to avoid these, or at least to introduce them very cautiously whenever VKA anticoagulants are being used. There is only weak evidence suggesting a real need for caution with the following herbs, but this is the minimal list most conventional doctors require their patients to avoid during chemotherapy:

- Astragalus
- Bromelain
- Curcumin
- Dong quai
- Evening primrose oil
- Flaxseed oil
- Garlic
- Ginger
- Ginkgo
- Omega-3 fish oil (EPA, DHA)
- Proteolytic enzymes
- St. John's wort
- Turmeric
- Vitamin E (including tocopherols and tocotrienols)

Having said all of that, it is important to note that these are all safe in modest or moderate doses. Even garlic and ginkgo, which are so commonly cited as high risk with anticoagulants, are actually quite safe in appropriate doses. In the words of Dr. Eric Yarnell, "The preponderance of evidence from clinical trials confirms that garlic does *not* significantly inhibit platelets or cause bleeding in humans, and does *not* interact with anticoagulant or antiplatelet drugs." Another phytochemistry authority, Dr. Kerry Bone, cites the published human clinical trial evidence to date and concludes that there are no clear interactions between ginkgo and anticoagulants.

In the case of vitamin E, a frequently cited "blood thinner agonist," a study investigating whether vitamin E enhances the pharmacologic effect of warfarin found that none of the subjects who received vitamin E had a significant change in the international normalized ratio (INR, a blood clotting scale), and thus it appears that vitamin E can safely be given to patients who require chronic warfarin therapy. So there is actually very little to worry about, provided there is general clinical prudence and careful monitoring.

Chemotherapy, Herbal Medicine, and Supplements

Often one of the most urgent questions patients have is about the safety and advisability of combining chemotherapy and herbal medicine. Unfortunately, careless use of language has led to an overly simplified view of the natural medicines' capacity to quench reactive oxygen species (ROS) and the idea that taking antioxidants will inhibit the oxidative effects of conventional chemotherapies. Nothing could be farther from the truth. In fact, compelling research now suggests that redox regulation may actually *promote* the oxidative stressors within the metabolically overactive cancer cells, while serving to protect healthy cells at the same time.

UNWARRANTED CONCERNS ABOUT ANTIOXIDANT INTERACTIONS

If the specific chemotherapy conducts its cytotoxic activity largely through ROS generation (as do most conventional chemotherapies), then higher doses of single antioxidants may conceivably interfere with the drug's antineoplastic activity. However, ROS are also responsible for many drug side effects, and in this case lower doses of an array of antioxidants may actually reduce the severity of such effects without interfering with the drug's antineoplastic activity. Indeed, these are sometimes prescribed by oncologists for this very reason. Antioxidants are often seen to be agonist or synergistic with chemotherapy drugs that induce apoptosis. Many antioxidants also stimulate apoptotic pathways, and this offers potential complementary prescribing. Redox regulators can regulate intentional and incidental cell damage, and this dichotomous or paradoxical balancing of oxidative stress and cell repair is a perfect example of the amphoteric, balancing, and normalizing capacity that herbs and natural medicines can exemplify.

A meta-analysis by Block et al. in 2007 of 19 randomized human trials (1,554 participants) showed similar or better survival rates for the antioxidant group than the control group, with none of the trials supporting the theory that antioxidant supplements diminish the effectiveness of chemotherapy. In 15 of 17 trials that assessed chemotherapy toxicities, including diarrhea, weight loss, nerve damage, and low blood counts, the antioxidant group showed lower rates of toxic response to a range of chemotherapy drugs.

"This study, along with the evolving understanding of antioxidant-chemotherapy interactions, suggests that the previously held beliefs about interference do not pertain to clinical treatment," said coauthor Robert Newman from MD Anderson Cancer Center. The researchers concluded that "the lack of negative impact of antioxidant supplementation on efficacy of ROS-generating chemotherapy in the studies reviewed, and the potential to diminish dose-limiting toxicity suggest that the clinical application of antioxidant supplementation during chemotherapy should be further explored."

Another follow-up study by Block in 2008 reviewed 33 clinical studies and verified that antioxidant supplementation during chemotherapy holds the potential for reducing dose-limiting toxicities. The antioxidants evaluated were glutathione, melatonin, vitamin A, an antioxidant mixture, N-acetylcysteine, vitamin E, selenium, L-carnitine, CoQ10, and ellagic acid. The majority (24) of the 33 studies reported evidence of decreased side effects from the concurrent use of antioxidants with chemotherapy. Nine studies reported no difference in toxicities between the two groups. One study on vitamin A reported a significant increase in toxicity in the people in the antioxidant group who continued to smoke tobacco. Five studies reported that the antioxidant group completed more full doses of chemotherapy or had less dose reduction than control groups. None of the studies demonstrated that antioxidants interfered with the cytotoxicity of chemotherapy. A 2018 meta-analysis of 174 peer-reviewed original articles comprising 93 clinical trials (and more than 18,000 patients), 56 animal studies, and 35 in vitro studies concluded, "Antioxidant [treatment] has superior potential of ameliorating chemotherapeutic induced toxicity. Antioxidant supplementation during chemotherapy also promises higher therapeutic efficiency and increased survival times in patients."

NEGLIGIBLE RISK FROM SUPPLEMENT INTERACTIONS

In the past 40 years or more, several hundred peer-reviewed in vitro and in vivo studies, including many human studies involving thousands of patients, have consistently shown that orthomolecular, targeted nutritional supplements do not interfere with therapeutic modalities for cancer. Furthermore, nonprescription antioxidants and other dietary nutrients enhance the effects of therapeutic modalities for cancer, decrease their side effects, and protect normal tissue.

There is negligible risk in taking most supplements while undergoing chemotherapy, and they offer a significant opportunity to maximize well-being throughout conventional treatment. Cancer patients are frequently malnourished, often despite being overweight, and their immune systems are highly compromised from chemotherapy, radiation, steroids, antibiotics, and pain medications. Antioxidants and other nutritional supplements can restore deficiencies and promote effective immune function. And as I've explained throughout this book, antioxidants—or redox regulators, as they are more correctly called—have direct antitumor effects, protect against the toxic effects of conventional cancer treatments, and contribute to enhanced longevity in patients. A multitude of plant constituents can regulate, stabilize, and normalize dozens of oncogenic pathways, with cancer cells being susceptible to inhibition and healthy cells being aided and supported at the same time.

It would be foolish and certainly untrue to say that herbs are always safe. Indeed, several of the herbs described in this book are actively *not* safe in the wrong hands or the wrong dose, for the wrong patient, or for the wrong reason. However, if we were to measure relative risk and known consequences or side effects of the cytotoxic herbs against those of licensed chemotherapy drugs, then the herbs would be much safer. Their use is restricted to qualified herbal practitioners for good reason, but aside from the cytotoxics, it is hard to imagine how any properly prescribed herb or nutrient could do anywhere near as much harm as any of the chemotherapy and immunotherapy drugs, or radiotherapy for that matter.

Research Showing Positive Benefits from Herbs

At this point, there are many herbs and nutrients documented as being safe and actively effective when combined with chemotherapy, including selenium, vitamin C, omega-3 fats (EPA, DHA), glutamine, astragalus, garlic, EGCG, quercetin, apigenin, curcumin, emodin, ginseng, vitamin D3, vitamin E, melatonin, and R+ lipoic acid.

Astragalus

In a meta-analysis of literature considering the safety and efficacy of astragalus-based Traditional Chinese Medicine herbal formulas when combined with chemotherapy versus chemotherapy alone for colorectal cancer, the addition of the herbal blend increased the tumor response rate, reduced adverse effects from the chemotherapy, and improved quality-of-life measurements. Repeated studies have demonstrated that astragalus is associated with increased benefits and reduced side effects from platinum-based chemotherapy in patients.

Astragalus is traditionally used as a blood builder, bone marrow tonic, nutritive adaptogen, and deep immune tonic to balance Th1 and Th2 functions and enhance phagocytosis.

Redox Regulators

Overall, research suggests that uncontrolled ROS formed during chemotherapy will create toxic aldehydes that arrest apoptosis—the opposite of what we want. Antioxidants (redox regulators) can reestablish this pathway by slowing aldehyde formation, which favors controlled cell death. Redox regulation favors apoptosis over necrosis in cancer cells with targeted cell death and less collateral damage. Holistic practitioners recommend a moderate dose of several key redox regulators during or concurrent with chemotherapy to maximize breadth of action and reduce risk from any one of them.

Redox Regulators to Use Concurrent with Chemotherapy

- Vitamin C to bowel tolerance
- Vitamin E succinate 400–800 IU
- Mixed carotenoids 50 mg (except for patients who smoke tobacco)
- Polyphenols and flavonoids 2 g (includes quercetin, resveratrol, green tea and turmeric/EGCG and curcumin as appropriate)
- Minerals: zinc 30–50 mg; selenium 100 mcg
- Omega-3 polyunsaturated fats: EPA 1,000 mg, DHA 500 mg

Turmeric, Curcumin, and Chemotherapy

Curcumin reduces chemotherapy- and radiotherapy-induced adverse reactions, mainly through antioxidative and anti-inflammatory effects. Curcumin can slow phase I detoxification pathways in the liver while promoting phase II pathways, thus reducing the risk of toxic intermediates accumulating, which accounts for the noted hepatoprotective effects.

STUDIES OF CURCUMIN IN CANCER TREATMENT

Below are noted just a few of the studies demonstrating safety and efficacy. There are hundreds more. Some of these are human studies and some are in vitro or animal studies, but they all point to the same effects overall, and this is supported by clinical practice.

In cell line studies, pretreatment with curcumin followed by 5-FU increased the susceptibility of human gastric cancer and colon cancer cells to the drug via suppression of the NF-κB signaling pathway, which may allow for lower doses of the drug and reduced adverse effects of drugs. Combined treatment of docetaxel and curcumin for 48 hours significantly inhibited the proliferation of and induced apoptosis in prostate cancer cells compared to the curcumin or docetaxel alone. Curcumin modulated COX-2, p53, NF-κB, phospho-Akt, PI3K, and tyrosine kinase receptors. Use of curcumin with docetaxel in prostate cancer may reduce cytotoxicity and overcome drug resistance.

Metformin (1,500–3,000 mg/day) is a widely used antidiabetic drug that also decreases the risk of many cancers. In vitro research suggests metformin and curcumin combined can induce apoptosis and inhibit metastasis and invasion in hepatocellular carcinoma and prostate cancer cells.

Curcumin (5 mg/kg) can enhance the absorption of doxorubicin and decrease drug efflux in vivo.

Cotreatment with curcumin and cisplatin has shown a potent synergistic effect in bladder cancer cell lines in vitro compared to curcumin or cisplatin alone. Celecoxib (Celebrex) is a nonsteroidal anti-inflammatory drug (NSAID), a selective inhibitor of COX-2 enzyme that induces inflammation. Celecoxib induces apoptosis and suppresses tumor angiogenesis in several types of cancer, but long-term use leads to cardiovascular toxicity. Combining curcumin and celecoxib reduces cancer cell growth in vitro better than celecoxib alone, and curcumin and celecoxib given together exhibited a synergistic inhibitory effect against human colorectal cancer cells. These findings suggest an opportunity to use lower doses of the drug and complement with a synergistic dose of curcumin.

WHAT ARE THE RISKS OF CURCUMIN?

Curcumin inhibits cytochromes 3A4, CYP1A2, CYP2A6, and CYP2D6 and may delay drug clearance, but these are cell line studies and the clinical relevance is not known.

A case report in the literature, reporting hepatotoxicity from turmeric with paclitaxel, describes a patient with lung cancer who experienced liver toxicity while undergoing active treatment with paclitaxel as well as turmeric at 15 grams daily. She also took multiple other supplements—including chlorella (520 mg/day), milk thistle (total of 13.5 mg silymarin/day), zinc sulfate (5.5 mg), and selenium (50 mcg). Upon review, the chlorella was found to be contaminated and tainted with a cyanobacteria producing 1.08 mcg of cyanotoxin microcystin-LR per gram of biomass. Notwithstanding this toxicity and all these variables, turmeric was determined to be the likely cause. This is unfortunately and misleadingly now entered into the literature as a case report of hepatotoxicity from turmeric with paclitaxel.

Contrasting with this case report, an interesting study in 2020 reviewed quality-of-life measurements and hematological parameters in 60 patients receiving paclitaxel chemotherapy for breast cancer. Turmeric given at the same time for 21 days resulted in clinically relevant and statistically significant improvement in global health status, symptom scores (fatigue, nausea, vomiting, pain, appetite loss, insomnia), and improvement in hematological parameters.

In summary, a wealth of research supports the use of curcumin in cancer, with both chemotherapy and radiotherapy, as well as in prevention and recovery programs. Studies have focused on the curcuminoids with their high degree of bioactivity, often dosing at ranges of 150–250 milligrams of curcuminoids per day. To achieve equivalent results using the whole root powder, assuming an average 5 percent curcuminoid content, would require upwards of 30–50 grams daily, which is probably unrealistic. In the case of turmeric, while I encourage the use of golden milk and other food applications to obtain a full spectrum of constituents, this is actually one of the times I strongly recommend people take a standardized isolate product as well, in order to approach the doses being used in the successful trials. Remember, too, that curcumin needs bioperine from black pepper and bromelain as adjuvants to promote absorption (see page 300).

Ashwagandha and Chemotherapy

Ashwagandha has demonstrated anticancer effects against several cancer cell lines, and in mouse studies it reduced neutropenia associated with chemotherapy. It supports bone marrow function, hemoglobin levels, and red blood cell count. It may alleviate chemotherapy-induced fatigue and improve quality of life. It has neuroprotective and anti-inflammatory properties that may reduce neuropathy, and it helps regulate blood sugar, insulin levels, and insulin sensitivity, which normalizes the terrain. Furthermore, it enhances chromosomal stability and is radio sensitizing. All of these outcomes make it safe and effective as an adjunct to chemotherapy, and there is no evidence of risk or harm.

In an open-label, nonrandomized trial on 100 women with breast cancer, patients received either taxotere, Adriamycin (doxorubicin), and cyclophosphamide or 5-fluorouracil (5-FU), epirubicin, and cyclophosphamide, and half the patients in each set were given ashwagandha at a dose of 2 grams every 8 hours throughout the course of chemotherapy. The quality-of-life and fatigue scores were evaluated before, during, and on the last cycles of chemotherapy. Significant benefit was seen in the patients taking the herb alongside the drugs when compared to the patients taking either chemotherapy cocktail without ashwagandha.

Green Tea and Chemotherapy

An extensive literature review published in 2016 considered dozens of trials examining green tea's synergy with chemotherapy and determined that the herb has a positive beneficial interaction with bleomycin, cisplatin, tamoxifen, paclitaxel, sulindac, celecoxib, curcumin, luteolin, docetaxel, and retinoids. They found green tea polyphenols had no effect on the pharmacokinetics or efficacy of the drug 5-FU. They had a negative interaction with only one drug in vitro—green tea polyphenols (super concentrated) neutralized the action and possible benefit of Velcade (bortezomib), a drug used to treat adults with multiple myeloma or mantle cell lymphoma. This is not an in vivo or clinical finding, but it may represent a possible risk and a possible contraindication. However, advice against green tea is not currently being given by doctors prescribing Velcade, so it is reasonable to assume the risk is negligible. Another study reported that EGCG reduced the bioavailability of sunitinib and suggested this finding has significant practical implications for tea drinking by patients on sunitinib. Advice against green tea is not currently being given by doctors prescribing sunitinib.

A study into green tea catechins in breast cancer reported a synergistic interaction with tamoxifen or raloxifene in the treatment of estrogen receptor–positive and estrogen receptor–negative breast cancer through estrogen receptor–dependent and estrogen receptor–independent mechanisms. This report also stated that no evidence of any adverse interaction of green tea catechins with aromatase inhibitors or fulvestrant has been found.

Green tea polyphenols have an overall positive interaction with many chemotherapy drugs, generally supporting antitumor activity and mitigating systemic toxicology.

342

CHAPTER 8

Diagnosis and Treatment Planning in Collaborative Oncology

In the immediate aftermath of a cancer diagnosis, there is a natural temptation to rush into aggressive treatment as quickly as possible. I have literally had patients be given a diagnosis on a Monday and start treatment by Friday. While this may at first glance look like great efficiency on the part of the medical system, what it usually means is a "one size fits all" treatment with no opportunity for individualized assessments and customizing a treatment plan. Although it may seem counterintuitive, the first thing to do upon diagnosis is to slow down, breathe deeply, and not rush into things without proper consideration. Start off with implementing lifestyle changes—cleaning up the diet, removing carcinogens from the home, reviewing any stress load, and developing stress-management strategies. All these will promote positive outcomes and proactive physiological enhancement as information is gathered and the best overall course of treatment is decided upon. This is not wasting time; this is building a strong foundation.

CHAPTER 8 CONTENTS

344 Whole-Person Custom Treatment Planning

344 Who Has the Disease?

348 Stages in Treatment Planning

348 Gather Information about the Diagnosis and the Terrain

349 Consider the Best Conventional Treatment Options

349 The Importance of Testing

350 Testing in Advance of Therapy

350 Blood Tests to Order

351 Tumor Markers

353 Pathology Testing on Excised Tissue

353 Specialty Testing for Cancer

354 Genetic Tests in Clinical Practice

359 Prioritizing Additional Tests

361 Addressing Cancer Directly

364 Address Free Radicals and Genetic Instability

365 Reduce Abnormal Gene Expression

366 Glycolytic Shift and the Cancer-Sugar Connection

367 Obesity and Cancer

368 Mitochondrial Rescue

369 Anabolic/Catabolic Balance

372 Induce Differentiation in Cancer Cells

372 Induce Apoptosis

374 Modulate Growth Factors

381 Stabilize Transcription Factors

385 Support the Immune System

386 Reduce Inflammation and Normalize Prostaglandin and Leukotriene Activity

389 Immune Evasion

390 Strengthen Connective Tissue, Promote Cell-to-Cell Communication

393 Inhibit Invasion and Metastasis

394 Decrease Vascular Permeability and Inhibit Angiogenesis

Whole-Person Custom Treatment Planning

It is quite easy to learn a list of herbal actions targeting particular pathology conditions. Rote learning—"take this herb for that disease"—may be quite effective for symptomatic treatments but will fall far short of the potential for herbs to make a deep and lasting difference in a person's health. The science of herbal medicine and herbal prescribing can be memorized, but the art of building a formula is something that comes with deep experience and long practice. This is not to say that beginner herbalists cannot be effective. The herbs can work their magic at many levels, but an experienced clinician will know how to mix and match remedies to create a customized plan where the whole is greater than the sum of the parts. It is this ability to repattern the herbal relationships in order to redirect the healing process, as required by the changing circumstances of the patient, that makes a great herbalist. Clinical herbal practitioners rarely use preblended proprietary formulas unless as a base to which to add other herbs; the proprietary formulas may be convenient as a part of a protocol, but they are unlikely to be sufficiently nuanced to do all that is required. With literally hundreds of herbs to choose from, the herbal practitioner can blend a truly unique, specific, and personal mix for each individual patient.

When I'm in my clinic, listening to a patient tell their story, trying to gather all the information I need to understand them and their situation, I hold some specific core questions in my mind as we talk, and later as I develop a treatment plan—essentially, "who, what, why, when, and where?" These are the key factors to take into consideration, aside from directly addressing symptoms of the cancer and its consequences.

Who Has the Disease?

Patient-focused treatment planning always starts with "who," and everything else takes off from there. Criteria may include their age, occupation, gender, core constitution and imbalances, and any comorbidities. It will also consider the physical, physiological, and psychological roots of the presenting problem. This is always important in successful clinical practice, but perhaps especially so in cancer care, where the urgency of the conventional medical services in the face of this particular diagnosis often precludes detailed assessment and analysis of the terrain in favor of prescribing aggressive drug therapies.

In clinical practice, this means that the assessment of underlying or foundational health parameters and the information gathered in the consultation is what informs and ultimately directs the individualized treatment. Two patients with the same apparent diagnosis may have quite different presentations and prognosis, and their needs might be quite different. A 75-year-old person with a stage III glioblastoma who is frail and debilitated from heart disease, and who is taking half a dozen prescription drugs already, is going to have a very different experience than a 30-year-old person with a stage III glioblastoma who has no other overt pathologies and is unmedicated. The younger person, for example, may have a more aggressive disease but also be more able to tolerate and recover from aggressive treatments. With a much longer future possibly ahead of them, they may also be more willing to attempt experimental drug treatments or other cutting-edge therapies. The same cytotoxic herbs may be indicated in both cases but in different doses and with different adjunctive herbs for each individual.

AGE

Very young children and the elderly have slower hepatic clearance rates than adults, with underperforming liver detoxification enzyme series, and often exhibit a prolonged half-life for drugs, and presumably for herbs as well. This may make them more sensitive to the effects of drugs or herbs, and possibly more susceptible to adverse effects, even after adjusting doses for body weight. Older people also tend to have lower levels of hydrochloric acid in the stomach. Not only does the acid serve to initiate the digestion of proteins, but it also helps trigger gastrin hormone that travels to all the organs of the gut to switch them on, wake them up, and prepare them for the food coming. Without adequate stomach acid, gastrin is low and there is a risk of overall digestive insufficiency, which may compromise the microbiome and affect digestion and absorption of drugs or herbs, as well as foods.

The greater the extreme of age (younger or older), the lower the dose of herbs that is required. Consider digestive support (bitter herbs, enzymes, pre- and probiotics, aperients). Look for ways to use herbs topically. Liquids and powders are preferred over capsules.

GENDER

Body mass index—or at least weight and general size—will probably have more influence on herbal dosing and pharmacokinetics than gender does. However, it is worth noting that women tend to detoxify through the liver slightly faster than men, and this may have some impact on dosing. For example, annual wormwood (*Artemisia annua*) induces cytochrome enzymes that degrade and eliminate it, so over a few days it is clearing too fast to be clinically effective and use should be paused. This on/off cycle should be shorter for women (5 days) than for men (7 days).

An area of clinical research that is sadly lacking in herbal medicine is the impact or significance of herbs in gender-transitioning individuals and whether this may impact some of the metabolic clearance pathways or have other implications for dosing strategies. Pharmacology and pharmacokinetic research and literature is still heavily dominated by gender duality, and the modern experience of gender fluidity has not been translated well to clinical research yet.

Obviously male and female bodies are different, and the hormonal milieu plays a significant role in health and disease for both sexes. Estrogen is a notable cell proliferant; it is no surprise that it fuels several kinds of cancer in men and women. Its job in the female body is to support proliferation of the endometrium preparatory to implantation of a fertilized egg, and in males it is essential for spermatogenesis as well as modulating libido and erectile function. Cancers of the breast, uterus, cervix, ovary, testes, prostate, bone, and lung, as well as melanoma, may all express estrogen receptors and use it to fuel progression. Testosterone, on the other hand, has a complex relationship with prostate cancer and doesn't simply drive it as is generally assumed. All prostate cells are highly testosterone dependent, but men with higher circulating levels of testosterone are not necessarily at greater risk of prostate cancer.

In clinical practice, outside of specific hormone-driven cancers or other reproductive diseases, there is generally no need for different formulas for men and women, although possibly different dosage schedules could be considered.

GENETICS

Since the near completion of mapping a human genome in 2003, and the filling in of missing details due to technological advances ever since then, much progress has been made in understanding the genetics of cancer and in developing new therapies for people with the disease. New drugs created based on countering the results of specific genetic mutations in cancer or overcoming immune resistance are proving to be game changers in some cancer patients. Being able to measure and treat these defects in specific cancers may open a whole new frontier in medicine. In some cases, gene testing can be predictive of cancer risk—for example, mutations of the tumor suppressor genes BRCA1 and 2 indicate a very high risk of developing breast or ovarian cancer (and it also indicates that siblings and children should be tested for the mutation).

Gene testing for hereditary risks and specific gene screening for use of monoclonal antibody and other immunotherapy drugs is offered through an oncologist. Genetic screening using buccal (cheek) swabs to assess metabolic capacities and risks is offered by holistic practitioners and functional medicine doctors and may include methylation capacity and immune resistance capacity, general detoxification and elimination capacity, specific drug metabolism and excretion capacity, and redox capacity.

Even if you cannot obtain most of these tests, it is reasonable to assume that in cancer, no matter where it starts, there is always some degree of genomic disturbance with activation of tumor-promoting genes and inhibition of tumor-suppressing genes. Most of the herbs, nutritional supplements, and health-promotion strategies described in the first part of this book are intended to work exactly in this nonspecific aspect of cancer—stabilize the genome, reassert mitochondrial functions, and reduce cancer progression overall, largely through immunomodulating and redox-regulating effects. This is the foundation of treatment and underpins the active treatment plan for acute care, which is where the cytotoxic herbs may be indicated as a sort of "herbal chemotherapy."

CONSTITUTION

The herbal practitioner is likely to work with some form of energetic or constitutional assessment tools, as well as biomedical sciences—whether this is through Traditional Chinese Medicine, Ayurvedic, or Western humoral and physiomedical principles—to assess the patient's core constitution and energetic imbalances. Although these three systems of medicine are all quite different, they are also all related historically. Each system includes the idea that heat in the body represents the life force or vitality, and cold in the body represents depletion or diminishment of that vital force. Remedies may be broadly considered as stimulants or relaxants according to the degree of heat or cold they engender, with further refinements of dryness or moisture woven through.

Hot and cold should be balanced in the body. Underpinning much traditional medicine is an attempt to reestablish that balance of anabolic (heating) and catabolic (cooling) cell metabolism. In the case of cancer, the tumor itself is usually considered to be in a hot state with a notable degree of metabolic activity, angiogenesis and increased blood supply, and inflammation. The host body, however, may be in a cold and depleted state, as the life force is redirected to the cancer.

These are not literal states where the thermometer will change—although fever certainly can happen in cancer and often represents activation of the immune system (which isn't necessarily a bad thing). Instead they are conceptual or metaphorical terms for a state of being that is not captured in the conventional cancer conversation in modern medicine. The herbal practitioner may think in terms of "cooling" the cancer to slow it down and set it back, while "warming" the body, in the sense of nourishing, building, restorative, and tonic strategies. This is not the place to explore the esoteric or energetic ways of herbal practice in detail—there are many other books about that—but we can reference these principles where it is useful in the process of developing a prescription.

Hot/Cold Constitution Assessment

A simple hot/cold assessment is just the beginning of constitutional evaluation, missing all the subtleties and nuances that help to differentiate patients and treatments in Ayurvedic, Traditional Chinese Medicine, and Western humoral medicine. But absent any of those formalized models of medicine, there are still fundamental principles of heat and cold in the body and strategies for regulating core constitutional imbalances that will be beneficial and valuable.

Hot/excess: Patient may be vigorous, irritable, or competitive; have a loud voice, strong opinions, a big appetite, strong thirst, or rapid digestion. Their diseases may be inflamed, throbbing, or swollen; their pulse may be bounding and full. Their tongue may be red, dry, and cracked; their skin may be dry, red, itchy. The hot person will benefit from cooling, calming, moistening, softening herbs, such as verbena, rose, milky oats, betony, cleavers, violet leaf, dandelion leaf, chickweed, mullein, marshmallow, hibiscus, and licorice.

Cold/deficiency: Patient may be listless, passive, pale, limp, or indecisive; have low appetite, little thirst, and slow digestion. Their pulse may be weak or thready, low, and slow; their tongue may be thick, wet, coated, or greasy looking; their skin may be cool, moist, or oily. The cold person will benefit from warming, stimulating, invigorating, uplifting herbs, such as ginger, turmeric, oregano, ginseng, leuzea, nettle leaf, cinnamon, clove, and tulsi.

Stages in Treatment Planning

Because we cannot do everything at once, it's useful to consider the treatment plan in stages or increments. There will be overlap, and some treatments may be long term while others may come and go over time, but this is a road map for developing a logical progression through a case.

Gather Information about the Diagnosis and the Terrain

At the outset, start by gathering as much specific information as possible about the patient's diagnosis. You will need to conduct a detailed intake interview, to review any reports and medical records that are available, to make an energetic or constitutional assessment, and possibly to request updated or additional testing if needed.

Stage, grade, and TNM classification. The stage or spread of the cancer, the grade or differentiation of cells, and the tumor node metastases (TNM) score are all ways of assessing progression and prognosis.

Comorbidities. Few patients present with cancer as the only diagnosed disease. Most will have some other preexisting condition like heart disease, diabetes, or arthritis or will develop problems during cancer treatment such as kidney damage from platinum-based chemotherapy or cardiomyopathy (heart muscle damage) from doxorubicin, and these may complicate the symptom picture and require additional healthcare strategies.

Blood work to assess terrain. Looking at biomarkers—the totals, range, and ratios—can reveal much about the state of metabolic functions and risk factors for progression of cancer.

Specialized blood work to assess cancer parameters. This may include antigens like CEA and CA125, as well as circulating tumor cells, inflammatory markers, and clotting factors.

Genetic testing. This and other specialty testing may be considered to further assess cancer parameters. This may reveal information about triggers and pathways that can be influenced through natural medicines, as well as specific genetic patterns that may make a patient a good candidate for targeted immunotherapies. These tests are done on slides of excised material and require a medical doctor to sign them out to the labs.

Consider the Best Conventional Treatment Options

You may meet a patient early in their journey and need to support them through surgery; or you may meet them in active treatment, receiving chemotherapy or other treatments, and with the herbal protocol needing to work around the drugs; or you may meet the patient later in their journey, when they have completed conventional treatment but are left with symptoms and with risk of recurrence. Each situation requires careful consideration of herb-drug interactions, as well as sequence or timing of herbal treatment around conventional care, for example using cytotoxic herbs in the days off chemotherapy and stopping them during active chemotherapy treatment days. This approach to understanding the body and its idiosyncrasies is described as functional medicine; it looks for imbalances, deficiencies and excesses, ratios and proportions.

In order to provide the optimal treatment plan, it's important to review all the existing blood work, pathology reports, and functional medicine tests available. Pharmacogenomic testing will help identify which gene sequences are expressed that might make one drug more effective than another. These tests may or may not all be readily available, but where they are, they can be used to direct and guide drug treatment and hence maximize benefits.

Key Questions for Planning Chemotherapy

- How do you determine if chemotherapy should be given?
- What drugs should be used, at what dosage, how frequently, and for how long?
- What else should be used to protect from collateral damage, improve recovery, enhance effectiveness, synergize, target specific pathways, and inhibit resistance?

The Importance of Testing

Possibly one of the greatest challenges that I experience in my clinical practice is that patients are making what are literally life-and-death decisions about treatment options without being fully informed of the implications and ramifications of each drug. Certainly, there is no magic crystal ball, no infallible test, and no guarantees of the outcomes, but there are numerous ways of assessing the health and healing capacities of the body, predictive tests for how a cancer may progress or how an individual may respond to a given treatment, and even simple run-of-the-mill blood work that isn't used to full advantage. While it may not always be possible to get specialty genetic testing or to access some of the newer drugs, it does not seem unreasonable that all cancer patients could be routinely tested for vitamin B12 and vitamin D status, copper, zinc, inflammatory markers, methylation markers, and fasting insulin. Just these simple blood tests alone can give much useful information to guide treatments and measure metabolic improvements. For practitioners who are not licensed to order blood work, it is important to collaborate with someone who can because it is highly likely that many basic screens will not be offered routinely.

Testing in Advance of Therapy

Testing pathology slides for single nucleotide polymorphisms (SNPs), gene mutations, and growth factors and doing live-cell tumor resistance and sensitivity testing can all help determine who is most at risk of cancer and which drugs at what dose would be most effective and carry the least side effects. To give just one example, overexpression of the Skp2 gene, measurable with genetic screening, results in loss of cell cycle inhibition leading to uncontrolled replication and is associated with poor prognosis in early breast cancer. Knowing this about your cancer might cause you to choose a more aggressive herbal plan, with higher-dose cytotoxics, or feel more urgency to do chemotherapy than someone without this genetic mutation. Additionally, high preoperative expression of Skp2 has been associated with resistance to the standard chemotherapy of cyclophosphamide/doxorubicin and 5-fluorouracil (CAF) therapy in many patients, but not with resistance to docetaxel. In patients with this mutation, a whole class of drugs may be less effective, despite being approved as a standard first-line treatment in breast cancer. This is important information and could change the entire course of a woman's life.

This way of assessing risk and targeting treatment is a rapidly developing branch of medicine, but what is known in the research world may take 10–20 years to become the standard of care in general practice. A good example of this is the drug Herceptin (trastuzumab), which was one of the very first monoclonal immunotherapy drugs approved by the FDA. This drug targets the receptor sites for epidermal growth factor (EGF) on cancer cells, which are often overexpressed due to an oncogenic gene mutation. Patients who test positive for the HER2/neu receptor site on their cancer cells are good candidates for the drug, and it has been approved in breast cancer since 1998. However, it took probably another 10 years before the test was routine in larger hospitals and facilities, and even now it may not be routinely offered to all women with breast cancer in some of the more remote medical clinics. Furthermore, the gene that mutates, and the receptor site protein it codes for, are recognized in various other cancers as well, notably gastric and intestinal, and yet is not tested or assessed anywhere outside of research settings, although patients testing positive could possibly be good candidates for Herceptin as well. In 5 years' time this may be the norm in stomach cancer, but not yet.

Blood Tests to Order

Blood work can be used to assess the terrain, identifying any disturbances within the internal environment that can be corrected, including nutritional status, pH, lipids, inflammation, glucose and insulin, hormonal imbalances, hypercoagulation, liver and kidney function, inflammatory status, and systemic toxic load.

ROUTINE BLOOD TESTS

This basic panel should be redone every 2 months while the patient is receiving active cancer care, and every 4–6 months for at least 2 years after completion of treatment.

- Complete blood count (CBC): red and white cells and differentials (anemia, neutropenia, bone marrow depletion)
- Chemistry panel: sodium, potassium, chloride, CO2, calcium, magnesium (electrolytes, pH balance, and hydration)
- Kidney panel: BUN, creatinine, eGFR, uric acid, urea (renal elimination capacity)
- Liver panel: AST, ALT, GGT, bilirubin (total), albumin, globulin, protein, LDH, alkaline phosphatase (liver stress/burden and liver functional capacity)
- Fasting glucose (blood sugar)

ADDITIONAL ROUTINE BLOOD TESTS

These should be requested at diagnosis and should need to be repeated only if results are out of range or the cancer progresses, or annually for ongoing monitoring. Note the many variables, such as availability and functionality of vitamin D receptors, binding of iron to tannins in food, elevation of ferritin in inflammation, and lipid ratios (not just absolute lipid numbers).

- Vitamin D: 25OH (anticancer, immune support, bone building, antidepressant)
- Iron, ferritin (especially if planning to use *Artemisia annua*)
- Homocysteine, B12, folate (methylation capacity)
- Lipids panel: cholesterol, HDL, LDL (including apolipoprotein A, apolipoprotein B, and lipoprotein A), triglycerides (cardiovascular risk screening)
- Fasting insulin, hemoglobin A1C (blood sugar at nadir, relative to the insulin, and blood sugar over several weeks)

SPECIALTY BLOOD TESTS

These are for assessing specific risks or drivers of cancer progression; they should be requested at diagnosis and should need to be repeated only if results are out of range or the cancer progresses.

- Zinc (should be high normal), copper, and ceruloplasmin (should be low normal; measures angiogenesis balance)
- Insulin-like growth factor 1 (stimulates cancer cells)
- Fibrinogen and D-dimer (markers of clotting risk)
- C-reactive protein and erythrocyte sedimentation rate (markers of inflammation)
- Estrogen, progesterone, testosterone, dihydrotestosterone, sex hormone binding globulin, DHEA (in reproductive cancers)

Tumor Markers

These should be requested at diagnosis and should need to be repeated only if results are out of range or the cancer progresses.

- Breast cancer: CA15-3, CA27-29

- Abdominal/visceral cancer (colon, rectum, prostate, ovary, or liver) as well as lung and thyroid: CEA
- Ovarian or peritoneal cancer: CA125
- Pancreatic cancer: CA19-9
- Prostate cancer: PSA, PAP
- Circulating tumor cells (CTC) of solid tumors

Note that except for CTC, none of these antigen markers is independently diagnostic, as they are actually indicating shedding of antigenic immune activating molecules that may be elevated for other reasons than cancer. These cancer markers are, more properly, markers of immune activation, and elevations may be due to nonmalignant causes. For example, prostate-specific antigen (PSA) can rise if there is a prostate or testicular infection, after long-distance running or biking, or from severe prostatitis or infection. Similarly, cancer antigen 125 (CA125) can be a biomarker of ovarian cancer and an indicator of malignancy, but it can be high in people who have pancreatitis or kidney or liver disease, making its accuracy as a cancer diagnostic tool somewhat limited. Carcinoembryonic antigen (CEA) is another biomarker that is elevated in patients with colorectal, breast, lung, or pancreatic cancer but is also raised in cigarette smokers. However, if there is known cancer in the body and the markers are elevated, then it can be a useful gauge of progression over time.

Another important consideration is that these markers should generally be zero or close to zero in someone who does not have, and has not had, cancer at all. However, in a patient who has recovered from cancer, these numbers, which may be very low immediately after completion of treatments, can then creep slowly up again and stabilize at a low or moderate level. For example, a patient that was diagnosed in 2013 with ovarian cancer had a CA125 over 3,000 at the time of diagnosis. It came down to 15 after adjunctive chemotherapy followed by surgery plus an extensive herbal and supplement program, and over the next 2 years it crept back up to the low 20s. The patient can set it back 3 or 4 points if it climbs over 25 by undergoing a deep and intensive detoxification program, and with this she has remained cancer-free for 9 years, but her CA125 has never gone back below 20. Another patient, a 64-year-old man with prostate cancer diagnosed 6 years ago with a PSA of 42, saw it go to zero after surgery and then rise back up to settle out between 8–10 ever since. It doesn't go higher and he doesn't have active cancer. This can be disconcerting to patients and may require careful counseling to alleviate fear.

A functional medicine doctor may go even further and run extensive genomic panels looking for genetically predisposed trends and patterns that may suggest areas of specific risks or concerns, so that customized and targeted protocols can be designed for each individual. A functional health report may test hundreds of genes in sets and groups that indicate specific areas of resistance and weakness to be addressed and can explain why some of our health conditions occur or persist even when we may live a relatively healthy lifestyle.

Pathology Testing on Excised Tissue

This is an opportunity to identify individual characteristics of the specific cancer and to gather clues to guide treatment planning. It requires properly prepared biopsy slides, and these will be stored for several years by the hospital in most cases. This does mean that if proper testing is not done initially, it may be possible to go back to the slides later and get more information. The slides are only useful for a year or so after they have been prepared, because if cancer is still present after that much time, then there is a high probability that it will have mutated quite a bit and no longer behave as the slides might suggest. Certainly, older biopsies of the primary tumor may not accurately reflect the behavior of subsequent metastases or recurrences. For example, a breast cancer that may be estrogen sensitive in the first instance may be hormone resistant if it recurs.

The following tests are fairly routine and should be easy to get done.

Mitotic index. S phase percentage and ki67—the higher these markers are, the more cells are actively replicating and the more aggressive the cancer is, which is not good news in principle, but it does indicate more likelihood of sensitivity to some conventional chemotherapies that are most active during the DNA synthesis phase (S phase) of the cell cycle.

BRCA1, BRCA2. These are genes that can be a factor in breast, ovarian, and other reproductive cancers; mutation leads to significant increased risk in the next generation and warrants family genetic counseling. These gene mutations in a woman can also cause higher prostate cancer risk in her sons.

ER+, PR+, HER2/neu+. These tests are routinely offered in breast cancer, but they should probably be done in all reproductive cancers. Note that ER-positive tumors may be less responsive to tamoxifen treatment if HER2/neu is also overexpressed.

Viral load. Testing for viruses such as herpes (HSV), Epstein Barr (EBV), human papilloma (HPV), and human immunodeficiency (HIV) may be warranted. These are especially significant in cervical, vulval, anal, and squamous cell carcinomas of the mouth and throat, easily transmitted by oral sex.

Specialty Testing for Cancer

Some of these tests will be routinely done in the original pathology report but others may be harder to get. They are helpful in assessing risks and prognosis in an individual, but even without these it is possible to address the foundations of health effectively and resist cancer.

CANCER CELL GENE TESTING

These tests will be increasingly available in the next 5–10 years. They will be used to refine and direct treatments so that individualized and targeted therapies will be the norm. But we are not there yet. Most are available only through private healthcare for now; hopefully this will change as their utility becomes better recognized by mainstream medicine.

Genomic testing. This looks at a wide profile of genes (the genome) as a screen for any abnormality of interest that can be targeted for treatment. Genomics includes the interactions of genes with each other and with the environment and is used in understanding complex diseases such as heart disease, asthma, diabetes, and cancer, which are caused by interactions of multiple genetic and environmental factors.

Genetic tests. These detect single gene mutations for establishing risk or cause of a cancer through inherited traits or conditions or through acquired epigenetic changes (such as BRCA1 and BRCA2).

Pharmacogenetics deals with individual patient variability in response to medications due to variation in single genes controlling specific drug receptors, transportation, and metabolism. This may be very significant in whether a treatment is likely to be effective in a particular patient.

Genetic Tests in Clinical Practice

Even without "proof" from tests, more or less every cancer starts as a genetic flaw or fault, and it is safe to assume that every cancer case shows some degree of dysregulation in inflammation, methylation, signal transduction and transcription, cell cycling, angiogenesis, and apoptosis—the basic cell (mis)behaviors in cancer. The specialty tests can be interesting when they are done, but it is clinically reasonable to proceed as if these genes are most or all somewhat deranged in most or all cancers, and to use natural agents accordingly.

EXAMPLES OF PREDICTIVE TESTING FOR DRUG RESPONSES

Tests for predicting response with 5-fluorouracil (5-FU). Dihydropyrimidine dehydrogenase (DPD) is a detoxifying enzyme that catalyzes the degradation of the chemotherapy drug 5-FU to an inactive metabolite for elimination. Overexpression of DPD correlates with resistance to 5-FU due to an accelerated degradation.

Thymidylate synthetase (TS) is involved in the early steps of DNA copying and is a molecular target of 5-FU. High expression correlates with resistance to 5-FU.

Thymidine phosphorylase (TP) promotes metabolism and excretion of 5-FU. High expression correlates with resistance to 5-FU.

Uridine phosphorylase (UP) catalyzes the formation of the active 5-fluorouracil-monophosphate metabolite from the inactive 5-FU. Downregulation of UP is associated with resistance to 5-FU.

Tests for predicting response with other anticancer drugs. Cyclooxygenase-2 (COX-2) is overexpressed in colorectal adenomas and tumors and this makes them more susceptible to specific COX-2 inhibitors.

Excision repair cross complementation 1 (ERCC1) repairs DNA damage, and overexpression of ERCC1 induces resistance to platinum-based drugs like oxaliplatin, cisplatin, and carboplatin that specifically work by inducing DNA damage.

Multidrug resistance–associated protein 2 (MRP2) helps transport drugs out of the cell. Overexpression of MRP2 confers resistance to several anticancer drugs like vinca alkaloids, anthracyclines, methotrexate, cisplatin, and carboplatin.

Vascular endothelial growth factor (VEGF) induces angiogenesis. High expression of VEGF in tumor cells is associated with poor response to hormone depletion with tamoxifen in breast cancer, but possibly better outcomes with bevacizumab (Avastin), which is targeted specifically against VEGF.

Test for predicting response to olaparib (an immunotherapy drug). People with BRCA1 and BRCA2 mutations may be genetically predisposed to some cancers, such as peritoneal cancer; pancreatic cancer; breast, ovarian, and fallopian tube cancer in women; and prostate cancer in men. These cancers associated with BRCA mutation are especially responsive to olaparib. If DNA copies with an error and it is noted and addressed, then the cell cannot divide during the repair process and may in fact undergo apoptosis if it cannot be adequately repaired. Cells use an enzyme called poly (ADP-ribose) polymerase (PARP) to repair DNA and allow cell replication to restart. The drug olaparib is a PARP inhibitor and thus indirectly prevents cell replication and drives apoptosis.

ONCOTYPE IQ GENOMIC INTELLIGENCE TESTING

This is a set of tests on preserved pathology slides that determines the relative risk of recurrence and predicts chemotherapy benefit, which informs the treatment choices—specifically for lung, prostate, colon, and breast cancer. In the US, all major insurance carriers including Medicare cover the costs for women with breast cancer who meet the criteria, as do the medical services plans of several Canadian provinces.

In breast cancer, the test is intended for use in newly diagnosed patients with stage I, II, or IIIa breast cancer who have node-negative or node-positive (1–3), estrogen receptor–positive (ER+), HER2-negative disease. The lower the Recurrence Score or DCIS Score, the lower the chances are that a woman's breast cancer will come back; the higher the Recurrence or DCIS Score, the greater the chances that breast cancer will come back, and this may impact clinical decisions about surgery, chemotherapy, and radiation.

In older men, prostate cancer usually grows very slowly and in men diagnosed over the age of 70 there is less than 5 percent chance that it will become life threatening. Aggressive treatment—through surgery, radiation, and hormones—brings significant side effects and overtreatment is a real concern. Oncotype assessment can discern the relative risk in the individual patient of aggressive cancer at the time of diagnosis, helping to identify who will benefit the most from immediate surgery or radiation therapy versus those who can more safely choose active surveillance. Similarly, in colon cancer stage II or stage III, the Oncotype DX Colon Recurrence Score test assesses the relative risk that the cancer will return, and that guides treatment choices.

PROSIGNA ASSAY: BREAST CANCER GENE SIGNATURE PROFILING

This test on preserved pathology slides is used to predict the risk of distant recurrence for postmenopausal women with up to three positive lymph nodes within 10 years of diagnosis of early-stage, hormone receptor–positive disease and after 5 years of hormonal therapy. The Prosigna assay can only be used on breast cancers diagnosed in postmenopausal women that:

- are stage I or stage II and lymph node-negative
- are stage II with one to three positive nodes
- are hormone receptor–positive
- are invasive
- have been treated with surgery and hormonal therapy

The Prosigna assay is performed on preserved tissue that was removed during the original biopsy or surgery. It looks at the activity of more than 50 genes to estimate the risk of distant recurrence of hormone receptor–positive breast cancer from 5–10 years after diagnosis and results are reported as a score from 0–100 that can be used to guide treatment choices.

MAMMAPRINT

The MammaPrint test on preserved pathology slides is used to predict the risk of recurrence within 10 years after diagnosis of stage I or stage II breast cancer that is hormone receptor–positive or hormone receptor–negative. The MammaPrint assay is recommended for patients with high-risk, hormone receptor–positive, HER2-negative, node-negative breast cancer to inform decisions regarding adjuvant systemic chemotherapy. It may also inform decisions in patients with HR-positive, HER2-negative cancer with up to three positive nodes and a high clinical risk.

FOUNDATION ONE CDX (F1CDX) PROFILING

This is a useful assay to be done before commencing immunotherapies, helping to identify targets for the plethora of new drugs being approved. This is a DNA test done on biopsy tissue and looking for substitutions, insertions, deletions, copy number alterations, and gene rearrangements in more than 300 genes, as well as genomic signatures including microsatellite instability (MSI) and tumor mutational burden (TMB). Currently FoundationOne profiling is offered for breast, colorectal, ovarian, prostate, non–small cell lung cancer, and melanoma and reviews dozens of gene abnormalities that would confer likely sensitivity to dozens of drug options, aiming for best fit. Some cancer care centers offer a more limited range of testing and a limited selection of drugs accordingly, but with ever increasing numbers of targeted drugs being developed, wide testing is recommended. Indeed, one of the clinical challenges now is the sheer plethora of new drugs and new tests being brought to medical practice, and the high hopes engendered from new pharmaceutical technologies despite the high level of side effects.

If a patient tests well for sensitivity to a certain drug, even if it is not yet approved for that particular cancer, it may be possible to obtain it from the drug companies under a "compassionate release" allowance. Drug companies want to trial their products widely in order to bolster applications for expanded licensing, so if the expected outcomes are good they want to know, and they may be willing to provide the drug at no cost for research purposes.

SALIVA/BUCCAL SWAB TESTING

None of these mouth swab tests is explicitly for cancer, but they are about understanding the terrain better. Relative risk of estrogen exposure, of detoxification capacities, and of immune deficiency can be measured and that will inform the choices around lifestyle, diet, and physiological enhancement. The lab I use offers several genomic panels that are especially useful in assessing the terrain in a cancer patient.

THE ESTROGENOMIC PROFILE

This evaluates single nucleotide polymorphisms (SNPs) or errors in genes that modulate estrogen metabolism. These cause downstream effects in cardiovascular function and heart disease, coagulation, bone health and osteoporosis, and inflammation. Some of these also increase susceptibility to breast cancer. Specific genes tested include those involved in:

- Estrogen metabolism—genes that code for phase I and phase II enzymes
- Hypercoagulation—genes that code for blood clotting
- Cardiovascular function—genes that code for heart functions
- Osteoporosis—genes that code for bone health

THE DETOXIGENOMIC PROFILE

This looks at a very extensive panel of genes and single nucleotide polymorphisms (SNPs) associated with impaired liver and detoxification capacity and greater risk from environmental toxins and adverse drug reactions. These include phase I liver detox cytochrome enzymes, the phase II detox glutathione-s-transferase enzymes, and N-acetyltransferase 1 and 2 (NAT1 and NAT2), which are cytosolic enzymes involved in activation or deactivation of many toxic compounds including pharmaceuticals and environmental carcinogens.

THE IMMUNOGENOMIC PROFILE

This looks at genes regulating immune functions and inflammatory activity. SNPs in these genes can affect cell mediated (Th-1) and humoral (Th-2) immunity, cause deficiencies and defects in immune defense, and both trigger and perpetuate chronic overactive inflammatory responses. These include interleukins as well as tumor necrosis factor-alpha (TNF-α).

SENSITIVITY AND RESISTANCE TESTING/FUNCTIONAL PROFILING

Sensitivity and resistance testing is premised on the fact that each cancer patient is unique and responses to therapy will be very different in individual patients, despite having apparently the same diagnosis or being given the same drug. Where the genomic testing assesses for mutations and other changes in multiple genes that might guide drug selection, especially the monoclonal antibody immunotherapy drugs, the sensitivity and resistance testing is quite different. It measures how cancer cells respond when they are exposed to drugs and drug combinations.

This really is the gold standard of chemotherapy assessments and should be the standard of care everywhere, although in fact it is offered only in a couple of specialty labs. If a patient goes to the doctor with a bad throat infection or a bad bladder infection, there is a good chance that a swab will be taken to culture in a laboratory and determine which antibiotic is going to be the most effective. This is more or less what is done in the sensitivity and resistance testing for cancer, and the expected response to the drugs chosen this way is much higher than simply taking the standard protocol on offer. This is a very elegant way of guiding treatment choice. It involves culturing fresh cells from the cancer, then exposing them to assorted chemotherapy cocktails to find those it responds to or not. It pinpoints the most effective chemotherapy regimen for an individual, whether or not it is approved for that particular cancer yet. Of all the tests suggested here, this is the only one that is done on fresh tissue—actual cancer cells, in real time—not on preserved slides or blood draws. Because this involves surgery to obtain a fresh sample, this is not something an herbalist is going to be able to order. However, the patient can certainly pursue this with their oncologist or seek private medical care, and perhaps in time it will come to be the norm.

ADDITIONAL TESTS

Thermographic imaging (thermography). Thermographic imaging measures areas of heat in tissues, which implies metabolic overactivity. Although mostly used in measuring breast health, it can also monitor other heat-generating pathologies (usually inflammation or growths). It is not invasive, and it can be helpful to establish a normal baseline measurement profile when there is no known pathology, then used to compare against over time and monitor changes. Remember that the technician is critical to the success of the readings; the level of objectivity that they are able to attain can make a substantial difference. Remember also that identification of hot spots is not a diagnosis of cancer. Dental infections, oral herpes infection, allergies, and head colds as well as hyperthyroidism, gastroesophageal reflux disease, and Barrett's esophagitis may all induce a heat gradient on the skin of the chest.

Mammograms. Mammogram technology has come a long way in the past 20 years. The amount of radiation exposure has been reduced substantially, and the accuracy of interpretation has also improved. Having said that, compression of breast tissue and exposure to radiation is never really a good thing, and this technology should be considered for diagnosis rather than for mass screening. Indeed, this was the intention when it was first introduced to medical practices, and even today if a positive finding is identified in a mammogram, the doctor will recommend that the patient have an ultrasound for confirmation.

Although it is true that early detection of cancer is always desirable, and screening mammograms may be able to offer this, there are adverse effects to consider as well—notably false alarms and overdiagnosis. A 2014 report in *JAMA* suggested, "Among 1,000 US women aged 50 years who are screened annually for a decade, 0.3 to 3.2 will avoid a breast cancer death, 490 to 670 will have at least 1 false alarm, and 3 to 14 will be overdiagnosed and be treated needlessly." This conclusion is astonishing as it actually suggests that up to four times as many women could be treated unnecessarily as would have their lives saved by mammograms.

Given the toxicity of chemotherapy and the long-term risks of conventional treatment, this means screening mammograms are highly unreliable. For all these reasons, I recommend reserving mammograms for use only if breast self-examination, ultrasound, or thermographic imaging has flagged a concern, or if there is some other reason, such as breast implants or scar tissue, that make it difficult to palpate and visualize without the mammogram.

Other assessment methods in development. The understanding and consequent treatment of cancer is constantly evolving. This is seen in testing, assessments, and evaluations as much as it is in treatments. For example, a study reported in the journal *Gut Microbiota* in 2021 presented evidence for a role for the microbiome in the development and progression of pancreatic ductal adenocarcinoma (PDAC) and suggested that a fecal test for specific microbiota may allow for early detection of PDAC.

A report in 2020 described a blood test capable of indicating asymptomatic cancer years before conventional diagnosis. In the Taizhou Longitudinal Study (TZL), 123,115 healthy subjects provided plasma samples for long-term storage and were then monitored for cancer occurrence. Preliminary results of PanSeer, a noninvasive blood test based on circulating tumor DNA methylation, on these plasma samples suggested that the test can detect cancer in 95 percent of asymptomatic individuals who were later diagnosed, suggesting that cancer may be noninvasively detected up to 4 years before expected.

In an exciting announcement in 2022, researchers described techniques to assess cervical cells collected during routine Pap smears that look for early warning signs of ovarian, breast, cervical, and uterine cancer. In the screening method, 14,000 epigenetic changes are checked for specific DNA signatures that predict risk of cancer.

Prioritizing Additional Tests

Given that it is unlikely everyone can access or afford many of the tests available, how do we prioritize for patients? There are some tests that should be done routinely to monitor progress and are not difficult or expensive to order. Others are done once and then not repeated unless the results are out of range. Mostly these are blood tests that can be ordered privately at a moderate but not exorbitant cost if the patient's insurance plan doesn't cover them. Genetic screening is more expensive and may be more difficult to get. The genetic tissue biopsy reviews require a medical doctor to sign the order, and this may not be possible. Many insurance plans in the US will happily pay for predictive testing because it costs them a lot of money if ineffective drugs are given (which is a big clue right there about how useful these tests are), and some provinces in Canada cover some of these, too (for example, British Columbia and Ontario pay for Oncotype testing in breast cancer).

CONCLUSIONS ABOUT TESTS

On a purely pragmatic level, there are only so many tests that can be done, and choosing the most useful tests is important. Certainly the basic blood chemistry and complete blood count are routine and easy to get, and many (maybe most) of the one-off, add-on blood tests suggested here can be readily obtained, even if they have to be paid for privately. The buccal swabs and urine or stool tests offered through private labs and assessing relative risks and resistance are perhaps a luxury or an optional layer of information about the body, the absence of which can be compensated for in the treatment planning regardless. The biopsy screening for genetic susceptibilities to specific drugs is a burgeoning field of medicine, and there are almost too many genes and too many drugs to keep up with. This is certainly the area for a skilled oncologist who can navigate between the testing availability, drug availabilities, and your personal proclivities to help decide what is useful and necessary. Sensitivity and resistance testing is the gold standard and the way of the future. If your cells react to a given drug, there is a reasonable probability to think that it will work in your body and may be worth the trade-off of side effects and other long-term consequences.

Managing the Patient Who Declines Chemotherapy

Some patients may be opposed to the drastic treatments available and choose to decline conventional care. This may present an opportunity to use higher doses of herbs, because the patient isn't already ill from chemotherapy or other drug therapies. Alternatively, it could mean a missed opportunity to use aggressive drug therapies for a short while to contain a critical state, then use herbs for recovery and rebalancing after the crisis is averted.

This is where the predictive testing techniques are so useful to give guidance and some way of assessing relative risk of progression or recurrence, and thus an indirect measure of the urgency of acute interventions. In general, the higher the risk profile of an individual, the more chemotherapy may be indicated, with herbal medicine being used strategically to mitigate side effects and protect the body but probably not sufficient to fight cancer alone. In stage I and grade 1 cancers, however, there is a much stronger argument to be made for using cytotoxic herbs judiciously, building terrain and supporting immune functions, and holding off from chemotherapy, at least in the first instance. It has absolutely happened in my clinical practice that I have been the person urging a patient to take chemotherapy when they were hesitant, but only when there was compelling evidence of unacceptably high risk of progression, or when tests had been done indicating a specific drug with a high likelihood of success.

If no chemotherapy is used, then it is easier to assess and evaluate symptoms of cancer because drug side effects are not adding to the presentation, and tolerance of herbs may be higher because the liver and kidneys are not so burdened. In the end, the decision to accept chemotherapy or not is always up to the patient, and you can support them with herbs and natural medicine regardless of the choices they make.

Addressing Cancer Directly

Cancer develops through three key steps or processes: initiation (what kicks it off or triggers the first DNA error), promotion (what allows that mistake to perpetuate), and proliferation or progression (what allows it to spread unchecked). At each stage, there is further loss of cell control and progressive growth of the cancer, and the diagnostic grade increases from 1 (well differentiated) to 4 (poorly differentiated).

Once cancer has been initiated, once gene defects are allowed to perpetuate and the cell is replicating unhindered, then a whole cascade of physiological responses may start to occur that promote cancer growth and proliferation. Growth-stimulating compounds cause unchecked proliferation until the point at which repetitive DNA errors give rise to self-stimulating cells. Cancer-promoting genes are overexpressed, tumor suppressor genes are underexpressed, and if neoplastic growth continues unchecked then a tumor will result. These cells have malignant features such as the ability to invade and metastasize, to mutate rapidly and accommodate or adjust when faced with adverse conditions (such as chemotherapy), and to induce the growth of new blood vessels (angiogenesis) and thus facilitate tumor growth.

Promotion of Cancer

- Oxidative stress and generation of free radicals
- Glycolytic shift
- Obesity, elevated insulin and IGF-1, deficient SHBG
- Inflammation and activation of toll-like receptors (TLRs)
- COX-2 and 5-, 12-, and 15-LOX overexpression
- Gene transcription instability and DNA mutation
- Mutation of regulatory proteins (p53, p21, p27)
- Upregulation of signal transduction (PTK, PKC, Ras proteins, and mTOR)
- Upregulation of signal transcription (NF-κB, AP-1, NRF2, PPAR)

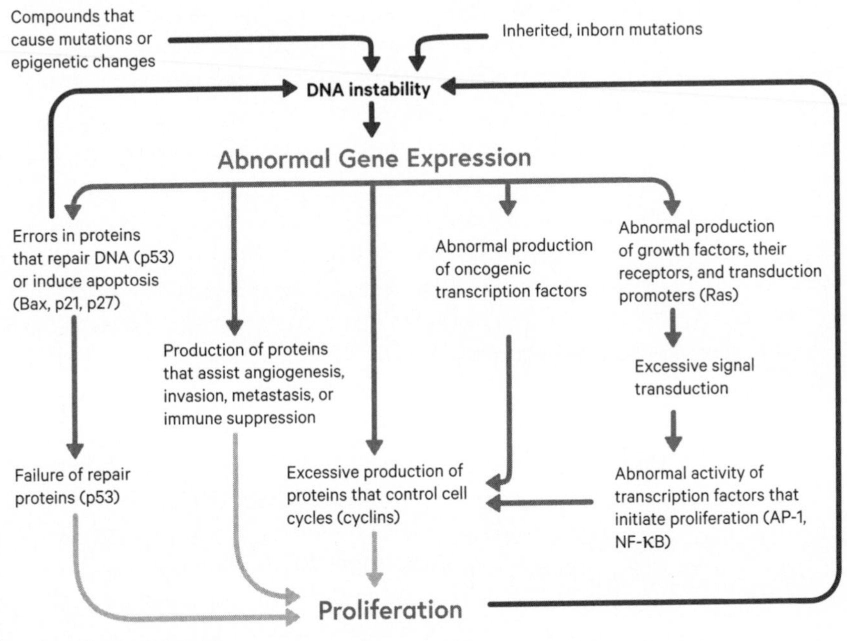

Diagram after Boik, 2001

Proliferation and Progression of Cancer

- Disruption of extracellular matrix and loss of cell-to-cell communication
- Loss of control of cell cycling (cyclin-dependent kinases)
- Growth factor upregulation and PTK or PKC receptor sites
- Immunosuppression and immune evasion
- Inflammation
- Failure of apoptosis
- Invasion and metastasis
- Angiogenesis
- Coagulopathies (clotting)

While physiological enhancement strategies may address the initiation phase and the beginning of promotion, it will take more directed and more potent pathological correction to address proliferation and progression. Pathological correction can be conceptualized as one side of the pyramid prescribing pattern (see page 318), comprising the effector agents, cytotoxics, and specific, targeted treatments with specific actions and doses.

Below I have described the cellular mechanisms and pathways in some detail, but please bear in mind that this is a vastly oversimplified summary of an indescribably complex process, with myriad moving parts and uncountable numbers of variables. In the interest of clarity and brevity, I have described just a few of the many control pathways and mechanisms—there are numerous others, including STAT and SPARK, the slug and snail genes, the sonic hedgehog pathway (yes, really!), and more.

As soon as oncologists think they have understood cancer, researchers discover something new that sends everyone back to the drawing board. The body is still revealing its mysteries to us. New hormones, new mechanisms, and even new tissues are still being discovered. For example, despite a few hundred years of brain tissue analysis—up to and including dissections, MRI, and CT scans—it was only in 2017 that researchers at the National Institute of Neurological Disorders and Stroke (NINDS) in the US discovered a complete lymphatic drainage system in the dura mater (outer wrapping) of the brain. Now it is named the glymph system as it represents an interface between lymph and glioma cells.

I have attempted below to explain the principal mechanisms of cancer development as they are currently understood; in a short time, this may be superseded by more detailed information. I have explained the key mechanisms of cancer, how it occurs, and how it progresses, as a means of illustrating the many opportunities for herbs and natural agents to guide cell behaviors toward health. It quickly becomes obvious that many agents are recommended again and again in multiple pathways, indicating their common mechanisms of action—very often fundamental redox-regulating or immunomodulating effects.

Major Metabolic Pathways to Target

- Redox balance—stabilize reactive oxygen species (ROS) and reduce genetic instability
- Cellular mitochondrial energy transfer—reverse glycolytic shift, lessen lactic acid and hypoxia
- Anabolic/catabolic balance—(1) regulate signal transduction: inhibit PTK and PKC receptor activities, regulate TGF-β signaling, inhibit Ras production and activation; and (2) regulate signal transcription: inhibit NF-κB and AP-1, stimulate nuclear factor erythroid 2-related factor 2 (NRF2), regulate apoptosis
- Cell cycling/replication—slow the rate of mitosis, induce differentiation, downregulate growth factors and their receptor sites
- Immune surveillance—enhance innate and acquired immune function, normalize TLRs
- Inflammatory response—support and regulate inflammation to attain resolution
- Connective tissue strengthening—stabilize extracellular matrix, restore CAM and gap junctions, enhance cell-to-cell communication, inhibit invasion and metastases
- Antiangiogenesis—resistance to vascular growth, vascular tissue integrity
- Coagulopathy—regulation of clotting and vascular endothelial health

Address Free Radicals and Genetic Instability

Understanding oxidation and its role in the progression of cancer requires a basic knowledge of how oxidation occurs at a cellular level. Electrons carry the negative charge in an atom and they orbit the protons and neutrons of the nucleus in pairs. If an atom donates an electron to fuel a metabolic process in the cell, then it has an unpaired electron looking for a mate, wanting to grab another electron from some other atom and the atom is unstable—a so-called free radical that creates oxidative stress.

Free radicals and reactive oxygen species (ROS) are highly reactive chemical forms that contain one (occasionally two) unpaired electrons. These unpaired electrons are continuously produced in the human body due to various metabolic functions such as chemical signaling, energy supply, detoxification, and immune reactions. ROS are generally considered cytotoxic because of the oxidative damage they can cause to cellular components. Antioxidants work by donating an electron to "quench" the free radical.

Redox (reduction and oxidation) reactions entail loss of an electron by one molecule and gain of an electron by another molecule. The redox state or redox potential refers to the dynamic balance between these two states. When an antioxidant donates an electron, it may itself become unstable and become an oxidizing agent and is, in turn, quenched by another antioxidant. This can continue in a cascade and is one reason why it is clinically helpful to provide an array of antioxidants. Complex plant-derived, flavonoid-based antioxidants exhibit a phenomenon called "resonance stabilization," in which they effectively share their electrons with the ROS, donating and then borrowing back repeatedly so that neither party ever remains oxidized long enough to cause cellular damage.

Cancer cells produce free radicals because of their rapid metabolism, and they thrive in this oxidative environment. The higher the level of oxidative stress, the more rapid the rate of DNA mutation; this can become a self-perpetuating cycle. Because of this, it is critically important to support redox regulation.

There is a dynamic balance of antioxidants and oxidants in healthy cells—where fluctuating concentrations of free radicals allow the body to activate or to deactivate many cell functions, including enzyme activity and gene expression—that is often lost in cancer cells.

Natural Agents That May Aid Redox Regulation

- R+ alpha-lipoic acid
- Coenzyme Q10
- Curcumin from turmeric
- MSM (methylsulfonylmethane)
- NAC (N-acetylcysteine)
- Omega-3 fats from fish oil (DHA, EPA)
- Polyphenol antioxidants (flavonoids)
- Resveratrol
- SAMe (S-adenosylmethionine)**
- Selenium
- Vitamins A, B6, B12, C, E, beta-carotenes, folic acid
- Zinc

**Avoid SAMe in people who are immunocompromised or who have bipolar disorder; SAMe may decrease the effects of levodopa used to treat Parkinson's disease.

Reduce Abnormal Gene Expression

Although your inborn, inherited DNA sequence is permanent, epigenetic (acquired) modifications can influence which genes are expressed or dormant, and these can be strongly affected by external factors. These acquired genetic changes are heritable, meaning that if this cell is allowed to go on and replicate, then the changes will perpetuate with it. Epigenetic changes to genes are mostly generated by adjustments of methyl molecules attached to DNA, and the greater the degree of methylation, the less the gene will express. Because epigenetic DNA mutations are functional, not structural, they are reversible. Normalizing methylation is the primary gene support required. Cancer-promoting genes are generally hypomethylated, so supplementing with methyl donor molecules will suppress them and inhibit cancer progression. These genes may also be activated by iron and copper accumulation, so testing for and chelating these minerals is helpful as well.

Metabolic Functions Controlled by Methylation

- Regulation of epigenetics—DNA copying and synthesis
- Biotransformation of endogenous and xenobiotic compounds
- Building neurotransmitters (norepinephrine, epinephrine, serotonin, melatonin)
- Metabolizing neurotransmitters (dopamine, epinephrine)
- Processing steroid hormones (estrogen, progesterone, testosterone)
- Building immune cells (T cells, NK cells)
- Production of cellular energy (CoQ10, carnitine, creatine, ATP)
- Production of the protective myelin sheath on nerves
- Building and maintaining cell membranes

TESTING FOR METHYLATION CAPACITY

The ability to carry out proper methylation may be assessed indirectly through homocysteine testing in blood. Homocysteine (a potentially toxic amino acid) should convert to methionine; failure to do this indicates poor methylation. It is often tested as part of a heart health workup; if elevated, it indicates increased risk of cardiovascular disease. However, in cancer it may indicate increased likelihood of epigenetic mutations due to methylation deficiency. Gene sequencing of a tissue sample (buccal swab) can assess for mutations in the gene that codes for the enzyme methylenetetrahydrofolate reductase (MTHFR). This is responsible for converting folic acid from the diet (found in leafy greens) into methylfolate (the active form), which then catalyzes the conversion of homocysteine to methionine. If this gene is mutated, it may be hard to get folic acid and affect DNA metabolism.

Natural Agents That May Promote Proper Methylation

- Betaine
- Curcumin from turmeric
- EGCG from green tea
- Folic acid
- Genistein from soy
- Luteolin (carrot, cabbage, artichoke, tea, celery, apple skin)
- Molybdenum
- R+ lipoic acid
- Resveratrol
- SAMe
- Vitamins B6, B12
- Zinc glycinate

> Cancer has only one prime cause. It is the replacement of normal oxygen respiration of the body's cells by an anaerobic, oxygen deficient cell respiration.
>
> DR. OTTO WARBURG, WINNER OF THE 1931 NOBEL PRIZE IN MEDICINE

Glycolytic Shift and the Cancer-Sugar Connection

It may not be as simple as Dr. Warburg implied in his famous quote (at right), but certainly a key behavior of cancer cells is the tendency to outgrow the blood supply and hence have low oxygen delivery. In response to this, cancer cells turn the Krebs cycle inefficiently and hence derive little energy that way. In a healthy cell, most of the adenosine triphosphate (ATP) or "energy currency" is made by the Krebs cycle and the sequential oxidative phosphorylation electron transfer chain that follows—both of which require oxygen to operate. Up to 36 molecules of ATP are made in this way using oxygen, in contrast to a net gain of just 2 molecules of ATP made by glycolysis without requiring anywhere near as much oxygen. As cancer progresses, the cells lose the ability to turn the Krebs cycle properly and develop a high rate of glycolysis and hence a high demand for sugar to make energy. This so-called "glycolytic shift" allows the cells to have a rapid metabolism in a low-oxygen environment. Glycolytic shift produces an excess of lactic acid and contributes to a local inflammatory environment and oxidative stress, which tends to promote cancer cell behavior.

Blood testing should be done for fasting glucose, fasting insulin, and elevation of serum IGF-1. Following a diet designed to stabilize blood sugar (an antidiabetic diet) is also an effective way to resist glycolytic shift.

PATHWAYS OF GLUCOSE METABOLISM

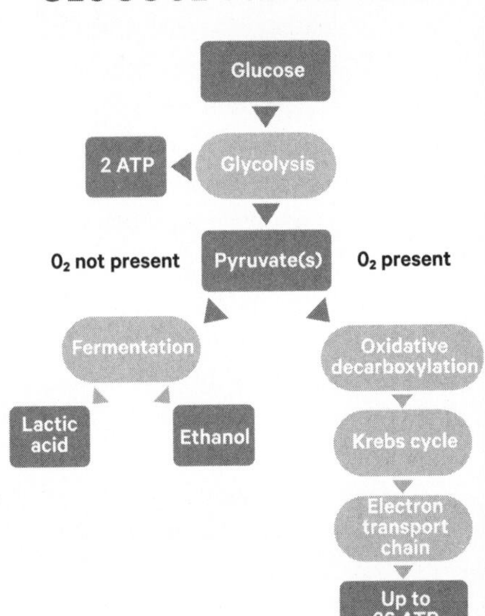

Obesity and Cancer

Excess body mass (obesity) leads to insulin resistance and elevated serum insulin and glucose levels. This will inhibit IGF-1 binding proteins and free up IGF-1 in the blood, which joins with insulin in encouraging cancer cells to take up sugar, metabolize faster, promote angiogenesis, and resist apoptosis.

Adipose (fat) cells regulate energy balance by taking up excess calories and releasing them very slowly. They also carry out conversion of testosterone into estrogen under the influence of aromatase enzyme. In obese patients, this can lead to an increased conversion of androgens into estrogens (estrone E1 and estradiol E2). Obese women have up to a 200 percent greater chance of breast cancer recurrence and 60 percent greater chance of dying from it than do women with a normal body mass index. Obesity is also a contributing factor in prostate and colon cancer.

Elevated serum insulin inhibits the liver from manufacturing sex hormone binding globulin (SHBG), a protein that binds to the hormones testosterone, dihydrotestosterone (DHT), and to a lesser extent estradiol and transports these hormones in the blood as biologically inactive forms. Specifically, pro-inflammatory cytokines and the hepatic steatosis (fatty liver) found in chronic insulin elevation and hyperglycemia will downregulate SHBG, such that plasma SHBG could be considered as a biomarker of the degree of inflammation in metabolic disorder.

A high SHBG level means that less free testosterone or estrogen is available to the tissues. Conversely, a low SHBG level means that more of the total testosterone is bioavailable and not bound to SHBG. Lower circulating levels of SHBG are found in obesity, type 2 diabetes, metabolic syndrome, nonalcoholic fatty liver disease, polycystic ovary syndrome (PCOS), and early puberty. Insulin resistance, even without obesity, results in lower SHBG levels.

SHBG can be supported with a diet high in plant fiber (legumes, vegetables, whole grains), flaxseed, fermented soy isoflavones, and kudzu. SHBG can also be modified by weight changes and by exercise. It increases significantly with weight loss of just 5 percent of starting weight and increases even more with 10 percent weight loss. It also increases significantly with a regular moderate-intensity exercise.

Foods or beverages rich in polyphenols lessen glycemic responses after eating, improve fasting hyperglycemia, and moderate acute insulin secretion and insulin sensitivity. Polyphenols, including flavonoids, phenolic acids, proanthocyanidins, and resveratrol, are found in many foods such as tea, coffee, wine, cocoa, cereal grains, soy, fruits, and berries.

Polyphenols may stabilize blood sugar by inhibition of carbohydrate digestion and glucose absorption in the intestine, stimulation of insulin secretion from the pancreas, modulation of glucose release from the liver, activation of insulin receptors and glucose uptake in the insulin-sensitive tissues, and modulation of intracellular signaling pathways and gene expression.

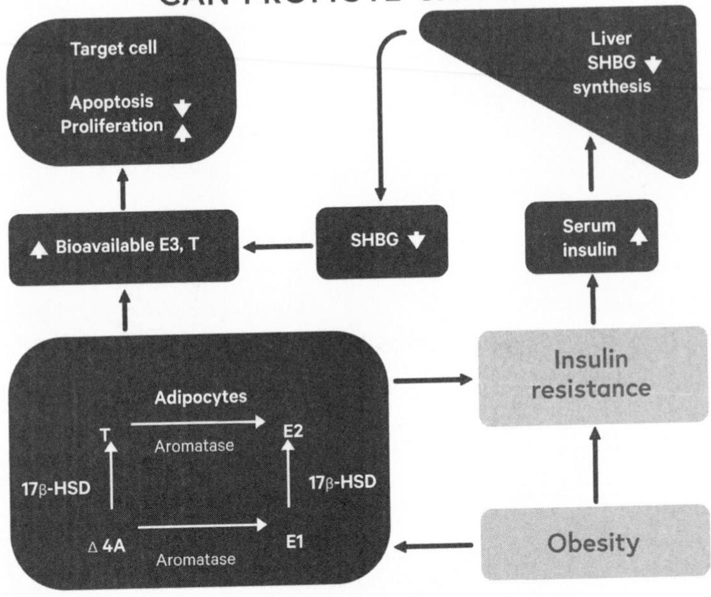

E1 = estrone, E2 = estradiol, E3 = estriol, T = testosterone, 17β-HSD = 17 beta-hydroxysteroid dehydrogenase, Δ 4A = delta-4 androstenedione

Natural Agents That May Lower Blood Sugar

- Barberry or Oregon grape root
- Bitter melon
- Burdock root
- Chromium
- Dandelion root
- Devil's club
- Fenugreek
- Flaxseed
- Goat's rue
- Grapeseed extract (oligomeric proanthocyanidins)
- Gurmar

Mitochondrial Rescue

This is the term given by naturopathic oncology specialist Dr. Neil McKinney to the elegant process he practices of reversing the glycolytic trend of cancer cells and reinstating the Krebs cycle and electron transfer chain, thus normalizing cellular energy production in stage I or II cancers and normalizing cell metabolism.

Natural Agents for Mitochondrial Rescue

- Berberine from barberry or Oregon grape
- B1 or thiamine (benfotiamine)
- B vitamins riboflavin (B2) and niacin (B3) as nicotinamide
- Coenzyme Q10
- Ellagic acid: 8 oz. of unsweetened pomegranate juice daily
- Gamma-tocopherol vitamin E succinate
- Indole-3-carbinal (I3C) and isothiocyanates from cruciferous vegetables

- L-carnitine
- Limonene
- Lipoic acid
- Lycopene
- Magnesium malate
- Oleic acid
- Omega-3 fats from fish oil
- Quercetin
- R+ alpha-lipoic acid
- Reishi mushroom
- Rhodiola root
- Selenium
- Silibinin from milk thistle
- Turkey tail mushroom
- Vanadium
- Vitamin D

Anabolic/Catabolic Balance

In normal healthy tissues, cells have a natural life span; they divide, mature, and die in a carefully calibrated sequence. Cell cycling (replication) and cell death (apoptosis) are tightly coupled, so that growth can occur when it's required and stop when it's completed (such as the normal cellular growth of a child or repair of an incision or a wound). One of the hallmarks of cancer is downregulation or inhibition of apoptosis and increased rate of replication so that anabolic and catabolic functions are no longer synchronous. Once a DNA error occurs and is not stopped, then it will perpetuate to daughter cells. Because cancer-promoting oncogenes are quick to mutate and hard for the immune system to recognize, replication and growth increase exponentially as cells divide and the daughter cells divide again. At about 28 doublings you have about a 2-millimeter heterogeneous mass of cells, still too small to be palpable but beginning to subvert cell behaviors and create its own microenvironment. This is not yet cancer in the fulminant sense, but it is strongly trending that way. These cells are still sensitive to terrain, and mitochondrial rescue practices can still revert them back to normal behaviors.

CONTROLLING CELL TURNOVER

A healthy cell spends most of its lifetime in the so-called gap or G0 phase. During this time it is metabolically active, conducting the activities of the tissue in which it occurs but not preparing for replication. Only when an active signal to divide is received will the cell progress into mitosis.

Cyclins. A specific family of proteins called cyclins control the signals that drive cell division (cycling) and govern the rate of cell turnover. They are activated by binding with cyclin-dependent kinases (enzymes), which themselves are regulated by cyclin-dependent kinase inhibitor proteins, including p21 and p27.

Cyclin-dependent kinase 1 (CDK1) orchestrates the first steps of the cell into mitosis and has been proposed as a tumor-specific anticancer target. CDK4 gene amplification results in loss of mitotic G1/S checkpoint control and contributes to melanoma, sarcoma, and glioblastoma. Cyclin D overexpression also results in loss of mitotic G1/S checkpoint control and contributes to breast, esophageal, and liver cancers. Two new immunotherapy CDK 4/6 inhibitor drugs have recently been approved: ribociclib (Kisqali) and palbociclib

(Ibrance). They are promising but cause severe side effects that are dose limiting.

Natural Agents That May Downregulate Cell Cycling

- Allicin from garlic
- Apigenin from parsley
- Berberine from barberry or Oregon grape
- Beta-carotene
- Beta-sitosterol
- Curcumin from turmeric
- EGCG from green tea
- Ellagic acid from pomegranate and berries
- Genistein from soy
- Ginger
- I3C and 3,3'-diindolylmethane (DIM)
- IP6 (inositol hexaphosphate)
- Limonene from citrus, lemongrass, and lemon verbena
- Lycopene from tomato
- NAC (N-acetylcysteine)
- Parthenolides from feverfew
- Perillyl alcohol
- Quercetin
- Reishi mushroom
- Silibinin from milk thistle
- Thymoqinone from nigella
- Vitamin A
- Zinc

TELOMERASE INHIBITION

Telomeres are sections of noncoding DNA at the end of each chromosome, the length of which indicates life expectancy and overall health status. Telomerase is a reverse transcriptase enzyme in cells that regulates the telomere length, and upregulation allows indefinite cell proliferation. This is a primary factor in almost all cancer cell types, and measuring it can even be used for predicting stage and prognosis.

Plant Compounds That Inhibit Telomerase

These act through various pathways, including pre- and posttranscriptional controls.

- Baicalein from Baikal skullcap
- Berberine from barberry
- Beta-lapachone from taheebo
- Diosgenin from fenugreek
- EGCG from green tea
- Gingerol from ginger
- I3C from cabbage
- Podophyllotoxin from mayapple
- Red rice yeast extract
- Silibinin from milk thistle
- Tanshinone IIA from dan shen (red sage root)

MUTATION OF REGULATORY PROTEINS (SUCH AS P21, P27, AND P53)

During cell replication, the cell can check itself for copying errors using a protein called p53 to conduct a DNA check—like a quality control scan. If errors are found in the copied DNA strand, then there is an opportunity to correct it or induce apoptosis.

P53 is both the name of a gene that is mutated early in many cancers and the name of the protein for which the gene codes. It is sometimes called the "guardian of the genome" because the protein acts as a sort of quality control supervisor in the cell. It scans a newly copied strand of DNA to see that it is accurate and responds to abnormal DNA by stimulating another gene called p21 to make proteins that prevent further cell division and a gene called p27 to initiate DNA repair, or another gene called Bax to initiate apoptosis if DNA cannot be repaired. Thus, p53 binds to multiple receptor proteins and stimulates several other regulatory genes, making it a nuclear transcription factor as well. Mutated p53 occurs in over half of all cancers and is generally associated with improved responsiveness to chemotherapy but worse overall prognosis.

P53 mutation is associated with eating a diet high in red meats, trans fats, and foods with a high glycemic load. It is functionally dependent on copper, so a good therapeutic goal is to keep copper in the lower twentieth percentile of normal lab range.

Natural Agents That May Inhibit p53 Mutation and/or Initiate Apoptosis via p53 Stimulation

- Apigenin from parsley
- Curcumin from turmeric
- EGCG from green tea
- Folate from leafy green vegetables
- Genistein from soy
- Ginsenosides from ginseng
- Luteolin
- Melatonin
- Milk thistle
- NAC (N-acetylcysteine)
- Oligomeric proanthocyandins (pycnogenol)
- Oridonin from *Rabdosia rubescens*
- Pawpaw seed
- Quercetin
- Resveratrol
- Selenomethionine
- Tocotrienols/vitamin E

Mutated p53 genes are hypomethylated in cancer cells, and methyl donors (folate, vitamin B12, SAMe) may reduce their overexpression. Retinoic acid, interferon alpha, and vitamin E may selectively disable mutated p53.

In addition to p53, both p21 and p27 genes are often underexpressed or mutated in many cancers. These genes code for proteins of the same name that control DNA repair and apoptosis in cell division, and mutation is associated with a worse prognosis.

Natural Agents That May Normalize p21 and p27

- Flavonoids including apigenin, genistein, EGCG
- Silymarin from milk thistle
- Sulforaphanes (broccoli or wasabi sprouts, cabbage family)
- Vitamins A, B3, B12, D3, E

HISTONE DEACETYLASE

Histones are components of DNA. Unwinding of DNA in preparation for cell division depends on histone deacetylase (HDAC), an enzyme that promotes many procancerous processes in the cell. Increased HDAC activity can be a driver of cancer, and inhibition of HDAC can reactivate silenced genes that control differentiation, cell cycling, apoptosis, angiogenesis, invasion, and metastases. Cancer cells appear to be more sensitive than normal cells to HDAC inhibitors, which disrupt the cell cycle and induce apoptosis via derepression of genes such as p21 and Bax.

Depakote (a valproic acid–based antiseizure medication) is now being investigated in cancer therapy for its HDAC-inhibition effects. If antiseizure medication is required for brain metastasis, this is one to consider for its secondary benefits.

Sulforaphane is an isothiocyanate found in cruciferous vegetables (cabbage family), most especially in sprouts (such as wasabi or broccoli sprouts). It acts as a potent inducer of phase 2 detoxification enzymes in the liver and also has epigenetic actions associated with inhibition of HDAC activity. In human subjects, a single ingestion of 68 grams of broccoli sprouts inhibited HDAC activity in circulating peripheral blood mononuclear cells 6 hours after consumption.

Natural Agents That May Modulate Histone Protein Deacetylation

- Butyrate (10 g/day)
- Baicalein from Baikal skullcap
- Biotin
- Curcumin from turmeric
- Diallyl disulfide from garlic
- Garcinol from *Garcinia cambogia*
- Grapeseed cyanidins
- Lipoic acid
- Apigenin from parsley
- Rosemary
- Silymarin from milk thistle
- Sulforaphane and other cruciferous isothiocyanates

Induce Differentiation in Cancer Cells

Cancer cells become progressively less differentiated than normal cells over time, indicating degeneration and loss of cell cycle control. In early stages it may be possible to reverse the damage and repair cellular processes. This is part of the mitochondrial rescue protocol and can also be useful in more progressed cancer that is still actively growing.

Natural Agents That May Induce Cell Differentiation

- Arctigenin from burdock root
- Berberine from Oregon grape or barberry
- Boswellic acid from Indian frankincense
- Bromelain from pineapple stem
- Butyrate (short-chain fatty acid)
- CAPE (caffeic acid phenethyl ester—a flavonoid complex from propolis)
- Emodin from rhubarb root, sheep sorrel root, and aloe
- Genistein from soy
- Inositol-6-phosphate (IP6)
- Melatonin
- Omega-3 fats from fish oil (EPA, DHA)
- Quercitin, apigenin, and luteolin (flavonoids)
- Resveratrol
- Vitamins A, D3

Induce Apoptosis

In Greek *apoptosis* means "to shed leaves." Just as that process is necessary for trees, so the elimination of unwanted or unnecessary cells is a requirement for healthy tissue function. Apoptosis, or programmed cell death, is the default position for normal healthy cells. Unless they receive regular and consistent signals from neighboring cells indicating "do not die," then normal healthy cells will self-destruct. Apoptosis is a controlled method of cell removal. In contrast to necrosis, where a large area dies off all at once, it affects scattered, individual cells, does not cause rupture of cell membranes, and does not induce inflammation. Leukocytes engulf and remove cells that have undergone normal apoptosis and no local cellular damage ensues.

In cancer cells, pro-cancer genes are mutated and generate antiapoptotic proteins that signal "do not die." In this way, cells gain some degree of longevity, if not immortality. "Do not die" signals may come from extracellular stimuli such as growth factors and hormones, or they may be self-induced through mutations of normal apoptosis regulators.

Natural Agents That May Promote Apoptosis

- Artemisinin from annual wormwood
- Baicalein from Baikal skullcap
- Berberine from barberry or Oregon grape
- Betulinic acid from chaga mushroom
- Boswellic acid from Indian frankincense
- CAPE from propolis
- Curcumin from turmeric
- EGCG and other catechins from green tea
- Garlic
- Genistein from soy
- Ginger
- I3C
- IP6
- Lemongrass and limonene
- Luteolin
- Melatonin
- Mistletoe
- Parthenolides from feverfew
- Quercetin
- R+ lipoic acid
- Reishi mushroom
- Resveratrol
- Taheebo
- Selenium
- Vitamins A, C, D3, E

Cancer cells resist apoptosis through overexpression of oncogenic genes such as c-Myc, which enhances cellular proliferation and suppresses p53, and antiapoptotic proteins such as Bcl-2 and survivin, as well as by downregulating proapoptotic proteins (caspases, Bad, Bax, etc.).

Tumor suppressive genes that function in healthy cells may mutate in cancer cells and no longer be able to carry out their intended functions. For example, Bcl-2 protein is normally found in the mitochondrial membrane, where it induces and regulates apoptosis, but mutation renders it unable to do so. High levels of mutated Bcl-2 are associated with most types of human cancer, and it appears to be a major contributor to both inherent and acquired resistance to current anticancer treatments. It can be tested in the tissue, and mutated Bcl-2 indicates an overall worse prognosis.

Natural Agents That May Reduce Mutated Tumor Suppressor Bcl-2 Gene Expression

- 3,3'-diindolylmethane (DIM)
- 6-gingerol from ginger
- Baicalein from Baikal skullcap
- Beta-lapachone from taheebo

- Beta-sitosterol, an adaptogenic dietary phytosterol
- Betulinic acid from chaga mushroom and birch
- Capsaicin from cayenne
- Carnosol from rosemary
- Echinocystic acid (EA) from Korean ginseng
- Eicosapentaenoic acid (EPA) from fish oil
- Forskolin from coleus
- Grapeseed extract
- Green tea extract (EGCG)
- Protocatechuic acid (PCA), a phenolic from hibiscus flower
- Lectin from mistletoe
- Parthenolide from feverfew
- Theophylline from green tea
- Turmeric

Modulate Growth Factors

Cancer cells quickly mutate to produce proteins called growth factors, and they also overexpress the cell surface receptors that respond to the growth factors and promote mitosis and malignant cell behaviors, thus creating a self-stimulating cycle. Some of these growth factors or their receptors can be tested for, but some or most of them are more or less always expected to be active, to a greater or lesser degree depending on the stage and grade of the cancer.

Growth Factors That Can Promote Cancer

- Epidermal growth factors (EGFs)
- Fibroblast growth factor (FGF)
- Insulin-like growth factors (IGFs)
- Platelet-derived growth factor (PDGF)
- Transforming growth factor-alpha (TGF-α)
- Transforming growth factor-beta (TGF-β)
- Vascular endothelial growth factor (VEGF)

Growth factors in interstitial fluids bind to receptor sites on the cell membranes, usually protein tyrosine kinase (PTK) receptors. They pass the signal from the extracellular domain through the transmembrane domain to the intracellular domain, where protein kinase C (PKC) receptors trigger the signal transduction phosphorylation cascade onward toward the nuclear membrane. Once in the nucleus, it activates transcription factors to initiate specific gene transcription and assembly of a new structural or functional protein.

By making the growth factors, and by overexpressing the receptor sites for them, cancer becomes an autotroph, supporting its own nutrition. It is these growth factors and their resulting oncogenic pathways that are mostly targeted by the new generation of cancer drugs, the immunotherapies that use targeted monoclonal antibodies and small molecules to knock out specific receptors.

SIGNAL TRANSDUCTION AND SIGNAL TRANSCRIPTION

Signal transduction requires a precisely calibrated, step-wise progression catalyzed and controlled by kinase enzymes. In many cases the receptor itself is an enzyme. This literally means it moves (kinesis or kinetic), and this spatial change triggers the next enzyme in the cascade. The PTK receptor type is predominant, and there is a whole family of these coded for by specific oncogenes. The extracellular portion of the PTK is activated by a growth factor, hormone, or other stimulating agent (the ligand), and this activates the intracellular portion to initiate phosphorylation or the process of signal transduction to carry the message across the cytoplasm to the nucleus.

This is all perfectly normal and natural; cells need a means of receiving messages from the environment and responding to them, and the receptor site and transduction pathways are how that is done. So far, so good. However, abnormally high PTK activity, whether from overly sensitive receptors or from excessive ligand binding, is a procancerous event, and proliferation, migration, and angiogenesis can be limited by using PTK inhibitors.

Because multiple protein kinase enzyme systems coexist and can be overexpressed or inhibited by multiple therapeutic agents, a broad-based, multifaceted approach is recommended. Natural therapeutic agents, such as polyphenols and especially flavonoids, are able to elicit such widespread and diverse results because they are inhibitors of multiple enzyme receptor and transduction systems.

Natural Agents That May Inhibit PTK or PKC Receptors

- Caffeic acid phenethyl ester (CAPE) from propolis
- Catechins from green tea, especially EGCG
- Curcumin from turmeric
- Emodin from rhubarb or sheep sorrel: use Essiac tea formula
- Flavonoids including apigenin, luteolin, quercetin, genistein
- Forskolin from coleus
- Hypericin (light activated) from St. John's wort
- Licorice
- Milk thistle
- Omega-3 fatty acids
- Parthenolide from feverfew
- Pomegranate
- Reishi mushroom
- Resveratrol
- Selenium
- Ursolic acid—triterpene from rosemary and tulsi
- Vitamin E (mixed tocopherols and tocotrienols)

EPIDERMAL GROWTH FACTOR 1

Also known as HER1 or ErbB1, this promotes cell proliferation, mobility, invasion, and metastases. High HER1 expression correlates with poor prognosis, notably in non–small cell lung cancer (NSCLC); prostate, brain, renal, pancreatic, and breast cancers; squamous cell carcinomas of the head and neck; and colon solid tumors. This receptor site is targeted by the first-generation monoclonal antibody drugs erlotinib (Tarceva) and gefitinib (Iressa), as well as the newer-generation immunotherapy cetuximab (Erbitux).

A papulo-pustular skin rash occurs in approximately two-thirds of patients treated with anti-EGFR drugs because skin cells also produce and respond to epidermal growth factors and inhibiting them means skin can no longer properly maintain itself and loses integrity. Although frequently tolerable and manageable, approximately 10 percent of patients require dose interruption and/or dose reduction due to severe rash. There is a strong association of cutaneous toxicity with favorable clinical outcomes to EGFR inhibitors, and this makes achievement of rash desirable.

EPIDERMAL GROWTH FACTOR 2 (HER2/NEU)

This tyrosine kinase receptor initiates cell proliferation and regulates angiogenesis; it may be mutated in up to 30 percent of breast cancers and in several other cancers, including NSCLC and ovarian, prostate, and gastric cancers. Overexpression correlates to poor prognosis. Trastuzumab (Herceptin) is a first-generation monoclonal antibody drug that acts as an antagonist for this receptor and is approved for HER2/neu-positive breast cancer in women where conventional chemotherapy has failed, or as an adjunct to conventional chemotherapy.

Natural Agents That Downregulate Epidermal Growth Factor 1 or 2

- Cacao procyanidins
- Curcumin from turmeric
- Cysteine (whey)
- EGCG from green tea
- Emodin from rhubarb or sheep sorrel
- Genistein from soy
- Grapeseed extract
- Honokiol from magnolia
- Licorice
- Lycopene from tomato
- NAC (N-acetylcysteine)
- Oleic acid from olives
- Quercetin
- Resveratrol
- Retinols
- Selenium
- Silibinin from milk thistle
- Thymoquinone from nigella
- Vitamin D3

Synergists and Potentiators of Trastuzumab

- High-dose turmeric and green tea
- DIM, I3C, sulforaphanes
- Vitamin D3
- Indian frankincense/boswellia (AKBA)
- EPA, DHA, and GLA
- Olives and olive oil

TRANSFORMING GROWTH FACTOR-BETA (TGF-β)

TGF-β is a multifunctional protein that controls proliferation and differentiation. It can stimulate or inhibit depending on the cell type and conditions. It is usually inhibitory in early-stage cancer, then cells develop resistance to TGF-β as cancer advances. In late-stage cancer, it can promote invasion and metastasis, partly through its immunosuppressive effects.

Natural Agents That May Inhibit Transforming Growth Factor-Beta*

- Berberine
- Boswellic acids from Indian frankincense (AKBA)
- CAPE from propolis
- Curcumin from turmeric
- Eicosapentaenoic acid (EPA)
- Flavonoids—luteolin, apigenin, genistein, quercetin, EGCG
- Garlic

- Ginkgo
- Resveratrol
- Selenium
- St. John's wort
- Vitamins A, C, D3, E

*Possibly most useful in inhibiting this pathway in stage 3 and 4 cancers. May be less useful in early-stage or well-differentiated cancer.

- Luteolin
- Milk thistle
- Oligomeric proanthocyanidins (OPCs) from grapeseed extract
- Mistletoe
- Pacific yew
- Pomegranate
- Resveratrol from Japanese knotweed

VASCULAR ENDOTHELIAL GROWTH FACTOR (VEGF)

VEGF induces endothelial proliferation and vascular permeability and is involved in angiogenesis. It is synergistic with platelet-derived growth factor (PDGF), is essential for wound healing, and is produced by epithelial cells, macrophages, and smooth muscle cells. VEGF stimulates the proliferation and migration of endothelial cells that initiate new blood vessel formation and induces the expression of metalloproteinases to weaken connective tissue and cell-adhesion molecules. The production of VEGF is considered essential for most cancer cell migration and for angiogenesis. A high VEGF expression level is associated with a worse outcome in a wide array of malignancies.

Natural Agents That May Inhibit Vascular Endothelial Growth Factor

- Baicalein from Baikal skullcap
- Cinnamon
- Annual wormwood
- Curcumin from turmeric
- Dong quai
- EGCG from green tea
- Genistein from soy
- Ginkgo
- Honokiol from magnolia seed cones
- I3C

Interestingly, psychosocial factors can also influence VEGF and cancer promotion. Greater support from friends and neighbors of presurgical patients with ovarian carcinoma appears to be associated with reduced level of VEGF and possibly less disease progression, according to researchers at the University of Iowa. The women with carcinoma who reported higher levels of social well-being had lower levels of VEGF. Women who reported greater helplessness or worthlessness had higher VEGF levels.

INSULIN-LIKE GROWTH FACTORS (IGFs)

In healthy individuals, these proteins are normally produced by the liver; they control repair of muscle and immune cells. However, tumors may also secrete IGFs for autostimulation of growth and for protection from apoptosis. The IGF proteins share many properties with insulin, except that they do not directly stimulate glucose uptake by cells unless blood sugar is unusually high. IGFs are important mitogenic factors involved in cell proliferation, differentiation, and metabolism.

The most metabolically significant insulin-like growth factor is type 1

(IGF-1), also called somatomedin C. It is encoded by the IGF-1 gene and acts as a hormone with several diverse effects. It is neurotrophic, nourishing and supporting of neurons. It induces protein synthesis in skeletal muscle and blocks muscle atrophy. It protects cartilage cells, activates osteoblasts, and is anabolic to bone. At high concentrations, it activates insulin receptors and complements the effects of insulin. All of these are useful and necessary functions for normal tissue repair, but they need to be controlled. If they are overactive, if IGF genes are mutated and the proteins are persistent, then cell derangement occurs.

Several components contribute to the cell-stimulating effects of insulin-like growth factor: the insulin-like growth factors themselves (IGF-1 and IGF-2), the type 1 and type 2 IGF receptors, and six known IGF binding proteins (IGFBP-1 through IGFBP-6) in blood. The IGFBPs can either augment or inhibit the bioavailability of free IGF ligand, hence controlling the interactions with the IGF receptors.

In plain English what this means is the more sugar you eat, the more easily sugar gets into the cancer cells and the better they are able to conduct glycolysis. There is a reason why natural health practitioners recommend very low-sugar and low-carbohydrate diets for cancer and why they talk about "starving the cancer." Cancer cells can use protein and fats for energy, like healthy cells, but it is not their preference and they readily mutate to produce more IGF-1 and less IGF-1 binding proteins to allow easier entry of sugar to the cells.

Natural Agents That May Inhibit Insulin-like Growth Factor 1 (IGF-1)

- Baicalein from Baikal skullcap
- EGCG from green tea
- Lycopene from tomato
- Silymarin from milk thistle (down-regulates IGF-1R)
- Vitamin D3
- Exercise, low-calorie diet, vegan diet, the hypoglycemic drug metformin

Natural Agents That May Induce IGF-1 Binding Protein Activity

Insulin-like growth factor 1 binding proteins inhibit the growth factor from binding to receptor sites and downregulate its effects.

- Dandelion, burdock, chicory: dried, roasted, and decocted to make a coffee substitute
- Flaxseed
- Oligomeric proanthocyanidins (OPCs)/pycnogenol
- R+ alpha-lipoic acid
- Vanadium
- Vitamin D3

MAMMALIAN TARGET OF RAPAMYCIN (MTOR)

mTOR is a multifunctional intracellular receptor site involved in cellular growth, proliferation, gene transcription, and cytoskeletal stability that ensures anabolic and catabolic cellular processes are tied to environmental cues, including nutrient levels and growth factors. It acts as a converging point for various signaling pathways and regulatory molecules relevant to hypoxia and angiogenesis, and it plays a significant role in integrating hypoxia and metabolite status of the cellular microenvironment with proangiogenic pathways. Upregulation of mTOR can drive cancer metabolism; this is a promising pathway for novel drug therapies.

The best-known inhibitor of mTOR is a drug called rapamycin, from which mTOR's name derives. Rapamycin was developed as an immunosuppressant, to block T cell activation, and has been licensed for use in autoimmune diseases and in preventing kidney graft rejection.

Rapamycin is generally not cytotoxic, acting instead as a cytostatic agent, and by downregulating immune responses, it can cause the upregulation of pro-oncogenic proteins and promote other tumorigenic events. These opposing effects make it challenging to predict clinical responses to rapamycin treatment. Newer-generation mTOR inhibitors include everolimus, temsirolimus, and ridaforolimus, but none of them are particularly successful in oncology yet.

MTOR AND IGF-1R

In the cytosol or intracellular domain, mTOR lies downstream of IGF-1 receptors. One key way in which sugar can drive cancer is that IGF-1 activates mTOR signaling, which causes anabolic cell responses. IGF-1 naturally occurs in the meat and milk of grass-fed herd animals but it is substantially higher if the animals are corn-fed. This obviously has implications in the modern diet where animals are kept in cages or feedlots and fed corn pellets, not eating their natural diet of grass. Compounding this IGF-1/mTOR upregulation from corn-fed meats or dairy is the lack of omega-3 fats and the overload of omega-6 fats in these foods. This will drive arachidonic acid pro-inflammatory pathways and cause oxidative stress.

Functional medicine doctors treating cancer may prescribe a diabetes drug called metformin that works to lower blood sugar by decreasing hepatic gluconeogenesis, by increasing the insulin sensitivity of body tissues, and by exerting an appetite suppressant effect, thereby reducing caloric intake. In 2017, it was the fourth most commonly prescribed medication in the US, with more than 78 million prescriptions and a wide margin of safety. It is originally derived from goat's rue, an herb still used very effectively by herbalists for lowering blood sugar.

Natural Agents That May Inhibit mTOR

- 3,3'-diindolylmethane (DIM)
- Curcumin from turmeric
- Diosgenin from wild yam
- EGCG from green tea
- Genistein from soy
- Pomegranate
- Resveratrol

RAS PROTEINS

Ras proteins, which are active at the onset of signal transduction, are often overexpressed in cancer cells. Ras proteins inside the cell membrane are activated by growth factor signaling (i.e., EGF, TGF-beta) and act as an on/off control point in growth signaling pathways that regulate genes that mediate cell proliferation.

Inhibition of mutated Ras gene expression and downregulation of Ras protein activity is a therapeutic goal. In a powerful example of positive feedback looping, PTK and PKC activation leads to downstream Ras protein activation, meaning that these mechanisms are mutually stimulating and rapidly become self-perpetuating. In light of these interactions, it is apparent that PTK and PKC inhibition also inhibits Ras protein expression. Ras proteins are critical initiators of many signal transduction pathways, and inhibiting this protein downregulates oncogenic behaviors.

Ras proteins are activated and made functional when they acquire a lipid tail and become embedded in the cell membrane. An effective way to inhibit Ras protein function is to inhibit production of the lipid tail. This lipid is an isoprene unit produced through the same pathway as cholesterol using a series of enzyme reactions initiated by the gatekeeper enzyme hydroxymethylglutaryl-coenzyme A reductase (HMGR). Inhibition of this enzyme by statin drugs lowers cholesterol but also leads to downregulation of Ras proteins through inhibiting formation of this lipid tail.

Another critical agent made by the same metabolic pathways as Ras is the laminin protein that forms the thin inner wall (lamina) of the nuclear membrane. Inhibiting this through HMGR depletion disrupts cancer cell reproductive ability. HMGR depletion also inhibits cancer by reducing cholesterol, which is required for building

METABOLISM OF FATS TO ANTICANCER TERPENES

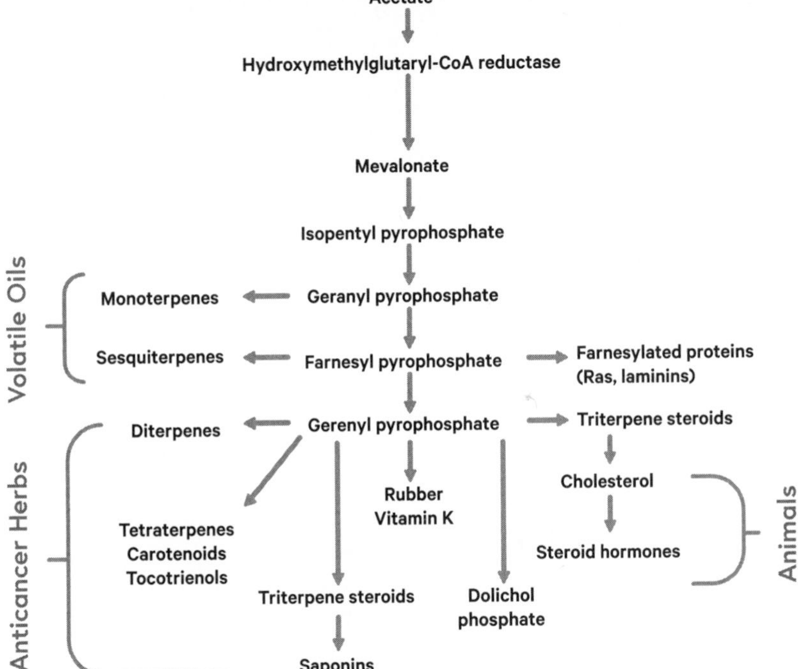

new cell walls. And one more important by-product of acetate metabolism is dolichol phosphate, which plays a critical role in the assembly of glycoproteins such as growth factors, enzymes, growth factor receptors, and membrane components. Synthesis of dolichol phosphate is required to enable transfer of insulin-like growth factor (IGF-1) receptors to the cell surface, where they can mediate IGF-1 activity. Inhibiting dolichol phosphate through HMGR depletion thus effectively disrupts cancer cell stimulus by IGF-1.

For all these reasons, the statin drugs are sometimes recommended as part of a cancer protocol. Unfortunately, they have a host of side effects and not everyone can use them. The supplement form of red yeast rice makes a mild form of a statin and works in the same manner to reduce cancer progression but without the side effects.

Natural Agents That May Downregulate Ras Proteins

- Garlic (organosulfur compounds—allicin, ajoene, diallyl disulfide)
- Lycopene from tomato
- Omega-3 fatty acids
- Parthenolide from feverfew
- Oridonin from *Rabdosia rubescens*
- Red yeast rice extract
- Sea buckthorn seed oil
- Taxanes from yew

Monoterpenes, such as those found in volatile oils, may inhibit HMGR at low doses and FTPase (farnesyl protein transferase, the enzyme that catalyzes farnesyl pyrophosphate to form Ras proteins) at higher doses and interfere with synthesis of IGF-1 receptors. Examples include:

- D-limonene, from orange and/or other citrus oils, found in the outer skin of the fruit
- Geraniol, found in the essential oils of rose geranium and lemongrass
- Perillyl alcohol, found in the essential oils of lavender and other plants

Stabilize Transcription Factors

Transcription factors are proteins that bind to the regulatory portion of a gene and initiate gene transcription (gene copying). They govern which portions of the DNA helix will unwind and how many copies will be made. They regulate inflammation, angiogenesis, cell invasion, and apoptosis. Their availability is determined by specific gene expression; thus, oncogenes may over- or underexpress certain transcription factors. Their activation is dependent on signal transduction of a message sent by a growth factor or other ligand docking in a cell surface receptor, a message received by cell-to-cell communication or by cell damage. Important pro-oncogenic transcription factors include activator protein 1 (AP-1), nuclear factor-kappa B (NF-κB), and nuclear factor erythroid 2-related factor 2 (NRF2).

The ability of NF-κB and AP-1 to bind to DNA and initiate gene transcription is controlled in part through redox status. An oxidative environment is required in the cytosol for NF-κB to be activated, but a reducing environment is required in the nucleus for NF-κB to bind to DNA. Thus the fluctuations of pH observed in healthy cells may serve a purpose in permitting and inhibiting different metabolic processes at different times. Overall, it is observed that antioxidants tend to inhibit NF-κB and AP-1 activation and thus are anticancerous. Hypoxia, as is seen in malignant tumors and in inflammation and wound healing, tends to promote AP-1 activation. In compensatory reoxygenation, free radicals are produced and NF-κB is stimulated.

NUCLEAR FACTOR-KAPPA B (NF-κB)

In a healthy cell, inflammation serves to permit and promote healing, and when resolution of the injury is reached it will switch off. In cancer cells, upregulation leads to loss of this control and chronic inflammation. Cancer cells thrive in the hypoxic, acidic environment generated by low levels of inflammation. Nuclear factor-kappa B (NF-κB) is actually a family of transcription factors that have crucial roles in inflammation, immunity, cell proliferation, and apoptosis. Activated NF-κB leads to inflammatory responses and cell proliferation. This response is mostly mediated by tumor necrosis factor (TNF)—an immune protein that in small amounts promotes angiogenesis but in higher amounts is toxic to cancer cells—as well as by collagenases, cell adhesion molecules (CAMs), and interleukins. NF-κB is also mediated through redox regulation.

ACTIVATOR PROTEIN 1 (AP-1)

AP-1 stimulates the expression of genes that drive the cell cycle. AP-1 works in direct relationship with NF-κB in controlling and regulating immune responses and is subject to most of the same promoting and inhibiting influences. AP-1 also promotes the transition of tumor cells from an epithelial to mesenchymal morphology, which is one of the early steps in tumor metastasis.

Natural Agents That May Inhibit AP-1 and/or NF-κB

- 6-gingerol from ginger
- Alpha-lipoic acid
- Artemisinin from annual wormwood
- Curcumin from turmeric
- Emodin from rhubarb and sheep sorrel
- Flavonoids—apigenin, CAPE, genistein, luteolin, EGCG, quercetin
- Isothiocyanates from the cabbage family
- Leukotriene inhibitors (fish oil and essential fatty acids)
- Melatonin
- (NAC) N-acetylcysteine
- Parthenolide from feverfew
- Proanthocyanidins
- Resveratrol
- Selenium
- Thymoquinone from nigella
- Ursolic acid
- Vitamins C, E succinate

NUCLEAR FACTOR ERYTHROID 2-RELATED FACTOR 2 (NRF2)

NRF2 is a transcription factor that integrates cellular stress signals and responds by switching on or off other transcription factors to fine-tune cellular responses to stressors or to gene copying signals, like a master switch. NRF2 triggers early responses against any deviations in redox metabolism by regulating the expression of antioxidant proteins, which protect against oxidative damage triggered by injury and inflammation. There are more than 100 genes regulated by NRF2. In healthy cells, potentially toxic molecules—such as reactive oxygen species (like hydrogen peroxide) and reactive nitrogen species (like nitric oxide)—are tightly controlled using NRF2. For this reason, activation of NRF2 is a promising pharmacological approach for chronic diseases that are associated with marked oxidative stress and inflammation—neurodegenerative, cardiovascular, and metabolic diseases—as well as cancer.

Natural Agents That May Induce NRF2

These are most useful in early-stage or well-differentiated cancer, as part of the mitochondrial rescue plan.

- Sulforaphane from cruciferous vegetables
- Curcumin from turmeric
- Resveratrol
- Quercetin
- Genistein from soy
- Andrographolide from andrographis

Due to its ability to cross the blood-brain barrier, sulforaphane protects against neurodegenerative disorders and against hypoxic-ischemic injury in part by upregulating NRF2 in neural tissues. In animal studies, sulforaphane reduced cognitive impairment in Alzheimer's disease and protected dopaminergic cells from neurotoxins in Parkinson's disease. Neurodegenerative diseases may be caused or induced by exposure to environmental toxins, and NRF2 plays a major role here through its potent induction of the intracellular antioxidant glutathione, as well as more than 20 other cytoprotective enzymes.

In the case of cancer, it is more complicated. Because NRF2 promotes cell survival under stress, it is reasonable to expect that increased NRF2 activity could be tumor promoting and protective for cancer cells. Indeed, mutations that occur in the gene coding for this transcription factor tend to enhance NRF2 activity and are generally associated with resistance to standard chemotherapy and poor survival from cancer. In these cases NRF2 inhibition is required to reduce the survival and proliferative advantage of cancer cells and also sensitize tumors to chemotherapy and radiotherapy. It is also significant that common oncogenes, such as KRAS, BRAF, and MYC, often mutated early in cancer cells, increase the transcription and activity of NRF2, resulting in an increase in cytoprotective activity in the cell and a decrease in reactive oxygen species (ROS) levels. Thus, oncogenes may promote tumorigenesis in part through creation of a more favorable intracellular environment by NRF2 or the survival of tumor cells.

Overall, studies suggest a protective role of NRF2 in the early stages of cancer, but in advanced stages, NRF2 overexpression helps cancer cells adapt and thrive. Dysplastic but not yet malignant cells are under tight controls in their microenvironment and have not yet reached a level of DNA damage that makes them autonomous. Therefore, enhancing NRF2 activity to lessen inflammatory and oxidative or mutagenic stress appears to be beneficial during premalignant states to normalize redox reactions in the cell and suppress carcinogenic changes. However, if cancer progresses, then NRF2 can cause malignant cancer cells to become more oxidized and resistant to treatment. NRF2 inhibitors can reduce the survival and proliferative advantage of cancer cells and also sensitize tumors to chemo- and radiotherapy.

Natural Agents That May Inhibit NRF2

These may be more effective as part of a strategy for later in the treatment planning or in high-grade (poorly differentiated) cancer.

- High-dose polyphenols—quercetin, EGCG, resveratrol, curcumin, apigenin, chrysin, luteolin, wogonin
- Naphthaquinones (such as plumbagin)
- Sesquiterpenes (such as parthenolide)

Thus it becomes apparent that NRF2 activation/inhibition needs to be carefully calibrated and balanced. Interestingly, both intermittent fasting and aerobic exercise, which are recommended as cancer-prevention strategies, serve to modulate and regulate NRF2 genes.

Various drugs (including steroids) and several natural agents (including the flavonoids luteolin and wogonin) have shown promise to inhibit NRF2 and sensitize cells to chemotherapy. However, none are target specific, and clinical implications are undetermined. Due to insufficient and incomplete data available, prudence suggests promotion of NRF2 genes and transcription activity in early-stage cancer, but withholding these agents during active chemotherapy, at least 1 or 2 days on either side of treatment—effectively pulse dosing them through the active chemotherapy stage and then increasing doses to a daily intake after chemotherapy is completed.

PEROXISOME PROLIFERATOR-ACTIVATED RECEPTORS (PPARS, INCLUDING ALPHA, GAMMA, AND DELTA TYPES)

PPARs are nuclear transcription factors that play an important role in the regulation of lipid and energy metabolism and immunity. Agonists of PPAR-γ are thus used to manage hyperglycemia associated with metabolic syndrome and type 2 diabetes. PPAR is a pleiotropic metabolism regulator, modulating innate immunity in various metabolic diseases. PPAR-α has an anti-inflammatory effect by activation of leukotriene B4. PPAR agonists are used to treat a number of conditions, such as dyslipidemia, type 2 diabetes, cardiovascular diseases, obesity, cancer, and other metabolic diseases.

Activation of PPARs by a ligand can suppress tumors by inducing apoptosis and generating antiproliferative actions in various cancer cell lines. For example, thymoquinone from nigella can activate and upregulate PPAR-γ while simultaneously downregulating Bcl-2 and Bcl genes involved in cell death and survival mechanisms in breast cancer cells.

Agonists of PPAR-α may restrict glycolysis and increase the production of ROS, causing oxidative stress in cancer cell mitochondria. This may induce cell cycle arrest, inhibit tumor growth, and resist metastasis.

Natural Agents That May Modulate PPARs

- Bitter melon
- Cannabis
- Grapes and wine
- EGCG from green tea
- Ginger
- Honokiol from magnolia
- Astragalus
- Thymoquinone from nigella
- Isoflavones from soy
- Oregano
- Rosemary
- Sage
- Thyme

Support the Immune System

Cancer subverts the immune system to its advantage, preventing recognition of faulty cells, promoting inflammation, and inhibiting healing. Unfortunately, so many of the conventional cancer treatments are myelosuppressive, and the bone marrow failure means neutropenia (white cell deficiency) and further immune weakness. Natural agents are used to stabilize bone marrow, to increase white cell count, and to normalize and renew immune functions.

Natural Agents That Provide Nonspecific Immune Support

- Arabinogalactans (polysaccharides from larch)
- Astragalus
- Bromelain
- Eleuthero
- Ginseng
- Glutamine
- Glutathione-sparing antioxidants (sulfur, silbinin and milk thistle, cruciferous vegetables)
- Melatonin
- Reishi, shiitake, cordyceps, and other mushrooms
- Selenium

Neutropenia is also an indication to use the nutritive and blood-building soups suggested in Chapter 5 for managing chemotherapy.

Flavonoids* as Immunomodulating Agents

- Inhibit eicosanoid-mediated inflammation
- Inhibit histamine-induced inflammation
- Inhibit PTK and PKC activity
- Inhibit cell motility

*Such as quercetin, genistein, and apigenin

Omega-3 Fats* as Immunomodulating Agents

- Reduce PGE2 and 4-series leukotrienes
- Reduce pro-inflammatory cytokines such as IL-1, IL-6, and TNF
- Modify gene expression leading to reduced expression of T cell stimulatory molecules

- Increase TGF-β and Fas membrane receptors that induce apoptosis in immune cells
- Inhibit PKC activity
- Increase plasma membrane fluidity
- Reduce ability of immune cells to present antigens to T cells and reduce ability of T cells to respond to antigen presentation

*Such as EPA and DHA

Reduce Inflammation and Normalize Prostaglandin and Leukotriene Activity

Inflammation is a nonspecific defensive response of the body to any tissue damage. It may be caused by pathogens, abrasions, chemical irritations, distortion or disturbances of cells, and extreme temperatures. Any injury to the body will immediately trigger a specific series of responses and a release of agents that induce immune responses at the site of damage:

- **Histamine.** This is released by neutrophils, macrophages, and mast cells.
- **Prostaglandins.** These are released by damaged cells; they intensify the effects of histamine and kinins.
- **Leukotrienes.** These inflammatory agents, produced by basophils and mast cells, help phagocytes adhere to pathogens.
- **Complement factor.** This protein of the immune system stimulates histamine release, attracts neutrophils, promotes phagocytosis, and destroys bacteria.

All of these immune fractions cause vasodilation and increased permeability, which allows for:

- **Fibrin formation.** The fibrinogen molecule is a soluble, large, and complex plasma glycoprotein that is converted by thrombin into fibrin during blood clot formation.
- **Phagocyte migration.** This is the margination and diapedesis or movement of white blood cells from vessels to tissues.
- **Pus or inflammatory exudate.** This forms as damaged cells and spent neutrophils die off.

Inflammation is characterized by the so-called cardinal symptoms of redness, swelling, heat, and pain. These are all necessary and useful to promote healing and resolution, but if they persist and become chronic they will lead to excessive production of pro-inflammatory mediators such as IL-1β, IL-6, TNF-α, and prostaglandin E2 (PGE2), promoting an inflammatory reaction cascade that becomes self-perpetuating.

Cancer is characterized by many of the same cell behaviors as chronic inflammation, and they share multiple signaling pathways. Several cancers are known to be preceded by chronic inflammation; for example, pancreatitis can lead to pancreatic cancer, and hepatitis C can lead to liver cancer.

Prostaglandins are synthesized under the control of cyclooxygenase-2 (COX-2), which should not be detectable in most normal tissues. It is induced

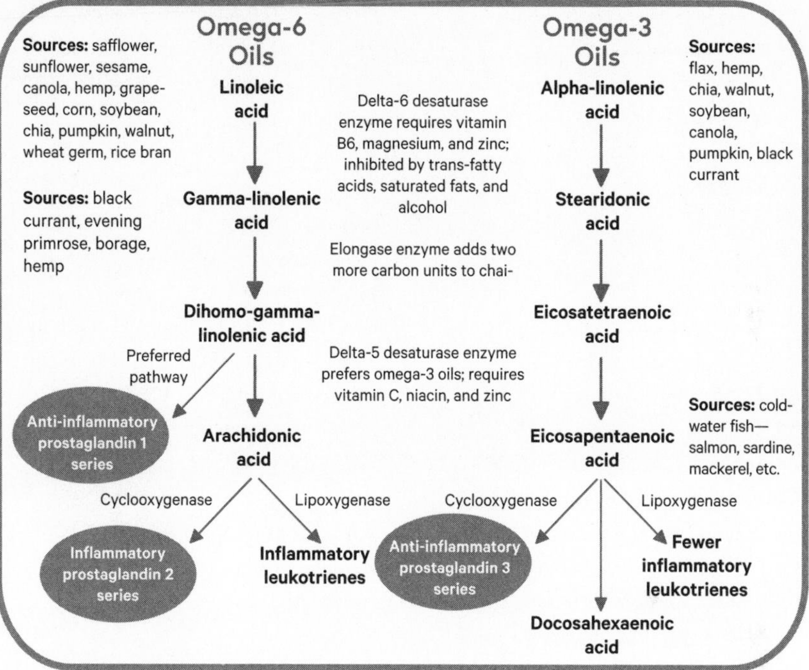

by stressors including inflammatory cytokines and growth factors, including transforming growth factor-beta (TGF-β) and beta-fibroblast growth factor (β-FGF), and prolonged activation of COX-2 is associated with carcinogenesis. In cancer, mutation of the transcription factors AP-1 and NF-κB may induce the activation of COX and promote inflammation. Modulation of COX-2 expression affects tumor growth, and treatment with COX-2 inhibitors, such as celecoxib or curcumin, reduces tumor growth. The delicate balance between activation of oncogenes and the inactivation of tumor suppressor genes, as well as expression of pro-inflammatory cytokines, can modulate the expression of COX-2 in tumors. A further complication is that conventional cancer therapies such as radiation, surgery, and chemotherapy can induce COX-2 and prostaglandin biosynthesis.

Cancer creates and thrives in an inflammatory environment—the low pH favors glycolysis and angiogenesis, and healing is delayed or impeded. The clinical aim is to modulate and regulate so that inflammation progresses in a controlled manner to allow resolution and repair.

Natural Agents That May Modulate Inflammation

- Bupleurum
- Evening primrose oil
- Ginger
- Indian frankincense
- Licorice

- Meadowsweet
- Omega-3 fish oil
- Rosemary
- Sarsaparilla
- Spearmint
- Turmeric
- Wild yam
- Willow
- Yucca

Curcumin has been shown to possess particular COX-2-inhibiting activity through the suppression of NF-κB. Thus, curcumin will be useful in the treatment of several cancers targeting angiogenesis since COX-2 expression stimulates angiogenesis. COX-2 inhibitors are particularly useful in the treatment of advanced breast cancers through inhibition not only of HER2/neu activity but also of aromatase activity.

TOLL-LIKE RECEPTORS (TLRS)

TLRs are a family of transmembrane receptors (proteins that cross or span the cell membrane) that recognize and respond to a broad range of microbial pathogens, including bacteria and viruses. They enable innate immunity (phagocytes, such as neutrophils, macrophages, and dendritic cells) by helping immune cells discriminate between pathogens and self. TLRs activate several downstream enzymes and proteins that lead to the synthesis of inflammatory cytokines, chemokines, matrix metalloproteinases, and other pro-oncogenic intracellular enzymes.

The expression of TLRs has been observed in many tumors, and their stimulation may result in tumor progression or regression, depending on the TLR and tumor type. Initially, TLR stimulation will induce immune responses and may be helpful. In sustained injury, however, they can promote chronic inflammation. This may cause TLRs on the cell surface to induce transcription factors, such as NF-κB and AP-1, that can drive oncogenic pathways.

There is now substantial evidence for the benefit of TLR agonists in early-stage cancer treatment, and several agents have been approved, such as BCG (bacillus Calmette-Guérin, an attenuated bacterial immunotherapy), MPL (monophosphoryl lipid A), and imiquimod (used for basal cell carcinoma).

TLRS, CHRONIC INFLAMMATION, AND OBESITY

The classic inflammatory response is an acute reaction to injury or infection and should progress fairly rapidly to resolution and restoration of function. However, the inflammatory process in obese individuals and in those with metabolic syndrome tends to be systemic, of low intensity, and more likely to become chronic. In particular, the toll-like receptor 4 (TLR4) signaling pathway is one of the main triggers of the obesity-induced inflammatory response and of the inflammatory processes in ischemia/reperfusion injury, neuropathic pain, neurodegenerative diseases, and cancer.

Antagonizing or inhibiting toll-like receptors lessens immune system stimulation and reduces immune activation and inflammation in later-stage cancers.

Natural Agents with TLR4 Antagonist Activity

- Celastrol, a pentacyclic triterpenoid from *Tripterygium wilfordii* (an herb used in TCM)
- Curcumin from turmeric
- Omega-3 fats (EPA, DHA)
- Ginsenosides from ginseng
- Sulforaphane and iberin from cruciferous vegetables
- Xanthohumol flavonoid from hops

Immune Evasion

The immune system attempts to detect and destroy malignant cells, and cancer cells have evolved various means of evading detection and disrupting normal immune responses and counterresponses, allowing the promotion and progression of the cancer.

One way in which cancer evades immune detection is by maintaining a relatively low pH in the tumor microenvironment, which suppresses anticancer immune responses. Tumors achieve this by regulating lactic acid secretion via modification of glucose/glutamine metabolisms and by promoting glycolytic shift. Cancer-generated lactic acid could thus be viewed as a critical, immunosuppressive metabolite in the tumor microenvironment, rather than simply a "waste product," and efforts should be made to clear it away through circulation and lymph drainage.

To evade immune surveillance, cancer cells may produce excessive amounts of immunosuppressive agents like PGE2 or immunosuppressive cytokines like TGF-β and IL-10.

Natural Agents That May Regulate Immunosuppression

- PSK and other mushroom-derived polysaccharides
- Proanthocyanidins
- Omega-3 fatty acids
- Monoterpenes like limonene
- Vitamin E
- Protein kinase inhibitors like genistein can block IL-10 signaling

The fibrin stroma around a malignant tumor may assist tumor progression by providing a physical support, by shielding it from immune attack, and by secreting fibrin degradation products that are angiogenic. Thus fibrinolytic agents may inhibit tumor progression but may also promote angiogenesis through provision of more even fibrin degradation by-products. Orally administered natural fibrinolytic agents, such as garlic, as well as proteolytic enzymes like bromelain, serrapeptase, and nattokinase appear to inhibit metastases into solid tumors without promoting angiogenesis.

Summary of the Effects of Proteolytic Enzymes on the Immune System*

IMMUNOSUPPRESSIVE

- Digestion of surface proteins
- Increased shedding of TNF receptors

IMMUNOSTIMULATING

- Increased antigen presentation by macrophages to increase T cell activation
- Direct stimulation of macrophage activity
- Increased cytokine production

- Digestion of immune complexes allows improved macrophage functioning overall
- Increased fibrinolysis improves circulation for immune cell delivery to affected parts

BOTH IMMUNOSUPPRESSIVE AND IMMUNOSTIMULATING

- Increased alpha-2 macroglobulin

*Boik, 2001

Strengthen Connective Tissue, Promote Cell-to-Cell Communication

Cells of similar form and function are held together as organs and tissues, packed in close proximity and communicating one with another as a coordinated whole. This is made possible by the extracellular matrix (ECM) in which they are embedded, which is, in effect, an entire, interconnected and body-wide communication and control system.

ECM is a complex of gelatinous connective tissue that surrounds all cells and through which all the electrolytes, metabolites, hormones, growth factors, enzymes, dissolved gases, trace elements, carbohydrates, fats, and proteins must filter in their passage to and from the cells. In it are also stored many metabolic compounds, including certain growth factors. It is made of proteoglycans and glycosaminoglycans (GAGs)—long, repeated sugar chains with embedded elastic, reticulin, and collagen fibers. The production and maintenance of the ECM is dynamic and the entire ECM of the body is replaced almost monthly. Since the GAGs are cellular products, it is through regulation of their production that cells regulate the structure and hence the function of the ECM. Cancer cells tend to manufacture hyposulfated and hence dysfunctional GAGs, creating a poorly constructed ECM with low integrity and favorable to migration and invasion of cancer cells.

TUMOR MICROENVIRONMENT (TME) AND THE ECM

Solid tumors are complex organlike structures that consist not only of tumor cells but also of vasculature, ECM, stromal, and immune cells. Often, this tumor microenvironment (TME) comprises the larger part of the overall tumor mass, and like the other components of the TME, the ECM in solid tumors differs significantly from that in normal organs.

Signaling between cells, transport mechanisms, metabolic functions, oxygenation, and immunomodulation are strongly affected by the ECM. Exerting regulatory control, the ECM not only influences invasion and growth of the tumor but also its response to therapy.

Protease enzymes that govern the relative fluidity of the ECM include collagenases and elastase, as well as enzymes that stimulate inflammation, cell proliferation, invasion, metastases, and angiogenesis. Hyaluronidase regulates hyaluronic acid levels and is quickly upregulated in cancer to facilitate breakdown of connective tissue and easier spread of cancer. In cancer, hyaluronidase is produced on the edges of tumors and partially "digests" ECM to allow easier cancer penetration and spread. One of the key values of echinacea in cancer is to impair hyaluronidase activity and slow the cancer spread through tissues.

A major group of collagenases that are active in cancer are the matrix metalloproteinases (MMPs). These are a family of at least 15 zinc-dependent enzymes that degrade the ECM. Curcumin from turmeric and EGCG from green tea can inhibit an MMP enzyme that is critical in angiogenesis. By stabilizing the ECM, it inhibits the stimulatory effects of growth factors stored in the ground substance matrix.

Aggressive or advanced cancers produce a loose vascular meshwork via MMP-2-mediated degradation of the laminins that can be inhibited by curcumin, resveratrol, and green tea. Heparanases break down heparan sulfate, a component of the ground substance of the ECM. Sulfated polysaccharides—including dextran sulfate and xylan sulfate, heparin (the drug), and fucoidin from sargassum seaweed—can inhibit the enzyme and thus inhibit invasion and metastases.

Natural Compounds That May Inhibit ECM Degradation

- Aescin from horse chestnut
- Apigenin and luteolin (flavones)
- Bilberry
- Bioflavonoids
- Boswellic acids
- Butcher's broom
- Chamomile
- Echinacea
- Fucoidin from kelp
- Glucosamine sulfate and other GAGs from bovine cartilage
- Gotu kola
- Passionflower
- Proanthocyanidins
- Propolis and caffeic acid phenethyl ester (CAPE)
- Resveratrol

Natural Compounds That May Inhibit Collagenase

- Curcumin
- EGCG from green tea
- Emodin
- EPA from fish oil
- Genistein
- Gotu kola
- Luteolin
- Proanthocyanidins and anthocyanidins
- Polysaccharide K (PSK) and other mushroom polysaccharides
- Quercetin
- Vitamins A, C

FIBROBLAST GROWTH FACTOR (FGF)

This is a family of growth factors stored in the ECM. Degradation of the ECM by cancer enzymes (such as hyaluronidase) releases the growth factor, and it contributes to proliferation and angiogenesis.

Natural Agents That May Stabilize Connective Tissue and Bind FGF

- Butcher's broom
- Echinacea
- Glycosaminoglycans
- Gotu kola
- Horse chestnut
- Horsetail

- Hyaluronic acid
- MSM
- Shark cartilage

GAP JUNCTIONS

These are openings between cells that allow direct exchange of molecules and ions. They contain special proteins called connexins that span the cell membrane and are coded for by a family of tumor-suppressing connexin genes that are mutated early in the development of cancer. Many tumor-promoting agents disrupt normal gap junction activity.

Natural Compounds That May Promote Normal Gap Junction Activity

- Apigenin
- Beta-carotene
- CAPE
- Genistein
- Glutathione
- Green tea
- Lycopene
- Resveratrol
- Selenium
- Vitamins A, C, D, E

CELL ADHESION MOLECULES

In healthy tissue, cells do not exist in isolation but communicate constantly among themselves to control and regulate metabolic activities, cell cycling, and apoptosis. Cell-to-cell communication occurs through glycoproteins called cell adhesion molecules (CAMs) on the outside of cells and through gap junctions or portals between cells that are spanned by connexin proteins, which allow a range of regulatory functions:

- Control intracellular and cell-to-cell communication
- Regulate organ architecture
- Regulate cell migration
- Regulate mitosis and apoptosis
- Regulate immune function

There are hundreds of CAMs on a cell, interlocking and enmeshing each cell with all the others in a tissue. Signals generated by CAMs travel to the nucleus and messages from the nucleus influencing CAM behavior travel back. In this way PTK, PKC, and other proteins that carry out that signal transduction can affect CAM function and activity. Cancer cells fail to maintain these intercellular connections and hence fail to receive contact inhibition signals and other regulatory signals from adjoining cells, so that a cancer cell can operate independently without constraint.

It is an abnormal level of epCAM (epithelial cell adhesion molecules) on cancer cells that is actually measured when doing blood work to assess for circulating tumor cells.

Natural Agents That May Normalize Cell Adhesion Functions

- Connective tissue herbal tonics, such as plantain or oat straw
- GAGs (glucosaminoglycans)
- Hyaluronic acid
- MCP (modified citrus pectin)
- MSM (methylsulfonylmethane)
- NAG (N-acetylglucosamine)
- Steroids and saponins (horse chestnut, horsetail, butcher's broom, gotu kola)
- Tangeritin (monoterpene in tangerine essential oil)

Inhibit Invasion and Metastasis

Metastasis is the movement of malignant cells from a primary tumor to a distant site, where they form a colony that becomes a new tumor. Metastatic cells travel through blood and lymphatic vessels, and the cells must penetrate the basement membrane and endothelial lining of the blood vessel in order to invade underlying tissue. Up to one billion malignant cells daily can be released from a primary tumor, and although a large percentage of them succeed in crossing the basement membrane, only a tiny fraction (perhaps 0.001 percent) of them ever succeeds in forming a new tumor. This appears to be a key control point and possible target of therapeutic intervention.

The process of cancer metastasis consists of a series of sequential interrelated steps, each of which is rate-limiting, since a failure at any of the steps arrests the process. Metastatic cells must complete all of these steps if a clinically relevant distant lesion is to develop. The outcome of the process is dependent on both the intrinsic properties of the tumor cells and the responses of the host. In principle, the steps or events in the pathogenesis of a metastasis are similar in all tumors, but the balance of these intrinsic and host-response interactions can vary among patients.

Transit of malignant cells into systemic circulation for distribution to distant sites is facilitated by weak-walled and poorly constructed blood vessels in the tumor, by increased hydrostatic pressure in an encapsulated tumor, and by increased proteolytic activity and decreased expression of CAMs within the tumor capsule.

Natural killer cells and macrophages attack the migrating cancer cells in the circulatory system. Agents that enhance immune function, such as PSK polysaccharide from turkey tail mushroom, can inhibit metastasis by this mechanism. Migrating cells may also be damaged or overwhelmed by mechanical forces in the tiny capillaries or by the relatively high oxygen concentrations in arterial blood.

Once the tumor cells have survived the circulation, they must halt in the capillary beds of distant organs—a process called cell arrest. Several factors contribute to this process, including disturbed CAM activity, vessel damage, platelet aggregation, and fibrin formation. Trauma and inflammation may damage capillary vessels and induce angiogenic factors that may permit easier spread of malignant cells. This can include the trauma of surgery and of chronic inflammation. Tumor cells manufacture excess fibrin and are "sticky" so that cells can more easily aggregate and form a cluster that is more likely to be arrested. Fibrinolytic (proteolytic) enzymes such as bromelain and papain can reduce this aspect of metastasis. Tumors may induce platelet aggregation and hence fibrin activity, clot formation, and easier cell arrest through the induction of prostaglandins and disturbance of the balance between prostacyclin (PG1) and thromboxanes. Aspirin and COX-2 inhibitors reduce this effect.

Arrested cells exit the blood vessel by penetrating the epithelial cells and basement membrane, a process called extravasation. Local trauma and inflammation can contribute to ease of cells exiting the blood vessel after arrest. Agents that act as connective tissue tonics and stabilizers may inhibit this process.

Proliferation within the organ completes the metastatic process. To continue growing, the micrometastasis must develop a vascular network and evade destruction by host defenses.

Blood Tests for Assessing and Monitoring Angiogenesis/ Metastatic Progression

- C-reactive protein (CRP)
- Copper, ceruloplasmin
- D-dimer
- ESR (erythrocyte sedimentation rate)
- Fibrinogen
- Insulin (fasting) and IGF-1
- LDH (lactate dehydrogenase)
- Leiden factor V
- Vitamin D3 (25 OH-VIT D)
- Zinc

Natural Agents That Are Antimetastatic

- Apigenin
- Beta-carotene, vitamin A
- Beta-sitosterol
- Bromelain
- Calcium-D-glucarate
- Coenzyme Q10
- Curcumin
- Echinacea
- EPA
- EGCG
- Flavonoids (catechin, quercetin, rutin)
- Indole-3-carbinol
- Larch arabinogalactan
- Maitake mushroom
- Melatonin
- Mistletoe
- Modified citrus pectin (MCP)
- Nigella
- R+ alpha-lipoic acid
- Resveratrol
- Ursolic acid

Decrease Vascular Permeability and Inhibit Angiogenesis

Angiogenesis, the formation of new blood vessels from existing ones, is seen in embryonic development, placenta formation, and wound healing and is a necessary prerequisite for tumor growth and metastases. The growth and survival of cells is dependent on an adequate supply of oxygen and nutrients and the removal of toxic products. Oxygen can diffuse from capillaries for only a very short distance, so the expansion of tumor masses beyond 1 millimeter in diameter depends on the development of a new blood supply, or angiogenesis.

As cancer grows, it requires more and more blood supply; activation of proangiogenic genes is common. The extent of angiogenesis is determined by the balance between promoting and inhibiting agents that are released by the tumor and host cells in the tumor microenvironment. The growth of many cancers is associated with upregulation of angiogenesis and loss of angiogenic controls. Many of these proangiogenic agents are stored in the ECM, and weakening of the matrix—by inflammation or cytokines, for example—can release them for activation.

Metabolic Factors That Promote Angiogenesis

- Angiogenin and angiotropin
- Collagenase
- COX-2, 5- and 12-LOX, NF-κB, AP-1
- Elastase
- Epidermal growth factor (EGF)
- Fibrin and plasmin
- Fibroblast growth factor (FGF)
- Heparinase
- Histamine
- Inflammatory eicosanoids (such as PGE2)
- Insulin-like growth factors 1 and 2 (IGF-1 and IGF-2), insulin and leptin
- Interleukin-1, interleukin-8, and possibly interleukin-6
- Kinins
- Lactic acid
- Platelet-activating factor (PAF)
- Platelet-derived growth factor (PDGF)
- Transforming growth factor-alpha (TGF-α) and TGF-β
- Tumor necrosis factor-alpha (TNF-α) at low concentrations
- Urokinase plasminogen activator (uPA)
- Vascular endothelial growth factor (VEGF)

COPPER AND ANGIOGENESIS

Copper is a cofactor in angiogenesis and acts as an obligatory on/off switch. Copper is incorporated into the structure of blood vessel walls and helps bind angiogenic molecules to the endothelial lining for activation. Copper is often elevated in cancer patients, possibly due to widespread use of copper piping in water systems, and may be a cause or a contributing factor in their diagnosis. Serum copper levels correlate with tumor incidence, tumor burden, malignant progression, and recurrence in several cancers, and high serum copper or ceruloplasmin (stored copper) is a prognostic indicator of metastases. Levels should optimally be in the lowest twentieth percentile. (In other words, if the lab range was 1–100, then the patient's level should be under 20.)

Natural Agents That May Chelate Copper

- Green tea
- Luteolin
- Molybdenum
- R+ lipoic acid
- Resveratrol
- Zinc glycinate

To effectively chelate copper, the lipoic acid, molybdenum, and zinc may need to be at a reasonably high dose to be markedly effective. I suggest zinc glycinate at 30 mg twice daily (never on an empty stomach), R+ lipoic acid at 300 mg three times daily, and molybdenum at 150 mcg three times daily until copper is in lowest 20 percent of range, then 150 mcg once or twice daily thereafter.

HYPOXIA AND ANGIOGENESIS

Benign tumors are sparsely vascularized, whereas malignant neoplasms are highly vascular and neovascularization is a significant and independent prognostic indicator in early-stage cancer. This understanding of increased vasculature bringing heat to an area has led to development of thermographic imaging techniques as another means of evaluating tumors.

In angiogenesis, vascular endothelial cells migrate from an angiogenic bud on a blood vessel toward the angiogenic stimulus (hungry cancer cells or an area of hypoxia). In wound healing, hypoxia occurs from a lack of blood circulation to the traumatized tissue. In tumors, hypoxia is a result of rapid metabolism, inflammation, and disordered vasculature. Hypoxia inhibits proper mitochondrial function and carboxylic acid (Krebs) cycling. This leads to increased lactic acid production and contributes to inflammation, which further promotes angiogenesis. New blood vessels growing into tumors are disordered and poorly constructed, with thin, weak vessel walls, and lack lymph vessels for drainage. This leads to increased hydrostatic pressure in the tumor capsule, which puts pressure on blood vessels, lessens incoming blood flow, and contributes to hypoxia.

Rapid tumor growth requires a high metabolic rate, and this may contribute to hypoxia in poorly perfused regions. Hypoxia activates a complex series of genes, mediated by hypoxia-inducible factor 1-alpha (HIF-1α), and leads to upregulation of glycolysis and hence the production of lactic acid.

Hypoxia-inducible factor 1 (HIF-1) is a nuclear transcription factor that is activated during times of low oxygen tension. HIF-1 induces the enzyme carbonic anhydrase 9, leading to upregulation of VEGF and MMPs and structural weakening of the extracellular matrix to allow easier passage of new blood vessels through it.

Carbonic anhydrase (CA) is a family of transmembrane proteins that is overexpressed in a wide variety of tumor types and is induced by hypoxia. It catalyzes the interconversion of carbon dioxide and bicarbonate and contributes to the low pH surrounding the tumor. Overexpression of CA contributes to angiogenesis, inhibition of apoptosis, and cell adhesion disruption. It has a strong association with poor outcomes.

Natural Agents That May Inhibit Carbonic Anhydrase

- Coumarins (highest in Fabaceae or pea family—e.g., clover, alfalfa)
- Piperine (alkaloid present in black pepper)
- Purple angelica (*Angelica purpurascens*)
- Isoflavones from kudzu
- Essential oil from summer savory (*Satureja hortensis*)
- Phenolics from peppermint, including eriodictyol, luteolin, hesperetin, apigenin, and rosmarinic acid
- White tea, certain honeys, seaweeds

MACROPHAGES AND ANGIOGENESIS

Macrophages are the predominant immune cell at tumor sites and can both induce and inhibit new blood vessel formation and tumor progression. This is parallel to their dual role in wound healing, where they promote angiogenesis in the earlier stages of healing but inhibit it in the late stage. In tumors, the inhibition stage is not reached and the tumor is akin to a nonhealing lesion with chronic, self-perpetuating inflammation.

Natural Agents That May Normalize Macrophage Activity

- Astragalus
- Echinacea
- Larch arabinogalactans
- Mushroom polysaccharides

TUMOR SUPPRESSOR GENE P53 MUTATION AND ANGIOGENESIS

An early mutation in cancer cells is often the p53 tumor suppressor gene, and, among other ramifications, it is also responsible for reduced production of the antiangiogenic factor thrombospondin.

ASSESSING ANGIOGENESIS

The rate or extent of angiogenesis can be evaluated from measuring:

- Serum VEGF, PDGF, β-FGF
- Circulating endothelial cells
- Circulating endothelial progenitors

The clinical aim is to degrade fibrin, reduce vascular permeability, regulate prostaglandin (PGE2) production, and reduce COX-2, VEGF, β-FGF, histamine, lactic acid, IGF-1; and chelate copper and iron.

Natural Agents That May Inhibit Angiogenesis

- Zinc via displacement of copper
- Several polyphenols, including epigallocatechin-3-gallate (EGCG) in green tea and resveratrol in red wine, inhibit angiogenesis through multiple mechanisms when administered orally

Natural Agents That May Inhibit Vascular Permeability

- Anthocyanidins
- Bilberry
- Butcher's broom
- Gotu kola
- Horse chestnut

Natural Agents That May Reduce Hypoxia and Lactic Acid

- Short-term benefits may be seen with ozone therapy, but this tends to become oxidative and tissue damaging over time.
- Redox regulators (flavonoids), specifically apigenin, luteolin, quercetin, and vitamin C, as well as lactofermented foods (sauerkraut, kimchi, kombucha) can promote removal of lactic acid from tissues.
- Mitochondrial repair strategies can reverse glycolytic shift and lower lactic acid production.

Natural Agents That May Inhibit Mast Cell Degradation and Histamine Release

Histamine released during injury or inflammation degrades ECM.

- Eleuthero, chamomile, nettle leaf, ephedra
- Flavonoids and vitamin C
- PTK and PKC inhibitors

CLINICAL STRATEGIES IN MANAGING BREAST CANCER

This diagram depicts some of the key metabolic pathways and processes that influence the development and progression of breast cancer. It illustrates the multiple mechanisms at play and how inducing or activating some pathways while inhibiting or downregulating others can contribute to resisting disease.

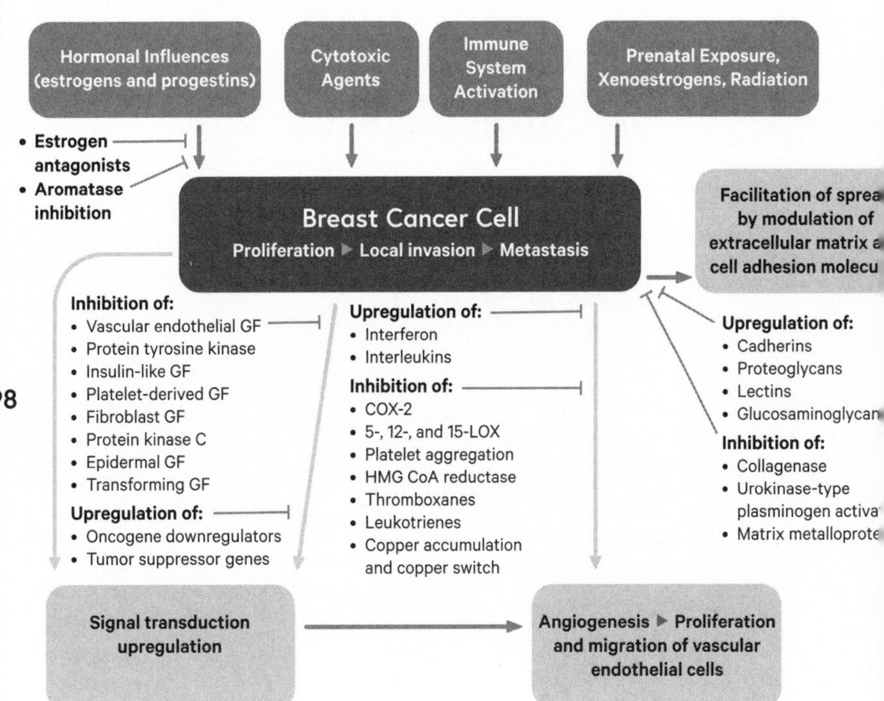

DOSING GUIDELINES FOR NATURAL SUPPLEMENTS FOR CANCER

The doses given below are only general recommendations. I am not suggesting that anyone should take *all* of the items listed below. The skillful practitioner will identify the priorities and develop a treatment plan that unfolds over time, addressing the most urgent concerns first, building resilience and strengthening the foundation, and ensuring that the most beneficial agents are used to the maximum efficacy and within safety ranges. By considering all of the actions of each therapeutic agent and by planning for synergies among herbs and supplements, the practitioner will be able to use the least number of agents to exert the greatest effect, knowing how to layer the actions of the herbs and the constituents of the herbs over time, as the circumstances of the patient change.

Supplement	Dose	Notes
3,3'-diindolylmethane (DIM)	200–400 mg	Take at bedtime for maximum liver impact.
Aescin (from horse chestnut)	40 mg three times daily	
Apigenin	3–10 mg/kg daily	
Artemisinin (from annual wormwood)	150–900 mg daily	See page 409 for more information on dosage.
Astragalus	9–30 g daily	
Baicalein (from Baikal skullcap)	500–1,500 mg daily	
Berberine (from Oregon grape or barberry)	250–400 mg three times daily	
Beta-carotene	5–15 mg daily	This dose is equivalent to 10,000–25,000 units of vitamin A activity.
Betaine	3–5 g twice daily	
Beta-lapachone	1.5–3 g daily of dried bark from the taheebo tree	
Beta-sitosterol	50–150 mg daily	
Biotin	Up to 10 mg daily	
Bromelain (from pineapple stem)	100–400 mg twice daily	
Burdock root	6 g daily	
Butyrate (short-chain fatty acid)	Up to 10 g daily	Especially effective with annual wormwood (see page 409)
Caffeic acid phenethyl ester (CAPE; from propolis)	300 mg two or three times daily	
Calcium-D-glucarate	500 mg daily	

Supplement	Dose	Notes
Carnosol (from rosemary)	500–1,500 mg daily	
Coenzyme Q10	100 mg three times daily	Absorbs best when taken with fats or oils
Curcumin (from turmeric)	500 mg–1 g daily	This dose is equivalent to 10–20 g of root powder.
Diosgenin	8 mg daily	
EGCG (from green tea)	200 mg two or three times daily	Possible hepatotoxicity with prolonged daily doses of more than 800 mg/day. Use a minimum of 400 IU of vitamin E succinate while taking higher-dose EGCG. Use caution when taking with Velcade (bortezomib) chemotherapy.
Ellagic acid	8 oz. unsweetened pomegranate, grape, or berry juices daily	
Emodin (from rhubarb or sheep sorrel)	Use Essiac Formula (see page 51)	
Evening primrose oil	1,000 mg daily	
Flavonoids, including apigenin, luteolin, quercetin, genistein	1–2 g daily	
Flaxseed	1 tsp.–1 tbsp. daily, soaked overnight	
Folic acid	400–800 mcg daily	
Forskolin (from coleus)	3–6 g of dried root twice daily	
Garlic (organosulfur compounds allicin, ajoene, diallyl disulfide)	1–2 cloves of fresh garlic daily	Chop fine, wait 10 minutes for activation of compounds, and swallow without chewing.
Genistein (isoflavone from legumes)	100 mg once or twice daily	
Glucosamine sulfate and other GAGs from bovine cartilage	500 mg two or three times daily	
Glutamine	Up to 15 g daily	
Glutathione	100 mg twice daily	
Honokiol (from magnolia bark)	60–150 mg daily	
Indian frankincense	2–3 g daily	

Supplement	Dose	Notes
Indole-3-carbinol (I3C)	200–600 mg daily	Take at bedtime for maximum liver impact. Found in cruciferous vegetables. Converts to DIM (active form) so take less I3C if also taking DIM.
Inositol-6-phosphate (IP6)	6–10 g daily	
Isothiocyanates	Eat lightly steamed cabbage-family vegetables several times a week.	
Larch arabinogalactan	1 tsp.–1 tbsp. daily in divided doses	Immunomodulatory starch from *Larix laricina* and *L. occidentalis*
Limonene	Eat organic Meyer lemons with peel; drink lemongrass tea with dried tangerine, lemon, and other citrus peels chopped into small pieces.	
Luteolin (found in carrot, cabbage, artichoke, celery, apple skin)	100 mg luteolin/10 kg body weight daily	
Lycopene	30 mg twice daily	
MCP (modified citrus pectin)	2 g twice daily (powder in water or cold herbal tea, taken away from food or drugs)	
Melatonin	To dream tolerance or up to 20 mg. Take at bedtime.	Start on 2–5 mg nightly for a week, then add 1 mg every 3 days, increasing until you notice overly vivid dreams, then reduce again by 0.5 mg. Dreams should normalize; this is your optimal dose. Do not use concurrently with corticosteroids or other medications used to suppress the immune system.
Molybdenum	150 mcg three times daily until copper is in lowest 20% of normal range, then 150 mcg twice daily thereafter	
MSM (methylsulfonylmethane)	500 mg twice daily	

Supplement	Dose	Notes
NAC (N-acetylcysteine)	500 mg twice daily	Do not use concurrently with platinum chemotherapies. Generally not recommended with other chemotherapy.
N-acetylglucosamine	500 mg twice daily	
Oleic acid	Eat 10 organic olives daily, and use olive oil in the kitchen.	
Oligomeric proanthocyanidins (OPCs)/pycnogenol	150 mg three times daily	Polyphenolics from *Pinus pinaster* or *Pinus maritima*, or from grape seed
Omega-3 fatty acids	EPA 500 mg and DHA 250 mg twice daily	
Parthenolide (from feverfew)	0.25–0.5 mg twice daily	
Quercetin	500 mg two or three times daily	
R+ alpha-lipoic acid	150–300 mg three times daily	Generally not recommended with chemotherapy
Red yeast rice extract	Fermented rice extract 500 mg–1 g, twice daily	
Resveratrol	1,500–2,000 mg daily	
SAMe (S-adenosylmethionine)	300–600 mg twice daily	
Sea buckthorn	5–45 g of dried berries or up to 5 g (1 tsp.) per day of pressed oil	
Selenium (selenomethionine)	100 mcg twice daily	Do not use selenomethionine in prostate cancer.
Silymarin (from milk thistle)	500 mg three times daily	
Sulforaphanes (found in broccoli and wasabi sprouts, cabbage family)	10–50 mg per day	A 1 oz. serving of broccoli sprouts provides 73 mg of glucoraphanin sulforaphane.
Tangeretin	Eat an organic tangerine including skin daily.	
Ursolic acid (triterpene from rosemary and tulsi)	150–250 mg twice daily	
Vanadium	50–100 mcg daily	
Vitamin A	600–900 mcg daily for a maximum of 3 months, then reduce dose or use beta-carotene	

Supplement	Dose	Notes
Vitamin B1 (thiamine or benfotiamine)	30–80 mg twice daily	
Vitamin B2 (riboflavin)	10–15 mg twice daily	Maximum daily intestinal absorption is approximately 20–25 mg
Vitamin B3 (niacin)	50–100 mg twice daily	
Vitamin B5 (pantothenic acid)	30–80 mg twice daily	
Vitamin B6 (pyridoxine)	50–100 mg twice daily	
Vitamin B7 (biotin)	20–40 mg twice daily	
Vitamin B9 (folate [folic acid])	200–400 mcg twice daily	Higher doses may mask functional B12 deficiency
Vitamin B12	200–400 mcg twice daily	
Vitamin C	To bowel tolerance	Acerola cherry extract preferred
Vitamin D3	2,000–5,000 IU twice daily	
Vitamin E (mixed tocopher-ols and tocotrienols)	400–800 IU daily	Can substitute vitamin E succinate
Vitamin K	100–120 mcg daily	
Whey (source of cysteine and immunoglobulins)	20–25 g daily	
Zinc glycinate	Regular daily dose of 10–15 mg. Can increase dose to 30–40 mg twice daily for 4–8 weeks if serum levels are low.	Always take with food in stomach.

CHAPTER 9

Materia Medica for Managing Cancer: The Cytotoxic Herbs

Big disease takes big medicine. This is what I tell my patients as I describe the extensive herbal and nutritional protocols I recommend, and possibly one of the reasons why some people do not get the results they seek with natural medicines is because they simply do not take enough. But, as well as requiring sufficient dosing, "big medicine" also refers to the more potent herbs—the activators or effectors, the cytotoxics.

Only qualified practitioners will be able to access these herbs and provide them to patients, and this is an appropriate safety measure, because if an herb can kill a cancer cell, it can probably also kill healthy cells, and specific dosing and monitoring are required. Cytotoxic herbs should be used for the shortest duration possible, meaning that a monitoring plan should be established to determine when to stop, based on measured reduction of cancer seen on scans or of cancer markers in the blood. If cancer is controlled but not gone, stable but not cured, then a low-dose cytotoxic rotation may be considered for a longer duration.

CHAPTER 9 CONTENTS

409 *Artemisia annua*

417 *Asimina triloba*

420 *Camptotheca acuminata*

422 *Catharanthus roseus*

423 *Chelidonium majus*

426 *Larrea divaricata, L. tridentata*

429 *Phytolacca decandra, P. americana*

432 *Podophyllum peltatum*

434 *Sanguinaria canadensis*

439 *Taxus brevifolia, T. baccata, T. wallichiana*

443 *Thuja occidentalis*

446 *Viscum album*

The Cytotoxic Herbs

Over the past few decades a multitude of new drugs have been approved for cancer treatment, many of which are derived directly from plants or based on them. Herbalists can use some of these same plants with cytotoxic constituents to retard cancer growth. These herbs can be toxic, and one of the biggest challenges for herbal prescribers is the difficulty in obtaining high-quality, reliable products, as well as the dearth of reliable clinical data.

The herbs we discuss in this chapter are not for the faint of heart. Some of them can cause significant side effects if used improperly, or even real damage in careless hands. If used judiciously, though, in carefully calibrated formulations, their cytotoxicity can be managed, directed, and used to good avail. For some of them, it is challenging to find contemporary references or dosing guidelines. In those cases, we need to go back to the older literature—notably the Eclectic physicians from the mid-nineteenth century, when these herbs were more routinely used, though remembering that they were not concerned about herb-drug interactions and co-prescribing in the way that we are today. For other herbs, it is hard to find dosing guidelines and references to the whole herb because the isolated constituent research has dominated the laboratories and the literature. All of these factors can make prescribing cytotoxic herbs decidedly tricky.

In the pyramid prescribing model described on page 318, the cytotoxic herbs are the activators or effectors. They have a narrow phytochemical target, often a narrow therapeutic index with relative toxicity at even a modest dose, and increased risk of side effects. They should be used with caution, in the lowest dose and for the shortest duration possible, but also in a sufficient dose to generate an effective clinical response. If you prescribe more than one at the same time, be aware of synergy and summation, or consider rotating them in and out of protocols periodically to reduce the possibility of toxin accumulation.

Using cytotoxics with chemotherapy, especially if the chemotherapy drug is derived from the herb, requires extra caution. Consider how you will know if a side effect is from the herb or the drug, as well as whether the herb will affect the drug. For example, Pacific yew extract may downregulate multidrug resistance and make taxol more effective, reducing side effects and possibly enabling a lower drug dose overall to achieve the same results. This sort of positive herb–drug interaction is immensely beneficial.

> Everything man needs to maintain good health can be found in nature; the true task of science is to find these things.
>
> PARACELSUS

Guidelines for Prescribing Cytotoxic Herbs

When working with cytotoxic herbs, there are a few key guidelines to follow.

Start low and go slow. In particularly fragile patients who have liver or kidney deficiency already, it may be useful to start with one cytotoxic herb and work up to an effective dose before commencing with another.

Anticipate side effects. Establish what side effects or abnormal test results could occur if an herb you want to use or a drug that is being taken were to have an adverse effect. This is the foundation of a safety monitoring plan that will be incorporated into routine blood work. Some herbal side effects may be relatively easy to identify, such as elevated liver enzymes in patients taking *Artemisia annua.* I have seen this in two patients in my practice—not enough to be definitive, but sufficient to make me alert to it. It is readily rectified by dose adjustments. However, for other herbs the means of monitoring may be less obvious. With symptoms such as nausea, skin rashes, or diarrhea, it may be virtually impossible to determine if they are due to the chemotherapy or the herbs. Stopping the herbs, monitoring for improvements, and restarting the herbs is the only definitive way to know, and this will only be effective with acute symptoms and cannot assess for relative risk of long-term organ or tissue damage.

Cross-reference to avoid interactions. Cross-reference the herbs you want to use with all drugs being used to assess for liver enzyme induction or inhibition. If an herb induces or inhibits specific known liver detoxification pathways, then it may be possible to assess which drugs also go through those pathways and could be affected as well. Unfortunately, the detoxification pathways of many of the drugs and most of the herbs are unknown, not to mention those of any foods or nutritional supplements or beverages the patient may be taking, so there is a natural and inevitable margin of error here.

Consider the maximum safe dose. For each cytotoxic herb in a formula, you'll use the maximum safe dose to determine proportions or ratios. The lower the allowable daily dose of an herb, the lower the proportion it will be in a cytotoxics blend.

Know when to avoid cytotoxic herbs altogether. Avoid cytotoxics in pregnancy and lactation and in anyone with known liver or kidney failure. The more progressed or advanced the cancer, the less tolerance a person may have for managing the herbs and any metabolic effects from cancer cell die-off.

INCORPORATING CYTOTOXIC HERBS

One major challenge for practitioners wishing to use these cytotoxic herbs is accessing high-quality and consistently reliable herbal medicines. Very few suppliers carry them, and making your own is not recommended, due to inconsistencies and irregularities from batch to batch (which makes it difficult to correctly calibrate doses). In some cases, I purchase a proprietary blended formula with several cytotoxic herbs in specified concentrations, which can then be supplemented or augmented by other herbs in a customized blend, if necessary.

This summary list below outlines the chemical mechanisms of action of some of the herbal constituents—those that have been researched in this way—and also outlines the traditional uses, the empirical clinical observations gleaned from generations of herbalists about where in the body some herbs may be more or less effective. This is a fine example of where the science of botanical pharmaceuticals can be skillfully woven through the practice of traditional and energetic herbal medicines, fine-tuning and focusing a treatment plan to suit each individual in their own cancer journey.

Specific Tissue Targets for Cytotoxic Herbs

Artemisia annua

- Broadly active against various types of cancer
- Modulation of the cell signal transduction pathway
- Initiation of apoptosis
- Inhibition of cancer proliferation, metastasis, and angiogenesis

Asimina triloba

- Broadly active against various types of cancer
- Especially useful in conjunction with conventional chemotherapy, where it can help inhibit multidrug resistance pumping and keep the chemotherapy in the target cells to inhibit mitosis, as well as causing less collateral damage to other cells

Camptotheca acuminata

- Broadly active against various types of cancer
- Quinoline alkaloids, notably camptothecin, have marked anticancer and antiviral effects
- Inhibition of topoisomerase I, induction of cell cycle arrest, and activation of caspase-3 and caspase-7, which induce apoptosis
- Used in making the chemotherapy drugs irinotecan and topotecan, which are inhibitors of topoisomerase I

Chelidonium majus

- Isoquinoline alkaloids inhibit the pro-cancerous mitotic cyclins A and B and the cyclin-dependent kinases CDK1 and CDK2, which all promote cell cycling (replication)
- Isoquinoline alkaloids also upregulate the anticancer CDK inhibitor protein called p27, which induces apoptosis
- Especially useful in cancers with a viral or bacterial component
- Used topically for skin cancers, warts, and virally induced cancers, such as squamous cell in mouth and throat, cervical cancer, melanoma, and lymphoma
- Specific focus to stomach, liver, gallbladder, pancreas, diaphragm, and omentum
- Used for hepatic congestion, jaundice, throbbing pain in right upper abdomen, bilious headaches (queasy, nauseous, dizzy), migraine, and supraorbital neuralgia

Larrea divaricata

- NDGA causes arrest of DNA copying in the S phase of cell replication and induces apoptosis
- Inhibits glycolysis and the electron transfer chain
- Flavones and flavanol glycosides contribute to an antioxidant effect
- May induce a reversal of multidrug resistance in cancer cells
- Used for virally induced cancers, such as squamous cell in mouth and throat, cervical cancer, melanoma, and lymphoma
- Used topically for skin cancers or for lesions on the skin from other types of cancer

Phytolaccca spp.

- Broadly active against various types of cancer
- Tropism to breast, throat, thyroid, lymphoma, ears, nose, and throat
- Nonspecific T lymphocyte inducer
- Leukocytic and anti-inflammatory
- Alterative/lymphatic decongestant for cysts, boils, acne, dry eczema, and psoriasis

Podophyllum peltatum

- Podophyllotoxin inhibits DNA topoisomerase II and inhibits tubulin polymerization, thus preventing DNA from copying and inhibiting mitosis
- Combining podophyllotoxin with etoposide enhances its efficacy in preclinical research
- Used for virally induced cancers, such as squamous cell in mouth and throat, cervical cancer, melanoma, and lymphoma
- Used for constipation or sluggish bowel, thick or greasy coating on tongue, halitosis, and mucus congestion (upper respiratory system), such as sinusitis, otitis, and mastoiditis

Sanguinaria canadensis

- Contains isoquinoline alkaloids, including sanguinarine and chelerythrine (also found in greater celandine), which are the most researched
- Antimicrobial and anti-inflammatory effects
- Used for leukemia, lymphoma, myeloma, and metastastic lymphatic spread
- Used topically for skin cancers or for lesions on the skin from other types of cancer

Taxus brevifolia

- Broadly active against various types of cancer
- Overstabilizes tubulin—prevents spindle formation and inhibits mitosis

- Inhibits multidrug resistance pumping
- Use with taxane drugs (paclitaxel, docetaxel)

Thuja occidentalis, T. plicata

- Alpha- and beta-thujone fractions are proapoptotic through the induction of ROS and p53 activation, leading to apoptosis
- Flavonols trigger caspase-3-mediated apoptosis as well
- Alpha- and beta-thujone fractions have antiproliferative, proapoptotic, and anti-angiogenic effects in vitro; in vivo assays showed that alpha- and beta-thujone inhibit neoplasia and inhibit the angiogenic markers including VEGF
- Used for pelvic and reproductive cancers, such as uterine, ovarian, bowel, bladder, prostate, and breast cancer
- Used for virally induced cancers, such as squamous cell in mouth and throat, cervical cancer, melanoma, and lymphoma

Viscum album

- Given as a subcutaneous injectable
- Inhibits cell replication, and the lectins inhibit agglutination of tumor cells
- Upregulates NK cells and macrophages; inhibits tumor growth and metastases
- Lectins have an immunomodulating activity
- Generally for all cancer as a nonspecific T lymphocyte inducer
- Used for brain cancer (primary or metastatic), lymphoma, hypertension, anxiety, and hysteria

Artemisia annua

Common names: Annual wormwood, Chinese wormwood, sweet Annie
Plant family: Asteraceae
Parts used: Leaves, flowering stems, especially from the top part of the plant

This is a highly aromatic annual herb of Asiatic and eastern European origin but now widely dispersed throughout the temperate regions and naturalized in the US. It is easy to grow and self-seeds readily. Energetically, it is considered bitter, acrid, and cooling, and it is traditionally used in TCM to clear "damp heat" or "summer heat." This traditional use led to research in the 1970s in treating malaria with the herb, and in vitro trials conducted in China by the World Health Organization in 1981 showed artemisinin and other compounds in the leaves to be effective against the erythrocytic stages of chloroquine-resistant and chloroquine-sensitive strains of *Plasmodium falciparum,* the parasite that causes malaria. Artemisinin and its derivatives have effectively treated malaria and cerebral malaria in human subjects ever since, without significant adverse reactions nor notable side effects. In 2015, Dr. Youyou Tu was awarded the Nobel Prize in Medicine and Physiology, as part of a team that developed artemisinin and derivatives as therapy against malaria. Unfortunately, but perhaps not surprisingly, some artemisinin-resistant malaria strains are becoming apparent now, a phenomenon that had not occurred in thousands of years of using the whole herb.

The principal constituents of note are found in the essential oil in the leaf—mainly sesquiterpenoids, including artemisinin and numerous related compounds and derivatives (artemisinin I, II, III, IV, and V, as well as artemisic acid, artemisilactone, artemisinol, epoxyarteannuinic acid, and others). The leaves have almost 90 percent of the total artemisinin in the plant, with the uppermost foliar portion of the plant (top one-third of growth at maturity) containing almost double that of the lower leaves, which has significant implications for harvesting guidelines and quality control of the raw herb.

Aside from their notable antimalarial activity and efficacy against schistosoma parasitic infection, artemisinin and its derivatives also demonstrate both in vitro and in vivo activities against various types of cancer, including modulation of the cell signal transduction pathway, initiation of apoptotic cell death, and inhibition of cancer proliferation, metastasis, and angiogenesis.

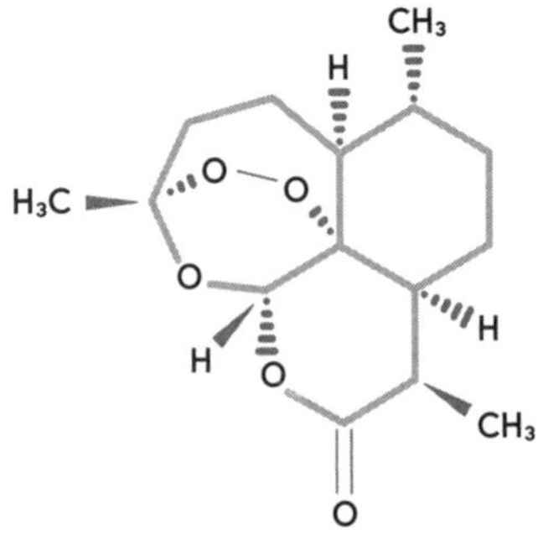

The molecular structure of artemisinin shows the endoperoxide bridge.

Artemisinin and its derivatives are unusual molecules with two oxygen atoms linked by an endoperoxide bridge. This is an unstable bond and can readily react with iron to form free radicals. In the case of cancer, the high replication rate of the cell requires significant supplies of iron. To this end, cancer cells overexpress soluble transferrin receptors (sTfR), which are proteins found in blood that deliver iron to cells for uptake. sTfR bind with iron to bring it into cancer cells, and artemisinin is taken up with the iron across the cell membrane, whereupon the endoperoxide bridge readily reacts with iron to create intracellular oxidative stress.

When the endoperoxide bridge of artemisinin dissociates, it causes or contributes to several cancer-inhibiting effects:

- Inhibition of intracellular Ras proteins and hence downregulation of oncogenic signal transduction
- Modulatory action on DNA damage and repair
- Decreased mitochondrial membrane potential in cancer cells, leading to 30–50% decrease in available cellular energy
- Inhibition of multidrug resistance pathways
- Induction of various cell death modes (apoptosis, autophagy, ferroptosis, necrosis)
- Inhibition of VEGF receptor expression; antiangiogenesis

All of these anticancer activities of artemisinin are exciting and encouraging, but in the whole herb there are also numerous other compounds that are therapeutically active. For example, more than 50 different phenolic compounds including flavonoids, coumarins, and phenolic acids have been isolated from leaves and found to have a major influence on bioactivity of the medicine. Flavonoids contribute to suppression of hepatic enzymes responsible for altering the absorption and metabolism of artemisinin in the body, giving a longer half-life than with isolated sesquiterpenes. They also promote beneficial immunomodulatory activity in parasitic and chronic infectious diseases and provide an array of redox-regulating opportunities, which modulate the oxidative stress induced by artemisinin.

The flavonoids act as a synergist, and artemisinin and its semisynthetic analogs are more effective in treating parasitic diseases (such as malaria) and cancer if delivered simultaneously with flavonoids. In studies, the sesquiterpenes significantly reduced production of prostaglandin E2 as well as production of inflammatory nitric oxide and secretion of cytokines. NO, PGE2, and cytokines were suppressed by the flavonoids casticin and chrysosphenol D. Researchers concluded that immune mediators of angiogenesis are inhibited by sesquiterpene lactones and flavonoids and that this synergy may be one of the mechanisms of anticancer activity of *Artemisia annua*.

In a study of 27 culinary herbs and 12 medicinal herbs, *Artemisia annua* was one of the four medicinal plants with the highest oxygen radical absorbance capacity (ORAC) level or redox capacity. All of these flavonoids and other polyphenolics combine to have a normalizing and supportive role in mediating inflammation.

There are also interesting studies considering artemisia, as a whole herb, in cancer care. For example, a 2019 study reported that, compared to artesunate isolate, a derivative of artemisinin, the dried whole leaf dose demonstrated notable therapeutic value in lung cancer. Another very interesting study in 2019 showed that an extract of an artemisinin-deficient *Artemisia annua* leaf preparation exhibited potent anticancer activity against triple-negative human breast cancer cells, confirming that at least several different compounds may contribute to the beneficial effects.

All the studies in cell lines or animals on isolates or semisynthetic derivatives, often using solvents not used in herbal medicine (methanol, benzene, and others), need to be interpreted carefully as they do not necessarily reflect clinical practices. However, when coupled with the long history of traditional use of *Artemisia annua*, the herbal clinician can appreciate both the cytotoxic effects of the sesquiterpenes and the redox-regulating effects of the polyphenols, and this determines the prescribing plan.

Capsules of standardized artemisinin are available, and these are useful for calibrating the correct dose (see below). Additionally, functional medicine doctors and naturopaths will sometimes use IV artesunate in acute care for cancer. This may be quite an effective emergency intervention in a crisis, but whole herb is needed for extracting the flavonoids, in a low-alcohol tincture (25–35% EtOH) or a simple tea if the patient is willing. In a tea, the flavonoids will extract into the water and the sesquiterpenes into the steam, which can be captured in a lid to condense back into the teapot or pan, but the tea is quite aromatic and bitter and not entirely palatable for many people.

Artemisinin is absorbed more quickly from tea preparations than from capsules. It is metabolized by hydrolysis to dihydroartemisinin. Upregulation of cytochrome detox enzymes CYP 2B6, CYP 2C19, and CYP 3A4 in the liver by exposure to artemisinin causes increased hepatic clearance of the herb, so plasma levels of artemisinin drop off after 5–7 days, and there is little to no systemic distribution from oral ingestion due to first pass through the liver. This may perhaps be an argument for considering an IV delivery. As noted previously, autoinduction is greatly diminished when taking whole herb alongside artemisinin, due to the presence of flavonoids and polyphenols. Taking artemisinin along with *Artemisia annua* will improve bioavailability.

The product I prescribe has 150 mg of artemisinin per capsule and 100 mg of an 8:1 whole herb extract—equivalent to 800 mg dried herb—which will yield the crucial flavonoids.

Adverse Reactions

Oral use. High doses of artemisia may cause abdominal pain, bradycardia, diarrhea, nausea, vomiting, decreased appetite, flulike symptoms, fever, liver enzyme elevations, and decreased reticulocyte count.

Topical use. Handling fresh artemisia may cause dermatitis, and possibly photosensitivity of the skin. It can be incorporated into salves and liniments, but subsequent sun avoidance is recommended.

Herb-Drug Interactions

Worldwide research into this herb is extensive now, and there is strong evidence for some significant anticancer activity. This does bring up the question of combining it with conventional chemotherapy, new immunotherapy drugs, radiotherapy, and/or antiangiogenics, and certainly there is research to be done in this area.

Artemisia can induce drug clearance, so pharmaceuticals that go through the same pathways risk being cleared more rapidly as well. For drugs with a narrow therapeutic index, this could mean they fall below a critical threshold and are no longer effective. The herbal prescriber needs to ascertain that drugs being taken concurrently won't be adversely affected by the herb, and to consider other cytotoxics if hepatic clearance induction is too risky.

Antacids. Artemisia interferes with antacids, sucralfate, proton pump inhibitors, and histamine receptor antagonists because it increases the production of stomach acid.

Clinical Pearls

Test for iron, ferritin, total iron binding capacity (TIBC), and soluble transferrin receptors (sTfR) before using artemisinin. Serum iron should be from 50–75% of the normal range. Ferritin should be from 25–50% of the normal range. TIBC and sTfR should be in 60–80% of normal range.

Pulse Dosing

Artemisinin induces cytochrome detox enzymes CYP 2B6, CYP 2C19, and CYP 3A4, but pulse dosing—taking breaks, with alternating weeks on and off—is expected to allow the enzymes to return to normal in between. Clinical research of this pulse dose posology is scanty, mostly predicated on one study of malaria patients and a lot of educated extrapolation. If nothing else, though, pulse dosing allows for better tolerance and compliance, because there is a weekly reprieve of die-off reactions triggered by wastes released into the bloodstream as cancer cells die.

Women upregulate liver functions faster than men when confronted with a cytotoxic agent to eliminate; this is probably a genetic benefit to protect the fetus from noxious agents. For prescribing artemisia, it means that ideally women would switch on and off every 5 days or so and men every 7 days. However, in clinical practice I have found the 5-day rotation is difficult to sustain, and patients tend to lose track. Seven days on and 7 days off is easier to manage and has better compliance.

The real challenge with dosing artemisia is that successful cytotoxicity results in cell death and metabolic waste released into lymph and systemic circulation, and this can lead to symptoms of a sort of mild Herxheimer reaction. Technically this is an acute febrile reaction mediated by cytokines—a severe fever that may be accompanied by headache, myalgia, bone pains, and rashes. In the case of artemisia, the fever may be minimal or absent, but symptoms of cytotoxity may include abdominal pain, diarrhea, nausea, vomiting, decreased appetite, malaise, and flulike symptoms. The challenge in using this herb is that you need to dose high enough to induce this cell die-off, and the patient needs to be able to tolerate the uncomfortable response in the body. Indeed, it is this response that indicates success and efficacy of the herb. Careful coaching of the patient is required to make them understand why this matters, and to encourage and support them to manage it. I suggest to my patients that they should not feel actively unwell (no fever, vomiting, or diarrhea), but in the week they are dosing artemisia, they should be able to feel it working in their body. They will feel under the weather, as if they were going to come down with a flu, perhaps wanting to rest more that week.

I also use these die-off reactions as a gauge for how much to take and for how long. Patients should start dosing at something quite moderate, like 150 mg of artemisinin twice daily in the first week. If this is well tolerated, then in the second cycle, the dose is increased by 150 mg daily, and in each cycle after that, a little more is taken until uncomfortable symptoms occur. This is the indication that there is sufficient herbal material to cause cell die-off, which is what we want. This individually established dose is repeated in week on/week off cycles for 2–3 months, or until cell die-off reactions are no longer felt, whichever comes first. At this point, the dose is increased by 150 mg daily again for 2 or 3 days; if there is no further die-off response, then it is time to stop the herb.

Pulse Dosing Artemisia

Pulse dose artemisia in alternating weeks, in increasing doses. Take it twice daily with 2 oz. grapefruit juice to slow the cytochrome activity that is induced by the artemisinin.

WEEK ONE

Artemisinin (ART) 150 mg (this will increase in each cycle) twice daily

Synergists (taken in two divided doses each day): butyric acid (up to 5 g); vitamin C (from acerola cherry) to bowel tolerance with vitamin K3; iron, if levels are low to bring it to 40–60% of normal range; DHA (500 mg), EPA (1 g or up to double this); proteolytic enzymes; lymphatic and hepatic support herbs

WEEK TWO

Cytotoxics blend

Redox-regulating support (flavonoids, polyphenols, carotenoids, zinc 50 mg daily, selenium 100 mg daily, NAC 500 mg daily)

WEEK THREE

ART 150 mg three times daily

Synergists, as listed for Week One

WEEK FOUR

Cytotoxics blend

Redox-regulating support (flavonoids, polyphenols, carotenoids, zinc 50 mg daily, selenium 100 mg daily, NAC 500 mg daily)

WEEK FIVE

ART 300 mg three times daily

Synergists, as listed for Week One

WEEK SIX

Cytotoxics blend

Redox-regulating support (flavonoids, polyphenols, carotenoids, zinc 50 mg daily, selenium 100 mg daily, NAC 500 mg daily)

WEEK SEVEN

ART 450 mg three times daily

Synergists, as listed for Week One

Synergists for Artemisia

Grapefruit juice. This will inhibit some of the same liver enzymes that the herb induces, especially in the first 2 or 3 days of each cycle; it allows a longer half-life and lower dosing. Caution is advised if the patient is also taking pharmaceuticals that go through these same pathways, as their clearance will be impacted as well.

Vitamin C and vitamin K3. Use vitamin C (from acerola cherry) to bowel tolerance (i.e., reduce dose if stool becomes loose or urgent) with vitamin K3 (in a 100:1 ratio). These vitamins operate synergistically as redox regulators to induce selective cancer cell death through several means, including intracellular hydrogen peroxide production leading to oxidative stress, DNA fragmentation, and cell membrane injury.

Omega-3 fatty acids (DHA and EPA). There is a delicate balance to be had between wanting the intracellular reactive oxygen species induced by the artemisinin endoperoxide bridge reaction with iron to kill the cell and needing to mitigate collateral damage in the tissues as those cells die off and release their contents, generating substantial regional oxidative stress.

Natural medicines offer a multitude of redox regulators, and in the effort to stop the cancer from mutating against specific agents, they can be alternated and switched out, in an attempt to run an endgame around the cancer. For this reason, the fish oils are taken in a relatively high dose in the week on, while the flavonoid and polyphenol-rich redox regulators are emphasized in the off week.

Use at least 500 mg DHA and 1 g EPA daily to modulate oxidative stress.

Iron. The only time to be actively supplementing iron in cancer is if you want to use artemisia and the patient has iron levels in the lowest 25% of the normal range. Generally with cancer treatment we want to see iron in the 15–25% of normal range. But iron levels that low may limit the action of artemisia, so if you are using the herb, take an iron supplement to bring iron levels to 40–60% of the normal range before using *Artemisia annua*.

If you supplement with iron, be careful to get the right form and take the right dose. It can be quite constipating in some people. Ferrous glycinate or ferrous gluconate will tend to be easier on the digestive system than ferrous sulfate—the most common type sold in drugstores. Dietary iron has two main forms: heme (derived from hemoglobin and hence found in meat, seafood, and poultry, but not in plants) and nonheme type (found in both plants and animals). Heme iron is the most easily absorbable form (15–35% bioavailability); nonheme iron derived from plants and iron-fortified foods is less well absorbed. Supplements may contain one or both types. Some of the richest sources of iron include lean meats, seafood, nuts, prunes, figs, beans, and leafy greens. Take calcium separately, as it can interfere with the absorption of iron.

Slow-release iron is recommended to decrease any potential gastrointestinal side effects (nausea, abdominal discomfort, or constipation). Leafy greens, prunes, and beans, themselves high in iron, will also reduce constipation. You can also take iron as an easily absorbed plant-based, liquid iron supplement. Doses vary from 10–50 mg of elemental iron daily, with constipation being somewhat dose dependent.

Consider taking vitamin C, as it can improve the absorption of iron. You can also use vitamin C to manage constipation that may be caused by higher iron intake. The required dose is different for everyone and changes over time (for example, there is a higher demand if the patient is fighting infection or has a severe burn). Because vitamin C is water soluble, the body cannot absorb more than it needs, and any excess will simply leave the body through the kidneys and intestines, where it will act as a diuretic and a laxative. This provides an easy way to gauge the right dose. Take enough to have the stool be soft but not loose; that is your best dose.

Proteolytic enzymes. These support macrophage (white blood cell) cleanup of dead cells and inflammatory debris remaining from effective *Artemisia annua* action. They include bromelain, serrapeptase, and nattokinase, and, if there is high risk of blood clots, the most potent is lumbrokinase.

Lymphatic and hepatic support. Herbs such as milk thistle, burdock, cleavers, calendula, and pokeroot will promote tissue detox. These strategies have been described in Chapter 2, as they relate to managing environmental stress and toxins, but the same principles are applicable here. When cytotoxic herbs such as *Artemisia annua* really work, there is cell die-off and a need to clear the morbid material from the tissues through lymph and liver for elimination.

Butyrate. This is a four-carbon short-chain fatty acid used as a synergist with artemisinin to multiply its effects. Butyrate is produced in the bowel during fermentation by gut flora of dietary fibers from legumes (beans, peas, and soybeans), fruits, nuts, cereals, and whole grains as well as being found in butter and cheese from grass-fed cows who have fermented plant fibers in their gut. Short-chain fatty acids contribute to around 70% of the energy requirements of colonic epithelial cells and 5–15% of the total daily calorie requirements of a person (another reason to eat your vegetables!).

Butyric acid purified from butyrate is an important regulator of colonocyte proliferation and apoptosis, gastrointestinal tract motility, and bacterial microflora composition. The names "butyric acid" and "butyrate" are commonly used interchangeably, even in scientific articles and studies. Technically, they have slightly different structures, but they're very similar in effect.

Butyrate in the gut maintains the integrity of the intestinal epithelia by upregulating the proliferation and turnover of epithelial cells, promoting the production of antimicrobial peptides, and enhancing barrier function.

Butyrate is also a potent inducer of cellular differentiation, mediated through its inhibition of histone deacetylase. Histone acetylation/deacetylation is an epigenetic control point that allows gene regulation. Histone deacetylase is required to enable a piece of DNA to copy, and inhibiting this nuclear enzyme prevents DNA transcription. In vitro studies of glioblastoma cell lines showed that butyrate induced a dose-dependent growth inhibition, with G1/S phase arrest. It also induced cellular senescence by upregulating and stabilizing the cell cycle regulator proteins p21, p27, and p53, and it inhibited tumor cell invasion.

Butyric acid is used for the treatment and prevention of various intestinal inflammations and diarrhea, functional gut disorders, dysbiosis, and post-surgery or post-chemotherapy conditions. The gut lining is continually challenged with physical and chemical stressors from food and digestive juices and maintains a low-grade inflammatory state in response. The first barrier of defense against bacterial invasion is production of mucins and defensins (antibacterial peptides). If this is not enough, then toll-like receptors (TLRs) are triggered, and they serve to induce gut-associated lymphoid tissue (GALT) and enterocytes (intestinal lining epithelial cells), some of which are specialized to transport bacterial antigens and present them to the immune cells in the gut wall. If immunological control is disrupted, the enterocytes experience inflammation and oxidative damage, which may cause or contribute to leaky gut syndrome, food allergies, and autoimmune diseases and eventually to bowel cancer.

Butyrate can act as an anti-inflammatory agent in the bowel through inhibition of pro-inflammatory cytokines. The current standard dose of butyric acid used in most studies is 150–300 mg, but this is significantly lower than even normal, healthy daily needs and is probably too low for anyone with active dysbiosis. Studies have shown that oral sodium butyrate supplementation at a dose of 4,000 mg daily for 4 weeks has no apparent ill effects.

However, more isn't always better. Butyrate has diverse and seemingly contradictory effects on cell proliferation, differentiation, and apoptosis and may be pro- or antitumorigenic according to variable factors like location, level of exposure, availability of other metabolic substrates, and intracellular milieu (the butyrate paradox). In normal intestinal epithelial cells, butyrate functions as the primary fuel for cell metabolism and as an energy source and food for normal, healthy colonocytes. As such, it can be considered a proliferative agent.

In cancer cells where the Warburg effect has caused glycolytic shift and the cell is not running the Krebs cycle much, then butyrate at a higher dose accumulates and functions as a HDAC (histone deacetylase) inhibitor, leading to an antiproliferative effect by histone acetylation that influences gene expression.

Although there are reports of doses of up to 10 or even 20 g daily being used, this is in no way practical, as the supplement product that practitioners can supply would require so many capsules it would be off-putting. In addition, at these high doses the main side effect is a body odor of rancid butter.

A dose of 150–300 mg two or three times daily is a "high normal" range that seems safe and well tolerated. Butyrate supplements should be given in divided doses through the day due to its rapid metabolism and short plasma half-life. Note that butyrate supplementation is not essential for successful use of artemisinin but may be a beneficial addition to the protocol if tolerated by the patient.

For people who like to eat their medicine, butyric acid is found in butter, and the distinctive smell of rancid butter is the result of the chemical breakdown of the butyric acid glyceride. Butter, ghee, raw milk, and Parmesan cheese are the best food sources. Fecal butyrate levels can vary greatly among individuals, but eating a diet high in resistant starches increases butyric acid levels and may help maintain colorectal health.

Asimina triloba

Common name: Pawpaw

Plant family: Annonaceae

Parts used: Seed, fruit, twigs

Pawpaw is the largest fruit native to North America, with a creamy, custardy texture and a flavor reminiscent of banana, mango, and pineapple. A fiber from the inner bark is used for making strong rope and string, and a yellow dye is made from the ripe flesh of the fruit. Pawpaw is the only temperate species among the 120 genera and more than 2,100 species in the family Annonaceae; the rest are tropical or subtropical. Several members of this family contain neurotoxic long-chain fatty acid derivatives known as acetogenins, including annonacin from the tropical soursop or graviola fruit (*Annona muricata*), which also shows anticancer activity.

What Makes It Medicinal

Pawpaw contains more than 50 acetogenins, found in all plant parts, but concentrated mostly in the seed. These are derivatives of long-chain (C-32 or C-34) fatty acids and are part of a large class of naturally occurring polyketides exhibiting potent anticancer activities. Polyketides are secondary metabolites from bacteria, fungi, plants, and animals. Polyketides have diverse biological activities and pharmacological properties and are the building blocks for a broad range of drugs.

Antiproliferative and inhibits multidrug resistance. Acetogenins from pawpaw polyketides are powerful inhibitors of the enzyme NADH ubiquinone oxidoreductase involved in cellular respiration and thus cause inhibition of ATP production, as well as inhibition of multidrug resistance. Acetogenins are especially effective in cases where chemoresistance is due to ATP-dependent efflux pumps. In commercial use, polyketide-based drugs are used as antibiotics, antifungals, cytostatics, anticholesterolemics, antiparasitics, animal growth promoters, and natural insecticides. Some well-known examples include erythromycin A (antibiotic), rapamycin (immune suppressant and mTOR inhibitor), lovastatin (anticholesterol), and resveratrol (redox regulating and chemoprotective).

The antiproliferative activity of pawpaw is higher in unripe seeds than in ripe ones and depends on acetogenin content. The leaves also contain toxic annonaceous acetogenins, making them unpalatable to most insects. The one notable exception is the zebra swallowtail butterfly, whose larvae feed on the leaves. This confers protection from predation throughout the butterfly's life, as trace amounts of acetogenins remain present, making the insects unpalatable to birds and other predators. The bark contains other acetogenins, including asimin, asiminacin, and asiminecin, but the seed is the most potent medicine.

Interestingly, at least in laboratory research, more than 30 known acetogenins seem to be selectively cytotoxic to one or only a few cancer cell lines. For example, squamotacin is selective for prostate cells only, while the 9-keto acetogenins are selective for pancreatic cells. In clinical practice, this is a strong argument for using whole herb extract to provide the full range of active compounds.

Clinical Applications of *Asimina triloba*

- Antitumor, pesticidal, antimalarial, antiparasitic, antiviral, and antimicrobial
- Shampoo for treating infestations of head lice, fleas, and ticks

Ointment for treatment of oral herpes (HSV-1) and other viral skin infections
Soak or lotion for scabies or chiggers

Adverse Effects

The pawpaw fruit is edible, but some people get stomach upset after eating it. Intravenous infusions of annonacin in rats showed neurotoxic effects at between 3.8 and 7.6 mg/kg per day for 28 days, but that is not a delivery method that herbalists would use, so it is difficult to extrapolate to oral consumption of seed extracts.

Neurotoxicity and symptoms of atypical Parkinsonism (postural instability, frontal lobe dysfunction, gait disturbance, accumulation of tau proteins in the midbrain, and poor response to treatment with L-dopa) has been associated with eating the fruit of *Annona muricata* (soursop), which contains annonaceous acetogenins, but this has not been reported in the fruit or seed of *Asimina triloba*. Possibly, this is due to more limited consumption of pawpaw, which is localized and seasonal, as the toxicity appears to be a cumulative, chronic problem caused by daily or almost daily consumption of the tropical species over several years. Researchers suggest that the neurotoxicity of soursop is caused by a synergy between the neurotoxic benzyltetrahydroisoquinoline alkaloids and the specific types of acetogenins that are peculiar to *Annona muricata*. They also suggest possible unknown genetic factors that predispose some people to atypical Parkinsonism. None of these findings have been reported from clinical use of pawpaw seed extract, but the possibility should not be discounted. Assessment may be challenging if pawpaw is being used concurrently with chemotherapies that may also contribute to neurological and central nervous system dysfunctions.

Dosing

The dried fruit pulp yields around 300 mcg of acetogenins per gram of dry weight. A typical dose for treating cancer would be 8–10 mg acetogenins twice daily, equivalent to approximately 30 g (1 oz.) of dried fruit twice daily. This is generally recognized as safe, with no abnormalities in liver, kidney, electrolyte, blood sugar, or bone marrow functions. A powdered seed product would be dosed much lower, as acetogenins are present in higher amounts in seed than fruit, and such products may be used in research but are not generally recommended for use in clinical practice.

Clinical Pearls

An analysis of acetogenin content of young pawpaw tree twigs showed up to 1,000 times variability, which suggests that when harvesting it is useful to collect materials from as many individual plants as possible to avoid a predominance of plants that are low or high producers.

A human trial in the early 2000s gave a standardized extract providing 17 mg acetogenins daily to patients with breast, lung, prostate, lymphatic, and colorectal cancers and determined that it was effective whether used alone or as an adjuvant with other treatments including IGF-1 and insulin potentiation. Tumor markers decreased, tumor size diminished, energy improved, weight stabilized, and metastases were inhibited, culminating in increased longevity. No abnormalities were found in liver, kidney, electrolyte, blood sugar, or bone marrow functions. Neither the fruit nor the seed of this plant are commercially available in tincture form; presumably a moderately high amount of alcohol would be required to extract the acetogenins. Due to the need for carefully calibrated doses with this herb, it is recommended to use a standardized extract where the acetogenin content has been reliably determined by lab analysis.

Camptotheca acuminata

Common names: Cancer tree, happy tree, xi shu
Plant family: Nyssaceae
Parts used: Seeds, leaves

This is a deciduous tree indigenous to southern China, reaching 75 feet high with a canopy about 40 feet wide. It takes its genus name from the Greek for "curved sheath," referring to the rather strange-looking small fruit pods that form a round cluster. The bark and leaves have long been used in Traditional Chinese Medicine for liver and stomach ailments, for common colds, and for treating symptoms of what we would now recognize as leukemia. The Dong people of southern China made a paste from fresh leaves or fruits or a powder from dry materials to treat many stubborn skin conditions, including boils and surface infections, and even possibly skin cancers. Its antiproliferative effect is helpful in treating psoriasis.

What Makes It Medicinal

Topoisomerase I and II are intracellular enzymes required for unwinding and rewinding of DNA to allow gene copying. The activity of both enzymes is particularly increased in rapidly dividing cells such as in cancer, and they are both useful targets for anticancer therapy. Topoisomerase inhibitor drugs currently approved for human use are irinotecan and topotecan, derived from the cancer tree (inhibitors of topoisomerase I), and etoposide and teniposide, derived from mayapple (inhibitors of topoisomerase II).

Research in the 1950s revealed that the seeds and leaves of cancer tree contain numerous quinoline alkaloids, notably camptothecin (CPT), which has marked anticancer and antiviral effects. Hydroxycamptothecin and methoxycamptothecin have also been identified in the seeds and leaves and appear to be active. CPT can be highly toxic, making it difficult to administer as an herbal medicine. Notwithstanding that, these alkaloids have been turned into commercial chemotherapy drugs called irinotecan (CPT-11) and topotecan, which are clinically active and less toxic than the parent compound. They work by inhibition of topoisomerase I, induction of cell cycle arrest, and activation of caspase-3 and caspase-7, which induce apoptosis.

An in vitro study of cell viability in 2014 found that an aqueous extract of cancer tree standardized to 0.28 mg/mL of CPT demonstrated comparable or even enhanced cytotoxicity, compared with purified CPT treatment alone. The aqueous extract of cancer tree also exhibited a synergistic effect on the cytotoxicity of cisplatin in human endometrial carcinoma cell lines. This is encouraging, as it suggests synergy among the constituents in the herbs and supports the traditional use of crude extracts. Some studies have suggested that polysaccharides in the fruit may be pharmacologically active as well, inhibiting proliferation of human oral carcinoma, pancreatic carcinoma, and gastric carcinoma cells in vitro. The sugars (long chains of glucose and mannose) have strong antioxidant activity and provide protection from oxidative damage, and they have potential synergistic antioxidative effect with vitamin C (ascorbic acid) in vitro. The fruit also contains triterpenes that suppress human hepatocellular carcinoma cell proliferation through inducing apoptosis.

The importance of sourcing. CPT accumulates to approximately 0.4 percent of the dry weight of young leaves. This level is 1.5-fold higher than that of the seeds and 2.5-fold higher than that of the bark, the two currently used sources of the drug. As the leaves mature, the concentration and absolute amount of CPT decreases rapidly. Harvesting seeds and bark is more damaging to a tree than taking leaves, so the preferred harvest is of young leaves. Once again, we are reminded of the critical importance of quality control throughout the supply chain and, as best as possible in an ideal world, getting to know the farmer who grows the herbs that you prescribe, as well as laboratory assessment of active constituents in the plant.

The Need for Preservation

The raw material for the chemotherapy drugs irinotecan (CPT-11) and topotecan is still only available from *Camptotheca acuminata* trees. The harvesting of *C. acuminata* for the pharmaceutical industry has decimated the population of the endemic trees in China. The tree is considered to be endangered by the government of China, and export is severely restricted. By some estimates, there may be fewer than 4,000 of the trees remaining in the wild in China. It takes years to grow a tree big enough to take a seed or bark harvest, and taking too many young leaves will be detrimental to the health of the tree in the long term. There is a movement to cultivate more of this tree for medicine; this will help maintain the supply.

Dosing

Although it is rather old now, a USDA Technical Bulletin from 1970 describes 10 studies with extracts of the fruit, involving 60 animals at dose levels from 44 to 800 mg of CPT/kg of body weight, in which all animals survived, implying a high degree of safety in the fruit.

Information on dosing the herb (whole leaf, fruit, or extracts thereof) is absent in the literature as the research has been focused on isolated constituents and semisynthetic analogs. The major dose-limiting toxicities seen with the drugs are neutropenia, anemia, and thrombocytopenia (low white cells, low red cells, and low platelets), as well as diarrhea and nausea. Liver enzyme elevation is commonly seen while taking the drugs but it usually corrects after drugs are finished.

An extract of seed, fruit, leaf, and root bark (taken from peripheral roots, so as not to harm the tree) made with 65% alcohol and 35% water is expected to yield alkaloids, triterpenes, and polysaccharides. A tincture made at 1:2 strength should be dosed at 1–2 mL daily, equivalent to 0.5–1 g of dried plant material. After 2 weeks test the liver enzymes, and if they are normal, then double the dose. Repeat liver enzyme tests monthly and consider doubling dose again if the liver remains stable and the cancer remains active.

Catharanthus roseus

Common names: Madagascar periwinkle, rosy periwinkle
Plant family: Apocynaceae
Parts used: Dried root, leaves, flowers, stalks

This is a small evergreen shrub, native to Madagascar. The first references to its use in medicine go back more than 4,000 years to early Mesopotamian folklore. It is now naturalized and cultivated in many countries, and many ethnobotanical (folk) uses have arisen. In India, the fresh juice is applied to bee and wasp stings. In the Philippines, a decoction of leaves is used for diabetes, abdominal cramps, and menorrhagia. In parts of Asia, the root is used for dysentery, and leaves and root are used for cancer. In Madagascar and the Caribbean, the leaves serve as emetics and the root as a purgative and vermifuge. Other folk traditions include using the flowers as an eye wash and the leaves for asthma and tuberculosis. It is considered a hemostatic (arresting bleeding) for easing heavy menses and is also used for muscle aching and rheumatism.

What Makes It Medicinal

There are more than 400 known alkaloids in this plant, of which two from the terpenoid-indole alkaloids grouping have become well-known anticancer drugs: vinblastine and vincristine. These have shown to be quite active against Hodgkin's disease, non-Hodgkin's lymphoma, testicular cancer, breast cancer, and choriocarcinoma. These drugs may have a cure rate of more than 90% in the treatment of testicular carcinomas, and in Hodgkin's disease the 5-year survival rate in people taking them can be as high as 98%. The semisynthetic drug vinorelbine is derived from several different catharanthus alkaloids and is used to treat non–small cell lung cancer. Hair loss, peripheral neuropathy, constipation, and hyponatremia are the major side effects of these drugs.

Other alkaloids in the plant can significantly reduce blood pressure, promote insulin production, and lower blood sugar. Ajmalicine, an alkaloid found in the roots, promotes cerebral blood flow. There is also an alkaloid called vinpocetine that enhances utilization of oxygen and sugars by the brain, and this improves learning capacity and memory.

Generally speaking, the anticancer alkaloids are present in the leaves, the antihypertensive alkaloids are found in the roots, and the antidiabetic flavonoids are found in the leaves and flowers. Madagascar periwinkle root also contains volatile and phenolic compounds with antioxidant activity.

The anticancer actions of vinblastine and vincristine are due to the alkaloids binding to tubulin in the mitotic spindle, thereby arresting cell replication and inducing apoptosis. The extent to which this occurs from ingesting simple tinctures of the herb is not known, but even tea leads to a decrease in white blood cells, so therapeutic action is expected and some caution is required; more is not always better. Antibacterial and wound-healing (vulnerary) actions of leaves and flowers can also be of use in cancer care.

Dosing

The traditional remedy of plant juice from pressed fresh leaves and stems is dosed at 10–20 mL daily. A tincture of *Catharanthus roseus* given once at a dose equivalent to 2,000 mg of alkaloids was not fatal to rats 14 days after ingestion, but the liver enzymes AST, ALT, and LDH as well as creatinine phosphokinase, urea, and creatinine were temporarily elevated in 300 mg and 2,000 mg daily doses.

The LD50 (lethal dose in 50 percent of subjects) for vinblastine in mice is 17 mg/kg given intravenously and for vincristine in mice is 5.2 mg/kg given by intraperitoneal injection. Extrapolating from this to clinical herbal practice is not easy, but it is clear that there is a very high safety record when using whole-plant extract.

Chelidonium majus

Common name: Greater celandine
Plant family: Papaveraceae
Parts used: Roots (for anticancer, antifungal, and antibacterial effects), foliage (for the liver and gallbladder and for antiviral effects); most herbalists use the whole plant

This is a very common English hedgerow plant that grows easily throughout temperate climate zones. Both the aerial parts and the root have traditional uses. The broken leaf or stem exudes a latex that is bright orange and slightly caustic. Traditionally used on warts and other small skin growths, it shows antiviral and antimitotic actions.

Internally, the plant is traditionally used as a stimulant with warming and drying (acrid) action and as an alterative, diuretic, diaphoretic, purgative, and vulnerary. It was especially indicated by Eclectic practitioners for people with sallow complexion, hepatic congestion, jaundice, throbbing pain in the right upper abdomen, and bilious headaches (queasy, nauseous, dizzy). It was also used for migraine, supraorbital neuralgia, bilious dyspepsia with headache, and other gastric and intestinal disturbance due to liver congestion and for hemorrhoids, hepatic and splenic congestion, and gastrointestinal disorders due to capillary engorgement of the viscera.

What Makes It Medicinal

Like other members of the poppy family, greater celandine contains a number of isoquinoline alkaloids, including coptisine (main alkaloid), chelidoxanthine, chelidonine, and berberine. Modern analytical research suggests that the alkaloids inhibit procancerous mitotic cyclins A and B and cyclin-dependent kinases CDK1 and CDK2, all of which would normally promote cell cycling (replication), and the alkaloids upregulate the anticancer CDK inhibitor protein p27, which induces apoptosis. Crude extracts of greater celandine, and purified compounds derived from them, have antiviral, anti-inflammatory, antitumor, and antimicrobial properties both in vitro and in vivo. All of these actions support the traditional uses as an alterative/blood purifier and anticancer agent.

The herb is considered to have tissue specificity for organs served by nerves from the solar plexus and with blood from the hepatic artery and the splenic artery. For treating cancer, I use this herb for all the subdiaphragmatic organs (stomach, pancreas, gallbladder, liver, kidneys, and spleen). I consider it an antimitotic and cytotoxic herb that is, helpfully, also a blood purifier, promoting liver detox pathways and bile production.

Specific Indications and Uses of *Chelidonium majus*

The Eclectic physicians of the middle to late 1800s in America prescribed herbs based not only on the chemistry and pharmacology of the plant, which they could see and measure, but also on the individual and unique needs of each patient. This became known as "specific medicine" and allowed for an understanding of constitution and phenomenology to guide the prescribing principles. This is illustrated well in the description of the patient who needed greater celandine found in *King's American Dispensatory*, written in 1898 by Harvey Wickes Felter and John Uri Lloyd:

"Full, pale, sallow tongue and mucous membranes; skin pale and sallow, sometimes greenish; hepatic congestion; jaundice, due to swollen bile ducts; sluggish hepatic action; cough, with hepatic pain; fullness, with tensive or throbbing pain in the right hypochondrium, and pain extending to right shoulder; melancholia, headaches, and gastric disorders, dependent upon faulty action of the liver."

Specific actions of the alkaloids. Alkaloids from the root are antimicrobial against *Staphylococcus aureus, Klebsiella pneumoniae, Mycobacterium smegmatis,* and *Candida albicans,* as well as antiviral against the measles virus, herpes virus, viral encephalomyocarditis, and influenza virus. Chelerythrine and sanguinarine are antimicrobial against gram-positive bacteria, anti-inflammatory in oral and mucous membrane infections, and antifungal against *Trichophyton mentagrophytes* and *T. rubrum, Microsporum canis, Epidermophyton floccosum,* and *Aspergillus fumigatus.* These alkaloids are of generally low toxicity, and the aerial parts of the plant can inhibit liver alanine aminotransferase and protect the liver from transiting toxins.

Pharmaceuticals Made from *Chelidonium majus*

An injectable pharmaceutical has been made from the alkaloids of greater celandine root, notably a thiophosphate derivative, called NSC-631570 or Ukrain, that enhances the quality of life and prolongs the life of patients with pancreatic cancer and exhibits antitumor and antigenotoxic activities in microdoses in liver cancer. It was developed more than 20 years ago and tested on patients with several different types of cancers. In lab studies, it kills cancer cells while leaving healthy cells alone. It has been controversial, exalted and reviled in equal measure, and is now undergoing research at Memorial Sloan Kettering Cancer Center in the US.

The drug works by inducing oxidative damage in cells and by inhibition of DNA, RNA, and protein synthesis. It exerts weak inhibition of tubulin polymerization, meaning dividing cells cannot build the spindles of the cytoskeleton properly and hence cannot arrange chromosomes correctly for cell division to proceed. In this way, it causes cell cycle arrest at the G2/M phase. It also supports total T cell count and T helper lymphocytes, decreases T suppressor cells, and activates splenic lymphocytes. In breast cancer and melanoma cells, it may have a synergistic effect when used with the chemotherapy drug bortezomib (Velcade). Human studies suggest it can help in palliative care and prolong survival in pancreatic cancer patients when administered with the chemotherapy drug gemcitabine.

In animal models, it restored pro-inflammatory functions of hypoxic macrophages. Ukrain exerted selective cytotoxic and cytostatic effects on tumor cells, simultaneously acting as an immune response modifier and showing good tolerance and lack of side effects even after long-term application.

It is not yet approved for general prescription in the US and it is uncertain how much we can extrapolate directly from the drug to the herbal extract, but certainly, once again, the new studies are confirming mechanisms of action for uses that have been long known.

Adverse Reactions

Adverse reactions may include soreness at injection site, nausea, diarrhea, dizziness, fatigue, drowsiness, thirst, frequent urination, and slight fever. Hematological side effects and tumor bleeding have been observed, but only with the injectable drug and not reported for the whole herb extract.

Clinical Pearls

Greater celandine root has anticancer action with some tissue specificity to the liver, gallbladder, and pancreas. It is indicated for hepatic and biliary tree dysfunctions such as fatty liver (NASH), cysts in the liver, fatty pancreas (NASP), gallstones, cholecystitis (gallbladder inflammation), or biliary dyskinesia (spasms and narrowing of the bile duct). It is especially useful in liver, gallbladder, and pancreatic cancers, as well as other subdiaphragmatic and abdominal cancers, and in skin cancers.

Greater celandine aerial parts (flowering tops and leaves) have antimicrobial and antifungal action with some specificity to oral mucosa and mucous membranes. There is a strong antimitotic and antiviral effect, making this useful as a topical application in warts and early-stage skin cancers. It is used as a gargle in squamous cell carcinomas of the mouth, which usually have a viral trigger (herpes, EBV, or HPV), and as a douche in cervical dysplasia or cervical cancer.

Toxicology and Safety

Numerous studies and case reports have suggested possible hepatotoxicity from isolated celandine alkaloids or combinations of them, although the in vivo relevance of these results is hard to determine. In studies on rats, doses of whole herb as high as 3 g/kg of body weight did not result in any symptoms of hepatic injury and did not alter liver function.

Notwithstanding that, case reports collected over 30 years include cholestasis and mild to severe liver impairments. No specific constituents have been directly linked to this, and it is suggested that drug interactions rather than intrinsic toxicity may be responsible. A 2017 meta-analysis of hepatotoxicity concluded that results of animal studies are ambiguous and any true toxicity due to DNA intercalating properties of sanguinarine and chelerythrine may be modulated and ameliorated by inducing or alleviating oxidative stress or adjustment of hepatic enzymes such as MAO and SOD.

This is particularly significant because one of the main traditional indications for celandine is to treat liver and biliary tract disorders, due to its cholagogue and hepatoprotective activities.

Dosing

A typical dose would be a tincture at 1:5 strength (45–65% EtOH) at 2–4 mL daily or up to 25 mL/week.

Larrea divaricata, L. tridentata

Common names: Chaparral, creosote bush, larrea
Plant family: Zygophyllaceae
Parts used: Aerial parts, leaves, twigs

This small shrub is from the Mojave, Sonoran, and Chihuahuan deserts and is commonly called creosote bush due to its distinctive smell. It has bright yellow flowers and the whole plant is covered in a sticky resin that deflects desert sun off the leaves and protects the plant from scorching. It has long been used by Indigenous people as a tea and a skin wash and is considered to be a very effective blood purifier, antiviral, antifungal, and anticancer agent. Modern research suggests it has benefits in treating human immunodeficiency virus (HIV), human papillomavirus (HPV or genital warts), cancer, and neurodegenerative diseases and for delaying cellular aging.

This plant expresses significant regionalism, which may affect medicinal uses. Plants growing in the Chihuahuan desert have normal paired chromosomes, while in the milder and slightly wetter climate of the Sonoran desert, each cell has four sets of chromosomes. Plants growing in the hotter and drier Mojave desert exhibit hexaploidy with six sets of chromosomes.

This phenomenon of polyploidy is known to have significant implications in some herbs (as with *Acorus calamus,* where the diploid type is safe and the polyploid type generates dangerous levels of neurotoxic asarone). The exact correlation of polyploidy in chaparral with the quantity and diversity of the production of secondary metabolites is currently under review. It may be that plants from specific regions have more or fewer benefits than those from different locations.

What Makes It Medicinal

Six polyphenolic lignans occur in the leaves of chaparral, and they exhibit strong growth-inhibitory activity against human breast cancer and human melanoma cell lines and weak activity against human colon cancer.

NDGA

The most widely researched medicinal constituent in *Larrea* species is the cyclic lignan molecule nordihydroguaiaretic acid (NDGA), a powerful phenolic antioxidant, and its derivatives. NDGA directly inhibits the function of two cell membrane PTK receptors that are often upregulated in cancer: the insulin-like growth factor 1 receptor (IGF-1R) and the HER2/neu receptor.

The leaves contain a significant level of resin, which comprises almost 50 percent NDGA and contains, as well, at least 19 flavonoids and a large quantity of essential oils (about 300 volatile compounds).

In vitro studies have shown that NDGA causes arrest of DNA copying in the S phase of cell replication and induces apoptosis. It inhibits glycolysis and the electron transfer chain. An additional 18 known flavones and flavanol glycosides contribute to an antioxidant effect as well.

Methylated NDGA derivatives may induce a reversal of multidrug resistance in cancer cells by inhibiting Sp1 transcription factor, which prevents overexpression of P-glycoprotein critical to efflux pumping.

Actions of Larrea

- Antioxidant
- Anti-inflammatory
- Antiallergy
- Hypolipidemic
- Antifungal
- Antiviral
- Hepatic stimulant
- Anticancer

Pharmacology of NDGA

- Anti-inflammatory—inhibits COX, which lowers the PGE2 series, and thromboxanes; inhibits LOX, which lowers leukotrienes
- Antiasthma—decreases histamine and slow-release substance of anaphylaxis in lungs; decreases bronchial spasm
- Anticancer—targeted cytotoxicity by blocking transcription specific genes, retards cancer cell growth and leads to cell cycle arrest and apoptosis

Flavonoids

- Inhibit aerobic glycolysis by bacteria and cancer cells through inhibition of mitochondrial NADH oxidases, succinoxidase, and folate dehydrogenase
- Inhibit lipid peroxidation and protect the liver from rancid fats

Volatile Oil

- Antibacterial
- Antiviral
- Antifungal

Polysaccharides

- Immunomodulating

Phytosterols

- Anti-inflammatory
- Alterative

Clinical Applications

- Hypercholesterolemia (lowers LDL and triglycerides, prevents peroxidation)
- Blood poisoning
- Chronic and subclinical infections
- Toxin accumulation
- Candida or chronic mold exposures
- Cancers, especially of the skin and the breast
- Increases cancer cell sensitivity to trastuzumab (Herceptin)

Addressing Safety Concerns

Chaparral was widely used during the 1950s as a food preservative and to preserve natural fibers. Subsequently, it was banned for food use after reports of renal and hepatotoxicity arose during the early 1960s from chronic exposure to NDGA. Prior to this there were no notable reports of hepatotoxicity from whole herb use.

In the 1990s, the FDA recorded multiple reports of hepatitis attributed to chaparral, most occurring within 1–12 months of commencing use and resolving within a few weeks to months of discontinuation. During this time frame the FDA received reports of several cases of mild elevations of serum liver enzyme concentrations, two cases of fulminant hepatitis requiring liver transplants, and four cases where there was progression to cirrhosis. *Larrea tridentata* was found in all preparations, and biochemical and microbial contamination was excluded. A causal relationship was indicated by the correlation between intake of chaparral and the onset of liver disease, a consistent pattern of hepatic damage, and the observation that reexposure to chaparral or an increased dose led to relapse or aggravation of clinical signs of liver disease. It was determined that the likely cause of hepatic injury was NDGA functioning as a dysregulator of cyclooxygenase and lipoxygenase pathways and generating a localized inflammatory response.

The American Herbal Products Association released a public statement in 1995 and updated it in 2004, stating, "Rare reports of serious liver disease have been associated with ingestion of chaparral. Seek advice from a healthcare practitioner before use and, in so doing, inform them if you have had, or may have had, liver disease, frequently use alcoholic beverages, or are using any medications. Discontinue use and see a doctor if vomiting, fever, fatigue, abdominal pain, loss of appetite, or jaundice (e.g., dark urine, pale stools, yellow discoloration of the eyes) should occur."

Health Canada released a similar statement in 2005, stating, "Consumers should stop ingesting retail products containing chaparral and seek medical attention if they have experienced symptoms such as nausea, vomiting, abdominal cramps, fever, fatigue or jaundice (e.g., dark urine, yellow discoloration of the eyes)."

Interestingly, there have been no new reports of larrea toxicity since the late 1980s. That may mean that the health warnings were effective in preventing long-term or high-dose use, and/or there may have been a contaminant in the supply chain in those years that is no longer present.

Chaparral-containing topical products, such as ointments, creams, and lotions, have not been associated with adverse effects and to date, Health Canada has received just one report of acute hepatitis associated with chaparral ingestion.

Methylation of NDGA renders it nontoxic, and attempts are being made now to create antiviral and anticancer drugs in this way.

Dosing

Tincture: 1–2 mL daily of 1:5 tincture (60% EtOH).

Patients should take it for 2 months on and 1 month off in rotation; monitor liver enzymes regularly.

Topical treatments: There is no restriction on using larrea topically. It can be included in lotions or creams, soaks or poultices, and can be used in a douche. Be cautious of strong alcohol on inflamed or abraded tissues, as it may sting and irritate. Dilute the tincture with water or make a decoction using 20 g of herb in 400 mL water.

Caveats

Avoid in individuals with known liver or renal compromise.

Clinical Pearls

This herbal extract is safe for topical use and can be used internally with care. It is especially indicated for cancers where there is a viral component—for example, as a gargle in squamous cell carcinoma of the mouth, or as a douche for cervical dysplasia with positive HPV screen.

Phytolacca decandra, P. americana

Common name: Pokeroot

Plant family: Phytolaccaceae

Part used: Root

Approach this herb with considerable caution; it can be toxic, in even quite modest amounts. Every year someone in the southern part of the US, where it grows wild, will become sick after eating the spring greens (a traditional dish). Even with two or three changes of water and repeated boiling, it can still cause severe digestive distress. Dosing requires particular care, as too much of this herb results in catharsis, cramping, and prostration. A particular concern is that poisoning can take some hours to become apparent, during which time more doses could be taken. It is useful here to start low and go slow.

The root contains:

- Triterpene saponins called phytolaccosides
- An alkaloid called phytolaccine
- A resin containing phytolaccic acid
- A lectin called pokeweed mitogen

Traditional applications include use as an alterative, antiphlogistic (tissue decongestant), and a drainage herb used for the lymphatic system to activate lymph glands and lymphocytes. It has long been recognized as a lymph system stimulant, used for lymphadenopathy (lymph node swelling) and chronic viral diseases.

Actions and Uses of Pokeroot

Pokeroot has some tropism for the skin and the epithelial (mucous membrane) glandular structures, especially those of the upper respiratory tract (throat, ears, sinuses), and the linings of the reproductive organs and glands. It also relieves congestion and edema and promotes free flow of lymph. If applied to the skin as a pressed juice, a strong decoction, or a poultice of the root, it is rubefacient, causing redness, heat, and possibly skin irritation or inflammation in sensitive individuals. It should be mixed with something innocuous as a carrier or diluent (e.g., almond oil, marshmallow root).

Specific Indications and Uses

This was a favorite herb of the Eclectics and they used it liberally:

> "Pallid mucous membranes with ulceration; sore mouth with small blisters on tongue and mucous membrane of cheeks; sore lips, blanched, with separation of the epidermis; hard, painful, enlarged glands; mastitis; orchitis; parotitis; aphthae; soreness of mammary glands, with impaired respiration; faucial, tonsillar, or pharyngeal ulceration; pallid sore throat, with cough or respiratory difficulty; secretions of mouth give a white glaze to surface of mouth, especially in children; white pultaceous sloughs at corners of mouth or in the cheek; and diphtheritic deposits."
>
> *King's American Dispensatory*, 1898

Pokeweed mitogen is a lectin (sugar/protein complex) that activates the acquired immune system. It is considered a polyclonal T cell activator because it reacts with the T cell surface nonspecifically and produces the same series of cellular events as does an antigen.

Unlike the situation with antigen stimulation, where only a small fraction of the cells are sensitive, pokeweed mitogen transforms a major portion of the T cells. Additionally, some B cells are affected, although their response appears to be T cell dependent. Pokeweed mitogen activates both T and B lymphocytes, but helper T cells are preferentially stimulated.

Therapeutic Actions

- Leukocytic (attracts white cells to an area where the herb is applied topically) for laryngitis, tonsillitis, mastitis, otitis, sinusitis, and inflammation or ulceration of mucous membranes; it can be helpful as a gargle and spit for the throat or an oil or tincture extract applied to the skin
- Lymph node and lymphocyte activator for lymphadenopathy and lowered immune states
- Alterative/lymphatic decongestant for cysts, boils, acne, dry eczema, psoriasis
- Anti-inflammatory, especially for autoimmune inflammations

(rheumatoid arthritis, lupus, polymyalgia rheumatica)

- Thyroid stimulant for hypothyrodism or goiter

Dosing

Tincture: 5–15 mL weekly of 1:10 tincture made with 65% EtOH. If using dried plant material to make the tincture, dose at the higher end of the range. If using fresh herb, dose at the lower end of the range, as it is more potent.

Start at a low dose and increase slowly over 2 or 3 weeks to establish tolerance. Bowel disturbance, cathartic action, and prostration can occur if dose is excessive.

Most herbals suggest using the dried herb for greater safety; Mills and Bone suggest a dose of up to 0.2 g of dried root per day or 0.15–0.7 mL/day of 1:5 tincture for adults, and they recommend avoiding the use of fresh plant tinctures because of potential toxic effects.

Topical application: One of the most effective ways to use pokeroot is to apply it topically, and so long as it is diluted properly it will be entirely safe. It is rubefacient (warming) and decongestant to underlying tissues.

Caveats

Pokeroot is classified by the *American Herbal Products Association's Botanical Safety Handbook* as class 3, meaning that it should be used only under supervision of a qualified practitioner.

Making Pokeroot Preparations

King's American Dispensatory reports that "this root loses its medicinal properties with age, consequently only recent material should be used for making the fluid preparations." Because it is impossible to know when you purchase a prepared tincture or oil product how old the herbs were when it was made, there is a concern about the risk of using older stock, as it would be a substandard product. For this reason, I like to make my own; it does take some work, though.

This plant grows prolifically in my apothecary garden, growing upwards of 10 feet high each year, with hollow stems over an inch in diameter, which I cut back to the ground every year for the winter. It is beautiful and imposing in the garden, with pretty, delicate flowers and gorgeous purple berries. I am always a little anxious that birds will take those berries and not only possibly poison themselves but also possibly spread seeds of this plant out into the forest, where it could become an invasive species, so I cut it down in fall just as the berries are ripening and burn that plant material.

Because it is such a big plant, it also has a big root, and it can take quite a bit of digging to unearth it. Once you have it out of the ground, cut the root material from the root crown (the part where the root and stem meet) and cut the aerial parts back to 8 inches or so above the crown, then plant the whole crown back into the ground and it will grow back. Scrub the roots very well in several changes of water and then cut them into small pieces. The easiest way is to use the slicing blade on a food processor; alternatively, you can use a very sharp knife, cleaver, or clippers (but that will tire out your hands).

Spread these pieces out on a clean cotton cloth on a baking sheet overnight to release some of their natural moisture so that they are less likely to mold if you use them to make an infused oil.

Pokeroot in Castor Oil

1. Chop 200 g of fresh root of pokeroot and allow to weep and wilt overnight.
2. Put it into a large glass jar and cover it with 1 L of castor oil.
3. Cover the top of the jar with fabric or a paper towel and an elastic band; do not seal a lid on the jar, as any moisture in the plant needs to escape.
4. Keep it at room temperature and stir daily for 2 weeks.
5. Strain off and discard the herb. Bottle the infused oil to use for castor oil packs (see page 119).

Podophyllum peltatum

Common name: Mayapple
Plant family: Berberidaceae
Part used: Root

For more than 100 years mayapple root has been known as one of the most stimulating and powerful alteratives and blood purifiers available. It is used in modest doses to relieve hepatic congestion, dyspepsia, and gallbladder dysfunction and in higher doses as a strong cholagogue and a slow but drastic purgative. It is also used for its antiviral, cytotoxic, and antineoplastic/antitumorigenic actions.

"May apple acts as a certain, but slow and gentle cathartic. It exerts a powerful influence upon the whole glandular system.

It acts as a gentle stimulant tonic, improves the appetite, and is particularly valuable in atonic dyspepsia, gastric and intestinal catarrh, and all atonic forms of indigestion, when the patient complains of dizziness, loss of appetite and heavy headache (or where) there is indisposition to exertion, the movements being heavy and sluggish, the tongue dirty and flabby, and the superficial veins, abdomen, and tissues in general, characterized by fullness. Podophyllum [may-apple] is specifically indicated by fullness of tissues, and particularly by fullness of superficial veins; oppressed full pulse; dirty yellowish coating of tongue and dizziness. It is contraindicated by pinched features and tissues, contracted skin and tongue.

By its slow and thorough action, yet permanent in its effects in restoring and maintaining the normal hepatic and intestinal secretions, podophyllum is one of the very best agents to overcome habitual constipation, and more especially if it be due to portal engorgement. The small dose should be given and continued until the evacuations become regular and normal."

King's American Dispensatory, 1898

In 1869, William Cook, a famous Eclectic doctor, cautioned that the fresh root of mayapple in higher doses is an acrid and excoriating poison, causing nausea, severe vomiting, burning of the esophagus, and violent catharsis, with severe twisting abdominal pain and watery (sometimes bloody) stools. He suggested that these symptoms may continue for up to 12 hours and may be followed by swelling, redness, dryness, and tenderness of the lips and mouth, tenderness and heat throughout the bowels, extreme prostration, with perhaps bloating of the face and other parts of the body—all of which may last for days, along with gastric tenderness, which may last for several weeks. He also notes that aging the root before using it in a preparation helps avoid these acute symptoms and suggests storing roots for 2 years before use.

What Makes It Medicinal

Mayapple contains a group of resinous lignan components, which can be extracted in high-alcohol tinctures. These include podophyllotoxins, which are functionally and structurally similar to alkaloids, with multiple rings, but lacking nitrogen. In both animal and human studies, these unique pseudoalkaloids have demonstrated antitumor activity. One of the podophyllotoxins, podophyllin, is licensed for use as a drug applied externally to treat venereal warts and herpes.

Two semisynthetic podophyllotoxin derivatives, etoposide and teniposide, are drugs used in the treatment of a variety of cancers. Etoposide acts primarily in the G2 and S phases of the cell cycle and arrests cell cycling by inhibiting DNA topoisomerase II, which causes irreparable damage to DNA. As a cell divides, tubulin polymerization required to form the spindle is a critical control point for inhibiting cell cycling. Etoposide does not inhibit tubulin polymerization; however, its parent compound, podophyllotoxin in the whole root, which has no inhibitory activity against DNA topoisomerase II, is a potent inhibitor of microtubule assembly. This is another example of the value of using whole herbs and whole herb extracts with certain chemotherapy drugs.

Clinical Pearls

According to the Eclectic physicians, mayapple is good for deep indolent ulcers, enlarged lymph glands, upper right abdominal aching, persistent sluggish bowel, fatty indigestion, and belching with nausea or headaches.

The root has been used as an escharotic to treat skin ulcers, for veterinary as well as human applications. It was used by Eclectic doctors as an escharotic, along with pokeroot and bloodroot, in a formula called Compound Tar Plaster, a forerunner of the infamous Black Salve (see page 435).

Dosing

The potency of each form is reflected by its relative dosage. The dose for the resinous podophyllin was traditionally given as ½–1 grain (30–65 mg) when taken as a mild cholagogue cathartic and up to 2 grains (130 mg) for gentle laxative and normalizing effects. From 2–4 grains (130–250 mg) of podophyllin may cause a drastic cathartic action with nausea and griping.

In 1869 William Cook recommended 5–10 grains (300–600 mg) of dried root as a strong single dose. He suggests that a cathartic dose (a good bit more than most people need) is obtained with 10–20 grains (600–1,200 mg). He also recommended that a dose not be repeated in less than 6 hours if the first one should fail to act, and it is generally best to wait 8 or 10 hours.

The *British Herbal Pharmacopoeia* suggests a daily dose of 0.12–0.6 g (120–600 mg) of dried root or 0.3–0.7 mL of a liquid 1:1 extract (made from dried root).

In my experience, an even lower dose is often effective. The dose above would be equivalent to 3–7 mL daily of 1:10 tincture (which I prefer to use). I suggest using a 1:10 made with 65% EtOH and dosing 10–20 drops (0.5–1 mL) twice daily.

Podophyllotoxin may be present in the root at concentrations of 0.3–1%. At the upper limit of 1% this would mean every 10 drops (0.5 mL) of a 1:10 tincture would yield 50 mg of dried herb equivalent and 0.5 mg of podophyllotoxin—well within the safety margins.

Caveats

Mayapple is classified by the *American Herbal Products Association's Botanical Safety Handbook* as 2b, meaning it should be avoided in pregnancy.

Sanguinaria canadensis

Common name: Bloodroot
Plant family: Papaveraceae
Parts used: Root, rhizome

This is a plant of the forest floor, blooming in the spring throughout the Appalachian Mountains in the eastern parts of the US and eastern Canada. It is slightly unusual in that it has only one large lobed leaf, up to 25 cm (10 in.) across, and it blooms before the leaves appear. The underground parts contain a red latex, hence the name. Indigenous peoples of North America called the herb "puccoon" and had many uses for it, including as a snuff to treat colds and sinus congestion, as a tea for sore throats, diphtheria, coughing blood, gastrointestinal bleeding, burns, and skin infections, and as an abortifacient, among other things.

Early settlers learned of this herb from Indigenous peoples and began to use it extensively, eventually recommending it as a bronchial muscle relaxant and stimulating expectorant for asthma, croup, and whooping cough, for its antibacterial action in pneumonia and tuberculosis, for gastrointestinal infections or bleeding, for jaundice and chronic liver disease, as an emmenagogue, and to treat rheumatism, suggesting anti-inflammatory properties. Dosing was 10–20 grains (about 0.75–1.25 g) daily.

Herbal practitioners today use bloodroot as an antimicrobial, a stimulating expectorant, a stimulant of mucous membranes, and an anticancer herb. It is recommended for atonic dyspepsia, pulmonary congestion, productive coughs, bronchitis and asthma, sinus discharge, catarrh and nasal polyps, or any red, swollen, purulent, or itchy mucous membranes. It is also used as a mouthwash for oral infections and gingivitis and topically for actinic keratosis and basal cell carcinoma.

The red latex found in the underground parts contains several long-chain alcohols (C26–C34), phytosterols, and triterpenes, but it is the array of alkaloids it contains that make it an especially interesting medicine. Bloodroot contains eight isoquinoline alkaloids at biologically relevant concentrations, including sanguinarine and chelerythrine (also found in greater celandine), which are the most researched. Actions attributed to these alkaloids include antimicrobial and anti-inflammatory effects.

Black Salve

Bloodroot has a long history of use in topical applications for skin ulcers and sores, and by the mid-1850s it was being prescribed in combination with zinc chloride in a product that became known as Black Salve. Sanguinarine is cytotoxic to animal cells, and if applied to the skin in sufficient concentration, it can cause tissue damage, localized necrosis, and formation of an eschar—a piece of dead tissue that sloughs off from the surface (different than a scab, which is composed of dried blood and inflammatory exudate).

Zinc chloride is corrosive and highly irritant, causing ulceration and burns on the skin. The two agents together were profoundly damaging and risked infection and scarring, quite aside from the pain endured. Needless to say, Black Salve is not recommended today!

Escharotics

In the 1800s, before there was effective anesthesia or antisepsis in surgery, it probably appeared safer and preferable to remove some cancers that were on or near the surface of the skin by "burning" them off with caustic salves, rather than undergoing the knife. These agents were called escharotics, after the term *eschar*—dead tissue that forms after a burn, an ulcerated insect or spider bite or fungal infection, and in gangrene. (As tissue repair and granulation occurs from the bottom of the injury toward the top, and the eschar serves as a protective layer, gradually loosening as healing happens, until it sloughs off.) Black Salve, which contains bloodroot, was one of the more effective and enduring escharotics. Indeed, people still ask about obtaining Black Salve today, and I am always quick to head them off. Now that surgery is safer and anesthesia is effective, it is not clinically justifiable to use escharotics for cancer anymore.

Having said that, some escharotics are still used in modern medicine; salicylic acid is keratolytic for treatment of genital and regular warts and of skin tags, and a drug called imiquimod is used for actinic keratosis and early-stage basal cell carcinoma (BCC). In some of these situations, however, there is a case to be made for using bloodroot topically for treating warts, actinic keratosis, and BCC instead of using imiquimod.

Imiquimod 5% cream causes a strong local inflammatory reaction, with redness, itching, and dryness, flaking, or scaling followed by blistering, crusting and scabbing, skin breakdown, and ulceration, as well as systemic reactions, such as fever, body aching, headache, and malaise. Even more worrying is that it causes lowering of hemoglobin and white blood cell count, even though it is being used topically. These reductions are not clinically significant in patients with normal blood levels, but a cancer patient who may be immunocompromised from chemotherapy and radiation, and who needs all the immune support they can get, may want to avoid using it. Imiquimod may also cause elevated liver enzymes, and there have been rare reports of worsening of autoimmune conditions. People who use immunosuppressing drugs are advised not to use imiquimod.

In the case of basal cell carcinoma, most people today undergo Mohs surgery, a complete excision to clear margins of any diseased tissue, with a success rate of 95+ percent. The technique was developed in the middle of the twentieth century by Dr. Frederick E. Mohs, and he often used a paste with bloodroot and zinc chloride for 24–48 hours prior to the surgery to induce immune responses. This is now replaced by the imiquimod (with all the collateral risks it entails).

Using Bloodroot for Actinic Keratosis and Basal Cell Carcinoma

Today herbal practitioners use bloodroot extract internally in drop doses, and topically as a salve, but not with the zinc chloride (as it was in Black Salve), which is too corrosive. In fact, today bloodroot is sometimes combined in a salve with zinc sulfate or zinc oxide, both of which are exceptionally healing and antimicrobial on the skin.

There is skin irritation, blistering, and broken skin when using bloodroot for actinic keratosis and BCC, as the herb triggers inflammatory and immune activation. But compared with imiquimod cream, the bloodroot is much safer! I have worked with both the herb and the drug in numerous patients, and bloodroot does not appear to have any adverse systemic effects on white blood cell count or on the liver enzymes.

Bloodroot in Dental Care and Oral Hygiene

Because of its antimicrobial actions, sanguinarine and bloodroot extract have been approved by the FDA for use in toothpastes or mouthwashes as an antibacterial or antiplaque agent. However, there is some concern that using bloodroot in dental care products may be associated with the development of leukoplakia (precursor to oral cancer), so this is not recommended for longer than a month without an equivalent time off.

The alkaloids of bloodroot and their effects are well researched, and some of the same alkaloids are found in greater celandine as well as related isoquinoline alkaloids in Oregon grape and barberry. In all these herbs, the alkaloids also exert antimicrobial action, but without the risk of mucosal irritation seen with bloodroot. I do use bloodroot in small doses (5% of total) in a mouthwash for infections, but I may suggest alternating months on and off for the bloodroot.

Bloodroot and Cancer Care

There is extensive current research available on sanguinarine and chelerythrine, but little to none on whole herb extracts. The extent to which we can reasonably extrapolate from isolates studied in cell cultures to the human experience of using whole herbs is uncertain but informed by history and traditional uses. In other words, we know that bloodroot has been used for at least 200 years to treat infections (including lung infections) and cancer, and modern research points to sanguinarine being a key active constituent.

Evidence suggests the combined alkaloids from bloodroot have up to four times greater antimicrobial effect against *Helicobacter pylori* than any individual alkaloid and up to 10-fold increased cytotoxicity against *Trypanosoma brucei,* indicating a marked synergistic effect. This suggests that whole herb extract may have greater effects than isolated constituents.

Sanguinarine causes disruption to the nucelotides of DNA and functions as a cytotoxic akin to the anthracycline chemotherapy drugs daunorubicin and doxorubicin. It induces DNA strand breaks and inhibits DNA strand repair through depletion of nuclear topoisomerase II, akin to the chemotherapy drug etoposide derived from mayapple. Sanguinarine binds the telomeres at the end of the chromosomes to prevent DNA unwinding and induces irreversible microtubule depolymerization in the cellular cytoskeleton, which inhibits cell proliferation and induces cell death. Sanguinarine also disrupts messenger RNA (mRNA), further interfering with protein synthesis and disturbing gene silencing and epigenetic regulation. Apart from its direct action on cellular nucleic acids, sanguinarine also exerts a cytotoxic effect via significant generation of reactive oxygen species (ROS).

Traditional use of bloodroot for cancer has been largely topical, but the antimicrobial and antiparasitic effects may indicate value in using it internally as well for pathogen-induced cancers.

Bloodroot and Heart Disease

Sanguinarine has a vasodilating effect by inhibiting alpha-1 and alpha-2 adrenoceptors and by inhibition of angiotensin II binding. Sanguinarine can slow the heart rate and increase the force of the beat in a similar way to the drug digoxin from foxglove. Protopine has vasodilating effects by elevating cAMP and cGMP.

Bloodroot and Inflammation

Protopine inhibits nitric oxide, reduces COX-2 expression, and impairs the production of prostaglandin E2, inflammatory interleukins IL-1β and IL-6, and TNF-α, and this generates a strong anti-inflammatory effect. Chelerythrine also has an anti-inflammatory action by inhibiting COX-2, 5-lipoxygenase, and PGE2 production.

Intercellular adhesion molecules (ICAM) and vascular cell adhesion molecules (VCAM) are key components of the inflammatory process by facilitating migration of neutrophils into tissues. Sanguinarine and isoliquiritigenin (a flavonoid from licorice) significantly downregulated VCAM-1 in vitro and this is likely to contribute to the anti-inflammatory effect.

Bloodroot and Infections

Sanguinarine is active against gram-negative and gram-positive bacteria and shows promise in treating methicillin-resistant *Staphylococcus aureus* (MRSA). Bloodroot alkaloids are active against *Mycobacterium aurum* (which causes tuberculosis) and have anthelmintic activity against schistosomiasis (snail-borne parasite) and other parasitic infections, including *Trypanosoma brucei,* the cause of sleeping sickness.

Dosing

As always, quality control is critical; knowing the source of the raw herb is optimal. In the case of sanguinarine, there are seasonal variations to consider. Plants contain the most alkaloid during flowering and early fruiting, so a spring harvest is preferred to fall.

Tincture: 0.3–2 mL three times daily of a 1:5 tincture made with 60% EtOH, equivalent to 60–400 mg of dried root three times daily. The emetic dose is between 1 and 2 grams dried herb or equivalent in tincture.

In 1869, Cook suggested the tincture be made with 6 oz. of dried root macerated in 1 quart of diluted alcohol (equivalent to 170 g in 946 mL); the ratio of alcohol to water not given. Today, we would suggest 60–65% alcohol to extract alkaloids well. Cook went on to recommend a dose of 5–15 drops as a stimulating expectorant. He also suggested a vinegar-based tincture (an anacetous tincture or acetracta) made with 4 oz. of bloodroot and a quart of distilled vinegar (113 g in 946 mL) as an expectorant but cautioned that this was "rather harsh to the respiratory membranes." Vinegar is an effective expectorant itself and was not infrequently used as the solvent to make expectorating remedies.

Taken as a powder of the root, the dose was suggested as 2–5 grains (0.13–0.32 g) three times a day for a tonic and alterative action and 1–2 grains (0.06–0.13 g) every 2 hours as an expectorant.

In more contemporary literature, the *British Herbal Pharmacopoeia* recommends bloodroot in combination with lobelia for bronchitis and asthma, with sage and cayenne to gargle for pharyngeal inflammations, with greater celandine topically for warts, and with slippery elm topically for chilblains.

Topical treatment: For topical use, Cook suggested 1 oz. of the vinegar tincture be diluted with 7 oz. of rose water to make a wash for ringworm, eczema, pimples, and other skin blemishes and eruptions.

Caveats

This herb is is classified by the *American Herbal Products Association's Botanical Safety Handbook* as 2b, meaning that it should be avoided in pregnancy, and 2d, meaning that it may cause nausea and vomiting. It is not recommended for use for longer than 1 month, and in Canada regulations prohibit it from being used in food articles.

Taxus brevifolia, T. baccata, T. wallichiana

Common names: Pacific yew (a.k.a. Western yew), Irish yew, Himalayan yew
Plant family: Taxaceae
Parts used: Bark, leaves, growth tips

Long revered as a symbol of longevity, but also feared because of its toxicity, yew is a potentially powerful medicinal plant to approach with great caution. The anticancer constituents in its bark are the source of several chemotherapy drugs; using the plant as part of a cytotoxic herbal protocol is worth considering.

Differences among Species

The genus *Taxus* is widespread across the northern hemisphere. It is important to know which species you're working with—and even, ideally, the actual percentage of different constituents—because some species are more toxic than others.

There are numerous subspecies and regional varieties of both Pacific and Irish yew.

Taxus brevifolia

Also known as Pacific yew, this small to medium-size evergreen tree is native to the Pacific Northwest, from southernmost Alaska south to central California, mostly in the Pacific Coast Ranges. Due to diminishing habitat and poor resource management, the Pacific yew is considered "near threatened" or on the edge of becoming endangered, as assessed by the International Union for Conservation of Nature (IUCN).

Taxus baccata

Taxus baccata (Irish yew) is native to western, central, and southern Europe, northwest Africa, northern Iran, and southwest Asia. It is slow growing but very long-lived, with the maximum girth probably being reached only after about 2,000 years. Some trees may be as much as 4,000 years old, making it the longest-living plant in Europe. The age of these trees is hard to determine accurately and is subject to much dispute, because the trunks often hollow out with age, making ring counts impossible.

Taxus wallichiana

Taxus wallichiana (Himalayan yew) is more prolific than Pacific yew and is a primary source material today for the manufacture of taxol. (Some is synthesized from Irish yew as well.) Himalayan yew is used in Ayurvedic and Unani medicine with apparent safety for its analgesic, antipyretic, anti-inflammatory, immunomodulatory, antiallergic, antibacterial, antifungal, antiplatelet, antispasmodic, anticonvulsant, and vasorelaxant effect.

All of these actions may be applicable in cancer care as well.

**The Life of a Yew,
the Length of an Age**

The lives of three wattles,
the life of a hound;

The lives of three hounds,
the life of a steed;

The lives of three steeds,
the life of a man;

The lives of three eagles,
the life of a yew;

The life of a yew, the length of an age;

Seven ages from Creation to Doom.

Attributed to Nennius, seventh-century historian (quoted from *Practical Magic in the Northern Tradition* by Nigel Pennick)

A Symbol of Death and Rebirth

Part of the yew's reputation for long life is due to the unique way in which the tree grows. Its branches grow out and then down into the ground to root themselves, and then they rise up around the old central growth as separate but cloned trunks. After a time, they cannot be distinguished from the original tree, and in this way there is an element of immortality in the tree. In addition, if a yew tree falls in the forest, another shoot will grow out of it. For these reasons, the yew has always been a symbol of death and rebirth, of passing over and being reborn, the new that springs out of the old.

In the old days, the people of the northern European regions worshiped underneath the yew tree, revering it for its age and powers. When the first Christian missionaries came to convert the "heathen" masses, they went to preach where the people already gathered for sacred service. For this reason, many of the oldest churches in northern Europe today have a huge old yew tree in their grounds, often much older than the church itself.

Toxicity

Most parts of the tree are toxic, except the bright red aril (fruit) surrounding the seed, which enables ingestion and seed dispersal by birds. Each species varies in its level of toxicity, with Irish yew being the most poisonous. The major toxins in yew are the alkaloidal taxines. The foliage remains toxic even when wilted or dried. Symptoms of overdose in humans are nausea, vomiting, abdominal pains, and dizziness; these are followed by bradycardia, ventricular arrhythmias and fibrillation, severe hypotension, and eventually death. A lethal dose of Irish yew leaf would be 0.6–1.3 g/kg (a total 36–78 g dose for a 60 kg [133-pound]adult), corresponding to 3–6.5 mg taxines/kg, but much smaller doses still cause serious illness.

What Makes It Medicinal

In addition to the toxic alkaloids in the needles, Pacific yew bark has as many as 27 different diterpene taxanes, some with potent anticancer activity. They are regulators of cell replication through decreasing the availability of tubulin to form spindles during mitosis, which inhibits cell replication. Taxol is one of the 27 diterpenes occurring in needles and bark and was first identified in the 1960s but not licensed for use until 1993 as a drug called paclitaxel. The bark of up to three mature trees was originally required to extract sufficient taxol for one person's treatment; this was quickly seen to be an unsustainable demand on the forest.

The average taxol concentration in the bark of Irish yew is about 0.055–0.008% of dry weight, while in Pacific yew it averages 0.01–0.02% or rarely up to 0.033%.

A semisynthetic taxane called docetaxel (Taxotere) was developed, as well as Abraxane, which is taxol bound to albumin for better bioavailability. These drugs are effective for many types of cancer, including ovarian, breast, and non–small cell lung cancer, but unfortunately initial benefits often do not last and drug resistance is common. Synthetic taxane drugs often cause undesirable side effects, and they induce multidrug resistance (MDR) by overexpression of the P-glycoprotein (Pgp) pump. This allows removal of chemotherapy from the target cell and is a major means of resistance to treatment. However, in the whole herb extract, some other diterpenes may act to inhibit multidrug resistance. In this way, co-prescribing taxol and yew extract will make taxol more potent and effective and may reduce side effects by keeping cytotoxic agents in the target cells.

Yew also contains flavonoids, including quercetin, which gives a redox-regulating effect, and plant sterols, which give an immunomodulating effect. Other potent chemical constituents may include immune-activating lignans and adaptogenic, anabolic phytoecdysteroids.

Dosing

There is a dearth of research on dosing yew, so herbal practitioners are left to do work-arounds to the best of their ability and based on evidence of relative safety of the whole herb. Even suggesting that it is safe for human consumption because animals eat it is dubious because the elk, moose, and deer that predominantly graze it are ruminants with a digestive system quite different from our own. Notwithstanding all of these variables, it is certainly an herb that the herbal practitioner will use in clinical practice, albeit with considerable caution.

Standardized dosing for the Pacific yew is not available, but it is substantially less toxic than Irish yew, as the cardiotoxic taxine alkaloids are almost absent. In one study, the LD50 of Pacific yew powder orally administered to rats could not be determined at doses up to 5 g/kg.

In mice, 100 and 200 mg/kg intraperitoneal doses of the extract from Himalayan yew was tolerated without apparent toxicity. In oral dosing, no toxicity was seen in mice given a single dose of 2 g/kg and observed for 7 days. This is equivalent to 120 g of leaves in one dose for a 60 kg (133-pound) person.

Using Irish yew is not recommended, and no standardized dose has been established for it.

There is only one commercial supplier of Pacific yew extract that I have found. They sell powdered branch tips in capsules at 300 mg each and suggest two capsules up to three times daily, equivalent to 1.8 g yew tip powder. They also make a tincture from fresh plant material at 1:1.7 ratio and give a suggested dose of 2 mL up to three times daily, equivalent to 3.36 g (3,360 mg) of dried herb daily. They do not explain the discrepancy in this recommendation in the company literature, but these are substantial doses and indicate a reasonable degree of safety.

Neither the tincture nor the powder of Pacific yew from this supplier are standardized, but using an average of 0.02% taxol by dry weight we can see that:

1 mL tincture at 1:1.7 = 585 mg dried herb equivalent per 1 mL of tincture

585 mg × 0.02% = 0.117 mg of taxol in every mL of tincture or 0.702 mg of taxol in 6 mL daily tincture dose

A 300 mg capsule has 0.06 mg of taxol per capsule so a daily dose of six capsules would yield 0.36 mg taxol.

Thus the supplier of this product is recommending a daily taxol dose range of 0.36–0.7 mg, given by mouth.

By way of comparison, when semisynthetic paclitaxel is given as a chemotherapy agent, doses range from 100–175 mg/m^2 given by intravenous injection over 3 hours.

Dosing the herb in capsule or tincture is not a direct equivalence because the drug is given by intravenous injection while the herb taken orally is subject to all the processes of the digestive system and hepatic metabolism before being released to systemic circulation. However, these calculations do serve to provide some assurance of safety with the herbal dosing.

I suggest starting at the lower dosage range, 1–2 g dried herb equivalent daily, and if that is well tolerated, without nausea, vomiting, abdominal pains, and dizziness, then you can increase to 3 or 3.5 g dried herb equivalent.

Clinical Pearls

As always, quality control is critical for good herbal medicine. There are seasonal changes in the concentrations of cardiotoxic taxine alkaloids in yew plants, with the highest concentrations during winter and the lowest in summer. Harvesting during summer is preferred, for a higher safety margin. Taxol content is also about 64 percent higher for male plants compared to female and is highest in older trees (over 110 years).

Metaphysical Meaning of Yew

One of the more interesting uses of this tree is in the esoteric realm, where its reputation for longevity and immortality, as well as myths and legends about its association with death, passing over, rebirth, and reincarnation, can be used as a conversation opener, an opportunity to explore the patient's fears and feelings. Sometimes, when talking with a patient about the taxol drug and how it works or talking about yew and how it works, both as a drug and as a metaphor or a spirit herb in the formula, it allows a deeper and more meaningful conversation to occur. In the apothecary garden at our farm, we have a tall, protective hedge of Irish yew for this very reason. It was a traditional hedging plant for medieval monastery gardens, but it also provides an opportunity for important conversations.

Aside from being ingested as medicine, yew can be used as a totem or amulet herb—a small sprig of the greenery perhaps kept close and contemplated, or an article made from yew wood, which is popular with wood turners and carvers for its interesting shapes and grains. It can be an ally herb for anyone who is dealing with cancer in some way or form, no matter if you take taxol or not. It can help, even as a flower essence, to break through expectations and conditioning, to face the fear and to get honest about what really matters. The yew tree helps to make the connection between our lovely but oh-so-short physical lives and the eternity we all return to.

Thuja occidentalis

Common names: Eastern arborvitae, northern white cedar (used interchangeably with *T. plicata* or western red cedar)
Plant family: Cupressaceae
Parts used: Young leaves and growing tips harvested in spring

This is a large and stately conifer from the northeastern Americas, now naturalized into Europe and widely planted around the world as an ornamental. Although nomenclature was unreliable in the 1500s and other trees could be contenders, it is believed to be the "tree of life" that was given by the indigenous people to save the lives of some sailors of Jacques Cartier's ill-fated voyage in the winter of 1536 when they were dying of scurvy. The decocted boughs of *Thuja occidentalis* contain appreciable amounts of vitamin C, as well as arginine, proline, and other amino acids that act as synergists in connective tissue to reduce the symptoms of vitamin C deficiency.

Ancient peoples of the Mediterranean cultures burned the aromatic wood of a local *Thuja* species (*T. orientalis*) along with sacrifices; indeed, the name "thuja" comes from the Latin form of the Greek word *thero* (to sacrifice). Other *Thuja* species were used in Egypt for embalming the dead, evidence of the strong antimicrobial action of this plant. In the Pacific Northwest, the indigenous species *T. plicata* is used interchangeably with *T. occidentalis* in medicine, with comparable research in both species.

The Grandmother of the Forest

The Indigenous peoples of the Pacific Northwest called *Thuja plicata* the grandmother of the forest, as it was often the oldest and the largest tree in the forest and provided for so many of their needs. The resin-infused wood is rot resistant and was used for building canoes, totem poles, and the ridgepole of the longhouse. The soaked and beaten bark fibers were used to make clothing and matting. Scored and steamed, hand-adzed planks were used to make the unique bentwood boxes of the region.

The idea of the thuja tree as a generous and benevolent grandmother, helping the people who love her, is borne out today in a more literal way by research by Dr. Suzanne Simard at the University of British Columbia. She established that these venerable old trees, with a huge photosynthetic capacity, are making a lot more sugars than they require for their own energy needs and are in fact "feeding" sugars via mushroom mycelia into the root systems of nearby seedlings that are still struggling to grow up above the competition on the forest floor.

Therapeutic Actions

- Astringent/cicatrant
- Stimulating expectorant
- Diuretic
- Antifungal
- Antiviral
- Moth and insect repellent
- Antineoplastic/antimitotic

Traditional Uses

The green spring tips have long been known for their antifungal and antiviral action. They can be boiled up to make a tea for washing dirty wounds, cleansing the sickroom, or used as a gargle for throat infections, and the steam can be inhaled for sinus and lung infections. Yew was traditionally used as a blood cleanser or depurative, especially for old, festering sores and for benign skin growths. It was considered a stimulating expectorant and decongestant remedy, used to treat acute bronchitis and other respiratory infections. It was also used as a diuretic and astringent to treat acute cystitis, bed-wetting in children, and incontinence. Thuja bough teas or extracts were recommended in gynecology for amenorrhea, leukorrhea, endometrial overgrowth, ovarian cysts, polyps, and uterine prolapse and were used as a douche for cervical dysplasia, yeast or bacterial overgrowth, herpes, and genital warts. Extracts were applied topically over stiff or painful joints or muscles as a counterirritant, improving local blood supply and warming the joint. Powdered cedar tips were used as a snuff or lavage for postnasal drip and for nasal polyps.

Thuja also has a long and established history in homoeopathic medicine, in which it is a key remedy for skin and genitourinary conditions with growths (such as warts, skin tags, fibroids, or uterine polyps), and especially as a depurative or blood cleanser where benign or malignant growths were considered to be a sign of blood dyscrasia. It is also recommended in homeopathy for people with low self-esteem and feelings of unattractiveness and worthlessness, for sharp left-sided headaches in the temple or forehead, and for a sensation that something is alive and moving in the abdomen, among other things.

What Makes It Medicinal

The main active ingredients are found in the oleoresin, which occurs at up to 4% in the leaf tips. It can be steam distilled and has particularly high levels of a monoterpene hydrocarbon called pinene, as well as monoterpene ketones such as carvone, (-)thujone, isothujone, and alpha- and beta-thujone.

These provide an antimicrobial action and promote granulation and tissue repair. They are antiparasitic, antifungal, and antiviral. There is some concern about neurotoxicity from prolonged dosing, so this means thuja should be taken in pulsed doses of 1 month on and 1 month off, alternating, and should be used only as an effector herb for specific conditions, not as a long-term tonic herb.

The essential oil also yields at least seven diterpenoids. There are thousands of different diterpene molecules found in plants, including, for example, the taxanes from Pacific yew and the ginkgolides from *Ginkgo biloba*. The diterpenes from thuja are poorly researched to date but are generally considered to offer anticancer action and to control rates of cell proliferation.

Large polysaccharides (sugars) may be extracted by boiling the leaf tips and may be partly responsible for enhanced immune surveillance.

Tannins provide the astringent and cicatrant properties that aid in wound healing and in treating prolapse, and flavonoids provide an antioxidant and anticancer effect.

Modern Research

A wealth of research available today validates the therapeutic claims of the past and explains the mechanisms of action of this herb. For the most part, the traditional uses and the Eclectic medical recommendations are entirely supportable and still relevant today.

Volatile oils high in terpenes are directly antibacterial, antiviral, and antifungal; tannins are astringent and cicatrizing; diterpenes and polysaccharides are immunomodulating and anti-inflammatory.

Actions and Uses Supported by Research

- Anti-inflammatory effects include downregulation of IL-6, TNF-α expression, and COX-2
- Antibacterial action is against both gram-negative and gram-positive bacteria
- Antifungal and antiviral, including against candida, HIV, and herpes virus
- Hepatoprotective, gastroprotective, and antiulcerogenic (reduces gastric acid production, promotes regeneration of the gastric epithelium)
- Antidiabetic, hypoglycemic
- Improve lipid profile (increased HDL fraction), antiatheromatous
- Antipyretic
- Redox regulating (radioprotective, antineoplastic)

The anticancer activity is due in part to the diterpenes that mediate stress responses and inflammation, but also due to a synergy of constituents that cause antioxidant or redox-regulating effects. In vitro studies show that alpha- and beta-thujone fractions are proapoptotic through the induction of ROS and p53 activation, leading to caspase-driven apoptosis. Flavonols from thuja trigger caspase-3-mediated apoptosis as well. Overall, the alpha- and beta-thujone fractions decrease the cell viability and exhibit a potent antiproliferative, proapoptotic, and antiangiogenic effects in vitro. In vivo assays showed that alpha- and beta-thujone inhibit neoplasia and inhibit angiogenic markers, including VEGF.

Dosing

Tincture: Up to 3 mL three times daily of 1:5 tincture made with 60% EtOH. Tincture should be taken 1 month on, 1 month off. A full dose of 9 mL at 1: 5 tincture daily is equivalent to 1.8 g dried herb daily.

The European Agency for the Evaluation of Medicinal Products (EMEA) gives the content of thujone in dried twigs as 7.6 mg/g, consisting of 85% alpha-thujone and 15% beta-thujone. The maximum daily dose is suggested as 1.25 mg thujone/kg body weight, equivalent to 68 mg thujone/

55 kg person per day, or 9 g per day of dried herb.

Topical treatment: It can be used topically as well, without limitation on unbroken skin, or in alternating-month doses in cases of open lesions. The green twigs can be macerated (soaked) into a carrier oil that is then used as the base of lotion, liniment, or salve. Alternatively, the distilled essential oil can be incorporated into a lotion, liniment, or salve. This plant extract may be used over any smaller skin cancers or surface lesions from systemic cancer, in a douche for dysplastic cervical cells, and for any fungal or viral infections of the surface of the body.

Toxicity

Thujone is a constituent of many commonly used herbs, such as wormwood, yarrow, thuja, and sage. This compound is mildly neurotoxic and its presence in liqueurs such as absinthe may have contributed to widespread toxicity and abuse syndromes in the early twentieth century.

The first sign of toxicity from thujone is a headache. Thujone inhibits the gamma-aminobutyric acid A (GABAA) receptors of the brain, causing excitation and convulsions in a dose-dependent manner. Care should be exercised when giving thujone-containing herbs in high doses to epileptics. These herbs include thuja (*Thuja* spp.), sage (*Salvia officinalis*), tansy (*Tanacetum vulgare*), wormwood (*Artemisia absinthium*), and some types of yarrow (*Achillea millefolium*). High and prolonged doses of the above herbs are hence best avoided, unless they are low-thujone varieties.

Metabolism of thujones is mainly through CYP2A6 enzymes in the liver, followed by CYP3A4 and CYP2B6. This could be affected by drugs or other herbs that induce or inhibit them, so care should be taken when prescribing thuja for internal use that potential drug interactions have been considered.

Clinical Pearls

There is variation in the composition of essential oils of *Thuja occidentalis* from different trees and different locations. It is recommended to harvest from several trees in a location and from several locations to avoid a single tree or location that may have particularly high or low concentrations.

Viscum album

Common name: Mistletoe
Plant family: Santalaceae/Loranthaceae
Parts used: Leaf, stem, flowers—harvested just before the berries form

This is a species of mistletoe native to Europe as well as western and southern Asia. It is a semiparasitic shrub that grows on the stems of various species of tree, from which it takes some nourishment, as well as having green leaves for photosynthesis. In Roman times, it was associated with peace, love, and understanding; the Romans hung it over doorways to protect the household. It was used in magical and mystical practices for millennia and still features in European mythology, legends, and customs. Mistletoe that grows on the black or water elm is considered the most efficacious in hermetic traditions.

It is important to point out that the information discussed here is pertaining to *Viscum album*, the European mistletoe, and not the American mistletoe, *Phoradendron leucarpum*, which is a totally different genus and species and is not considered safe for human ingestion.

Why Do We Kiss under the Mistletoe at Christmas?

The story goes that long, long ago, by a deceit of Loki, the joker or trickster of Norse tradition, Balder's blind brother accidentally shot him with an arrow made of mistletoe. Balder was restored to life at the request of the other gods and goddesses who loved him, and mistletoe was forgiven for the misdeed and afterward given into the keeping of the goddess of love. It was ordained that everyone who passed under it should receive a kiss, to show that the tree was forgiven, and the branch had become an emblem of love, and not of hate.

Traditional Indications

The leaves and young twigs of mistletoe have a long history of folk use as an antispasmodic, cardiac relaxant, narcotic, nervine, vasodilator and hypotensive, cytostatic, and diuretic. Mistletoe is traditionally used to lower blood pressure and heart rate, ease anxiety, and promote sleep.

In low doses it can also relieve panic attacks and headaches and improves the ability to concentrate. It is prescribed as an antispasmodic nervine for seizures, hysteria, and tension.

Traditional Clinical Applications of Mistletoe

- Hypertension with dizziness and headaches
- Nervous tachycardia (racing heart), valvular insufficiency, feeble pulse
- Cardiac hypertrophy, edema, dyspnea (shortness of breath), orthopnea (breathlessness on lying down)
- Seizure disorders—epilepsy, Tourette's, palsies, torticollis, paralysis
- Anxiety and hysteria

Modern Research

This herb contains cytotoxic lectins (carbohydrate-binding proteins on cell surfaces that mediate many immunological activities), including viscumin, which binds to sugar residues of the cell surface and may be taken up into the cell by endocytosis. Viscumin strongly inhibits protein synthesis in the cell, which in turn inhibits cell replication, and the lectins inhibit agglutination of tumor cells. Mistletoe upregulates NK cells and macrophages, and it inhibits tumor growth and metastases. Overall, mistletoe lectins have an immunomodulating activity that enhances the host defense system against tumors and have prophylactic and therapeutic effects on tumor metastasis. Mistletoe also contains cytotoxic polypeptides and polysaccharides that stimulate nonspecific immune cells.

Anticancer Actions of Mistletoe Lectins, Peptides, and Polysaccharides

- Increase numbers of leukocytes, eosinophils, and granulocytes
- Increase phagocytic and cytotoxic actions of macrophages

- Increase neutrophil production and maturation
- Enhance cellular and humoral immune response
- Increase thymic weight and thymocyte activity
- Increase production of cytokines
- Increase natural killer cell activity
- Induce IL-1, IL-6, TNF, interferon
- Selectively reduce COX-2 levels
- Induce DNA repair
- Increase apoptosis
- Inhibit angiogenesis

Mistletoe and Cancer

Mistletoe extract, given in small doses and repeated regularly, has been a regular feature of complementary cancer treatment in Germany for decades and is among the most frequently used integrative oncological drugs in several European countries. The remedy is made from fresh leafy mistletoe shoots and berries from different host trees, which impart unique chemistry to the medicine.

There are several subtypes, depending on the host tree, which influences the chemistry. According to one well-established German brand, mistletoe can be harvested from fir, maple, almond, birch, hawthorn, ash, apple, pine, and oak, and each may target different cancers. There has been some preliminary research suggesting a correlation between mistletoe grown on ash with treatment of metastatic tumors, on apple with treatment of breast cancer, and on oak with treatment of gastrointestinal tumors and tumors of the male sex organs, but this is not yet validated by wider trials.

When mistletoe first became known as a remedy for cancer, it was given by mouth in the form of extracts, tinctures, or teas. Over the past several decades, however, it has become popularized in Europe and North America in a form potentized as a homeopathic complex and given by subcutaneous injection for many different cancers. I am not licensed to do this in my own practice, but I have referred patients for it and seen the good results many times now.

The intention of treatment is improvement of quality of life and reduced side effects associated with conventional anticancer strategies. This is achieved through several pathways of immunomodulation. It also reduces the leukocytopenia produced by radiation and chemotherapy. Treatment can be started before standard therapies (surgery, chemotherapy, and radiotherapy) and is then used intermittently in intervals between cycles of chemotherapy. A complete course of treatment may be several months up to as long as 5 years.

A randomized, controlled clinical trial of injectable mistletoe extract involving breast, ovarian, and non–small cell lung cancer patients showed decreased side effects of chemotherapy and improved quality of life. In one meta-analysis, 22 of 26 assessed studies reported a benefit—most notably, improvements in fatigue, sleep, exhaustion, energy, nausea, vomiting, appetite, depression, anxiety, ability to work, and emotional and functional well-being in general. Less consistently, it reported improvements in pain, diarrhea, general performance, and side effects of conventional treatments.

Mistletoe lectins induce production of granulocyte-macrophage colony-stimulating factor (GM-CSF) to elevate neutrophils in blood, induce interleukin-5 and interferon gamma, and have an immune-potentiating effect.

Dosing

Notwithstanding the fact that injectable versions are potent, reliable, and effective, it is not always possible to obtain them, in which case the tincture and tea are useful. Preparations of the fresh plant (tincture) or freshly dried plant (tea) should be used; mistletoe loses its properties on keeping. As with other cytotoxic herbs, it's best to start low and work up.

Tea: 2–6 g three times daily of dried herb decocted.

Tincture: The recommended dose varies a lot in different reference books. The *British Herbal Pharmacopoeia* suggests a low dose of just 0.5 mL three times daily of 1:5 tincture made with dried plant material and 45% alcohol. The respected herbalist Kerry Bone, in his book *A Clinical Guide to Blending Liquid Herbs*, suggests a much higher dose of 3–6 mL daily of 1:2 extract made with dried plant material, alcohol content not specified. Clearly the herb is not acutely toxic in moderate doses. However, if you ingest an excessive amount there may be vomiting, catharsis, bloody stool and bowel spasms, collapse, and convulsions, but this should never occur if it is properly prescribed by a qualified herbalist.

Adverse events from injectable mistletoe are dose dependent and primarily confined to reactions at the injection site and mild, transient fever and flulike symptoms, which may actually be considered a positive sign of an immune response and activation of interferon.

Taken by mouth, mistletoe therapy may be administered concurrently with conventional treatment (such as chemotherapy, radiotherapy, or corticosteroids). Although there is some controversy and not all studies entirely agree, the preponderance of evidence suggests that mistletoe extract has a positive impact on quality of life and can reduce side effects of conventional therapies.

Clinical Pearls

This herb is recommended for people who are anxious, fretting, worried and restless, twitching, and clutching. It lowers the blood pressure, relaxes the heart, and eases tension headaches. The Eclectics suggest taking it as a sleeping aid and muscle relaxant with valerian, a warming and circulation-stimulating herb to offset the cooling properties of mistletoe.

CHAPTER 10

Case Histories

The cases that follow are illustrative of the range of patients and presentations a clinician can see in a typical day and the range of herbs and nutraceutical options to choose from. Though the same items may repeat in different protocols, there may be differences in dose (such as melatonin at 10 mg per night in the beginning of treatment as an antiangiogenic, or at 1 mg per night for someone in remission but with lingering sleep onset delay), or there may be differences in type (such as magnesium citrate/glycinate/oxide being a muscle relaxant especially helpful in kidney stones, anxiety, and constipation, respectively). Because the herbs are polyvalent, working in multiple physiological pathways simultaneously, they are rarely specific to a particular type of cancer but can be applied across all malignant proliferative states, and often for prevention as well. Turmeric and green tea, for example, are going to be used in almost all cancer cases, unless the patient is taking certain specific chemotherapy or other contraindicated drugs.

Some of the supplements and nutritional agents I recommended in these cases are single agents, in which case I have given optimal doses. A few are proprietary blends or mixes for which I have deliberately not given exact formulations or brands because in different countries there will be different items available, and these are simply meant to be guidelines. See Resources, on page 529, for a list of the brands I use the most in my clinic, but note that they may not be available everywhere. If not, these lists of ingredients will help inform other choices.

CHAPTER 10 CONTENTS

452 **Breast Cancer**
452 Case Summary
453 Initial Treatment Planning
454 Initial Tincture Formula
455 Tea Formula
456 Poke Oil Breast Rub
457 Bach Flower Remedy Mixture
458 Daily Smoothie Recipe
459 Clinical Progression
459 Case Update and Revised Protocol
461 Adjusted Daily Tincture Formula
461 Tea Formula
461 Castor Oil Pack
462 Discussion

463 **Bladder Cancer**
463 Case Summary
463 Additional Health Factors
466 Blood Work Review
466 Treatment Options
467 Initial Treatment Planning
468 Initial Tincture Formula
468 Daily Tincture Formula
469 Daily Herbal Powder
470 Daily Tea Blend
471 Extra-Strength Tea for Acute Urinary Tract Infection
472 Herbal Castor Oil Pack
472 Case Update and Revised Protocol
474 Liver Tonic
474 Daily Tincture
475 Discussion

476 **Lung Cancer**
476 Other Health History of Note
477 Suggested Schedule of Blood Testing
478 Initial Tincture Formula
479 Soup Blend
479 Tea Formula
481 Specific Cytotoxic Anticancer Herbs
481 Case Update and Revised Protocol
482 Daily Tincture Formula
482 Herbal Tea for Swelling and Inflammation
485 A Warm Wax Herbal Treatment
486 Discussion

Breast Cancer

Ms. H. is one of the few patients I have seen in my clinic who elected to do a minimal surgery only and no other conventional treatments. Understandably, most people are too fearful not to do the maximum treatment they are offered; I am often seeing them partway through or after completion of conventional therapies. Ms. H. never did do the recommended chemotherapy and radiation treatments. Her case is thus illustrative of how sometimes it isn't necessary to poison or burn the body in order to heal.

She was 48 years old at the time of diagnosis in 2011, an artist, perimenopausal, single, with no children. When we began, our focus was entirely on her breast cancer, but over the past 10 years this has become a background concern and treatment has been adjusted to consider menopause, allergies, thyroid deficiency, and, most recently, dermoid cysts. I will discuss here the initial protocol (2011, shortly after diagnosis), some highlights of treatment over time, and the current protocol to illustrate how they changed to follow the patient's changing health circumstances.

Case Summary

Ms. H. presented with a left breast infiltrating (invasive) ductal carcinoma, grade 1, stage I, T1, N0, M0, found on a routine annual exam taking place 4 years since her previous mammogram. It was moderately sensitive to estrogen and progesterone and negative for HER2/neu mutations. She was offered chemotherapy followed by radiation and then 5–10 years of tamoxifen and declined them all. She elected to undergo a lumpectomy only, and to date that is the only medical intervention she has had.

In the 2 years prior to diagnosis, Ms. H. had been quite uncomfortable with symptoms of perimenopause: hot flashes, brain fog, irritability, and insomnia. Progesterone cream helped a lot, but she stopped hormone treatment when the breast cancer was diagnosed. Subsequently, she developed marked menopause symptoms, with hot flashes and sleep disturbance, painful atrophic vaginitis with vulvar/perineal irritation and inflammation, and an overactive bladder. Thus, in the treatment planning, we needed to keep estrogens low enough to avoid feeding the cancer but high enough to manage menopause with tolerable symptoms.

She had experienced significant stress and distress in the previous 4 years with multiple bereavements and car accidents. She had a whiplash injury, which continued to cause chronic neck pain, managed by exercise and osteopathic care. She also had a personal and family history of depression.

I recommended some simple things to help the neck and the pain, primarily a heating pad or hot packs on the neck (flaxseed or buckwheat in a pillow that can be microwaved), a contour neck pillow at night, regular stretching, neck rolls and shoulder rolling, and an herbal liniment for pain and muscle spasms.

To help with pain and sleep, I suggested warm baths by candlelight at bedtime with Epsom salts (1 cup) and essential oil of lavender for relaxation (10–15 drops). Epsom salt is properly known as magnesium sulfate and it is a powerful muscle relaxant; it also aids detoxification through the skin.

I encouraged her to consider what stressors she could avoid, and I counseled her on how to develop a stress-management tool kit. I also included condor vine in her tincture formula to support healthy appetite and parasympathetic tone.

Initial Treatment Planning

When we first met, the lumpectomy had not yet been done, so the first order of business was to prepare her for surgery: to build up the immune system and liver dextoxification functions, manage inflammation, and promote tissue repair. We also discussed the importance of ensuring that she was signing up to a sentinel node biopsy and not a lymph node dissection, and we reviewed testing and assessment options both within and outside the medical system. I asked her to arrange for more informative blood work from her doctor, and we agreed she would follow the initial herbal protocol for 6 weeks, then we would review all the new test results and make adjustments as required. After that we would develop a monitoring plan for the next 3, 6, and 12 months.

Overall Case Management Plan

- Start taking herbal cytotoxics blend and lymphatic support herbs.
- Start taking mitochondrial rescue protocol.
- Get blood work and other specific testing set up.
- Address diet—do a modified Clean and Green Detox Diet (page 41) and prehabilitation plan.

Before Surgery

- Stop herbal remedies and supplements 4–6 days before the procedure.

After Surgery

- Start recovery and rehabilitation (use herbs for pain and tissue repair as required).
- Recommence using herbal items and supplements (targeted anticancer and recovery protocol) 4–6 days after the procedure.
- Continue with mitochondrial rescue for 2 months after surgery.
- Support the liver to promote detoxification pathways.
- Manage stress and support restful sleep.
- Start taking immune tonics and anti-inflammatories.
- Strengthen connective tissue and inhibit angiogenesis.
- Start *Artemisia annua* on an alternate-week schedule.
- Continue with herbal cytotoxics blend and lymphatic support herbs.

Initial Tincture Formula

All tinctures are 1:2 strength.

+ 15 mL licorice
+ 15 mL astragalus
+ 15 mL cat's claw
+ 15 mL schisandra
+ 15 mL gotu kola
+ 10 mL rhodiola
+ 10 mL Baikal skullcap
+ 5 mL condor vine
+ 2 drops lemongrass essential oil

Mix all tinctures. Take 7.5 milliliters (1½ tsp.) twice daily in hot water or in tea.

Licorice is an adrenal-sparing adaptogen. It is used for managing stress and supporting the immune system, and it has moistening and soothing properties for irritated mucous membranes (sinuses and vaginal lining, in this case). It modulates inflammation and is often included in formulas to sweeten and disperse other herbs.

Astragalus is a deep immune tonic for repair and rejuvenation in bone marrow and lymph nodes, normalizing immune responses at the deepest level to resist cancer.

Cat's claw is an immunostimulant, usually used short term to boost overall immune functions. It is hard to get high-grade herb as it is in short supply, and I may not choose this herb today.

Schisandra is an adaptogen with some tropism to the liver, and hence specifically indicated here for surgical drugs in the system, being detoxified and eliminated by hepatic cells.

Gotu kola has myriad anticancer actions of its own but is especially called for when surgery will necessitate connective tissue repair and scar formation. Its cerebral tonic properties are also useful for any postoperative cognitive dysfunction that may occur.

Rhodiola is an adaptogen with some tropism to cardiac muscle tissue and to cardiac function. It is astringent, drying, and toning to tissue and especially indicated for loss of tone in the cardiovascular system (regurgitant heart valves, varicose veins, hemorrhoids, flushing). It is also stimulating, and higher doses can cause palpitations.

Baikal skullcap root is a mediator of inflammation and promotes tissue repair, and inhibits cancer.

Condor vine is used specifically for loss of appetite due to anxiety or nerves. It is a digestive tonic nervine in a similar way to hops but without the astringency, or to chamomile without the anti-inflammatory action. It supports mood and promotes parasympathetic tone. Possibly the closest equivalent to substitute if condor vine is unavailable would be damiana or maybe blue vervain.

Lemongrass is rich in limonene, a monoterpene hydrocarbon prevalent in the volatile oil of many plants, and pleasant tasting, so it can mask a lot of other things in a blend. It has marked anticancer activity and also reduces dyspepsia and gastric reflux.

Tea Formula

This tea blend was formulated with a focus on the symptoms of menopause and hormone regulation, hence the black cohosh, chasteberry, and red clover. Taheebo is an antifungal and antiviral immunostimulant, and reishi is a deep immune tonic, aiding in building white cells. Rose is astringent and cooling, heals bereavement, loss, and sadness, and supports grieving (the patient had experienced several bereavements shortly before diagnosis). Calendula has antioxidant and vulnerary (wound-healing) properties, supports lymph drainage, and is a bitter digestive stimulant.

DECOCTION BLEND

+ 50 g black cohosh root
+ 50 g chasteberry
+ 50 g taheebo*
+ 50 g reishi fruiting body

INFUSION BLEND

+ 50 g red clover tops
+ 50 g calendula flowers
+ 50 g rose petals
+ 25 g lemongrass leaves
+ 25 g hawthorn leaf and flower

Put 2 heaping tablespoons of the decoction blend in a pan with 2–3 cups of cold water. Cover, bring to a boil, and simmer for 10 minutes. Turn off the heat. Add 2 heaping tablespoons of the infusion blend. Steep overnight. Strain and drink through the next day. Can be gently rewarmed, but do not boil the tea. For simplicity or convenience, add the Initial Tincture (opposite page) to the tea.

*Note: I created this formula more than a decade ago. Today, taheebo is endangered; usnea may be a suitable substitute.

PROTOCOL ANALYSIS FOR MS. H., BREAST CANCER PATIENT

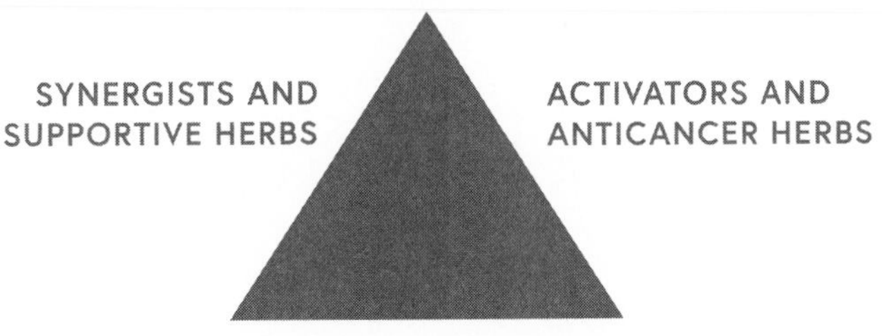

Foundation Herbs for Prehabilitation and Physiological Enhancement

Stress management, sleep support, immune tonics: licorice, astragalus, schisandra, rhodiola, taheebo, reishi, flower essences
Hormone balancing: black cohosh, vitex, red clover
Tonic, astringent: rose petals, lemongrass, hawthorn tops
Digestive support: condor vine

Synergists and Supportive Herbs

Connective tissue tonics, anti-angiogenics: gotu kola, horse chestnut, blueberry leaf
Immunomodulators, inflammodulators: Baikal skullcap, curcumin (turmeric), licorice, cat's claw
Lymph support: red root, pokeweed, cleavers, calendula
Liver support: silymarin (milk thistle)
Antioxidants: CoQ10, green tea, quercetin, resveratrol, selenium, zinc, omega-3 fats, vitamin C

Specifics: Activators and Anticancer Herbs

Cytotoxics: Chinese wormwood, Pacific yew, Madagascar periwinkle, pawpaw, pokeroot, mistletoe, camptotheca, lemongrass
Anticancer: MCP, IP6, melatonin

Poke Oil Breast Rub

Pokeroot is believed to act as a tissue decongestant by promoting lymphatic drainage. Fresh pokeroot is a mild rubefacient, drawing blood to the tissue where it is applied, which in turn creates more lymph. In this way, pokeroot supports a lymphatic flushing effect, acts as a decongestant, and promotes lymphatic drainage,* which activates lymphocytes against pathogens. Castor oil is deeply penetrating and carries the pokeroot deeper into the tissues. The essential oils are lymphatic decongestant, antimitotic, anti-inflammatory, and vulnerary.

+ 150 mL pokeroot-infused grapeseed oil
+ 50 mL castor oil
+ 1 mL each essential oils of benzoin, mandarin, lemongrass, cedarwood, bay laurel

Mix all ingredients. Pour 1 teaspoon of the oil into the hand and gently massage over the breast using smooth strokes to move from the nipple radiating outward, following the direction of lymph flow. Be sure to get up into the armpit as well.

*Note: This will not cause the cancer to spread, as the lymph system only works if it is flowing and lymphocytes get recruited to the battlefield. Cancer is a living tissue, with blood and lymph flowing in and out, and stray cells do escape—hence the reason for using cytotoxic herbs or chemotherapy for a systemic effect. Flushing the lymph through the system will have the advantage of activating lymphocytes and increasing the immune response.

Bach Flower Remedy Mixture

These are potentized extracts of (mostly) flowers into pure water, and they are prescribed for psycho-emotional or psychospiritual reasons, not for physical states.

+ 8 drops each of the following Bach Flower Remedies: rock rose, mimulus, cerato, hornbeam, and star of Bethlehem
+ 25 mL spring water
+ 25 mL brandy

Mix all the ingredients. Take 4 drops of the blend four times daily, either under the tongue or in a glass of water and sipped.

Rock rose: Helps when you experience fears, such as terror or fright that makes you feel frozen and unable to move or think clearly.

Mimulus: Helps when you feel fear that you recognize or can name, such as fear of illness or fear of being a burden.

Cerato: Helps you trust your own judgment in decision-making and to follow your gut feelings.

Hornbeam: Helps when you feel that you do not have sufficient mental or physical strength to carry the burden that life has placed on you.

Star of Bethlehem: Helps when you experience serious news, loss of someone dear, personal disaster, fright, or great distress; helps when the distress and unhappiness feel unbearable.

Daily Smoothie Recipe

+ 1–2 tablespoons green superfood powder
+ ½–1 cup blueberries or other fruit (fresh or frozen)
+ ½–1 cup almond milk, rice milk, kefir, or water
+ ½ cup live, natural, organic yogurt
+ 1–5 g buffered vitamin C powder
+ 1–2 tablespoons coconut powder (good calories, helps taste)
+ Optional: ½ avocado, ½ banana, 1 tablespoon nut butter (as a thickener)
+ Raw cocoa powder to taste
+ 1–2 scoops whey protein powder (high lactoferrin, lactoalbumin, and lactoglobulin), to provide at least 20 g protein

Blend the ingredients well. Add water to get the preferred consistency. The proteins in whey are fragile, so add the whey protein powder to the blender last, then blend for only 1 minute longer. Pour over ice. If not drinking immediately, store in the fridge or a chilled thermos flask for up to 6 hours.

DAILY SUPPLEMENT RECOMMENDATIONS

- CoQ10: 100 mg
- Green tea extract (standardized EGCG): 50 mg
- IP6 (inositol hexaphosphate): 5 g
- Melatonin: 3–6 mg at bedtime
- Milk thistle (standardized at 70% silymarin): 1 g
- Multivitamin and mineral without iron or copper
- Probiotic blend (50 billion bacteria)
- Quercetin: 2 g
- Resveratrol: 2 g
- Selenium: 200 mcg
- Vitamin D3: 4,000 IU
- Zinc citrate: 60 mg (for the first month, then 30 mg daily)

PROPRIETARY CAPSULE FORMULAS		
Action	**Dose**	**Blend**
Anti-inflammatory, anticancer	3 capsules twice daily	Indian frankincense, feverfew, magnolia bark, andrographis, Baikal skullcap, ginger, bromelain, BioPerine
Antioxidant, anticancer	3 capsules twice daily	Turmeric, green tea, quercetin, grape seed and skin, tulsi, rosemary
Immune and bone marrow tonic, anticancer	3 capsules twice daily	Astragalus, dong quai, millettia, cordyceps, atractylodes, echinacea, cat's claw
Immune tonic, anticancer	3 capsules twice daily	Red reishi, turkey tail, chaga, shiitake, and poria mushrooms; Baikal skullcap root extract and baicalein; milk thistle
Promote detox pathways in the liver	2 capsules at bedtime	Broccoli seed extract and cabbage sprouts, 3,3'-diindolylmethane (DIM), wasabi, calcium-D-glucarate, N-acetylcysteine, pomegranate

ALTERNATE-WEEK DAILY SUPPLEMENTS

Week One

- Artemisinin: 300 mg twice daily (building up to 600 mg twice daily), taken in 3–4 oz. of grapefruit juice
- Butyren (butyric acid): 1,500 mg twice daily
- Vitamin C: to bowel tolerance
- Omega-3 fats from fish oil: 1,000 mg EPA, 450 mg DHA
- Evening primrose oil: 1,500 mg

Week 2

- Cytotoxic blend: Pacific yew, Madagascar periwinkle, pawpaw, pokeroot, mistletoe, and camptotheca, tincture blend, dosed at ½ tsp. twice daily in water

Clinical Progression

Ms. H. remained on a full-dose herbal and supplement regimen for around 2 years, with some adjustments to address allergies, stress, and menopause along the way. This included the artemisia cycling for 6 months and the cytotoxic blend for 18 months. After that, we began to reduce doses and dropped some of the more expensive proprietary herbal capsule products (the anti-inflammatory and the bone marrow and blood-building formulas).

Case Update and Revised Protocol

The patient has remained cancer-free for 10 years. She has used thermograms and ultrasound for regular breast monitoring. She has generally kept up a healthy lifestyle and diet and has continued to follow a wellness program of herbs and nutritional supplements throughout. Over the years, other health challenges have occurred and some continue to be of concern:

- Consistently low neutrophils with seemingly normal immune function, experiencing one or two colds annually like most adults. Not responsive to herbal and dietary strategies.
- Nonspecific thyroiditis with mildly elevated thyroglobulin and episodic, intermittent swelling of the thyroid and feeling of congestion in the throat. Managed with diet, herbs, and supplements.
- Severe allergic rhinitis (hay fever–type symptoms) from several foods identified by ELISA blood testing and also from pollens, grass, weeds, and animal dander. Strict trigger avoidance has reduced the food reactions, and desensitizing shots for pollens, grass, weeds, and animal dander have been quite successful.
- Bilateral dermoid (ovarian) cysts developed after completion of menopause. Surgery in 2021 during which the bowel was damaged, leading to substantial abdominal infection and inflammation, lung collapse, thrombosis, and septicemia. After repeated surgery to clean it up, she is now in recovery.

Originally her oncologist had requested annual checkups for 10 years—twice as long as usual because he was distrustful of the natural remedies she chose over the conventional approaches. He recently told her she no longer needs to go back and he has closed her file. She continues to have other health challenges, and herbal medicine continues to have much to offer her.

This case illustrates the importance of taking a substantial protocol as soon as possible after diagnosis and then maintaining good health practices. The full dosing protocol in this case was sustained for more than 2 years, with some minor adjustments, and then continued in lesser doses as a long-term maintenance strategy. This does not preclude other conditions arising, but if the terrain is healthy and resilient, then recovery from disease is more likely.

The overall clinical picture shows a patient with a tendency to abnormal growths and swellings (thyroid gland, ovarian cysts), with a deficient immune response and a past history of cancer. In the classic sense of cancer being considered, in part, a toxic overload, this clinical picture represents considerable risk as it indicates significant congestion and stagnation of the tissues. Over time the protocol was adjusted to provide more focus on thyroid support, detoxification pathways, and removal of morbid wastes, using alterative herbs—those with a blood-cleansing or depurative action—to promote detoxification of cells, tissue, and organs. More recently the postsurgical complications have been a priority, but they are expected to resolve in time.

Detoxification and tissue cleansing. Burdock, blue flag, stillingia, sarsaparilla, pokeroot, and larrea are all traditional herbs for deep blood cleansing and depurative effects, eliminating toxins stored in cells. This is a priority in the plan, because drug residues from the recent health crisis may be compromising detoxification pathways, which could then increase exposure to metabolic or xenobiotic toxins. As with most herbs, there are other beneficial secondary effects that cause these herbs to be particularly indicated in this patient. Blue flag and pokeroot are also thyroid stimulants. Sarsaparilla is also an adaptogen with hormone-balancing and anti-inflammatory properties. Burdock also has complex sugars that balance glucose uptake and metabolism and support the gut microbiome. Pokeroot has immune-potentiating lectins. Larrea has anticancer and cytotoxic properties.

Lymphatic support. Cleavers, red root, and calendula are herbs that support movement of lymph from tissues to lymph vessels and back to the systemic circulation, activating and stimulating lymphocytes and supporting detoxification and tissue drainage.

Pelvic decongestants. Ginger and yarrow flower assist with pelvic circulation and moving waste matter from the pelvic organs.

NEW SUPPLEMENT RECOMMENDATIONS

- Green tea extract (EGCG): 50 mg daily
- Iodine (potassium iodide): 10 mg daily
- Milk thistle (standardized to 70% silymarin): 1 g daily
- Omega-3 fish oil: 1,000 mg EPA, 450 mg DHA daily
- Turmeric (standardized to 95% curcumin): 2 g daily
- Quercetin: 2 g daily
- Resveratrol: 2 g daily

Continued on page 46

Adjusted Daily Tincture Formula

This tincture was extensively revised after the abdominal infection and repeated surgeries to focus on immune health, tissue repair, and detoxification. The following tinctures are 1:2 strength, except where indicated. The indicated amounts add up to 100 milliliters, or a week's supply at the recommended dosage below.

+ 15 mL burdock
+ 15 mL cleavers
+ 10 mL blue flag
+ 10 mL red root
+ 10 mL stillingia
+ 10 mL yarrow flower
+ 10 mL calendula
+ 5 mL sarsaparilla
+ 5 mL ginger
+ 5 mL pokeroot (1:10)
+ 5 mL larrea (1:5)

Take 5 milliliters (1 tsp.) twice daily in hot water, 15 minutes before meals.

Tea Formula

+ 100 g red clover
+ 100 g nettle leaf
+ 75 g plantain
+ 50 g goldenrod
+ 50 g orange peel
+ 25 g artichoke leaf

Put 3 tablespoons of the herb mix into a pot and pour on 3 cups of boiling water. Cover and steep overnight. Strain and drink through the next day. Can be gently rewarmed, but do not boil the tea. For simplicity you can add the Adjusted Daily Tincture Formula (see above) to the herbal tea.

Allergies. Nettle leaf is nutritive and full of chlorophyll for building blood. More specifically for Ms. H., it is also an antihistamine agent that reduces symptoms of allergy and hay fever. She has been drinking some variant of a hay fever herbal tea blend with nettle leaf, plantain, and goldenrod for a few years now and it has helped with her symptoms.

Detox and blood cleansing. The red clover contains phytoestrogens to inhibit cancer and support menopause symptoms, as well as being a traditional detoxification and blood-purifying herb. The artichoke leaf is a liver stimulant and promotes elimination of metabolic wastes.

Castor Oil Pack

To reduce tissue congestion, I formulated an abdominal castor oil pack (see page 119 for instructions on how to make a castor oil pack) with essential oils targeted to lymph drainage and congestion (cypress, fennel, grapefruit). This mix can also be rubbed daily into swollen lymph nodes and over the thyroid gland.

+ 100 mL pokeroot-infused castor oil
+ 6 drops each essential oils of cypress, grapefruit, fennel, and ho wood

- Vitamin D3: 4,000 IU daily
- Liver detox blend: alpha-lipoic acid, N-acetyl-cysteine, turmeric (95% curcuminoids), milk thistle (80% silymarin), broccoli sprout concentrate, artichoke leaf, taurine, glycine, L-glutamine, L-methionine, chlorella, ascorbyl palmitate (fat-soluble vitamin C)
- Thyroid support: ashwagandha extract, L-tyrosine, *Coleus forskohlii* (root), folate, vitamin A, vitamin B6, iodine, selenium glycinate, zinc glycinate

Optional Extras

- Hormone-balancing blend: chasteberry, Japanese knotweed, black cohosh, DIM, chrysin, calcium-D-glucarate, rosemary, resveratrol, grapeseed extract, green tea extract (EGCG), vitamin B6, vitamin B12, folate, magnesium, and calcium
- Maca: two 500 mg capsules once per day, as needed (adaptogen)
- Five-mushroom formula: two capsules daily with meals
- MCHC (microcrystaline hydroxyapatite) : 1,000 mg elemental calcium daily with boron, silicon, vitamin D, and vitamin K as cofactors (for strong bones)

Discussion

Ten years after her original diagnosis, this patient is no longer being monitored or tracked by the medical system for cancer. I organize regular blood work and she remains committed to healthy diet and lifestyle choices. Were this patient newly diagnosed today, she would probably be offered the Oncotype testing and would almost certainly come back showing low risk of recurrence and less urgency of treatment than was determined by the oncologist in 2012. This is a good illustration of the usefulness of the testing, because most patients are not willing or able to resist the pressure to fully engage with all the chemotherapy and radiation options available. In this case, Oncotype testing wasn't available when she needed it, and she had to make best guesses as to the relative risk of recurrence.

Also factoring into that decision was the fact that she was prepared to commit fully to taking anticancer herbs and supplements, playing an active role in her treatment. Patients who choose this path, who step away from conventional treatments and do not attend the conventional cancer centers, are not counted in the statistics of cancer morbidity and mortality in the same way. Additionally, if they regain health and remain healthy, there is no data to document that information. This remains an omission in the literature and hence is not included in the consideration of treatment options in conventional cancer care.

In this case, the decision to use only minimal conventional interventions (lumpectomy) and follow through on a comprehensive holistic treatment and then a strong maintenance plan was clearly the right one. Despite the recent setback of an ovarian cyst surgery gone bad, this patient has remained cancer-free and has not required aggressive treatments like chemotherapy or radiotherapy to date.

Bladder Cancer

Mr. E. is a retired business professional in his early 70s with a low-stress, country lifestyle and with strong community support. He is in a relationship but lives alone with his dog. He exercises regularly, mostly eats well, and has a long-term regular meditation practice.

Case Summary

Mr. E. was diagnosed with transitional cell carcinoma (TCC) of the bladder in October 2015. No local spread was observed on scans, so he was treated with conservative (bladder-sparing) surgery that removed three high-grade tumors. The surgeon also removed 8 right and 10 left inguinal nodes, and all were found to be negative for cancer spread. No further pathology report was available.

As a precaution Mr. E. was given BCG infusions into the bladder in summer 2016; this is a form of immunotherapy using bacillus Calmette-Guérin, classically used to inoculate against tuberculosis. It generates an immune response in the bladder lining cells and is considered the first line of therapy in bladder cancer that has not yet invaded the underlying muscle wall. It can be quite effective, with an estimated 66 percent of patients disease-free at 3 years after treatment, but the risk of side effects is significant. Over 80 percent of patients experience dose-dependent local and systemic side effects, including arthritis or arthralgia, cystitis, epididymitis, prostatitis, lung infections, liver toxicity, fever, and sepsis.

Indeed, for Mr. E. a follow-up series of BCG infusions in early 2017 resulted in severe urinary tract infections and treatment could not be completed. His doctor recommended that he have his bladder removed, but surgery for this was commenced and then terminated because there was too much internal scar tissue from a previous lower bowel surgery for Crohn's disease and formation of a J pouch (artificial rectum).

When he presented in my clinic in the fall of 2017, he was still considered to have carcinoma in situ. He was minimally symptomatic, with some pain in the left midback (flank) if not well hydrated and a deep aching in the bladder with urination. The fact that there were multiple original lesions and that it had not completely resolved after BCG did put him into a higher risk category for possible progression, so further treatment was expected.

Additional Health Factors

Mr. E.'s case was complicated by several comorbidities and a number of pharmaceutical medications, all of which needed to be considered when prescribing herbs. Indeed, it is highly likely that the immunosuppressive drug he was taking for Crohn's disease may have been compromising his immune system and increasing the risk of cancer.

His case provides an illustration of the unfortunate reality that people often have many health issues going on at once; if you don't address some or all of them, their cancer is unlikely to get better and their quality of life will still be compromised as they struggle with their other conditions (which are often worsened by conventional cancer therapy). In the case of Mr. E., he was actually quite stable and functional, and his conditions were well managed by the drugs he was taking, so I was not in a rush to suggest he stop taking his current prescriptions. Nonetheless, herbs could be used alongside the pharmaceuticals to manage symptoms, address cancer cells, and support him through the process so his other health concerns could remain stable.

Crohn's disease. This had resulted in bowel resection and creation of a J pouch (artificial rectum). He was medicated with adalimumab (Humira), a monoclonal antibody that is an immunosuppressive and possibly contributed to increased vulnerability to bladder infections and also increased the risk from BCG given for the bladder cancer. Adalimumab is a tumor necrosis factor (TNF) blocker, and for children and adults taking it there is an increased chance of getting lymphoma, two types of skin cancer (basal cell and squamous cell), or other cancers. Despite that, Mr. E. was reluctant to stop the drug, as it was successfully managing bowel symptoms.

We discussed the importance of diet in managing inflammatory bowel disease and he was quite receptive to this. Helpfully, the kind of diet I suggested for cancer was largely applicable to Crohn's as well—lots of fresh vegetables and whole fruit, fish, eggs, limited whole grains, no sugar or refined carbohydrates.

Arrhythmia and high blood pressure. An obstruction in transmission of nerve impulses around the heart (right bundle branch block) caused an occasional momentary arrhythmia but was otherwise asymptomatic and not medicated. His blood pressure was slightly elevated, until he cleaned up his diet and lost 30 pounds.

We discussed the importance of maintaining healthy weight and blood pressure, as well as stress-management practices. Helpfully, as with the dietary recommendations, several of the suggestions I gave him for treating cancer are also indicated in a healthy heart protocol—coenzyme Q10, vitamin E, resveratrol, flavonoids—and were able to do double duty for him.

Chronic upper digestive aching. This was aggravated by stress. No formal diagnosis was given but symptoms were managed with rabeprazole (a proton pump inhibitor) at 20 mg daily. I had some concerns about this drug, as the proton pump inhibiting (PPI) drugs are not intended for long-term use. Prescribing guidelines recommend that they should only be used for 2–4 weeks for regular indigestion, while patients with the more severe gastroesophageal reflux disorder might need to take them for up to 2 months but should not use them longer. Long-term use of high-dose PPIs may produce vitamin B12 deficiencies, and use of PPIs for 5 years or more has been correlated with a more than 60 percent increase in the risk of osteoporosis-related hip fractures due to impaired calcium absorption. Another significant complication from PPI drugs is that lowering stomach acid has negative impacts on gut flora and the microbiome, which increases the risk of *Clostridium difficile* infections, a specific concern in this case where antibiotics were required regularly for bladder infections, adding to his risk profile. I suggested that we work toward cessation of this drug over several weeks or even a few months, introducing appropriate herbs first, then reducing the dose and frequency of drug use.

Benign prostate hyperplasia. This caused delayed onset of urinary flow and altered flow dynamics. He had been medicated with tamsulosin (Flomax) daily for the past 15 years. The dose had been reduced from 3 pills to 1 pill per day, but flow diminished after his bladder procedures, so the dose had been increased back up to 2 per day when he came to my clinic. Tamsulosin is generally well tolerated and without significant complications, so I advised him to continue using it as needed. Herbs like saw palmetto (*Serrenoa repens*) might have reduced need for tamsulosin, but that would take away from the focus on cancer—sometimes clinical practice requires picking your battles.

Once his cancer treatment regimen was established and he was able to comply with the diet and supplement recommendations I'd given him, then we would address his other concerns and conditions.

General Prostate Health Recommendations

- Always heed the urge to urinate and never delay this.
- Try sitting on the toilet to urinate, rather than standing, to see if this relieves pressure on the gland. Allow yourself to relax.
- Avoid heavy consumption of alcohol because it irritates the bladder and, reflexively, the prostate gland.
- Eat a handful of pumpkin seeds daily to provide zinc and essential fatty acids that are the precursors to the prostaglandins made by the prostate gland. Or use pumpkin seed butter as a spread or in sauces, salad dressings, and dips.
- Avoid sitting for long periods, especially on cold or damp surfaces.
- Exercise daily, especially walking, running, dancing, in-line skating, ball games, or racket sports where the hips and pelvis are moving (sports like kayaking, horseback riding, and golf are not so effective at promoting pelvic circulation).

Migraines. Severe migraines every few weeks had been a long-standing concern. They were managed with self-prescribed nonsteroidal anti-inflammatories, as needed, and he was not seeking specific help with this.

Kidney stones. He had experienced kidney stones 8 years prior. Although this was not an active concern at the time of attending my clinic, I encouraged him to keep well hydrated, to avoid large amounts of oxalate-rich foods (spinach, chard, lamb's quarters, rhubarb, strawberries, chocolate) and to take magnesium citrate (250 mg) daily. I also recommended a low-oxalate diet to protect the bladder from irritation.

Back stiffness, deep aching, and tightness. This was managed with occasional massage or acupuncture. My assessment was that this was related to the internal scarring (adhesions) from chronic inflammation and surgeries. Organs in the abdomen are supported by muscles outside the peritoneal cavity, and those muscles are more or less slung off the deep muscles of the back. Adhesion of organs causes pulls and strains on muscles that all ultimately transmit to the spine. I suggested regular body work (deep tissue massage), weekly if possible, as well as sauna or other heat applications, stretching, and yoga. I also prescribed castor oil packs for the bladder, which could be incidentally helpful for adhesions as well.

Blood Work Review

Very little blood work had been done. This patient lives on a remote island with limited medical services, and although he was very proactive and engaged in his own care, he had not known to ask for more extensive reviews, nor had the local doctors offered any. He was not under direct care of an oncologist, and the urologist attended only to the actual bladder symptoms. He did, however, show a low red blood cell count and hemoglobin just barely in range and had symptoms of being borderline anemic—tired, lethargic, breathless on exertion, fast pulse, feeling the cold.

Aside from routine metabolic chemistry, liver, and kidney function screening, I also suggested some specialty urine testing. Molecular markers in urine may aid in predicting cancer progression to muscle invasion and recurrence, and hence in guiding treatment choices and assessing urgency of interventions. Hyaluronic acid (HA) is a glycosaminoglycan that promotes tumor metastasis. Hyaluronidase (HAase) promotes tumor growth, invasion, and angiogenesis. Both HA and HAase levels in urine are cutting-edge, noninvasive tests to measure diagnostic markers for bladder cancer. Another promising urine test for monitoring bladder cancer is quantitative measurement of telomerase, which has the potential to replace cytology as a noninvasive biomarker for disease diagnosis and follow-up.

Mr. E. did subsequently get an extensive metabolic chemistry assessment that found no significant abnormalities except elevated D-dimer, but unfortunately he was unable to access any of the specialty prognostic cancer tests suggested.

Treatment Options

After the canceled bladder removal, Mr. E.'s urologist recommended that he have more BCG infusions with additional infusion of mitomycin chemotherapy and electrical stimulation (Dr. Stasi protocol). The mitomycins are a family of drugs derived from the bacteria *Streptomyces caespitosus* or *Streptomyces lavendulae*. Mitomycin can cause a severe bone marrow depression and increase the risk of serious infection or bleeding. It may cause hemolytic uremic syndrome (a potentially life-threatening condition that injures red blood cells, causing anemia and kidney problems). There is evidence of better outcomes and fewer side effects if there is a period of pretreatment dehydration (no fluids for 8 hours prior to treatment), urinary alkalinization, confirmation of complete bladder drainage prior to instillation, and a higher mitomycin concentration (40 mg/20 mL). One study showed the severe irritative side effects and subsequent systemic complications can be prevented with prophylactic isoniazid (an antitubercular and antimycobacterial) given for 3 days, beginning the morning of treatment, but accessing this option may be hard.

We discussed Mr. E.'s medical options: Take more BCG and try to get the antibiotic preceding it, take the BCG and mitomycin and do the dehydration and alkalizing protocol, or do none of these. I pointed out to him that if BCG had not been sufficient to cause complete regression in the past, and given that it was so poorly tolerated, the chances of it being really effective for him now were slim to none. There are other drug options to consider—epirubicin, doxorubicin, and valrubicin are approved by the US FDA for the treatment of BCG-refractory bladder carcinoma in situ in patients who cannot undergo radical cystectomy. Gemcitabine has initially been shown to have promising results as well, in the context of BCG failure. In an ideal situation this is where we would have the patient give a tissue sample and have sensitivity and resistance testing done to find out what they might respond to before bombarding them with any random drug. In the case of Mr. E. the bigger challenge would have been accessing the drug(s) that tested as likely contenders. The testing can be done privately if desired and if it is affordable for the patient, but still you need to get the drugs administered, and if they are "off label," that may be next to impossible in many countries. His doctors were unwilling to pursue this option and in the end Mr. E. declined all chemotherapy options.

Initial Treatment Planning

The clinical challenge with this patient was to focus on his cancer, bladder health, and quality of life, while also noting and addressing the other health issues. He was taking an immunosuppressive drug that was impairing immune responses and an antacid that could impair downstream digestive functions and nutrient uptake. I was not concerned about the prostate drug, as the side effects are minimal, but I did hope to address the other underlying health concerns.

Chronic Upper Digestive Aching

- Stay on rabeprazole for now.
- Implement diet changes first and introduce herbs slowly.
- Consider focused herbal treatment and drug withdrawal prior to recommencing BCG (desirable to get the gut microbiome stable and healthy before taking an immunosuppressive).

Benign Prostate Hyperplasia

- Stay on tamsulosin for now.
- Implement lifestyle changes now as outlined above and introduce herbs later as needed.

He did subsequently undergo a green-light therapy for prostate enlargement, a sort of laser ablation procedure; it was very successful. He no longer needs medication for this.

Crohn's Disease

- Stay on adalimumab for now.
- Implement a grain-free, dairy-free diet.
- Take probiotics to support the microbiome.
- Eat naturally fermented foods (not pasteurized), such as sauerkraut and kimchi.
- Discuss issue of immunosuppression with urologist and oncologist in context of BCG—is there a better way to address the bowel?

Initial Tincture Formula

The main area of concern was the bladder wall health and resisting cancer, but we needed to look at the big picture as well as address specific issues. To get started I used a program of herbs to exert some general damage control, using balancing, fortifying, and tonifying herbs. We especially focused on supporting the liver and kidneys because they are the major organs of detoxification and remove toxins that may be stressors from the tissues. Some of the herbs were chosen to build the immune system and enable the body to mount a defense and immune response more effectively. Some herbs were intended to be more directly toxic to cancer cells or more like "herbal chemotherapy."

Daily Tincture Formula

The following tinctures are all 1:2 strength. The amounts listed below add up to 100 milliliters, which is enough for about 1 week.

+ 20 mL ashwagandha
+ 15 mL astragalus
+ 10 mL reishi mushroom
+ 10 mL crataeva
+ 10 mL burdock root
+ 10 mL Baikal skullcap
+ 5 mL Oregon grape
+ 5 mL propolis
+ 5 mL feverfew
+ 5 mL kava
+ 5 mL gotu kola

Take 7.5 milliliters (1½ tsp.) in hot water twice daily before meals.

Ashwagandha, astragalus, and reishi are all adaptogens and immune tonics with anticancer action. Nutritive and balancing to the immune system, these are addressing the underlying autoimmune condition as well as the cancer.

Crataeva (also known as varuna) is a bladder tonic and relaxant, anti-inflammatory, and diuretic. Indeed, the name *varuna* comes from Varun (the god of water) in Sanskrit mythology. This herb is recommended in Ayurveda for the treatment of various urinary problems including kidney stones, spasms, and pain in the ureters and bladder.

Burdock root is rich in fructo-oligosaccharides that feed good gut flora (prebiotic) and is used as blood-sugar balancer and a bowel function normalizer. It is also a bitter digestive stimulant and alterative. Not all the constituents will come out in solvents, so the tincture is only 25% alcohol, and ideally the patient would be taking capsules or drinking burdock decoction as well.

Baikal skullcap and propolis are both rich in flavonoids and provide redox regulation and immunomodulation. Baikal skullcap is anti-inflammatory. Propolis provides a rich polyphenol complex, including CAPE, which has anticancer activity.

Oregon grape alkaloids inhibit multidrug resistance pumping, augmenting the cytotoxic and redox-regulating effects of other natural compounds. It is also a bitter digestive stimulant and alterative.

Feverfew has anticancer sesquiterpenes in the volatile oil from the flowers; it is anti-inflammatory and reduces the severity and frequency of migraines. It is also a bitter, carminative digestive aid.

Kava has a particular relaxing and soothing action in the urinary system and acts as a tissue relaxant and antispasmodic. It may incidentally ease prostate symptoms as well.

Gotu kola is a connective tissue tonic to heal and tone the epithelial lining cells of the bladder. It also has marked anticancer actions.

Daily Herbal Powder

When mixed with water, this powder creates a soothing, mucilaginous, demulcent gel that coats the back of the throat, the tonsils and larynx, the esophagus, the stomach, and all the length of the small and large intestines. It soothes any burning and irritation, reduces local inflammation, soaks up bacteria toxins and acid wastes that irritate the skin, and promotes healing of tissue. For Mr. E., this powder was aimed at reducing the need for the proton pump inhibitor, protecting and healing any inflammation in the gut, and supporting a healthy microbiome.

+ 100 g marshmallow root powder
+ 50 g slippery elm bark powder
+ A pinch of cinnamon

Combine the marshmallow, slippery elm, and cinnamon and mix well. Stir 1 teaspoon to 1 tablespoon of the mixture into ½ cup of cold water. Take it as a gruel in the morning, and follow with ½ glass of water, then wait at least 30 minutes before eating.

Daily Tea Blend

This blend is nutritive and mineral rich, soothing, flushing, and healing to the kidneys and bladder. It supports heart rate and rhythm and reduces vascular tension and blood pressure. The amounts below add up to 300 grams, which is enough to last a month.

+ 100 g hawthorn leaf and flower
+ 75 g stinging nettle leaf
+ 50 g cornsilk
+ 50 g horsetail
+ 50 g linden

Put 3 heaping tablespoons of the blend in a pot, pour on 2–3 cups of boiling water, cover, and let steep for at least 30 minutes. Drink warm or cold.

PROTOCOL ANALYSIS FOR MR. E., BLADDER CANCER PATIENT

Foundation Herbs for Prehabilitation and Physiological Enhancement

Stress management: rhodiola, schisandra, gotu kola
Gut lining, hyperacidity, microbiome: slippery elm, marshmallow root
Immune tonics: astragalus
Cardiovascular health: hawthorn, linden, rhodiola

Synergists and Supportive Herbs

Connective tissue and bladder wall tonics: gotu kola, plantain, horsetail, varuna
Immunomodulators, anti-inflammatories: boswellia, turmeric, omega-3 fats, feverfew, Baikal skullcap, astragalus, mushrooms
Liver support and detoxification: milk thistle, schisandra, celandine, burdock, Oregon grape, turmeric, artichoke leaf, kutki, sulforaphane, DIM
Prostate support: pumpkin seed oil, saw palmetto (*Serrenoa repens*) fruit, stinging nettle root, rye flower pollen, evening primrose oil
Kidney restoratives: nettle seed, corn silk, gotu kola, goshajinkigan
Bladder relaxant: kava
Antioxidants: green tea, zinc, lipoic acid, turmeric, omega-3 fats

Specifics: Activators and Anticancer Herbs

Cytotoxics: Pacific yew, Madagascar periwinkle, pawpaw, pokeroot, mistletoe, camptotheca, Chinese wormwood
Anti-inflammatory, pelvic decongestant: ginger
Anticancer: MCP, vitamin D

SYNERGISTS AND SUPPORTIVE HERBS

ACTIVATORS AND ANTICANCER HERBS

FOUNDATION HERBS

DAILY SUPPLEMENT RECOMMENDATIONS

- Green tea extract (EGCG): 400 mg daily
- Zinc complex with L-malic acid, molybdenum bisglycinate, vitamin B2 (riboflavin), taurine, vitamin B6 (pyridoxine hydrochloride), zinc bisglycinate: 60 mg total zinc
- Modified citrus pectin: 4 g daily
- R+ alpha-lipoic acid: 800 mg daily, taken away from turmeric
- Vitamin D3: 4,000 IU daily
- Curcuminoid complex: 2 g daily
- Omega-3 fats: EPA 1,500 mg, DHA 750 mg
- DIM complex: 200 mg daily
- Probiotic blend: 50 billion bacteria daily
- Optional prostate tonic: borage oil, pumpkin seed oil, saw palmetto (*Serenoa repens*) fruit liposterolic extract, stinging nettle root extract, rye flower pollen extract, plant sterols (beta-sitosterol, campesterol, stigmasterol), cranberry (*Vaccinium macrocarpon*) fruit, tocopherols, lycopene, zinc citrate, selenium

SPECIALTY CYTOTOXIC AGENTS

Cytotoxic blend: Pacific yew, Madagascar periwinkle, pawpaw, pokeroot, mistletoe, and camptotheca, dosed at ¼ tsp. twice daily in water

- Artemisinin taken cyclically, 1 week on and 1 week off, in increasing doses, to 300 mg twice daily

Extra-Strength Tea for Acute Urinary Tract Infection

In this recipe, bearberry leaf is a disinfectant in the kidneys and bladder, as is thyme, and echinacea is an immunostimulant. They have synergy together to support the immune system in resisting urinary tract infections. Corn silk has demulcent mucilage and vulnerary allantoin that heals any inflammations or ulcerations in the urinary tract. Marshmallow also provides demulcent mucilage and reduces irritation and inflammation. It's already in the daily powder formula (page 469), but here is an extra allowance for burning urinary tract inflammation.

DECOCTION HERBS

- 40 g bearberry leaf
- 20 g corn silk
- 10 g echinacea

INFUSION HERBS

- 20 g marshmallow root
- 10 g thyme

Simmer 3 tablespoons of the decoction herbs in 500 milliliters of water for 10–15 minutes. This will create a strong brew. Remove it from the heat and add 1 tablespoon of the infusion herbs. Allow that to steep for an additional 5–10 minutes. Strain and consume 2–3 cups throughout the day. Use as needed.

Herbal Castor Oil Pack

Castor oil applied over the skin will be rubefacient (warming and reddening); anticancer and anti-inflammatory frankincense and lavender essential oils are carried into the tissue below.

+ 250 mL castor oil
+ 12 drops essential oil of frankincense
+ 20 drops essential oil of lavender

Apply three to six times weekly, for 30–60 minutes each time.

Case Update and Revised Protocol

Mr. E. did get more extensive blood work done, including, at my request, testing for some clotting factors. I was concerned about the chronic inflammatory state and increased risk of thrombosis. His D-dimer result was alarmingly high, but even before he could tell me that, he actually had a deep vein thrombosis after a flight from Australia. This was despite having used aspirin prophylactically. He then commenced using a blood thinner and remains on rivaroxaban (Xarelto), an anticoagulant, to date.

He experienced acute onset of nonviral hepatitis of unknown origin in February 2020, immediately after returning from a month in Mexico, and was acutely ill at the time of diagnosis. No drugs were given but he used an herbal tincture from my office.

By April 2020 the blood work showed liver enzymes at half what they were in February but still markedly elevated. They have subsequently regained normal levels. However, erring on the side of caution, we decided not to use the hepatostimulating *Artemisia annua* for a while, focusing on the cytotoxic tinctures in the daily blend.

A bladder scope in December 2019 showed some abnormal cells but no visible cancerous lesions. In 2020 he underwent surgery for a lodged kidney stone. After a couple of bladder infections, he began a continuous prophylactic antibiotic, which has caused an antibiotic-induced dysbiosis and flare-up of Crohn's symptoms (frequent, loose stools, up to 10 times in 24 hours).

Another bladder scope in April 2020 showed atypical cells but no visible tumor. CT and MRI scans of the liver showed spread of bladder cancer to the pelvis, lungs, and diaphragm with no evidence of lesions in the liver. He was offered chemotherapy and declined. In late 2020 Mr. E. had another CT scan that showed substantial reduction in size of the pelvic and subdiaphragmatic lymph nodes and stability with no change in the lung nodes. In late 2021 a follow-up CT scan showed no change, and he remains stable and well.

RESULTS FROM BLOOD WORK IN EARLY 2021

Iron and ferritin (stored iron) were low, although, interestingly, the hemoglobin was back in range and red cell count was normal. Recommendation: Try to cook in cast-iron pans, eat organic red meat and bone broths, and eat as many greens as possible. This does not mean taking an iron supplement (usually not recommended in cancer) but instead supplying sufficient naturally sourced, dietary iron to maintain normal blood levels.

Borderline high monocytes were noted. Monocyte macrophages are the main scavenger cells of the immune system and elevation indicates chronic infection, an autoimmune disorder, cancer, or all three. Recommendation: Use a range of mushrooms. The best way is in soup (stewing them in a cotton bag or thin sock, if they are woody).

Creatinine was elevated and glomerular filtration (kidney function) was low, indicating slow progression of kidney decline. C-reactive protein was elevated in September 2020, showing inflammation, but has not been retested since. INR was normal, but D-dimer was not retested. Liver enzymes were all normal.

GOSHAJINKIGAN POWDER

Mr. E. began to notice neuropathy in 2019; 2 teaspoons of powdered goshajinkigan formula in water daily has completely reversed it. Neuropathy and this formula are discussed in more detail beginning on page 222.

NEW SUPPLEMENT RECOMMENDATIONS

- Green tea extract (EGCG): 400 mg daily
- Zinc complex with L-malic acid, molybdenum bisglycinate, vitamin B2 (riboflavin), taurine, vitamin B6 (pyridoxine hydrochloride), zinc bisglycinate: 60 mg total zinc
- Modified citrus pectin: 4 g daily
- R+ alpha-lipoic acid: 800 mg daily, taken away from turmeric
- Vitamin D3: 4,000 IU daily
- Curcuminoid complex: 2 g daily
- Omega-3 fats: EPA 1,500 mg, DHA 750 mg
- Probiotic blend: 50 billion bacteria daily

LIVER DETOX SUPPORT BLENDS	
Alpha-lipoic acid, N-acetylcysteine, turmeric extract, milk thistle extract, broccoli sprout concentrate, artichoke, taurine, glycine, L-glutamine, L-methionine, chlorella, fat-soluble vitamin C	2 capsules twice daily
3,3'-diindolylmethane (DIM), calcium-D-glucarate, flaxseed extract, 5-methyltetrahydrofolate (from calcium 5-MTHF), vitamin B6 (pyridoxine HCl and pyridoxal-5-phosphate), vitamin B12 (methylcobalamin)	2 capsules twice daily

Liver Tonic

This formula is antimicrobial, antiparasitic, and anti-inflammatory. The tinctures listed below are all 1:2 strength.

+ 30 mL milk thistle
+ 20 mL schisandra
+ 20 mL nettle seed
+ 15 mL andrographis
+ 15 mL kutki*
+ 10 mL licorice
+ 10 mL turmeric

Take 10 milliliters twice daily in water for 2 weeks, then 7.5 milliliters in water twice daily for 2 more weeks. Retest liver enzymes and viral load each month.

*Also known as picrorhiza, this herb is critically endangered in the wild. Only certified sustainable sources should be used.

Daily Tincture

I prescribed a new formula for him in 2021, still addressing bladder cancer, kidney health, and immune strength as the main focus. This is not expected to "cure" him of anything but to keep his condition stable, to sustain kidney and liver functions, to reduce side effects of drugs, and to enhance quality of life. All tinctures are 1:2 strength.

+ 15 mL gotu kola
+ 15 mL astragalus
+ 10 mL milk thistle
+ 10 mL schisandra
+ 5 mL rhodiola
+ 5 mL ginger
+ 5 mL corn silk
+ 5 mL mistletoe
+ 5 mL thuja
+ 5 mL greater celandine

Take 10 milliliters (2 tsp.) in hot water twice daily before meals.

Nettle seed rebuilds kidney function. (It also serves as a substitute for crataeva, which is hard to source now. Nettle seed is also more nutritive and restorative and less of a dredging or kidney/prostate/bladder detox herb.)

Gotu kola is a connective tissue tonic and anticancer herb.

Astragalus is an immunomodulator and tonic.

Milk thistle and schisandra are liver tonics and support detoxification pathways.

Rhodiola and schisandra are adaptogens to support normal immune responses.

Ginger stimulates pelvic circulation and removes stagnation and congestion.

Corn silk has saponins and sugars that are immune activating and mucilage for a soothing and moistening effect.

Mistletoe, thuja, and greater celandine are cytotoxics and direct anticancer agents.

SPECIALTY CYTOTOXIC AGENTS

Cytotoxic blend: Pacific yew, Madagascar periwinkle, mistletoe, pawpaw, pokeroot, and mayapple, dosed at ½ teaspoon twice daily

ADDITIONAL ITEMS

These are to keep on hand for use as needed.

- Proprietary formula for acute bladder infections: berberine hydrochloride, thyme extract, cinnamon extract, oregano extract, neem extract, kinnikinnick extract
- DGL (deglycyrrhizinated) licorice root lozenges for gastric reflux and heartburn

Discussion

This patient has been battling ill health with good grace for a long time. His body is worn out and beaten up, and he is getting tired. In the meantime, though, he is now almost 2 years beyond what the doctors predicted and still getting up and enjoying his days. He is in no particular pain and still feels he can keep the cancer in a manageable state for a good while longer. My job is to support that and do everything I can to keep him in good shape, but not to be unrealistic with false hope. I am more or less following his lead at the moment—he still wants to fight, so I am still prescribing cytotoxics and immunostimulants and also actively addressing the incipient kidney failure because that will adversely impact the whole body. It is unusual to keep a patient on the cytotoxic blends, but he was stable for many months, until spring of 2022, when he began losing ground again. A short course of chemotherapy (gemcitabine) has stabilized him again.

This case illustrates how herbs and other natural agents can only do so much and cannot always turn the tide—just as chemotherapy or radiation isn't guaranteed to do so. For a practitioner, this is one of the most difficult times, because our training and instinct are all about helping people survive and thrive. When they choose to let go with grace and deliberation, it is our challenge to support that and know that it, too, is healing. By the time Mr. E. wrote the quote below, in early 2021, he had already outlived the expectations of his doctors by a couple of years. At the time of this writing, in the fall of 2022, he is still enjoying walks in the woods and the company of friends, and the herbs continue to play a role in supporting him to do that.

Note from a Cancer Patient

The health protocol that Chanchal suggested for me, I believe, has kept my system healthy and strong, allowing me to work on my healing from many different aspects. Thank you!

Receiving this diagnosis took the wind out of my sails initially, and I quickly realized that if I wanted it to be something different, then it was up to me to change it. I went about this by drawing on many years of self-healing, visualizations, and meditation.

First of all, I had to accept the prognosis: I have only 6 to 8 months to live!

I worked through the emotions related to this reality and during that time knew that the best way for me to deal with this prognosis, and in fact my life, was in the present moment. In that moment I committed to myself and to what was best for my best highest good, and to treat each moment as precious and honor it for what it was and do whatever felt right to change my situation and ultimately to live the rest of my life from that place. Coupled with my belief that gratitude is an essential component of my everyday life, and that cancer has been the most profound teacher in my life, I could move forward living each day as it comes with no expectation that it will be different or the same, while being grateful for the opportunity this situation had brought into my life.

The following quote from the Dalai Lama encapsulates my experience perfectly: "I am open to synchronicity, and I do not let expectations hinder my path." —Mr. E.

Lung Cancer

Mrs. R. is married, retired, and a nonsmoker and had been in generally good health until her cancer diagnosis. She was 65 when she was diagnosed in 2015 with adenocarcinoma in the right lower lung lobe. It was removed surgically and determined to be pT3, N0, M0. She immediately went into treatment with cisplatin and vinorelbine, which was completed shortly before she attended my clinic for the first time. She had completed four cycles but required a dose reduction to manage side effects, and she presented with marked fatigue and debility, although she was much better than she had been when in active treatment. She was expecting to go back for a follow-up CT scan to assess the success of chemotherapy.

Other Health History of Note

Elevated blood pressure. This was managed with hydrochlorothiazide and may have been overmedicated as the levels were tending to be low on recent readings. I had some misgivings about this drug, as new research from 2018 suggests that it can have unintended or unexpected consequences that could be quite significant. Hydrochlorothiazide is one of the most frequently used diuretic and antihypertensive drugs and is a known photosensitizing agent that has been previously linked to lip cancer. A retrospective study in Denmark examining the association between hydrochlorothiazide use and the risk of basal cell carcinoma (BCC) and squamous cell carcinoma (SCC) found that hydrochlorothiazide use is associated with a substantially increased risk of nonmelanoma skin cancer, especially squamous cell carcinoma. Additionally, it is associated with elevated blood sugar, probably due to cellular magnesium and potassium depletion.

Generally poor stress management. She was anxious and had occasional palpitations. We discussed breath awareness and meditation and the critical importance of getting outdoor activity on a regular basis.

Frequent urination and urge incontinence. I recommended practicing pelvic floor muscle exercises, and we also discussed surgical lifts and pelvic physiotherapy options.

Initial Treatment Planning

- Focus on recovery from surgery and chemotherapy, as well as residual cancer risk.
- Start an herbal and nutritional protocol to address vital force and restore the capacity to heal—build core strength; initiate and promote deep tissue healing; restore resilience to the system.
- Support the adrenal glands and capacity for repair and tissue healing, using balancing, fortifying, and tonifying herbs.
- Support the liver and kidneys—major organs of detoxification.
- Support the spleen (lymphatic system)—for tissue detox and decongestant.
- Stabilize and normalize bone marrow function and immune responses; increase resistance to cancer.
- Take cytotoxic herbs for 6 months to address stray remaining cancer cells.
- Get further testing to establish baselines and to measure cancer drivers.
- Follow a cancer-prevention diet.
- Follow the initial protocol for 3 weeks and then have a follow-up visit to discuss the results of new tests and make adjustments as required.
- Develop a monitoring plan for the next 3, 6, and 12 months (after first follow-up visit).

Suggested Schedule of Blood Testing

Basic Tests Needed Regularly

Repeat every 4 weeks for 6 months, then every 8 weeks for 6 months.

- Blood cell count—red and white cells and differentials
- Liver profile—AST, ALT, GGT, LDH, ALP, bilirubin, protein, albumin, globulin
- Kidney function—electrolytes (sodium, potassium, calcium, chloride), creatinine, BUN, urea

One-Time Tests for Cancer Drivers and Inhibitors

These assess terrain and relative risk and are repeated only if they're out of normal range.

- Zinc, copper, ceruloplasmin
- Vitamin D (25 OH)
- Vitamin B12, iron, ferritin, homocysteine, magnesium, selenium, hemoglobin A1c
- Fasting glucose, fasting insulin

One-Time Tests for Probability of Cancer-Driven Blood Clots

These are repeated only if they're out of normal range.

- Fibrinogen, D-dimer

One-Time Tests for Cardiovascular Health

These are repeated only if they're out of normal range.

- Total cholesterol, triglycerides, HDL, LDL, lipoprotein A, apolipoprotein A and B

Initial Tincture Formula

Mrs. R. is quite small and frail, so this is a building, nourishing, invigorating, and stimulating tonic. All tinctures are 1:2 strength. The amounts below add up to 100 milliliters, which is about enough for a week's supply.

+ 20 mL astragalus
+ 15 mL ashwagandha
+ 10 mL Baikal skullcap
+ 10 mL greater celandine
+ 10 mL larrea
+ 10 mL vervain
+ 10 mL gotu kola
+ 10 mL rhodiola
+ 5 mL ginseng
+ 2 drops ginger essential oil

Take 7.5 milliliters (1½ tsp.) twice daily in hot water or in tea.

Astragalus is an immune tonic.

Ashwagandha is an adaptogen for supporting energy and recuperation.

Baikal skullcap is an anti-inflammatory immune tonic.

Greater celandine and larrea are cytotoxics that can address stray cancer cells in tissues or in circulation.

Vervain is a tonic nervine for debility, depression, fear, anxiety, and self-doubt.

Gotu kola supports oxygenation of the brain and improves mental energy, as well as being a connective tissue tonic for lung repair.

Rhodiola and ginseng are adaptogens for supporting energy and recuperation. Rhodiola supports oxygenation.

Ginger is warming and diffusive.

Soup Blend

I would have preferred to use cordyceps mushrooms for better gaseous exchange in the lungs, but what was available and affordable for this patient was reishi and chaga mushrooms, dried and cut. Long, slow decoctions, like how soup stocks are made, is an ideal way to extract mushrooms.

+ 75 g chaga*
+ 75 g red root
+ 75 g reishi
+ 75 g taheebo

Put 4 tablespoons of the blend in 3 cups of water, cover, and simmer for 1 hour on very low heat. Strain and reserve the liquid, using it as a base for making soup. Alternatively, put the herbs and mushrooms in a clean cotton bag, tie it off, and add it directly to a soup stock in progress. This way, they can extract into the stock as it simmers.

*Chaga is high in oxalates; people with a history of kidney stones should use caution.

Tea Formula

The amounts below add up to 400 grams, which is enough to last about a month.

+ 150 g Essiac blend (burdock root, rhubarb root, sheep sorrel, and slippery elm)
+ 75 g oat seed
+ 75 g calendula
+ 50 g nettle
+ 25 g lemongrass
+ 25 g orange peel

Put 4 heaping tablespoons of the blend in a pot. Add 3–4 cups of boiling water. Steep overnight. Strain and drink through the next day. Can be gently rewarmed, but do not boil the tea. For simplicity you can add the Initial Tincture Formula (opposite page) to the herbal tea.

PROTOCOL ANALYSIS FOR MRS. R., LUNG CANCER PATIENT

Foundation Herbs for Prehabilitation and Physiological Enhancement

Adaptogens for stress management: milky oats, ashwagandha, rhodiola
Tonic nervines: vervain, ashwagandha, gotu kola
Liver support: milk thistle

Synergists and Supportive Herbs

Connective tissue strengthening and lung tonics: gotu kola, plantain, horsetail, bryony, cordyceps
Immunomodulators and inflammomodulators: turmeric, Baikal skullcap, taheebo, cat's claw, mushrooms
Lymph support: calendula
Detox: Essiac blend, dandelion, artichoke, I3C
Energy tonics/stimulants: rhodiola, ginseng, gotu kola, leuzea
Antioxidants: green tea, resveratrol, quercetin, grapeseed, CoQ10, selenium, zinc, vitamin E
Antiarthritics: bryony, turmeric, omega-3 fats

Specifics: Activators and Anticancer Herbs

Cytotoxics: Pacific yew, Madagascar periwinkle, pawpaw, pokeroot, mistletoe, camptotheca, lemongrass, orange peel, celandine, chaparral, Chinese wormwood
Oxygenators: gotu kola, rhodiola, cordyceps
Anticancer: melatonin, vitamin D, MCP

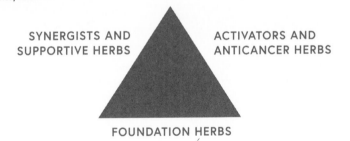

SYNERGISTS AND SUPPORTIVE HERBS

ACTIVATORS AND ANTICANCER HERBS

FOUNDATION HERBS

DAILY SUPPLEMENT RECOMMENDATIONS

- Probiotics blend: 50 billion bacteria
- High-potency multivitamin and mineral without iron or copper
- Vitamin D3: 6,000 IU
- Cordyceps mushroom: 2 g
- Turkey tail mushroom: 2 g
- B-complex vitamins:100 mg
- Omega-3 fish oils: 1,200 mg EPA, 500 mg DHA
- Modified citrus pectin: 3 g (take on an empty stomach)
- Green tea extract (EGCG): 500 mg
- Vitamin E succinate: 600 IU
- Zinc gluconate: 50 mg
- Selenium: 100 mcg
- Curcumin: 2 g
- Grapeseed extract: 1 g
- Resveratrol: 1 g
- Quercetin: 1,500 mg
- CoQ10: 100 mg

Supplements for Bedtime

- Milk thistle (silymarin): 1 g
- Melatonin: 4 mg
- Probiotics blend: 50 billion bacteria
- Indole-3-carbinol (I3C): 500 mg
- Proprietary capsule formula with *Rhaponticum carthamoides* (leuzea), *Ajuga turkestanica,* shilajit, *Cissus quadrangularis, Epimedium* spp., and *Cordyceps sinensis.* This powerful blend is designed to promote lean muscle development and strength, to optimize recovery time from physical demands, to enhance physical performance and endurance, to support bone density, and to restore energy reserves.

Specific Cytotoxic Anticancer Herbs

ALTERNATE-WEEK DAILY SUPPLEMENTS

Week One

- Artemisinin: 300 mg twice daily (building up to 600 mg or more twice daily), taken in 3–4 oz. of grapefruit juice
- Butyren (butyric acid): 1,000 mg twice daily
- Vitamin C: to bowel tolerance

Week 2

- Cytotoxic blend: Pacific yew, Madagascar periwinkle, mistletoe, pawpaw, pokeroot, and camptotheca, tincture blend, dosed at ½ tsp. twice daily in water

Case Update and Revised Protocol

Irregular heartbeat. Mrs. R. had episodes of racing heart and irregular beats; atrial flutter and fibrillation with frequent preatrial contractions and occasional preventricular contractions were confirmed by a 24-hour Holter monitor. Her doctor prescribed 12.5 mg atenolol (a beta-blocker) to calm and relax the heart, and it seemed to help quite a bit.

Mistletoe is indicated for this cardiac condition and may have cytotoxic effects as well. Hawthorn flower and leaf, linden, motherwort, and lemon balm tea would have been optimal here, but she was already taking a lot of items and the symptoms were managed with the drug, so we elected to make no changes for the time being and to review it in a few months.

Acute arthritis. This began in 2016, affecting smaller joints of the hands and feet, knees, and wrists. Pain was managed with naproxen initially and subsequently ibuprofen 200–400 mg.

I changed her herbal protocol entirely in response to the arthritis, which was acute, severe, and disabling. The cancer was apparently gone, so we continued to keep some herbs for immune and liver support and lung tonics, but the arthritis was now affecting her quality of life, so we prioritized it in the planning. Within a few weeks of starting this new plan, the symptoms were well managed with herbs and diet, and analgesic medications were no longer required.

Daily Tincture Formula

Tinctures are all at 1:2 strength unless otherwise indicated. The amounts below add up to 100 milliliters, which should be enough for a 10-day supply.

+ 15 mL Solomon's seal
+ 15 mL willow
+ 10 mL ashwagandha
+ 10 mL pleurisy (*Asclepius tuberosa*) root
+ 10 mL barberry
+ 10 mL devil's claw
+ 10 mL burdock
+ 10 mL yucca
+ 5 mL greater celandine (1:10)
+ 5 mL bryony (1:10)
+ 2 drops ginger essential oil

Take 5 milliliters (1 tsp.) twice daily in hot water or in tea.

Herbal Tea for Swelling and Inflammation

Mixing 75 grams of each of the dried, whole-leaf herbs below will yield 300 grams—a month's supply.

+ cleavers
+ meadowsweet
+ dandelion leaf
+ nettle leaf

Mix all the herbs. Put 4 tablespoons of the mix in a pot and cover with 3 cups of boiling water. Steep for at least 30 minutes. Drink 3 cups daily.

Antiarthritic Herbs for Hands and Feet

- Barberry and bryony are alteratives with tropism to the synovial joints, removing acid wastes and inflammatory debris.
- Burdock and devil's claw are also alteratives with tropism to the synovial joints, but less depurative than barberry, and more restorative and tonic to the tissues.
- Solomon's seal root contains saponins, phytohormones, glycosides, flavonoids, esters, and alkaloids. It has antibacterial and antifungal activities and has historically been used for analgesic, antipyretic, and

anti-inflammatory effects. It is an antioxidant and cytotoxic, induces apoptosis, shows prominent anticancer activity in breast cancer cells by inducing the phosphorylation of Bcl-2, and has anti-inflammatory action through inhibition of cyclooxygenase-1 and cyclooxygenase-2. It is also indicted for spinal and bone joint pain and inflammation.
- Willow and meadowsweet have anti-inflammatory and analgesic salicylates, and yucca has anti-inflammatory saponins.

Herbs for Anticancer Action
- Greater celandine has antimitotic actions and is hepatic.

Lung Tonics
- Pleurisy root (*Asclepius tuberosa*)
- Bryony (*Bryonia* spp.)

PLEURISY ROOT

Pleurisy root (*Asclepius tuberosa* and related species) has long been known for its bark, which was used to make a fiber and woven into twine or cloth. The seed floss was used for stuffing in pillows and mattresses, for candle wicks, and for fibers to make cloth. Today the floss is used for cleaning up oil spills at sea.

The root was extolled by early white settlers in the eastern US for diaphoretic, diuretic, laxative, tonic, carminative, expectorant, and respiratory antispasmodic properties. It was specifically indicated for intercostal neuralgia and rheumatism, as well as in pericardial pains and to lessen arterial tension. The name "pleurisy root" refers to the traditional use of the plant to treat inflammation of the lining of the lungs and the pleura and to relieve bronchial and pulmonary spasms. Pleurisy root stimulates the vagus nerve to induce perspiration, bronchial dilation, and expectoration. It is considered a warming and stimulating respiratory tonic for enhancing functional lung capacity.

> While it is serviceable even where the temperature is high, [pleurisy root] does its best work where the temperature is but moderately exalted, and when the skin is slightly moist, or inclined to moisture, and where the pulse is vibratile and not too rapid.
>
> *King's American Dispensatory*, 1898

Traditional Uses for Pleurisy Root
- In a salve for itching and flaking skin conditions
- For diarrhea and loose stools
- As a galactogogue
- As a gargle for sore throats
- As an anthelmintic for tapeworm

BRYONY

Bryony (*Bryonia dioica, B. alba, B. cretica* subsp. *dioica*) is an English hedgerow plant in the cucumber family and climbs and vines like a cucumber or melon. The genus *Bryonia* comprises 12 species, many of which have folk uses in love potions and spells, and several of which are used in folk medicine. *B. dioica* is from western Europe and *B. alba* from eastern Europe but there is geographic overlap and the two species are used interchangeably.

The genus name derives from the Greek *bryo*, meaning "shoot" or "sprout," in reference to the vigorous new stem growth in spring.

The root is the medicinal part, and it can get as large as an adult's leg. Primary actions are anti-inflammatory, antinociceptive (pain reducing), and antioxidant, partly due to a high phenolic and flavonoid content. There are at least seven unique triterpene glycosides, known as the bryoniosides A–G (1–7), and several unique tetracyclic terpenes collectively called the cucurbitacins. There are also immune-potentiating lectins and resins.

Bryony is known to be hypotensive, cathartic to hydrogogue, counterirritant, diaphoretic, and antirheumatic and to promote platelet aggregation. Flavonoids including lutonarin, saponarin, iso-orientin, and isovitexin provide for notable antioxidant action.

Cytotoxicity testing has shown a general lack of significant toxicity. However, due to the cathartic resins the tincture is made at 1:10 strength and the dose is restricted to 0.5 milliliter three times daily or 10 milliliters weekly at maximum.

Supplement Recommendations for Mrs. R.

- Omega-3s: EPA 1,750 mg, DHA 875 mg daily
- Green tea extract (EGCG): 500 mg daily
- Zinc complex with L-malic acid, molybdenum bisglycinate, vitamin B2 (riboflavin), taurine, vitamin B6 (pyridoxine hydrochloride), zinc bisglycinate: 50 mg total zinc daily
- Boswellia complex with boswellia gum oleoresin, celery seed, ginger, turmeric: two capsules twice daily
- Resveratrol: 1.5 g daily
- Quercetin: 2 g daily
- Vitamin B6: 100 mg daily
- Methylsulfonylmethane (MSM): 2 g daily
- Glucosamine sulfate (GLS): 1 g daily
- Vitamin D3: 3,000 IU daily
- Vitamin K2: 150 mcg daily
- N-acetylglucosamine (NAG): 750 mg daily
- L-glutamine: 5 g daily

WARM WAX HAND TREATMENTS

Warm wax treatments are approved by the Arthritis Foundation in the US to help relieve sore, painful joints caused by arthritis. Wax treatments provide moist heat, increase blood circulation, and ease stiffness due to joint inflammation. Warm wax treatments will ease stiffness and soreness in the hands or feet and provide quick short-term relief that makes it easier for the affected people to then exercise, which will also in turn significantly relieve the pain.

It is not only those with rheumatoid arthritis who will benefit from this. The antiestrogen drugs, especially tamoxifen and the aromatase inhibitors, are particularly known to cause small joint pain (hands, feet, elbows, and ankles). The penetrating heat of warm wax treatments is soothing and comforting.

Many books and teachers in the twentieth century suggested using paraffin wax, but I have a hard time with that. I understand that it is a well-established practice and has a history of "safe use," but somehow I find it hard to endorse using a petrochemical as a medicine. You can substitute beeswax and you can even infuse herbs into it by placing them into a muslin or thin cotton bag with a tight drawstring and immersing it for 15–30 minutes in the warm wax or in a warm base oil that can be added to the wax. Beeswax is great because it melts at a temperature of 144–147°F (62–64°C), has traces of propolis (which adds to the anti-inflammatory effects), and is widely available. If you don't use any animal products, then shea butter or cocoa butter will also work.

A Warm Wax Herbal Treatment

+ 500 g beeswax
+ 30 g licorice root powder
+ 25 g frankincense resin
+ 25 g kelp powder
+ 20 g cayenne powder

1. Place the wax into a glass bowl over simmering water (double boiler). Combine the herbs in a muslin bag and add it to the wax. Warm gently until the wax is completely melted.
2. Allow the wax to cool until the surface films very slightly. It should be around 125°F (52°C).
3. Wash your hands or other body part to be treated, and coat lightly with almond or grapeseed oil; this will make it easier to remove the beeswax.
4. Use your hands to coat the affected part with several layers of warm semiliquid beeswax. Leave it on for about 30 minutes. When the wax on the body part starts to cool, dip a cloth in very hot water and lay it over the beeswax coating to keep it flexible.
5. When you are done, peel off the beeswax and return it into its container for reuse. Move the affected parts gently to keep circulation going after the wax is removed.
6. Cool and store the wax to reuse it up to five or six times. Be careful to just melt it each time and not to scorch it.

Discussion

Mrs. R. remains cancer-free. Her rheumatoid arthritis is in remission and she is mobile, active, and mostly pain-free. Her blood pressure is well managed with beta-blocker medication and usually measures 130–140/80 (10 points lower than what was reported in fall of 2020). An ECG was normal, as was a stress test. She has not chosen to address her blood pressure with herbs.

I have recommended getting a bone density test, as the last one was in 2015, and I have encouraged her to book a couple of sessions or a series with a personal trainer to create a custom plan for a safe and effective workout routine.

Current Medications

- Ramipril: 15 mg (for blood pressure)
- Atenolol: 25 mg (to regulate the heart)
- Aspirin: 81 mg (to thin the blood)
- Low-dose naltrexone: alternate days (for the cancer). This is a mood-elevating and antidepressant agent with marked anticancer effects. It was prescribed to her by a naturopath.

This patient remains largely well, moderately medicated for the blood pressure and tolerating the drugs well. The low-dose naltrexone is still used for its anticancer activity. Her autoimmune inflammatory symptoms have eased and she is feeling overall well. This case illustrates the need to follow the patient as they present each time, adjusting and adapting the protocols to suit the need. Your job is not done once the cancer is in abeyance. Now comes the long-term plan for healthy living, and herbs and nutrition are key factors. All the ideas and suggestions proposed in Chapters 1 and 2 about prevention, resistance, and resilience are just as relevant after cancer as they are before.

ACKNOWLEDGMENTS

It may be a cliché but it is nevertheless true that a book is not written by one person alone. In the case of this book, there were many people who helped to make it happen.

First of all, I would like to thank my wonderful, patient editor Carleen Madigan, who convinced me I could write this book and who has corralled my sprawling manuscript into a coherent story.

I owe a big debt of gratitude to expert readers Dr. Eric Yarnell and Dr. Uwaya Erdman, who were invaluable in pointing out all my errors and omissions, and to my husband, Dr. Thierry Vrain, who always encouraged and supported me.

None of this would be possible without some wonderful teachers and mentors along the way—Hein Zeylstra, Simon Mills, Kerry Bone, Donnie Yance, David Winston, Dr. Jillian Stansbury, Jonathan Treasure, Dr. Eric Yarnell, Dr. Nic Rowley, and Dr. Neil McKinney, among others. I am grateful for your years of friendship and support.

Above all, I want to thank all the many patients in my clinic over the past two decades who have invited me to help them manage their cancer journeys and to support them with herbs.

References and Background Reading

Primary Reference Texts

Beuth, Joseph, and Moss, Ralph. *Complementary Oncology*. Thieme Publications, 2006.

Boik, John. *Natural Compounds in Cancer Therapy: A Textbook of Basic Science and Clinical Research*. Oregon Medical Press, 2001.

Bone, Kerry. *A Clinical Guide to Blending Liquid Herbs*. Churchill Livingstone Press, 2003.

Bone, Kerry. *Functional Herbal Therapy*. Aeon Books, 2021.

Bone, Kerry, and Mills, Simon. *Principles and Practice of Phytotherapy*. Churchill Livingstone Press, 2013.

British Herbal Medicine Association. *British Herbal Compendium*. Volume 1. British Herbal Medicine Association, 1992.

British Herbal Medicine Association. *British Herbal Pharmacopoeia*. British Herbal Medicine Association, 1996.

Bruneton, Jean. *Pharmacognosy: Phytochemistry of Medicinal Plants*. Intercept Books, 1999.

Gardner, Zoë, and McGuffin, Michael, eds. *American Herbal Products Association's Botanical Safety Handbook*. CRC Press, 2013.

LeMole, G., Mehta, P., McKee, D. *After Cancer Care*. Rodale Books, 2015.

McKinney, Neil. *Naturopathic Oncology: An Encyclopedic Guide for Patients and Physicians*. Liaison Press, 2010.

Mills, Simon, and Bone, Kerry. *The Essential Guide to Herbal Safety*. Churchill Livingstone, 2005.

Parmar, Gurdev, and Kaczor, Tina. *Textbook of Naturopathic Oncology*. Medicatrix Holdings Press, 2020.

Priest, A. W., and Priest, L. R. *Herbal Medication: A Clinical and Dispensary Handbook*. L. N. Fowler & Co., 1983.

Stansbury, Jill. *Herbal Formularies for Health Professionals*, Volumes 1–5. Chelsea Green Publishing, 2018–2021.

Tisserand, R., Balacs, T. *Essential Oil Safety: A Guide for Health Care Professionals*. Churchill Livingstone, 1995.

Weiss, Rudolph. *Herbal Medicine*. Arcanum Press, 1988.

Yance, Donald. *Herbal Medicine, Healing & Cancer*. Keats Publishing, 1999.

References from the Eclectic Physicians

Cook, W. H. *The Physio-Medical Dispensatory*, Cincinnati (1869). Reprinted by Eclectic Medical Publications, 1985.

Ellingwood, F. *American Materia Medica, Therapeutics and Pharmacognosy*, 11th edition (1919). Reprinted by Eclectic Medical Publications, 1994.

Felter, H. W., and Lloyd, J. U. *King's American Dispensatory*, Vols. 1 and 2, 18th edition (1898). Reprinted by Eclectic Medical Publications, 1983.

Jones, Eli. *Cancer: Its Causes, Symptoms and Treatments*. Therapeutic Publishing Company 1911. Reprinted by Isha Books, New Delhi, 2013.

An Introduction to Holistic Cancer Care

DeMartino, P. C., Miljković, M. D., Prasad, V. "Potential Cost Implications for All US Food and Drug Administration Oncology Drug Approvals in 2018." *JAMA Internal Medicine* 181, no. 2 (2021): 162–67.

Diamandopoulus, G. T. "Cancer: An Historical Perspective." *Anticancer Research*, no. 16 (1996): 1595–602.

Gallucci, B. B. "Selected Concepts of Cancer as a Disease: From the Greeks to 1900." *Oncology Nursing Forum*, no. 12 (1985): 67–71.

Greenwald, P., Kramer, B., Weed, D., eds. *Cancer Prevention and Control*. National Cancer Institute. Marcel Dekker Inc., 1995.

Islami, F., Goding Sauer, A., Miller, K. D., et al. "Proportion and Number of Cancer Cases and Deaths Attributable to Potentially Modifiable Risk Factors in the United States." *Cancer Journal for Clinicians* 68 (2018): 31–54.

Kardinal, C., Yarbro, J. "A Conceptual History of Cancer." *Seminars in Oncology* 6 (1979): 396–408.

Keene, M. R., Heslop, I. M., Sabesan, S., Glass, B. D. "Complementary and Alternative Medicine Use in Cancer: A Systematic Review." *Complementary Therapies in Clinical Practice* 35 (2019): 33–47.

Makary, M. A., Daniel, M. "Medical Error—The Third Leading Cause of Death in the US." *The British Medical Journal* 353 (2016): i2139.

Verrax, J., et al. "The Association of Vitamins C and K3 Kills Cancer Cells Mainly by Autoschizis, a Novel Form of Cell Death. Basis for Their Potential Use as Coadjuvants in Anticancer Therapy." *European Journal of Medicinal Chemistry* 38, no. 5 (May 2003): 451–57.

Witt, C. M., et al. "A Comprehensive Definition for Integrative Oncology." *JNCI Journal of the National Cancer Institute Monographs* 52 (2017).

World Health Organization. https://www.who.int/health-topics/cancer.

Chapter 1: Understanding Cancer

Alagawany, M., Abd El-Hack, M., Farag, M., Gopi, M., Karthik, K., Malik, Y., Dhama, K. "Rosmarinic Acid: Modes of Action, Medicinal Values and Health Benefits." *Animal Health Research Reviews* 18, no. 2 (2017): 167–76.

Anwar, S., Shamsi, A., Shahbaaz, M., et al. "Rosmarinic Acid Exhibits Anticancer Effects via MARK4 Inhibition." *Scientific Reports* 10, (2020): 10300.

Bower, J. E., Ganz, P. A., Aziz, N., Olmstead, R., Irwin, M. R., Cole, S. W. "Inflammatory Responses to Psychological Stress in Fatigued Breast Cancer Survivors: Relationship to Glucocorticoids." *Brain Behavior and Immunity* 21, no. 3 (March 2007): 251–58.

Campbell, K. L., McTiernan, A. "Exercise and Biomarkers for Cancer Prevention Studies." *Journal of Nutrition* 137, no. 1 (January 2007): 161S–69S.

Caoimhe Twohig-Bennett, C., Jones, A. "The Health Benefits of the Great Outdoors: A Systematic Review and Meta-analysis of Greenspace Exposure and Health Outcomes." *Environmental Research* 166 (October 2018): 628–37.

Carlson, A. J., Hoezel, F. "Apparent Prolongation of the Life Span of Rats by Intermittent Fasting." *Journal of Nutrition* 31 (1946): 363–75.

Carrillo-Vico, A., et al. "Melatonin: Buffering the Immune System." *International Journal of Molecular Science* 14 (2013): 8638–83.

Cole, S. W., Hawkley, L. C., Arevalo, J. M., Sung, C. Y., Rose, R. M., Cacioppo, J. T. "Social Regulation of Gene Expression in Human Leukocytes." *Genome Biology* 8, no. 9 (2007): R189.

Dantzer, R. "Cytokine-Induced Sickness Behavior: Where Do We Stand?" *Brain Behavior and Immunity* 15, no. 1 (March 2001): 7–24.

Dauchy, R. T., et al. "Circadian and Melatonin Disruption by Exposure to Light at Night Drives Intrinsic Resistance to Tamoxifen Therapy in Breast Cancer." *Cancer Research* 74, no. 15 (August 1, 2014): 4099–110.

Davis, D. L., Bradlow, H. L. "Can Environmental Estrogens Cause Breast Cancer?" *Scientific American* 273, no. 4 (October 1995): 166–170, 172.

De Cabo, R., Mattson, M. P. "Effects of Intermittent Fasting on Health, Aging, and Disease." *New England Journal of Medicine* 381 (2019).

Del Bianco, A., PhD, Demers, P., PhD. "Occupational Cancer Is the Leading Cause of Workplace Fatalities." Occupational Cancer Research Centre, York University, Toronto, 2013. http://www.occupationalcancer.ca/wp-content/uploads/2012/05/Del-Bianco_Fatalities_PIP_May2012.pdf.

Fischer, N., Seo, E. J., Efferth, T. "Prevention from Radiation Damage by Natural Products." *Phytomedicine* 47 (2018): 192–200

Godar, D. E., Subramanian, M., Merrill, S. J. "Cutaneous Malignant Melanoma Incidences Analyzed Worldwide by Sex, Age, and Skin Type over Personal Ultraviolet-B dose Shows No Role for Sunburn but Implies One for Vitamin D3." *Dermato-Endocrinology* 9, no. 1 (2017).

Harvie, Michelle N., Howell, Tony. "Could Intermittent Energy Restriction and Intermittent Fasting Reduce Rates of Cancer in Obese, Overweight, and Normal-Weight Subjects? A Summary of Evidence." *Advances in Nutrition* 7, no. 4 (July 2016): 690–705.

Ikeda, A., et al. "Social Support and Cancer Incidence and Mortality: The JPHC Study Cohort." *Cancer Causes Control* 24, no. 5 (2013): 847–60.

Johnsen, E. L. "Vascular Endothelial Growth Factor and Social Support in Patients with Ovarian Carcinoma." *Cancer* 95, no. 4 (August 2002): 808–15.

Kemeny, M. E., Schedlowski, M. "Understanding the Interaction between Psychosocial Stress and Immune-Related Diseases: A Stepwise Progression." *Brain Behaviour and Immunology* 21, no. 8 (2007): 1009–18.

Khan, Aiman Q., et al. "Roles of UVA Radiation and DNA Damage Responses in Melanoma Pathogenesis." *Environmental and Molecular Mutagenesis* 59, no. 5 (2018): 438–60.

Kloog, I., Haim, A., Stevens, R. G., Barchana, M., Portnov, B. A. "Light at Night Co-distributes with Incident Breast but not Lung Cancer in the Female Population of Israel." *Chronobiology International* 25, no. 1 (2008): 65–81.

Kotte, D., Li, Q., Shin, W. S., and Michalsen, A., eds. *International Handbook of Forest Therapy*. Cambridge Scholars Publishing, 2019.

Kroenke, C. H., et al. "Social Networks, Social Support, and Burden in Relationships, and Mortality after Breast Cancer Diagnosis in the Life After Breast Cancer Epidemiology (LACE) Study," *Breast Cancer Research and Treatment* 137, no. 1 (2013): 261–71.

Lee, J. H., Yoo, S. B., Kim, N. Y., Cha, M. J., Jahng, J. W. "Interleukin-6 and the Hypothalamic-Pituitary-Adrenal Activation in a Tumor Bearing Mouse." *International Journal of Neuroscience* 118, no. 3 (March 2008): 355–64.

Lin, G.-J., et al. "Modulation by Melatonin of the Pathogenesis of Inflammatory Autoimmune Diseases." *International Journal of Molecular Science* 14 (2013): 11742–66.

Lissoni, P., et al. "Five Years Survival in Metastatic Non-small Cell Lung Cancer Patients Treated with Chemotherapy Alone or Chemotherapy and Melatonin: A Randomized Trial." *Journal of Pineal Research* 35, no. 1 (August 2003): 12–15.

Loeb, L. A., Harris, C. C. "Advances in Chemical Carcinogenesis: A Historical Review and Prospective." *Cancer Research* 68, no. 17 (2008): 6863–72.

Lowell Center for Sustainable Production. University of Massachusetts, Lowell. https://www.uml.edu/research/lowell-center.

Lutgendorf, S. K., Cole, S., Costanzo, E., Bradley, S., Coffin, J., Jabbari, S., Rainwater, K., Ritchie, J. M., Yang, M., Sood, A. K. "Stress-Related Mediators Stimulate Vascular Endothelial Growth Factor Secretion by Two Ovarian Cancer Cell Lines." *Clinical Cancer Research* 9, no. 12 (October 1, 2003): 4514–21.

Meerlo, P., Sgoifo, A., Suchecki, D. "Restricted and Disrupted Sleep: Effects on Autonomic Function, Neuroendocrine Stress Systems and Stress Responsivity." *Sleep Medicine Review* 12, no. 3 (June 2008): 197–210.

Mentella, Maria Chiara, et al. "Cancer and Mediterranean Diet: A Review." *Nutrients* 11, no. 9 (2019): 2059.

Miller, G., Roehrig, C., Hughes-Cromwick, P., Lake, C. "Quantifying National Spending on Wellness and Prevention." *Advances in Health Economics and Health Services Research* 19 (2008): 1–24.

Morita, E., et al. "Psychological Effects of Forest Environments on Healthy Adults: Shinrin-yoku (Forest-Air Bathing, Walking) as a Possible Method of Stress Reduction." *Public Health* 121 (2007): 54–63, E.

Palesh, O., Butler, L. D., Koopman, C., Giese-Davis, J., Carlson, R., Spiegel, D. "Stress History and Breast Cancer Recurrence." *Journal of Psychosomatic Research* 63, no. 3 (September 2007): 233–39.

Park, B., et al. "The Physiological Effects of Shinrin-yoku (Taking in the Forest Atmosphere or Forest Bathing): Evidence from Field Experiments in 24 Forests across Japan." *Environmental Health and Preventative Medicine* 15, no. 1 (January 2010): 18–26.

Patterson, Ruth E., Sears, Dorothy. "Metabolic Effects of Intermittent Fasting." *Annual Review of Nutrition* 37 (2017): 1, 371–93.

Pollan, M. *How To Change Your Mind: What the New Science of Psychedelics Teaches Us about Consciousness, Dying, Addiction, Depression, and Transcendence.* Random House Publishers, 2018.

Raffaghello, L., Lee, C., Safdie, F. M., Wei, M., Madia, F., Bianchi, G., Longo, V. D. "Starvation-Dependent Differential Stress Resistance Protects Normal but Not Cancer Cells against High-Dose Chemotherapy." *Proceedings of the National Academy of Science USA* 105, no. 24 (June 17, 2008): 8215–20.

Rajapakse, N., Silva, E., Kortenkamp, A. "Combining Xenoestrogens at Levels below Individual No-Observed-Effect Concentrations Dramatically Enhances Steroid Hormone Action." *Environmental Health Perspectives* 110, no. 9 (September 2002): 917–21.

Reiche, E., Nunes, S., Morimoto, H. "Stress, Depression, the Immune System, and Cancer." *The Lancet, Oncology* 5, no. 10 (October 2004): 617–25.

Russel, J. Reiter, et al. "Melatonin, a Full Service Anti-cancer Agent: Inhibition of Initiation, Progression and Metastasis." *International Journal of Molecular Science* 18, no. 4 (2017): 843.

Sephton, S. E., Sapolsky, R. M., Kraemer, H. C., Spiegel, D. "Diurnal Cortisol Rhythm as a Predictor of Breast Cancer Survival." *Journal of the National Cancer Institute* 92, no. 12 (June 2000): 994–1000.

Shih W. L., Fang, C. T., Chen, P. J. "Anti-viral Treatment and Cancer Control." *Recent Results in Cancer Research* 193 (2014): 269–90.

Song, C., Ikei, H., Miyazaki, Y. "Physiological Effects of Nature Therapy: A Review of the Research in Japan." *International Journal of Environmental Research and Public Health* 13, no. 8 (August 3, 2016).

Srinivasan, V., et al. "Melatonin, Environmental Light, and Breast Cancer." *Breast Cancer Research and Treatment* (May 31, 2007).

Steingraber, S. *Living Downstream: An Ecologist's Personal Investigation of Cancer and the Environment.* Da Capo Press, 2010.

Thaker, P. H., Sood, A. K. "Neuroendocrine Influences on Cancer Biology." *Seminars in Cancer Biolo*gy 18, no. 3 (2008): 164–70.

Twohig-Bennett, C., Jones, A. "The Health Benefits of the Great Outdoors: A Systematic Review and Meta-analysis of Greenspace Exposure and Health Outcomes." *Environmental Research* 166 (October 2018): 628–37.

Verkasalo, P. K., et al. "Sleep Duration and Breast Cancer: A Prospective Cohort Study." *Cancer Research* 65, no. 20 (October 15, 2005): 9595–600.

Watson, C. S., et al. "Xenoestrogens Are Potent Activators of Nongenomic Estrogenic Responses." *Steroids* 72, no. 2 (February 2007): 124–34.

Witek-Janusek, L., Gabram, S., Mathews, H. L. "Psychologic Stress, Reduced NK Cell Activity, and Cytokine Dysregulation in Women Experiencing Diagnostic Breast Biopsy." *Psychoneuroendocrinology* 32, no. 1 (January 2007): 22–35.

Yang, Y., Li, T., Frenk, S. M. "Social Network Ties and Inflammation in U.S. Adults with Cancer." *Biodemography and Social Biology Journal* 60, no. 1 (2014): 21–37.

Zhao, Chan-Na, et al. "Potential Role of Melatonin in Autoimmune Diseases." *Cytokine & Growth Factor Reviews* 48 (August 2019): 1–10.

To calculate how long you need to get adequate vitamin D production and maximum safe sun exposure before burning: "Calculated Ultraviolet Exposure Levels for a Healthy Vitamin D Status and No Sunburn," NILU. https://fastrt.nilu.no/VitD-ez_quartMEDandMED_v2.html.

Chapter 2: Nutrition and Lifestyle Choices to Inhibit Cancer

Anand, P., Kunnumakkara, A. B., Sundaram, C., et al. "Cancer Is a Preventable Disease That Requires Major Lifestyle Changes." Published correction appears in *Pharmaceutical Research* 25, no. 9 (September 2008): 2200.

Anderson, O. S., KaSant, K. E., Dolinoy, D. C. "Nutrition and Epigenetics: An Interplay of Dietary Methyl Donors, One-Carbon Metabolism and DNA Methylation." *Journal of Nutritional Biochemistry* 23, no. 8 (August 2012): 853–59.

Baier, A., Szyszka, R. "Compounds from Natural Sources as Protein Kinase Inhibitors." *Biomolecules* 10, no. 11 (2020): 1546.

Beaver, Laura M., et al. "3,3'-Diindolylmethane, but Not Indole-3-Carbinol, Inhibits Histone Deacetylase Activity in Prostate Cancer Cells." *Toxicology and Applied Pharmacology* 263, no. 3 (2012): 345–51.

Besedovsky, Luciana, Lange, Tanja, Born, Jan. "Sleep and Immune Function." *Pflugers Archives* 463, no. 1 (2012): 121–37.

Clifton, K., Ma, C., Fontana, L., Peterson, L. L. "Intermittent Fasting in the Prevention and Treatment of Cancer." *A Cancer Journal for Clinicians* 71 (2021): 527–46.

Dion, C., Chappuis, E., Ripoll, C. "Does Larch Arabinogalactan Enhance Immune Function? A Review of Mechanistic and Clinical Trials." *Nutritional Metabolism Journal* 13 (2016): 28.

Divella, Rosa, at al. "Anticancer Effects of Nutraceuticals in the Mediterranean Diet: An Epigenetic Diet Model." *Cancer Genomics & Proteomics* 17, no. 4 (2020): 335–50.

Evdokimova, S. A., Nokhaeva, V. S., Karetkin, B. A., Guseva, E. V., Khabibulina, N. V., Kornienko, M. A., Grosheva, V. D., Menshutina, N. V., Shakir, I. V., Panfilov, V.I. "A Study on the Synbiotic Composition of *Bifidobacterium bifidum* and Fructans from *Arctium lappa* Roots and *Helianthus tuberosus* Tubers against *Staphylococcus aureus*." *Microorganisms* 9, no. 5 (April 26, 2021): 930.

Fabre, Bibiana, et al. "Prostate Cancer, High Cortisol Levels and Complex Hormone Interactions." *Asian Pacific Journal of Cancer Prevention* 17 (2016): 3167–71.

Filocamo, A., Nueno-Palop, C., Bisignano, C., Mandalari, G., Narbad, A. "Effect of Garlic Powder on the Growth of Commensal Bacteria from the Gastrointestinal Tract." *Phytomedicine* 19, nos. 8–9 (June 15, 2012): 707–11.

Fu, Y-P., Feng, B., Zhu, Z-K., Feng, X., Chen, S-F., Li, L-X., Yin, Z-Q., Huang, C., Chen, X-F., Zhang, B. Z., Jia, R-Y., Song, X., Lv, C., Yue, G-Z., Ye, G., Liang, X-X., He, C.L., Yin, L-Z., Zou, Y-F. "The Polysaccharides from *Codonopsis pilosula* Modulates the Immunity and Intestinal Microbiota of Cyclophosphamide-Treated Immunosuppressed Mice." *Molecules* 23, no. 7 (July 20, 2018): 180.

Kim, Mi-Sun, Sung, Hwa-Jung, Park, Jong-Yi, Sohn, Ho-Yong. "Evaluation of Anti-oxidant, Anti-microbial and Anti-thrombosis Activities of Fruit, Seed and Pomace of *Schizandra chinensis* Baillon." *Journal of Life Science* 27, no. 2 (February 28, 2017): 131–38.

Ladas, E. J., et al. "A Randomized, Controlled, Double-Blind, Pilot Study of Milk Thistle for the Treatment of Hepatotoxicity in Childhood Acute Lymphoblastic Leukemia (ALL)." *Cancer* 116, no. 2 (2010): 506–13.

Maier, Monica L. Vermillion, et al. "3,3'-Diindolylmethane Exhibits Significant Metabolism after Oral Dosing in Humans." *Drug Metabolism and Disposition* 49, no 2 (August 1, 2021): 694–705.

Maino Vieytes, C. A., Taha, H. M., Burton-Obanla, A. A., Douglas, K. G., Arthur, A. E. "Carbohydrate Nutrition and the Risk of Cancer." *Current Nutrition Report* 8, no. 3 (September 8, 2019): 230–39.

Mentella, M. Chiara, et al. "Cancer and Mediterranean Diet: A Review." *Nutrients* 11, no. 9 (September 2, 2019): 2059.

Moro, T. M. A., Clerici, M. T. P. S. "Burdock (*Arctium lappa*) Roots as a Source of Inulin-Type Fructans and Other Bioactive Compounds: Current Knowledge and Future Perspectives for Food and Non-food Applications." *Food Research International* 141 (March 2021): 109889.

Munakarmi, Suvesh, Chand, Lokendra, Shin, Hyun B., Jang, Kyu Y., Jeong, Yeon J. "Indole-3-Carbinol Derivative DIM Mitigates Carbon Tetrachloride-Induced Acute Liver Injury in Mice by Inhibiting Inflammatory Response, Apoptosis and Regulating Oxidative Stress." *International Journal of Molecular Sciences* 21, no. 6 (2020): 2048.

Park, Hyoung Joon, et al. "*Schisandra chinensis* Prevents Alcohol-Induced Fatty Liver Disease in Rats." *Journal of Medicinal Foods* 17, no. 1 (January 2, 2014): 103–10.

Perego, M., Tyurin, V. A., Tyurina, Y. Y., Yellets, J., Nacarelli, T., Lin, C., Nefedova, Y., Kossenkov, A., Liu, Q., Sreedhar, S., Pass, H., Roth, J., Vogl, T., Feldser, D., Zhang, R., Kagan, V. E., Gabrilovich, D. I. "Reactivation of Dormant Tumor Cells by Modified Lipids Derived from Stress-Activated Neutrophils." *Science Translational Medicine* 12, no. 572 (December 2, 2020): eabb5817.

Peterson, C. T., Vaughn, A. R., Sharma, V., Chopra, D, Mills, P. J., Peterson, S. N., Sivamani, R. K. "Effects of Turmeric and Curcumin Dietary Supplementation on Human Gut Microbiota: A Double-Blind, Randomized, Placebo-Controlled Pilot Study." *Journal of Evidence-Based Integrative Medicine* 23 (January–December 2018): 2515 690X18790725.

Singh, A. A., Patil, M. P., Kang, M. J., Niyonizigiye I., Kim, G. D. "Biomedical Application of Indole-3-Carbinol: A Mini-Review." *Phytochemistry Letters* 41 (2021).

Slattery, M. L., Curtin, K., Ma, K., et al. "Diet, Activity, and Lifestyle Associations With p53 Mutations in Colon Tumors." *Cancer Epidemiology, Biomarkers and Prevention* 11, no. 6 (June 2002): 541–48.

Tai, Shu-Yu, Huang, Shu-Pin, Bao, Bo-Ying, Wu, Ming-Tsang. "Urinary Melatonin-Sulfate/Cortisol Ratio and the Presence of Prostate Cancer: A Case-Control Study." *Scientific Reports* 6 (2016): 29606.

Trojanová, I., Rada, V., Kokoska, L., Vlková, E. "The Bifidogenic Effect of *Taraxacum officinale* Root." *Fitoterapia* 75, nos. 7–8 (December 2004): 760–63.

Valerio, F., de Candia, S., Lonigro, S. L., Russo, F., Riezzo, G., Orlando, A., De Bellis, P., Sisto, A., Lavermicocca, P. "Role of the Probiotic Strain *Lactobacillus paracasei* LMGP22043 Carried by Artichokes in Influencing Faecal Bacteria and Biochemical Parameters in Human Subjects." *Journal of Applied Microbiology* 111, no. 1 (July 2011): 155–64.

Zick, S. M., Sen, A., Feng, Y., Green, J., Olatunde, S., Boon, H. "Trial of Essiac to Ascertain Its Effect in Women with Breast Cancer (TEA-BC)." *Journal of Alternative and Complementary Medicine* 12, no. 10 (2010): 971–80.

SOY

Cassidy, A., et al. "Factors Affecting the Bio-availability of Soy Isoflavones in Humans after Ingestion of Physiologically Relevant Levels from Different Soy Foods." *Journal of Nutrition* 136, no. 1 (January 2006): 45–51.

Kennedy, A. R. "The Bowman-Birk Inhibitor from Soybeans as an Anticarcinogenic Agent." *American Journal of Clinical Nutrition* 68, 6 suppl. (December 1998): 1406S–12S.

Kilkkinen, A., Pietinen, P., Klaukka, T., Virtamo, J., Korhonen, P., Adlercreutz, H. "Use of Oral Antimicrobials Decreases Serum Enterolactone Concentration." *American Journal of Epidemiology* 155, no. 5 (March 1, 2002): 472–77.

McMichael-Phillips, D. F., Harding, C., Morton, M., et al. "Effects of Soy Protein Supplementation on Epithelial Proliferation in the Histologically Normal Human Breast." *American Journal of Clinical Nutrition* 68 suppl (1998): 1431S–35S.

Messina, Mark. "Soy, Soy Phytoestrogens (Isoflavones), and Breast Cancer." *American Journal of Clinical Nutrition* 70, no. 4 (October 1999): 574–75.

Miura, A., Sugiyama, C., Sakakibara, H., Simoi, K., Goda T. "Bioavailability of Isoflavones from Soy Products in Equol Producers and Non-producers in Japanese Women." *Journal of Nutrition & Intermediary Metabolism* 6 (2016): 41–47.

Okabe, Yuki, Shimazu, Tsukasa, Tanimoto, Hiroyuki. "Higher Bioavailability of Isoflavones after a Single Ingestion of Aglycone-Rich Fermented Soybeans Compared with Glucoside-Rich Non-Fermented Soybeans in Japanese Postmenopausal Women." *Journal of the Science of Food and Agriculture* 91, no. 4 (March 2011): 658–63.

Tsangalis, D., Wilcox, G., Shah, N., Stojanovska, L. "Bioavailability of Isoflavone Phytoestrogens in Postmenopausal Women Consuming Soya Milk Fermented with Probiotic Bifidobacterial." *British Journal of Nutrition* 93, no. 6 (2005): 867–77

Wu, A. H., Wan, P., Hankin, J., Tseng, C. C., Yu, M. C., Pike, M. C. "Adolescent and Adult Soy Intake and Risk of Breast Cancer in Asian-Americans." *Carcinogenesis* 23, no. 9 (September 2002): 1491–96.

Wu, A. H., Yu, M. C., Tseng, C. C., Pike, M. C. "Epidemiology of Soy Exposures and Breast Cancer Risk." *British Journal of Cancer* 98, no. 1 (2008): 9–14.

Chapter 3: Preparing for Surgery and Enhancing Recovery

Altinyay, Ç., et al. "Antimicrobial Activity of Some *Alnus* Species." *European Review for Medical and Pharmacological Sciences* 19 (2015): 4671–74.

Antal, O., et al. "Lipidomic Analysis Reveals a Radiosensitizing Role of Gamma-Linolenic Acid in Glioma Cells." *Biochimica et Biophysica Acta* 1851 (2015): 1271–82.

Bar-Yosef, S., et al. "Attenuation of the Tumor-Promoting Effect of Surgery by Spinal Blockade in Rats." *Anesthesiology* 94 (2001): 1066–73.

Ben-Eliyahu, S., Page, G. G., Yirmiya, R., Shakhar, G. "Evidence That Stress and Surgical Interventions Promote Tumor Development by Suppressing Natural Killer Cell Activity." *International Journal of Cancer* 80, no. 6 (March 15, 1999): 880–88.

Bito, T., Okumura, E., Fujishima, M., Watanabe, F. "Potential of Chlorella as a Dietary Supplement to Promote Human Health." *Nutrients* 12, no. 9 (August 20, 2020): 2524.

Bosse, J. P., Papillon, J., Frenette, G., et al. "Clinical Study of a New Anti-keloid Agent." *Annals of Plastic Surgery* 3, no. 1 (1979): 13–21.

Burzykowski, Tomasz, Coart, Elisabeth, Saad, Everardo D., et al. "Evaluation of Continuous Tumor-Size–Based End Points as Surrogates for Overall Survival in Randomized Clinical Trials in Metastatic Colorectal Cancer." *JAMA* 2, no. 9 (September 4, 2019): e1911750.

Castellani, L., Gillet, J. Y., Lavernhe, G., Dellenbach, P. "Asiaticoside and Cicatrization of Episiotomies" [article in French]. *Bulletin de la Fédération des Sociétés de Gynécologie et Dóbstétrique* 18, no. 2 (1966): 184–86.

Cesarone, M. R., Incandela, L., De Sanctis, M. T., et al. "Flight Microangiopathy in Medium- to Long-Distance Flights: Prevention of Oedema and Microcirculation Alterations with Total Triterpenic Fraction of *Centella asiatica*." *Angiology* 52, suppl. 2 (2001): S33–37.

Charlotte, F. J. M., et al. "Vascular Density in Colorectal Liver Metastases Increases after Removal of the Primary Tumor in Human Cancer Patients." *International Journal of Cancer* 112, no. 4 (November 20, 2004): 554–59.

Concerto, C., Infortuna, C., Muscatello, M. R. A., Bruno, A., Zoccali, R., Chusid, E., Aguglia, E., Battaglia, F. "Exploring the Effect of Adaptogenic Rhodiola Rosea Extract on Neuroplasticity in Humans." *Complementary Therapies in Medicine* 41 (December 2018): 141–46.

Damaj, M. I., Patrick, G. S., Creasy, K. R., Martin, B. R. "Pharmacology of Lobeline, a Nicotinic Receptor Ligand." *Journal of Pharmacology and Experimental Therapeutics* 282, no. 1 (July 1997): 410–19.

Das, U. N., Rao, K. P. "Effect of y-Linolenic Acid and Prostaglandins E1 on Gamma-Radiation and Chemical-Induced Genetic Damage to the Bone Marrow Cells of Mice." *Prostaglandins Leukotrienes and Essential Fatty Acids* 74 (2006): 165–73.

Davar, D., et al. "Fecal Microbiota Transplant Overcomes Resistance to Anti–PD-1 Therapy in Melanoma Patients." *Science* 371, no. 6529 (February 5, 2021): 595–602.

Decker, M. W., Majchrzak, M. J., Arnerić, S. P. "Effects of Lobeline, a Nicotinic Receptor Agonist, on Learning and Memory." *Pharmacology, Biochemistry & Behaviour* 45, no. 3 (July 1993): 571–76.

De Simone, R., Ajmone-Cat, M. A., Carnevale, D., et al. "Activation of α7 Nicotinic Acetylcholine Receptor by Nicotine Selectively Up-Regulates Cyclooxygenase-2 and Prostaglandin E2 in Rat Microglial Cultures." *Journal of Neuroinflammation* 2, no. 4 (2005).

Dimpfel, W., Schombert, L., Panossian, A. G. "Assessing the Quality and Potential Efficacy of Commercial Extracts of *Rhodiola rosea* L. by Analyzing the Salidroside and Rosavin Content and the Electrophysiological Activity in Hippocampal Long-Term Potentiation, a Synaptic Model of Memory." *Frontiers in Pharmacology* 9 (May 24, 2018): 425.

Do Nascimento, K. C., et al. "Immunohistochemical Localization of the NM23 Protein in Salivary Gland Neoplasms with Distinct Biological Behavior." *Virchows Archives: European Journal of Pathology* (November 8, 2006).

Eldred-Evans, David, Tam, Henry, Smith, Andrew P. T., Winkler, Mathias, Ahmed, Hashim U., "Use of Imaging to Optimise Prostate Cancer Tumour Volume Assessment for Focal Therapy Planning." *Current Urology Reports* 21, no. 10 (2020): 38.

Flaig, T. W., Glodé, M., Gustafson, D., van Bokhoven, A., Tao, Y., Wilson, S., Su, L-J., Li, Y., Harrison, G., Agarwal, R., Crawford, E. D., Lucia, M. S., Pollak, M. "A Study of High-Dose Oral Silybin-Phytosome Followed by Prostatectomy in Patients with Localized Prostate Cancer." *Prostate* 70, no. 8 (June 1, 2010): 848–55.

Goto, E., et al. "Low-Concentration Homogenized Castor Oil Eye Drops for Noninflamed Obstructive Meibomian Gland Dysfunction." *Ophthalmology* 109 (2002): 2030–35.

Grady, H. "Immunomodulation through Castor Oil Packs." *Journal of Naturopathic Medicine* 7 (1998): 84–89.

Hanin, Leonid. "Paradoxical Effects of Tumor Shrinkage on Long-Term Survival of Cancer Patients." *Journal of Frontiers in Applied Mathematics and Statistics* (2020). https://doi.org/10.3389/fams.2020.00027.

Ikeda, M., et al. "Surgery for Gastric Cancer Increases Plasma Levels of Vascular Endothelial Growth Factor and Von Willebrand Factor." *Gastric Cancer* 5, no. 3 (2002): 137–41.

Jiang, W. G., Hiscox, S., Bryce, R. P., Horrobin, D. F., Mansel, R. E. 'The Effects of N-6 Polyunsaturated Fatty Acids on the Expression of Nm-23 in Human Cancer Cells." *British Journal of Cancer* 77 (1998): 731–38.

Kadu, B., et al. "An Overview: Natural Herbs as an Athero-Thrombolytics." *European Journal of Biomedical and Pharmaceutical Sciences* 8, no. 8 (2021): 148–55.

Keaton, D., Myatt, D. "Effects of Castor Oil on Lymphocytes Subsets." Presented at AANP Conference; September 2–6, 1992, The Buttes, Tempe, Arizona.

Kotekar, N., Shenkar, A., Nagaraj, R. "Postoperative Cognitive Dysfunction—Current Preventive Strategies." *Clinical Interventions in Aging* 13 (2018): 2267–73.

Kursinszki, L., Szőke, E. "HPLC-ESI-MS/MS of Brain Neurotransmitter Modulator Lobeline and Related Piperidine Alkaloids in Lobelia inflata L." *Journal of Mass Spectrometry* 50, no. 5 (2015).

Lazzeroni, M., Guerrieri-Gonzaga, A., Gandini, S., Johansson, H., Serrano, D., Cazzaniga, M., Aristarco, V., Puccio, A., Mora, S., Caldarella, P., Pagani, G., Pruneri, G., Riva, A., Petrangolini, G., Morazzoni, P., DeCensi, A., Bonanni, B. "A Presurgical Study of Oral Silybin-Phosphatidylcholine in Patients with Early Breast Cancer." *Cancer Prevention Research* 9, no. 1 (January 2016): 89–95.

Leach, M. "A Critical Review of Natural Therapies in Wound Management." *Ostomy Wound Management* 50, no. 2 (February 2005).

Lv, L., Shao, Y. F., Zhou, Y. B. "The Enhanced Recovery after Surgery (ERAS) Pathway for Patients Undergoing Colorectal Surgery: An Update of Meta-analysis of Randomized Controlled Trials." *International Journal of Colorectal Disease* 27, no. 12 (2012): 1549–54.

Ma, G. P., et al. "Rhodiola rosea L. Improves Learning and Memory Function: Preclinical Evidence and Possible Mechanisms." *Frontiers in Pharmacology* (December 4, 2018).

Maissa, C., Guillon, M., Simmons, P., Vehige, J. "Effect of Castor Oil Emulsion Eyedrops on Tear Film Composition and Stability." *Contact Lens and Anterior Eye* 33 (2010): 76–82.

Marshall, J. C., Lee, J. H., Steeg, P. S. "Clinical-Translational Strategies for the Elevation of Nm23-H1 Metastasis Suppressor Gene Expression." *Molecular Cell Biochemistry* 329 (2009): 115–120.

McCutcheon, A. R., Ellis, S. M., Hancock., R. E. W., Towers, G. H. N. "Antibiotic Screening of Medicinal Plants of the British Columbian Native Peoples." *Journal of Ethnopharmacology* 37, no. 3 (1992): 213–23.

Menendez, J. A., Vellon, L., Colomer, R., Lupu, R. "Effect of y-Linolenic Acid on the Transcriptional Activity of the Her-2/neu (erbB-2) Oncogene." *Journal of the National Cancer Institute* 2 (2005): 1611–15.

Miroddi, M., Navarra, M., Quattropani, M. C., Calapai, F., Gangemi, S., Calapai, G. "Systematic Review of Clinical Trials Assessing Pharmacological Properties of *Salvia* Species on Memory, Cognitive Impairment and Alzheimer's Disease." *CNS Neuroscience Therapies* 20, no. 6 (June 2014): 485–95.

Miyake, J. A., Benadiba, M., Colquhoun, A. "Gamma-Linolenic Acid Inhibits Both Tumor Cell Cycle Progression and Angiogenesis in the Orthotopic C6 Glioma Model through Changes in VEGF, Flt1, ERK1/2, MMP2, Cyclin D1, pRb, p53 and p27 Protein Expression." *Lipids, Health and Disease* 8 (March 17, 2009): 8.

Ohba, T., et al. "Protective Effects of *Huperzia serrata* and Its Components against Oxidative Damage and Cognitive Dysfunction." *PharmaNutrition* 13 (September 2020): 100203.

Panahi, Y., Darvishi, B., Jowzi, N., Beiraghdar, F., Sahebkar, A. "*Chlorella vulgaris*: A Multifunctional Dietary Supplement with Diverse Medicinal Properties." *Current Pharmaceutical Design* 22, no. 2 (2016): 164–73.

Pooli, A., Johnson, D. C., Shirk, J., Markovic, D., Sadun, T. Y., Sisk Jr., A. E., Mohammadian Bajgiran, A., Afshari Mirak, S., Felker, E. R., Hughes, A. K., Raman, S. S., Reiter, R. E. "Predicting Pathological Tumor Size in Prostate Cancer Based on Multiparametric Prostate Magnetic Resonance Imaging and Preoperative Findings." *Journal of Urology* 205, no. 2 (February 2021): 444–51.

Ray, S., Chattopadhyay, N., Mitra, A., Siddiqi, M., Chatterjee, A. "Curcumin Exhibits Antimetastatic Properties by Modulating Integrin Receptors, Collagenase Activity, and Expression of Nm23 And E-Cadherin." *Journal of Environmental Pathology, Toxicology and Oncology* 22, no. 1 (2003): 49–58.

Retsky, M., Demicheli, R., Hrushesky, W. J. "Does Surgery Induce Angiogenesis in Breast Cancer? Indirect Evidence from Relapse Pattern and Mammography Paradox." *International Journal of Surgery* 3, no. 3 (2005): 179–87.

Romanelli, M. N., et al. "Central Nicotinic Receptors: Structure, Function, Ligands, and Therapeutic Potential." *ChemMedChem* 2 (2007): 746–67.

Sati, Sushil Chandra, et al. "Bioactive Constituents and Medicinal Importance of Genus *Alnus*." *Pharmacognosy Reviews* 5, no. 10 (2011): 174–83.

Schmidt, J. M., Greenspoon, J. S. "*Aloe vera* Dermal Wound Gel Is Associated with a Delay in Wound Healing." *Obstetrics and Gynecology* 78, no. 1 (July 1991): 115–17.

Schreiter, D., Rabald, S., Bercker, S., Kaisers, U. X. "The Significance of Perioperative Immuno-nutrition" [article in German]. *Laryngorhinootologie* 89, no. 2 (February 2010): 103–13.

Scott, M. J., Fawcett, W. J. "Oral Carbohydrate Preload Drink for Major Surgery—The First Steps from Famine to Feast." *Anaesthesia* 69, no. 12 (October 2014): 1308–13.

Seifert, M., Welter, C., Mehraein, Y., Seitz, G. "Expression of the nm23 Homologues nm23-H4, nm23-H6, and nm23-H7 in Human Gastric and Colon Cancer." *Journal of Pathology* 205, no. 5 (April 2005): 623–32.

Sengupta, S., et al. "Modulating Angiogenesis: The Yin and the Yang in Ginseng." *Circulation* 110 (2004): 1219–25.

Sevin, P. "Some Observations on the Use of Asiaticoside (Madecassol) in General Surgery." *Progress in Medicine* 90 (January 10, 1962): 23–24.

Skarping, I., et al. "Neoadjuvant Breast Cancer Treatment Response; Tumor Size Evaluation through Different Conventional Imaging Modalities in the NeoDense Study." *Acta Oncologica* 59, no. 12 (2020): 1528–37.

Stassen, P. "The Use of Asiaticoside in Traumatology." *Revue Medicale du Liege* 19 (1964): 305–8.

Sun, Q. Q., Xu, S. S., Pan, J. L., Guo, H. M., Cao, W. Q. "Huperzine-A Capsules Enhance Memory and Learning Performance in 34 Pairs of Matched Adolescent Students." *Acta Pharmacologica Sinica* 20, no. 7 (July 1999): 601–3.

Terrando, N., et al. "Resolving Postoperative Neuro-inflammation and Cognitive Decline." *Annals of Neurology* 70, no. 6 (December 2011): 986–95.

Vieira, C. "Pro- and Anti-inflammatory Actions of Ricinoleic Acid: Similarities and Differences with Capsaicin." *Naunyn Schmiedebergs Archives of Pharmacology* 364, no. 2 (August 2001): 87–95.

Vieira, C., et al. "Effect of Ricinoleic Acid in Acute and Subchronic Experimental Models of Inflammation, Mediators." *Inflammation* 9 no. 5 (2000): 223–28.

Wang, Yi, Qin, Zhiqiang, Wang, Yamin, Chen, Chen, Wang, Yichun, Meng, Xianghu, Song, Ninghong. "The Role of Radical Prostatectomy for the Treatment of Metastatic Prostate Cancer: A Systematic Review and Meta-analysis." *Bioscience Reports* 38, no. 1 (February 28, 2018): BSR20171379.

Xu, N., et al. "Neuroprotective Effect of Salidroside against Central Nervous System Inflammation-Induced Cognitive Deficits: A Pivotal Role of Sirtuin 1-Dependent Nrf-2/HO-1/NF-κB pathway." *Phytotherapy Research* 33, no. 5 (2019).

Yang, Y. F., Li, P. Z., Liang, X. B., Han, X. L., Li, Y. P., Cong, J. "Study on the Prognostic Factors of Colorectal Cancer after Radical Resection and on Suggested Model for Prediction" [article in Chinese]. *Zhonghua Liu Xing Bing Xue Za Zhi* 26, no. 3 (March 2005): 214–17.

Yarnell, E. "The Musculoskeletal Aspects of *Lobelia inflata* and Beyond." *Naturopathic Doctor News & Review* (November 23, 2005). https://ndnr.com/pain-medicine/the-musculoskeletal-aspects-of-lobelia-inflata-and-beyond/.

Zurek, A. A., Yu, J., Wang, D. S., Haffey, S. C., Bridgwater, E. M., Penna, A., Lecker, I., Lei, G., Chang, T., Salter, E. W., Orser, B. A. "Sustained Increase in α5GABAA Receptor Function Impairs Memory after Anesthesia." *Journal of Clinical Investigation* 124, no. 12 (December 2014): 5437–41.

Chapter 4: Managing Pain with Botanicals

Alhassen, Lamees, Nuseir, Khawla, Ha, Allyssa, Phan, Warren, Marmouzi, Ilias, Shah, Shalini, Civelli, Olivier. "The Extract of *Corydalis yanhusuo* Prevents Morphine Tolerance and Dependence." *Pharmaceuticals* 14, no. 10 (2021): 1034.

Besharat, S., Besharat, M., Jabbari, A. "Wild Lettuce (*Lactuca virosa*) Toxicity." *BMJ Case Reports* 2009 (2009): bcr0620080134.

Elzinga, S., Fischedick, J., Podkolinski, R., Raber, J. C. "Cannabinoids and Terpenes as Chemotaxonomic Markers in Cannabis." *Natural Products Chemistry & Research* 3 (2015): 181.

Fields, D. "Map the Other Brain." *Nature* 501 (2013).

Fields, R. Douglas. "New Culprits in Chronic Pain." *Neuroscience* (2009). https://www.scientificamerican.com/article/new-culprits-in-chronic-pain.

Fischedick, J. T. "Identification of Terpenoid Chemotypes among High (–)-trans-D9-Tetrahydrocannabinol-Producing *Cannabis sativa* L. Cultivars." *Cannabis and Cannabinoid Research* 2, no. 1 (2016): 34–47.

Gatti, A., et al. "Palmitoylethanolamide in the Treatment of Chronic Pain Caused by Different Etiopathogenesis." *Pain Medicine* 13, no. 9 (2012): 1121–30.

Gromek, D., Kisiel, W., Klodzińska, A., Chojnacka-Wójcik, E. "Biologically Active Preparations from *Lactuca virosa* L." *Phytotherapy Research* 6, no. 5 (September/October 1992): 285–87.

Harsha, S. N., Anilakumar, K. R. "Effects of *Lactuca sativa* Extract on Exploratory Behavior Pattern, Locomotor Activity and Anxiety in Mice." *Asian Pacific Journal of Tropical Disease* 2, suppl. 1 (2012): S475–79.

Heshmatian, B., Nasri, S., Asghari, Mehrabad J., Mahmoudi, Far F. "Antinociceptive Effects of Hydroalcoholic Extract of *Lactuca sativa longifolia* Leaves in Male Mice." *Horizons of Medical Sciences* 16, no. 2 (2010): 5–11.

Hesselink, J. M. K. "Evolution in Pharmacologic Thinking around the Natural Analgesic Palmitoylethanolamide: From Nonspecific Resistance to PPAR-α Agonist and Effective Nutraceutical." *Journal of Pain Research* 6 (2013): 625–34.

Hesselink, J. M. K. "New Targets in Pain, Non-Neuronal Cells, and the Role of Palmitoylethanolamide." *Open Pain Journal* 5 (2012): 12–23.

Hesselink, J. M. K., Hekker, T. A. "Therapeutic Utility of Palmitoylethanolamide in the Treatment of Neuropathic Pain Associated with Various Pathological Conditions: A Case Series." *Journal of Pain Research* 5 (2012): 437–42.

Jabbari, A., Besharat, S., Besharat, M. "Wild Lettuce Toxicity: Case-Series." *Journal of Medicinal Plants* 9, no. 36 (2010): 175–79, 198 ref. 5.

Kriplani, P., Guarve, K., Baghael, U. "*Arnica montana* L.—A Plant of Healing: Review." *Journal of Pharmacy and Pharmacology* 69, no. 8 (August 2017): 925–45.

Lyss, G., Schmidt, T. J., Merfort, I., Pahl, H. L. "Helenalin, an Anti-inflammatory Sesquiterpene Lactone from *Arnica*, Selectively Inhibits Transcription Factor NF-κB." *Journal of Biological Chemistry* 378 (1997): 951–61.

MacCallum, C. A., Russo, E. B. "Practical Considerations in Medical Cannabis Administration and Dosing." *European Journal of Internal Medicine* 49 (March 2018): 12–19.

Minnella, Enrico Maria, et al. "Multimodal Prehabilitation Improves Functional Capacity before and after Colorectal Surgery for Cancer: A Five-Year Research Experience." *Acta Oncologica* 56, no. 2 (2017): 295–300.

Mohammad, A. "Traditional Use Of Kahu (*Lactuca scariola* L.): A Review." *Global Journal of Research on Medicinal Plants & Indigenous Medicine* 2, no. 6 (June 2013): 465–74.

Mullins, M. E., Horowitz, B. Z. "The Case of the Salad Shooters: Intravenous Injection of Wild Lettuce Extract." *Veterinary and Human Toxicology* 40, no. 5 (October 1998): 290–91.

Paladini, A., et al. "Palmitoylethanolamide, a Special Food for Medical Purposes, in the Treatment of Chronic Pain: A Pooled Data Meta-analysis." *Pain Physician Journal* 19 (2016): 11–24.

Rotermann, M., Langlois, K. "Prevalence and Correlates of Marijuana Use in Canada, 2012." *Health Reports* 26, no. 4 (2015): 10–15.

Russo, E. "The *Cannabis sativa* versus *Cannabis indica* Debate: An Interview with Ethan Russo, MD." *Cannabis and Cannabinoid Research* 1, no. 1 (2016).

Schauer, G. L., et al. "Toking, Vaping, and Eating for Health or Fun: Marijuana Use Patterns in Adults, U.S., 2014." *American Journal of Preventative Medicine* 50, no. 1 (2016): 1–8.

Sugier, D., Sugier, P., Jakubowicz-Gil, J., Winiarczyk, K., Kowalski, R. "Essential Oil from *Arnica montana* L. Achenes: Chemical Characteristics and Anticancer Activity." *Molecules* 24, no. 22 (2019): 4158.

Sugier, P., Jakubowicz-Gil, J., Sugier, D., Kowalski, R., Gawlik-Dziki, U., Kołodziej, B., Dziki, D. "Chemical Characteristics and Anticancer Activity of Essential Oil from *Arnica montana* L. Rhizomes and Roots." *Molecules* 25, no. 6 (2020): 1284.

Ujváry, István. "Psychoactive Natural Products: Overview of Recent Developments." *Annali dell'Istuto superiore di sanita* 50, no. 1 (2014): 12–27.

Wang, K. Y., Tull, L., Cooper, E., Wang, N., Liu, D. "Recombinant Protein Production of Earthworm Lumbrokinase for Potential Antithrombotic Application." *Evidence-Based Complementary and Alternative Medicine* (2013): 783971.

Wesołowska, A., Nikiforuk, A., Michalska, K., Kisiel, W., Chojnacka-Wójcik, E. "Analgesic and Sedative Activities of Lactucin and Some Lactucin-Like Guaianolides in Mice." *Journal of Ethnopharmacology* 107, no. 2 (September 19, 2006): 254–58.

Wightman, E. L., Jackson, P. A., Spittlehouse, B., Heffernan, T., Guillemet, D., Kennedy, D. O. "The Acute and Chronic Cognitive Effects of a Sage Extract: A Randomized, Placebo Controlled Study in Healthy Humans." *Nutrients* 13, no. 1 (2021): 218.

Chapter 5: Thriving during Chemotherapy and Radiation

American Cancer Society. "Treatments and Side Effects." https://www.cancer.org/treatment/treatments-and-side-effects.

Berger, A., Henderson, M., Nadoolman, W., Duffy, V., Cooper, D., Saberski, L., Bartoshuk, L. "Oral Capsaicin Provides Temporary Relief for Oral Mucositis Pain Secondary to Chemotherapy/Radiation Therapy." *Journal of Pain and Symptom Management* 10, no. 3 (1995): 243–48.

Biswal, B. M., Sulaiman, S. A., Ismail, H. C., Zakaria, H., Musa, K. I. "Effect of *Withania somnifera* (Ashwagandha) on the Development of Chemotherapy-Induced Fatigue and Quality of Life in Breast Cancer Patients." *Integrated Cancer Therapy* 12, no. 4 (July 2013): 312–22.

Block, K., et al. "Making Circadian Cancer Therapy Practical." *Integrative Cancer Therapies* 8, no. 4 (2009): 371–86.

Bone, K. "The Underestimated Value of Bitter Herbs." *Dynamic Chiropractic* 30, no. 11 (May 20, 2012).

Chaput, G., Ibrahim, M., Towers, A. "Cancer-Related Lymphedema: Clinical Pearls for Providers." *Current Oncology* 27, no. 6 (2020): 336–40.

Chen, Jhong-Yuan, Wang, Yi-Hsiu, Hidajah, Atik Choirul, Li, Chung-Yi. "A Population-Based Case-Control Study on the Association of *Angelica sinensis* Exposure with Risk of Breast Cancer." *Journal of Traditional and Complementary Medicine* 10, no. 5 (2020): 454–59.

de Vogel, Johan, et al. "Green Vegetables, Red Meat and Colon Cancer: Chlorophyll Prevents the Cytotoxic and Hyperproliferative Effects of Haem in Rat Colon." *Carcinogenesis* 26, no. 2 (February 2005): 387–93.

Ferruzzi, Mario G., Blakeslee, Joshua. "Digestion, Absorption, and Cancer Preventative Activity of Dietary Chlorophyll Derivatives." *Nutrition Research* 27, no. 1 (2007): 1–12.

Gupta, C., Dhan, P. "Therapeutic Potential of Milk Whey." *Beverages* 3, no. 3 (2017): 31.

Hadad, S., Iwamoto, T., Jordan, L., Purdie, C., Bray, S., Baker, L., Jellema, G., Deharo, S., Hardie, D. G., Pusztai, L., Moulder-Thompson, S., Dewar, J. A., Thompson, A. M. "Evidence for Biological Effects of Metformin in Operable Breast Cancer: A Pre-operative, Window-of-Opportunity, Randomized Trial." *Breast Cancer Research and Treatment* 128, no. 3 (August 2011): 783–94.

Hamada, S., Kataoka, T., Woo, J., Yamada, A., Yoshida, T., Nishimura, T., Otake, N., Nagai, K. "Immunosuppressive Effects of Gallic Acid and Chebulagic Acid on Ctl-Mediated Cytotoxicity." *Biological & Pharmaceutical Bulletin* 20, no. 9 (1997): 1017–19.

Inglis, Julia E., et al. "Nutritional Interventions for Treating Cancer-Related Fatigue: A Qualitative Review." *Nutrition and Cancer* 71, no. 1 (2019): 21–40.

Johnson, J. B., John, S., Laub, D. R. "Pre-treatment with Alternate Day Modified Fast Will Permit Higher Dose and Frequency of Cancer Chemotherapy and Better Cure Rates." *Medical Hypotheses* 72, no. 4 (April 2009): 381–82.

Kamarudin, M. N. A., Sarker, M. M. R., Zhou, J-R., et al. "Metformin in Colorectal Cancer: Molecular Mechanism, Preclinical and Clinical Aspects." *Journal of Experimental Clinical Cancer Research* 38 (2019): 491.

Karimi, G., Vahabzadeh, M., Lari, P., Rashedinia, M., Moshiri, M. "'Silymarin,' a Promising Pharmacological Agent for Treatment of Diseases." *Iranian Journal of Basic Medical Science* 14, no. 4 (July 2011): 308–17.

Kim, J. W., Han, S. W., Cho, J. Y., Chung, I. J., Kim, J. G., Lee, K. H., Park, K. U., Baek, S. K., Oh, S. C., Lee, M. A., Oh, D., Shim, B., Ahn, J. B., Shin, D., Lee, J. W., Kim, Y. H. "Korean Red Ginseng for Cancer-Related Fatigue in Colorectal Cancer Patients with Chemotherapy: A Randomised Phase III Trial." *European Journal of Cancer* 130 (May 2020): 51–62.

Lauriola, M., Enuka, Y., Zeisel, A., et al. "Diurnal Suppression of EGFR Signalling by Glucocorticoids and Implications for Tumor Progression and Treatment." *Nature Communications* 5 (2014): 5073.

Lemke, Emily A. "Ginseng for the Management of Cancer-Related Fatigue: An Integrative Review." *Journal of the Advanced Practitioner in Oncology* 12, no. 4 (May 2021): 406–14.

Levi, F. "Chronotherapeutics: The Relevance of Timing in Cancer Therapy." *Cancer Causes Control* 17, no. 4 (May 2006): 611–21.

Lien, K., Georgsdottir, S., Sivanathan, L., Chan, K., Emmenegger, U. "Low-Dose Metronomic Chemotherapy: A Systematic Literature Analysis." *European Journal of Cancer* 49, no. 16 (2013): 3387–95.

Linn, B., Amos, H. "Rapid Loss of ATP by Tumor Cells Deprived of Glucose: Contrast to Normal Cells." *Biochemical and Biophysical Research Communications* 82, no. 3 (June 14, 1978): 787–94.

Liu, Y., et al. "The Efficacy and Toxicity Profile of Metronomic Chemotherapy for Metastatic Breast Cancer: A Meta-analysis." *PLOS ONE* open access (2017). https://journals.plos.org/plosone/article?id=10.1371/journal.pone.0173693.

Mallik, R., Chowdhury, T. A. "Metformin in Cancer." *Diabetes Research and Clinical Practice* 143 (2018): 409–19.

Morazzoni, P., Petrangolini, G., Bombardelli, E., Ronchi, M., Cabri, W., Riva, A. "SAMITAL®: A New Botanical Drug for the Treatment of Mucositis Induced by Oncological Therapies." *Future Oncology* 9, no. 11 (2013): 1717–25.

Morgan, M. "Bitter Herbs: Improve Digestive Function & Potentially More." *MediHerb: A Phytotherapist's Perspective*, no. 44 (December 2015).

Najafi, T. F., Bahri, N., Tohidinik, H. R., Feyz, S., Bloki, F., Savarkar, S., Jahanfar, S. "Treatment of Cancer-Related Fatigue with Ginseng: A Systematic Review and Meta-analysis." *Journal of Herbal Medicine* 28, art. no. 100440 (2021).

Pawar, D., Neve, R. S., Kalgane, S., Riva, A., Bombardelli, E., Ronchi, M., Petrangolini, G., Morazzoni, P. "Samital Improves Chemo/Radiotherapy-Induced Oral Mucositis in Patients with Head and Neck Cancer: Results of a Randomized, Placebo-Controlled, Single-Blind Phase II Study." *Supportive Care in Cancer* 21, no. 3 (March 2013): 827–34.

Peres, Natália da Silva Leitão, et al. "Medicinal Effects of Peruvian Maca (*Lepidium meyenii*): A Review." *Food and Function* 11, no. 1 (2020): 83–92.

Pourmohamadi, K., Ahmadzadeh, A., Latifi, M. "Investigating the Effects of Oral Ginseng on the Cancer-Related Fatigue and Quality of Life in Patients with Non-Metastatic Cancer." *International Journal of Hematology-Oncology and Stem Cell Research* 12, no. 4 (October 1, 2018): 313–17.

Raffaghello, L., Lee, C., Safdie, F. M., Wei, M., Madia, F., Bianchi, G., Longo, V. D. "Starvation-Dependent Differential Stress Resistance Protects Normal but Not Cancer Cells against High-Dose Chemotherapy." *Proceedings of the National Academy of Science USA* 105, no. 24 (June 17, 2008): 8215–20.

Ramachandran, B., Jayavelu, S., Murhekar, K., Rajkumar, T. "Repeated Dose Studies with Pure Epigallocatechin-3-gallate Demonstrated Dose and Route Dependant Hepatotoxicity with Associated Dyslipidemia." *Toxicology Reports* 3 (March 5, 2016): 336–45.

Sadeghian, M., Rahmani, S., Zendehdel, M., Hosseini, S. A., Zare, Javid, A. "Ginseng and Cancer-Related Fatigue: A Systematic Review of Clinical Trials." *Nutrition and Cancer* 73, no. 8 (2021): 1270–81.

Safdie, Fernando M., et al. "Fasting and Cancer Treatment in Humans: A Case Series Report." *Aging* 1, no. 12 (December 2009).

Salehi, B., et al. "Plant-Derived Bioactives in Oral Mucosal Lesions: A Key Emphasis to Curcumin, Lycopene, Chamomile, Aloe vera, Green Tea and Coffee Properties." *Biomolecules* 9 (2019): 106.

Saraei, P., Asadi, I., Kakar, M. A., Moradi-Kor, N. "The Beneficial Effects of Metformin on Cancer Prevention and Therapy: A Comprehensive Review of Recent Advances." *Cancer Management and Research* 11 (2019): 3295–313.

Simsek, C., Esin, E., Yalcin, S. "Metronomic Chemotherapy: A Systematic Review of the Literature and Clinical Experience." *Journal of Oncology* (March 20, 2019): 5483791.

Solak, B. B., Akin, N. "Health Benefits of Whey Protein: A Review." *Journal of Food Science and Engineering* 2 (2012): 129–37.

Tewari, I., Shukla, P., Sehgal, V. K. "Carcinogenic Herbs: A Review." *International Journal of Research in Medical Sciences* 7, no. 2 (February 2019): 652–58.

Vaňková, Kateřina, et al. "Chlorophyll-Mediated Changes in the Redox Status of Pancreatic Cancer Cells Are Associated with Its Anticancer Effects." *Oxidative Medicine and Cellular Longevity* 2018, article 4069167 (July 2018).

Wang, E., Braun, M. S., Wink, M. "Chlorophyll and Chlorophyll Derivatives Interfere with Multi-Drug Resistant Cancer Cells and Bacteria." *Molecules* 24, no. 16 (2019): 2968.

Xu, R., et al. "Experimental Therapeutics, Molecular Targets, and Chemical Biology: Inhibition of Glycolysis in Cancer Cells: A Novel Strategy to Overcome Drug Resistance Associated with Mitochondrial Respiratory Defect and Hypoxia." *Cancer Research* 65 (January 15, 2005): 613–21.

Yanan, Luo Y., et al. "Peptoid Nanotubes: Bioinspired Peptoid Nanotubes for Targeted Tumor Cell Imaging and Chemo-Photodynamic Therapy." *Nano, Micro, Small Journal* 15, no. 43 (2019): 1970231.

Yue, Grace Gar-Lee, Wong, Lok-Sze, Leung, Hoi-Wing, Gao, Si, Tsang, Julia Y. S., Lin, Zhi-Xiu, Law, Bonita, Tse, Gary, Lau, Clara Bik San. "Comprehensive Preclinical Evidences to Disprove the Paradoxical Perception of Angelica sinensis in Promoting Breast Cancer Growth" (May 9, 2018). Available at SSRN: https://ssrn.com/abstract=3247849 or http://dx.doi.org/10.2139/ssrn.3247849.

Zhu, Hongni, You, Jeishu, Wen, Yi, Jia, Lei, Gao, Fei, Ganesan, Kumar, Chen, Jianping. "Tumorigenic Risk of *Angelica sinensis* on ER-Positive Breast Cancer Growth through ER-Induced Stemness in Vitro and in Vivo." *Journal of Ethnopharmacology* 280 (2021): 114415.

TRIPHALA

Kinoshita, S., Inoue, Y., Nakama, S., Ichiba, T., Aniya, Y. "Antioxidant and Hepatoprotective Actions of Medicinal Herb, *Terminalia catappa* L. from Okinawa Island and Its Tannin Corilagin." *Phytomedicine* 14, no. 11 (2007): 755–62.

Lu, K., Chakroborty, D., Sarkar, C., et al. "Triphala and Its Active Constituent Chebulinic Acid Are Natural Inhibitors of Vascular Endothelial Growth Factor—A Mediated Angiogenesis." *PLOS ONE* 7, no. 8 (2012): e43934.

Mukherjee, P. K., et al. "Clinical Study of 'Triphala'—A Well Known Phytomedicine from India." *Iranian Journal of Pharmacology and Therapeutics* 5, no 1 (January 2006): 51–54.

Peterson, C. T., Denniston, K., Chopra, D. "Therapeutic Uses of Triphala in Ayurvedic Medicine." *Journal of Alternative and Complementary Medicine* 23, no. 8.

Peterson, C. T., Pourang, A., Dhaliwal, S., Kohn, J. N., Uchitel, S., Singh, H., Mills, P. J., Peterson, S. N., Sivamani, R. K. "Modulatory Effects of Triphala and Manjistha Dietary Supplementation on Human Gut Microbiota: A Double-Blind, Randomized, Placebo-Controlled Pilot Study." *Journal of Alternative and Complementary Medicine* 26, no. 11 (November 26, 2020): 1015–24.

Phetkate, Pratya, Kummalue, Tanawan, U-Pratya, Yaowalak, Kietinun, Somboon. "Significant Increase in Cytotoxic T Lymphocytes and Natural Killer Cells by Triphala: A Clinical Phase I Study." *Evidence Based Complementary and Alternative Medicine* 2012 (2012): 239856.

Russell, L., Mazzio, E., Badisa, R., et al. "Differential Cytotoxicity of Triphala and Its Phenolic Constituent Gallic Acid on Human Prostate Cancer LNCap and Normal Cells." *Anticancer Research* 31, no. 11 (2011): 3739–45.

Sandhya, T., Lathika, K. M., Pandey, B. N., Mishra, K. P. "Potential of Traditional Ayurvedic Formulation, Triphala, as a Novel Anticancer Drug." *Cancer Letters* 231, no. 2 (2006): 206–14.

Shi, Y., Sahu, R. P., Srivastava, S. K. "TriphalaIinhibits Both in Vitro and in Vivo Xenograft Growth of Pancreatic Tumor Cells by Inducing Apoptosis." *BMC Cancer* 8, article 294 (2008).

Srikumar, R., Jeya Parthasarathy, N., Sheela Devi, R. "Immunomodulatory Activity of Triphala on Neutrophil Functions." *Biological and Pharmaceutical Bulletin* 28, no. 8 (2005): 1398–1403.

HEART HEALTH

Bharani, A., Ganguly, A., Bhargava, K. D. "Salutary Effect of Terminalia arjuna in Patients with Severe Refractory Heart Failure." *International Journal of Cardiology* 49, no. 3 (May 1995): 191–99.

Cheng, F., Jiang, W., Xiong, X., Chen, J., Xiong, Y., Li, Y. "Ethanol Extract of Chinese Hawthorn (*Crataegus pinnatifida*) Fruit Reduces Inflammation and Oxidative Stress in Rats with Doxorubicin-Induced Chronic Heart Failure." *Medical Science Monitor* 26 (November 24, 2020): e926654.

Dwivedi, S., Agarwal, M. P. "Antianginal and Cardioprotective Effects of Terminalia arjuna, an Indigenous Drug, in Coronary Artery Disease." *Journal of the Association of Physicians of India* 42 (1994): 287–89.

Madeddu, Clelia, et al. "Pathophysiology of Cardiotoxicity Induced by Nonanthracycline Chemotherapy." *Journal of Cardiovascular Medicine* 17, suppl. 1 (May 1, 2016): S12–18.

NEPHRITIS

Atanu, Bhattacharjee, Shashidhara, Shastry Chakrakodi, Aswathanarayana. "Phytochemical and Ethno-Pharmacological Profile of *Crataeva nurvala* Buch-Hum (Varuna): A Review." *Asian Pacific Journal of Tropical Biomedicine* 2, no. 2, suppl. 2012 (2012): S1162–68.

Bopana, Nishritha, Saxena, Sanjay. "Crataeva nurvala: A Valuable Medicinal Plant." *Journal of Herbs, Spices & Medicinal Plants* 14, nos. 1–2 (2008): 107–27.

Khattar, Vandana, Wal, Ankita. "Utilities of *Crataeva nurvala*." *International Journal of Pharmacy and Pharmaceutical Sciences* 4, no. 4 (2012): 21–26.

Kumar, D., Sharma, S. Kumar, S. "Botanical Description, Phytochemistry, Traditional Uses, and Pharmacology of *Crataeva nurvala* Buch. Ham.: An Updated Review." *Future Journal of Pharmaceutical Sciences* 6, no. 113 (2020).

Qadi, M., et al. "Antibacterial, Anticandidal, Phytochemical, and Biological Evaluations of Pellitory Plant." *BioMedical Research International* (2020): art. ID 6965306.

Shakil, M., et al. "The Effects of New Polyherbal Unani Formulation AJMAL06 on Serum Creatinine Level in Chronic Renal Failure." *Pakistan Journal of Pharmaceutical Science* 29, suppl. 2 (March 2016): 657–61.

Shirwaikar, Annie, Manjunath, Setty M., Bommu, Praveen, Krishnanand, B. "Ethanol Extract of Crataeva nurvala Stem Bark Reverses Cisplatin-Induced Nephrotoxicity." *Pharmaceutical Biology* 42, no. 7 (2004): 559–64.

Treasure, J. "Urtica Semen Reduces Serum Creatinine Levels." *Journal of the American Herbalists Guild* 4 (2003): 22–25.

Varalakshmi, P. Shamila, Y., Latha, E. "Effect of *Crataeva nurvala* in Experimental Uurolithiasis." *Journal of Ethnopharmacology* 28, no. 3 (1990): 313–21.

Velazquez, D. V., Xavier, H. S., Batista, J. E., de Castro-Chaves, C. "*Zea mays* L. Extracts Modify Glomerular Function and Potassium Urinary Excretion in Conscious Rats." *Phytomedicine* 12, no. 5 (May 2005): 363–69.

Yarnell, E. "*Urtica* spp. (Nettles)." *Journal of the American Herbalists Guild* 4 (2003): 8–14, 23.

Yarnell, E., Abascal, K. "Herbs for Relieving Chronic Renal Failure." *Journal of Alternative & Complementary Therapies* (February 2007).

Zhang, S., et al. "Total Coumarins from *Hydrangea paniculata* Show Renal Protective Effects in Lipopolysaccharide-Induced Acute Kidney Injury via Anti-inflammatory and Antioxidant Activities." *Frontiers of Pharmacology* (December 14, 2017).

NEUROPATHY

Cascella, M., Muzio, M. R. "Potential Application of the Kampo Medicine Goshajinkigan for Prevention of Chemotherapy-Induced Peripheral Neuropathy." *Journal of Integrative Medicine* 15, no. 2 (2017): 77–87.

Flatters, S. J. L., Dougherty, P. M., Colvin, L. A. "Peripheral Neuropathy (CIPN): A Narrative Review." *British Journal of Anaesthesia* 119, no. 4 (October 2017): 737–49.

Imai, R., et al. "Goshajinkigan, a Traditional Japanese Medicine, Suppresses Voltage-Gated Sodium Channel Nav1.4 Currents in C2C12 Cells." *BioResearch Open Access* 9, no. 1 (2020).

Lee, G., Grovey, B., Furnish, T., et al. "Medical Cannabis for Neuropathic Pain." *Current Pain and Headache Report* 22, no. 8 (2018).

Lee, G., Kim, S. K. "Therapeutic Effects of Phytochemicals and Medicinal Herbs on Chemotherapy-Induced Peripheral Neuropathy." *Molecules* 21, no. 9 (2016): 1252.

Mizuno, K., et al. "Goshajinkigan, a Traditional Japanese Medicine, Prevents Oxaliplatin-Induced Acute Peripheral Neuropathy by Suppressing Functional Alteration of TRP Channels in Rat." *Journal of Pharmacological Science* 125, no. 1 (2014): 91–98.

Mücke, M., Phillips, T., Radbruch, L., Petzke, F., Häuser, W. "Cannabis-Based Medicines for Chronic Neuropathic Pain in Adults." *Cochrane Database of Systematic Reviews* no. 3 (2018): art. no. CD012182.

Pachman, D. R., et al. "Chemotherapy-Induced Peripheral Neuropathy: Prevention and Treatment." *Clinical Pharmacology & Therapeutics* 90, no. 3 (2011).

Ushio, S., et al. "Goshajinkigan Reduces Oxaliplatin-Induced Peripheral Neuropathy without Affecting Antitumor Efficacy in Rodents." *European Journal of Cancer* 48, no. 9 (June 2012): 1407–13.

Windebank, A. J., Grisold, W. "Chemotherapy-Induced Neuropathy." *Journal of the Peripheral Nervous System* 13, no. 1 (2008).

SKIN RASH

Ilnytska, O., et al. "Colloidal Oatmeal (*Avena sativa*) Improves Skin Barrier through Multi-Therapy Activity." *Journal of Drugs in Dermatology* 15, no. 6 (2016).

Kurtz, E. S., Wallo, W. "Colloidal Oatmeal: History, Chemistry and Clinical Properties." *Journal of Drugs in Dermatology* 6, no. 2 (January 31, 2007): 167–70.

Nagore, E., Insa, A., Sanmartín, O. "Antineoplastic Therapy—Induced Palmar Plantar Erythrodysesthesia ('Hand-Foot') Syndrome." *American Journal of Clinical Dermatology* 1, no. 4 (2000): 225–34.

Reynertson, K., et al. "Anti-inflammatory Activities of Colloidal Oatmeal (*Avena sativa*) Contribute to the Effectiveness of Oats in Treatment of Itch Associated with Dry, Irritated Skin." *Journal of Drugs in Dermatology* 14, no. 1 (2015).

CLEAVERS

Atmaca, H., Bozkurt, E., Cittan, M., Tepe, H. D. "Effects of *Galium aparine* Extract on the Cell Viability, Cell Cycle and Cell Death in Breast Cancer Cell Lines." *Journal of Ethnopharmacology* 186 (2016): 305–10.

Bokhari, J., et al. "Evaluation of Diverse Antioxidant Activities of *Galium aparine*." *Spectrochimica Acta Part A: Molecular and Biomolecular Spectroscopy* 102 (2013): 24–29.

Ilina, T., Kashpur, N., Granica, S., et al. "Phytochemical Profiles and *In vitro* Immunomodulatory Activity of Ethanolic Extracts from *Galium aparine* L." *Plants* (Basel) 8, no. 12 (2019): 541.

Neelam, S., Khan, Z. "Antioxidant Activity of *Galium aparine* L. from Punjab, Pakistan." *Pakistan Journal of Botany* 44, special issue (March 2012): 251–53.

CALENDULA

Pommier, P., Gomez, F., Sunyach, M. P., D'Hombres, A., Carrie, C., Montbarbon, X. "Phase III Randomized Trial of *Calendula officinalis* Compared with Trolamine for the Prevention of Acute Dermatitis during Irradiation for Breast Cancer." *Journal of Clinical Oncology* 22, no. 8 (April 15, 2004): 1447–53.

Schneider, F., Danski, M. T., Vayego, S. A. "Usage of *Calendula officinalis* in the Prevention and Treatment of Radiodermatitis: A Randomized Double-Blind Controlled Clinical Trial." *Revista da Escola da Enfermagem USP* 49, no. 2 (April 2015): 221–28.

Sharp, L., Finnilä, K., Johansson, H., Abrahamsson, M., Hatschek, T., Bergenmar, M. "No Differences between Calendula Cream and Aqueous Cream in the Prevention of Acute Radiation Skin Reactions—Results from a Randomised Blinded Trial." *European Journal of Oncology Nurses* 17, no. 4 (August 2013): 429–35.

CHLOROPHYLL

Suryawanshi, R. P., Sudhir, S., Kamat, S. "Studies on Similarities in Chemical Structure of Chlorophyll and Hæme." *World Journal of Pharmaceutical Research* 6, no. 3 (2017): 1661–70.

Xu, X. F., et al. "Effects of Sodium Ferrous Chlorophyll Treatment on Anemia of Hemodialysis Patients and Relevant Biochemical Parameters." *Journal of Biological Regulators and Homeostatic Agents* 30, no. 1 (December 31, 2015): 135–40.

Yuniarti, E., et al. "Effect of Wheat Grass Juice (*Triticum aestivum* L.) against the Erythrocytes and Hemoglobin in Male Mice (*Mus musculus* L.) Anemia Induced by Sodium Nitrite." *Journal of Physics: Conference Series* 1317. The 3rd International Conference on Mathematics, Sciences, Education, and Technology. October 4–5, 2018.

NOVEL DRUGS AND OTHER TREATMENTS

Begley, C. Glenn, et al. "Drug Repurposing: Misconceptions, Challenges, and Opportunities for Academic Researchers." *Science Translational Medicine* 13, no. 612 (September 22, 2021).

Brodie, S. A., Brandes, J. C. "Could Valproic Acid Be an Effective Anticancer Agent? The Evidence So Far." *Expert Review of Anticancer Therapies* 14, no. 10 (2014): 1097–100.

Commonweal. "Beyond Conventional Cancer Therapies (BCCT)." www.commonweal.org.

Morrow, M. "Cimetidine for Cancer Treatment." *Life Extension Magazine,* July 2002. https://www.lifeextension.com/magazine/2002/7/cover_cimetidine.

Pantziarka, P., Bouche, G., Meheus, L., Sukhatme, V., Sukhatme, V. P. "Repurposing Drugs in Oncology (Redo)-Cimetidine as an Anti-cancer Agent." *ecancermedicalscience* 8 (2014): 485.

Tołoczko-Iwaniuk, N., et al. "Celecoxib in Cancer Therapy and Prevention—Review." *Current Drug Targets* 20, no. 3 (2019): 302–15.

Wawruszak, A., Halasa, M., Okon, E., Kukula-Koch, W., Stepulak, A. "Valproic Acid and Breast Cancer: State of the Art in 2021." *Cancers* 13 (2021): 3409.

RADIOTHERAPY

Baliga, M. S., Rao, S. "Radioprotective Potential of Mint: A Brief Review." *Journal of Cancer Research and Therapies* 6 (2010): 255–62.

Farrugia, Carrie-Jo E., Sutton Burke, Elizabeth, Haley, Mariah E., Bedi, Komul T., Gandhi, Mona A. "The Use of Aloe vera in Cancer Radiation: An Updated Comprehensive Review." *Complementary Therapies in Clinical Practice* 35 (2019): 126-30.

Ganasoundari, A., Zare, S. M., Devi, P. U. "Modification of Bone Marrow Radiosensensitivity by Medicinal Plant Extracts." *British Journal of Radiology* 70, no. 834 (June 1997): 599–602.

Garg, A. K., Buchholz, T. A., Aggarwal, B. B. "Chemosensitization and Radiosensitization of Tumors by Plant Polyphenols." *Antioxidants & Redox Signaling* 7, nos. 11, 12 (November–December 2005): 1630–47.

Hazra, B., Ghosh, S., Kumar, A., Pandey, B. N. "The Prospective Role of Plant Products in Radiotherapy of Cancer: A Current Overview." *Frontiers in Pharmacology* 2 (2011): 94.

Kalekhan, F., Kudva, A. K., Raghu, S. V., et al. "Traditionally Used Natural Products in Preventing Ionizing Radiation-Induced." *Anti-cancer Agents in Medicinal Chemistry* 22, no. 1 (2022): 64–82.

Lee, T. K., et al. "Radioprotective Potential of Ginseng." *Mutagenesis* 20, no. 4 (July 2005): 237–43.

Okunieff, P., et al. "Curcumin Protects against Radiation-Induced Acute and Chronic Cutaneous Toxicity in Mice and Decreases mRNA Expression of Inflammatory and Fibrogenic Cytokines." *International Journal of Radiation, Oncology, Biology, and Physics* 65 (2006): 890–98.

Palatty, P. L., et al. "Topical Application of a Sandalwood Oil and Turmeric Based Cream Prevents Radiodermatitis in Head and Neck Cancer Patients Undergoing External Beam Radiotherapy: A Pilot Study." *British Journal of Radiology* 87, no. 1038 (June 2014): 20130490.

Rao, S., et al. "An Aloe vera-Based Cosmeceutical Cream Delays and Mitigates Ionizing Radiation-Induced Dermatitis in Head and Neck Cancer Patients Undergoing Curative Radiotherapy: A Clinical Study." *Medicines* (Basel) 4, no. 3 (June 24, 2017): 44.

Yarnell, E., Abascal, K. "Radiosensitizing Herbs–Parts 1 and 2." *Journal of Alternative and Complementary Therapies* 17, no. 6 (December 2011), and 18, no. 1 (February 2012).

Yogi, Veenita, Singh, O. P., Varsha, Mandloi, Ahirwar, Manish. "Role of Topical Aloe vera Gel in the Recovery of High-Grade, Radiation-Induced Sermatitis." *Clinical Cancer Investigation Journal* 7, no. 5 (2018): 167–70.

HONEY

Afrin, S., et al. "Therapeutic and Preventive Properties of Honey and Its Bioactive Compounds in Cancer: An Evidence-Based Review." *Nutrition Research Reviews* 33, no. 1 (2020): 50–76.

Carter, D. A., Blair, S. E., Cokcetin, N. N., et al. "Therapeutic Manuka Honey: No Longer So Alternative." *Frontiers in Microbiology* 7 (April 20, 2016): 569.

Eteraf-Oskouei, T., Najafi, M. "Traditional and Modern Uses of Natural Honey in Human Diseases: A Review." *Iran Journal of Basic Medical Science* 16, no. 6 (2013): 731–42.

Fogh, S. E., et al. "A Randomized Phase 2 Trial of Prophylactic Manuka Honey for the Reduction of Chemoradiation Therapy–Induced Esophagitis during the Treatment of Lung Cancer: Results of NRG Oncology RTOG 1012." *International Journal of Radiation Oncology* 97, no. 4 (March 15, 2017): 786–96.

Münstedt, K., Momm, F., Hübner, J. "Honey in the Management of Side Effects of Radiotherapy or Radio/Chemotherapy-Induced Oral Mucositis. A Systematic Review." *Complementary Therapies in Clinical Practice* 34 (February 2019): 145–52.

Tsiapara, A. V., et al. "Bioactivity of Greek Honey Extracts on Breast Cancer (MCF-7), Prostate Cancer (PC-3) and Endometrial Cancer (Ishikawa) Cells: Profile Analysis of Extracts." *Food Chemistry* 116, no. 3 (2009): 702–8.

Waheed, M. "Honey and Cancer: A Mechanistic Review." *Clinical Nutrition* 38, no. 6 (December 2019): 2499–503.

Chapter 6: Materia Medica: A Directory of Herbs for Cancer

Yarnell, E. Herb-drug interactions reference checker on the website Bot Med Rocks, https://www.botmed.rocks.

ALOE VERA

Lissoni, P., Rovelli, F., Brivio, F., Zago, R., Colciago, M., Messina, G., Mora, A., Porro, G. "A Randomized Study of Chemotherapy versus Biochemotherapy with Chemotherapy Plus *Aloe arborescens* in Patients with Metastatic Cancer." *In Vivo* 23, no. 1 (January–February 2009): 171–75.

Mohammed, A., Paranji, N., Singh, A., Sanaka, M. R. "*Pseudomelanosis coli*, Its Relation to Laxative Use and Association with Colorectal Neoplasms: A Comprehensive Review." *Journal of Gastroenterology and Hepatology Open* 5, no. 6 (May 4, 2021): 643–46.

ANDROGRAPHIS

Chauhan, Ekta Singh, Kriti, Sharma, Renu, Bist. "*Andrographis paniculata*: A Review of Its Phytochemistry and Pharmacological Activities." *Research Journal of Pharmacy and Technology* 12, no. 2 (2019): 891. doi: 10.5958/0974-360X.2019.00153.7.

He, C. L., et. al. "Xiang-Qi-Tang and Its Active Components Exhibit Anti-inflammatory and Anticoagulant Properties by Inhibiting MAPK and NF-κB Signaling Pathways in LPS-Treated Rat Cardiac Microvascular Endothelial Cells." *Immunopharmacology and Immunotoxicology* 35, no. 2 (2013): 215–24.

Islam, Muhammad Torequl, et al. "Andrographolide, a Diterpene Lactone from *Andrographis paniculata* and Its Therapeutic Promises in Cancer." *Cancer Letters* 420 (2018): 129–45.

Li, L., Yue, G. G.-L., Lee, J. K.-M., et al. "Gene Expression Profiling Reveals the Plausible Mechanisms Underlying the Antitumor and Antimetastasis Effects of *Andrographis paniculata* in Esophageal Cancer." *Phytotherapy Research* 32 (2018): 1388–96.

Liaqat, Hamaira. "*Andrographis paniculata*: A Review of Its Anti-cancer Potential." *Journal of Medicinal & Aromatic Plants* 10, no. 5 (2021).

Malik, Z., Parveen, R., Parveen, B., Zahiruddin, S., Khan, M. A., Khan, A., Massey, S., Ahmad, S., Husain, S. A. "Anticancer Potential of Andrographolide from *Andrographis paniculata* (Burm.f.) Nees and Its Mechanisms of Action." *Journal of Ethnopharmacology* 272 (2021): 113936.

Sharma, P., Shimura, T., Banwait, J. K., Goel, A. "Andrographis-Mediated Chemosensitization through Activation of Ferroptosis and Suppression of B-catenin/Wnt-Signaling Pathways in Colorectal Cancer." *Carcinogenesis* 41, no. 10 (October 2020): 1385–94.

Vetvicka, Vaclav, Vannucci, Luca. "Biological Properties of Andrographolide, an Active Ingredient of *Andrographis paniculata*: A Narrative Review." *Annals of Translational Medicine* 9, no. 14 (2021): 1186.

Widjajakusuma, E. C., Jonosewojo, A., Hendriati, L., Wijaya, S., Ferawati, Surjadhana, A., Sastrowardoyo, W., Monita, N., Muna, N. M., Fajarwati, R. P., Ervina, M., Esar, S. Y., Soegianto, L., Lang, T., Heriyanti, C. "Phytochemical Screening and Preliminary Clinical Trials of the Aqueous Extract Mixture of *Andrographis paniculata* (Burm. f.) Wall. ex Nees and Syzygium Polyanthum (Wight.) Walp Leaves in Metformin Treated Patients with Type 2 Diabetes." *Phytomedicine* 55 (March 1, 2019): 137–47.

Zhao, Yinghui, Chuanxin, Wang, Ajay, Goel. "A Combined Treatment with Melatonin and Andrographis Promotes Autophagy and Anti-cancer Activity in Colorectal Cancer." *Carcinogenesis* 43, no. 3 (2022).

Zhao, Yinghui, Chuanxin, Wang, Ajay, Goel. "Andrographis Overcomes 5-Fluorouracil-Associated Chemoresistance through Inhibition of DKK1 in Colorectal Cancer." *Carcinogenesis* 42, no. 6 (2021): 814–25.

Zhao, Yinghui, Souvick, Roy, Chuanxin, Wang, Ajay, Goel. "A Combined Treatment with Berberine and Andrographis Exhibits Enhanced Anti-cancer Activity through Suppression of DNA Replication in Colorectal Cancer." *Pharmaceuticals* 15, no. 3 (2022): 262.

BAIKAL SKULLCAP

Cheng, Chien-Shan, et al. "*Scutellaria baicalensis* and Cancer Treatment: Recent Progress and Perspectives in Biomedical and Clinical Studies." *American Journal of Chinese Medicine* 46, no. 1 (2018): 25–54.

Gharari, Z., Bagheri, K., Khodaeiaminjan, M., Sharafi, A. "Potential Therapeutic Effects and Bioavailability of Wogonin, the Flavone of Baikal Skullcap." *Journal of Nutritional Medicine and Diet Care* 5, no. 2 (2019): 39.

Goldberg, V. E., Ryzhakov, V. M., Matiash, M. G., Stepovaia, E. A., Boldyshev, D. A., Litvinenko, V. I., Dygaĭ, A. M. "Dry Extract of *Scutellaria baicalensis* as a Hemostimulant in Antineoplastic Chemotherapy in Patients with Lung Cancer" [article in Russian]. *Eksperimental'naia i Klinicheskaia Farmakologiia* 60, no. 6 (November–December 1997): 28–30.

Hussain, Imran, et al. "*Scutellaria baicalensis* Targets the Hypoxia-Inducible Factor-1α and Enhances Cisplatin Efficacy in Ovarian Cancer." *Journal of Cellular Biochemistry* 119, no. 9 (September 2018): 7515–24.

Khan, Asifa, et al. "Phytocompounds Targeting Metabolic Reprogramming in Cancer: An Assessment of Role, Mechanisms, Pathways, and Therapeutic Relevance." *Journal of Agricultural and Food Chemistry* 69, no. 25 (2021): 6897–928.

Liu, Defu, et al. "Targets and Potential Mechanism of *Scutellaria baicalensis* in Treatment of Primary Hepatocellular Carcinoma Based on Bioinformatics Analysis." *Journal of Oncology* (February 12, 2022): 1–19. doi: 10.1155/2022/8762717.

Smol'ianinov, E. S., Goldberg, V. E., Matiash, M. G., Ryzhakov, V. M., Boldyshev, D. A., Litvinenko, V. I., Dygaĭ, A. M. "Effect of *Scutellaria baicalensis* Extract on the Immunologic Status of Patients with Lung Cancer Receiving Antineoplastic Chemotherapy" [article in Russian]. *Eksperimental'naia Klinicheskaia Farmakologiia* 60, no. 6 (November–December 1997): 49–51.

Yimam, M., Burnett, B. P., Brownell, L., Jia, Q. "Corrigendum to 'Clinical and Preclinical Cognitive Function Improvement after Oral Treatment of a Botanical Composition Composed of Extracts from *Scutellaria baicalensis* and *Acacia catechu*.'" *Behavioral Neurology* 2016 (2016): 7240802.

Zhou, Xian, et al. "Drug-Herb Interactions between *Scutellaria baicalensis* and Pharmaceutical Drugs: Insights from Experimental Studies, Mechanistic Actions to Clinical Applications." *Biomedicine & Pharmacotherapy* 138 (2021): 111445. doi: 10.1016/j.biopha.2021.111445.

BUPLEURUM

Kim, Byeong Mo. "The Role of Saikosaponins in Therapeutic Strategies for Age-Related Diseases." *Oxidative Medicine and Cellular Longevity* 2018 (April 2018).

Lei, Z., Zou, G., Gao, Y., Yao, Y., Peng, C., Shu, J., Yang, M. "A New Triterpenoid and a New Flavonoid Glycoside Isolated from *Bupleurum marginatum* and Their Anti-inflammatory Activity." *Natural Product Research* 34, no. 24 (December 2020): 3492–98.

Yan, J., Luo, Q., Long, F., et al. "Malconenoside A, a New Phenolic Glycoside from *Bupleurum malconense*." *SAGE Journal Natural Product Communications* (September 13, 2021).

Zhang, X., Liu, Z., Chen, S., Li, H., Dong, L., Fu, X. "A New Discovery: Total *Bupleurum saponin* Extracts Can Inhibit the Proliferation and Induce Apoptosis of Colon Cancer Cells by Regulating the PI3K/Akt/mTOR Pathway." *Journal of Ethnopharmacology* 283 (January 30, 2022): 114742.

CACAO

Baharum, Z., Akim, A. M., Hin, T. Y., Hamid, R. A., Kasran, R. "*Theobroma cacao*: Review of the Extraction, Isolation, and Bioassay of Its Potential Anti-cancer Compounds." *Tropical Life Science Research* 27, no. 1 (2016): 21–42.

Greenberg, J. A., et al. "Chocolate Intake and Heart Disease and Stroke in the Women's Health Initiative: A Prospective Analysis." *American Journal of Clinical Nutrition* 108, no. 1 (July 2018): 41–48.

Jalil, A. M., Ismail, A. "Polyphenols in Cocoa and Cocoa Products: Is There a Link between Antioxidant Properties and Health?" *Molecules* 13, no. 9 (September 16, 2008): 2190–219.

Miller, K. B., Hurst, W. J., Payne, M. J., Stuart, D. A., Apgar, J., Sweigart, D. S., Ou, B. "Impact of Alkalization on the Antioxidant and Flavanol Content of Commercial Cocoa Powders." *Journal of Agriculture and Food Chemistry* 56, no. 18 (September 24, 2008): 8527–33.

Montagna, M. T., et al. "Chocolate, 'Food of the Gods': History, Science, and Human Health." *International Journal of Environmental Research and Public Health* 16, no. 25 (2019): 4960.

Pereira, T., et al. "Randomized Study of the Effects of Cocoa-Rich Chocolate on the Ventricle-Arterial Coupling and Vascular Function of Young, Healthy Adults." *Nutrition* (2019): 63–64, 175–83.

Rimbach, G., Melchin, M., Moehring, J., Wagner, A. E. "Polyphenols from Cocoa and Vascular Health—A Critical Review." *International Journal of Molecular Sciences* 10, no. 10 (2009): 4290–309.

CALENDULA

Cruceriu, D., Balacescu, O., Rakosy, E. "*Calendula officinalis*: Potential Roles in Cancer Treatment and Palliative Care." *Integrative Cancer Therapies* 17, no. 4 (December 2018): 1068–78.

Cruceriu, D., Diaconeasa, Z., Socaci, S., Socaciu, C., Rakosy-Tican, E., Balacescu, O. "Biochemical Profile, Selective Cytotoxicity and Molecular Effects of *Calendula officinalis* Extracts on Breast Cancer Cell Lines." *Notulae Botanicae Horti Agrobotanici Cluj-Napoca* 48, no. 1 (2020): 24–39.

Hernández-Rosas, N. A., et al. "Polyphenols Profile, Antioxidant Capacity, and *In vitro* Cytotoxic Effect on Human Cancer Cell Lines of a Hydro-Alcoholic Extract from *Calendula officinalis* L. Petals." *TIP Revista Especializada en Ciencias Químico-Biológicas* 21, suppl. 1 (2018): 54–64.

Kondziołka, J., Wilczyński, S. "Overview of the Active Ingredients in Cosmetic Products for the Care of Skin That Has Been Exposed to Ionizing Radiation—Analysis of Their Effectiveness in Breast Cancer Radiotherapy." *Clinical Cosmetic and Investigational Dermatology* 14 (2021): 1065–76.

CORYDALIS

Chang, S., Yang, Z., Han, N., Liu, Z., Yin, J. "The Antithrombotic, Anticoagulant Activity and Toxicity Research of Ambinine, an Alkaloid from the Tuber of *Corydalis ambigua* var. *amurensis*." *Regulatory Toxicology and Pharmacology* 95 (2018): 175–81.

Dai, Wen-Ling, Liu, Xin-Tong, Bao, Yi-Ni, Yan, Bing, Jiang, Nan, Yu, Bo-Yang, Liu, Ji-Hua. "Selective Blockade of Spinal D2DR by Levocorydalmine Attenuates Morphine Tolerance via Suppressing PI3K/Akt-MAPK Signaling in a MOR-Dependent Manner." *Experimental & Molecular Medicine* 50, no. 11 (2018): 148

Hu, J., Xie, J., Hu, J., Zhang, Y., Wang, J., Chen, R. "Effect of Some Drugs on Electroacupuncture Analgesia and Cytosolic Free Ca2+ Concentration of Mice Brain" [article in Chinese]. *Zhen Ci Yan Jiu* (Acupuncture Research) 19, no. 1 (1994): 55–58.

Ito, C., Itoigawa, M., Tokuda, H., Kuchide, M., Nishino, H., Furukawa, H. "Chemopreventive Activity of Isoquinoline Alkaloids from Corydalis Plants." *Planta Medica* 67, no. 5 (July 2001): 473–75.

Lalanne, L., Ayranci, G., Kieffer, B. L., Lutz, P. E. "The Kappa Opioid Receptor: From Addiction to Depression, and Back." *Frontiers in Psychiatry* 5 (2014): 170.

Lin, M. T., Chueh, F. Y., Hsieh, M. T., et al. "Antihypertensive Effects of DL-Tetrahydropalmatine: An Active Principle Isolated from Corydalis." *Clinical and Experimental Pharmacology and Physiology* 23 (1996): 738–42.

Liu, J., He, Z., Li, S., Huang, W., Ren, Z. "Network Pharmacology-Based Analysis of the Effects of *Corydalis decumbens* (Thunb.) Pers. in Non-Small Cell Lung Cancer." *Evidence Based Complementary and Alternative Medicine* (August 21, 2021): 4341517.

Trang, Tuan, et al. "Pain and Poppies: The Good, the Bad, and the Ugly of Opioid Analgesics." *Journal of Neuroscience* 35, no. 41 (October 14, 2015): 13879–888.

Wang, L., Zhang, Y., Wang, Z., et al. "The Antinociceptive Properties of the *Corydalis yanhusuo* Extract." *PLOS One* 11, no. 9 (2016): e0162875.

Xie, G., et al. "Chemical Constituents and Antioxidative, Anti-inflammatory and Antiproliferative Activities of Wild and Cultivated *Corydalis saxicola*." *Industrial Crops and Products* 169 (2021).

Xuan, B., Wang, W., Li, D. X. "Inhibitory Effect of Tetrahydroberberine on Platelet Aggregation and Thrombosis." *Zhongguo Yao Li Xue Bao* (*Acta Pharmacologica Sinica*) 15, no. 2 (March 1994): 133–35.

Zhang, J., et al. "A Review of the Traditional Uses, Botany, Phytochemistry, Pharmacology, Pharmacokinetics, and Toxicology of *Corydalis yanhusuo*." *Natural Product Communications* 15, no. 9 (September 2020).

Zhang, Y., Wang, C., Guo, Z., Zhang, X., Wang, Z., Liang, X., Civelli, O. "Discovery of N-Methyltetrahydroprotoberberines with κ-Opioid Receptor Agonists-Opioid Receptor Agonist Activities from Corydalis yanhusuo W. T. Wang by Using Two-Dimensional Liquid Chromatography." *Journal of Ethnopharmacology* 155, no. 3 (September 29, 2014): 1597–602.

DAN SHEN

Chun-Yan, Su, et al. "*Salvia miltiorrhiza*: Traditional Medicinal Uses, Chemistry, and Pharmacology." *Chinese Journal of Natural Medicines* 13, no. 3 (2015): 163–82.

Fan, G., Zhu, Y., Guo, H., Wang, X., Wang, H., Gao, X. "Direct Vasorelaxation by a Novel Phytoestrogen, Tanshinone IIA Is Mediated by Nongenomic Action of Estrogen Receptor through Endothelial Nitric Oxide Synthase Activation and Calcium Mobilization." *Journal of Cardiovascular Pharmacology* 57, no. 3 (March 2011): 340–47.

He, Y., et al. "Salvianolic Acid B Attenuates Epithelial-Mesenchymal Transition in Renal Fibrosis Rats through Activating Sirt1-Mediated Autophagy." *Biomedicine & Pharmacotherapy* 128 (2020): 110241.

Jiang, Z., Gao, W., Huang, L. "Tanshinones, Critical Pharmacological Components in *Salvia miltiorrhiza*." *Frontiers in Pharmacology* 10 (March 14, 2019): 202.

Wang, L., Ma, R., Liu, C., et al. "*Salvia miltiorrhiza*: A Potential Red Light to the Development of Cardiovascular Diseases." *Current Pharmaceutical Design* 23, no. 7 (2017): 1077–97.

Zhou, S., Shao, W., Duan, C. "Observation of Preventing and Treating Effect of *Salvia miltiorrhiza* Composita on Patients with Ischemic Coronary Heart Disease Undergoing Non-heart Surgery." *Zhongguo Zhong Xi Yi Jie He Za Zhi* (Chinese) 19, no. 2 (February 1999): 75–76.

ECHINACEA

Abouelella, Amira, Shahein, Yasser, Tawfik, Sameh, Zahran, Ahmed. "Phytotherapeutic Effects of *Echinacea purpurea* in Gamma-Irradiated Mice." *Journal of Veterinary Science* 8, no. 4 (December 2007): 341–51.

De Rosa, N., Giampaolino, P., Lavitola, G., Morra, I., Formisano, C., Nappi, C., Bifulco, G. "Effect of Immunomodulatory Supplements Based on *Echinacea angustifolia* and *Echinacea purpurea* on the Posttreatment Relapse Incidence of Genital Condylomatosis: A Prospective Randomized Study." *Biomedical Research International* 2019 (April 11, 2019): 3548396.

Driggins, S., et al. "The Inhibitory Effect of *Echinacea purpurea* and *Echinacea pallida* on BT-549 and Natural Killer Cells." *MedCrave Online Journal Cell Science & Report* 4, no. 3 (2017).

Espinosa-Paredes, Daniel Abraham, et al. "Echinacea angustifolia DC Extract Induces Apoptosis and Cell Cycle Arrest and Synergizes with Paclitaxel in the MDA-MB-231 and MCF-7 Human Breast Cancer Cell Lines." *Nutrition and Cancer* 73, nos. 11–12 (2021): 2287–2305.

Khalaf, A. A., Hussein, S., Tohamy, A. F., et al. "Protective Effect of *Echinacea purpurea* (Immulant) against Cisplatin-Induced Immunotoxicity in Rats." *DARU Journal of Pharmaceutical Science* 27 (2019): 233–41.

McGrowder, D. A., et al. "Medicinal Herbs Used in Traditional Management of Breast Cancer: Mechanisms of Action." *Medicines* 7, no. 8 (2020): 47.

Moradian, F., et al. "Effect of *Echinacea purpurea* Extract on the Expression of VEGF-A Gene and Antiproliferative, Induction of Apoptosis, Inhibition of Cell Migration, and Colony Formation on Gastric Cancer Cell Line AGS." Preprint. doi: 10.21203/rs.3.rs-41158/v1.

Park, Jin-Hong, et al. "Cytotoxicity of Extracts and Fractions from *Echinacea pupurea* L. on Human Cancer Cells." *Korean Journal of Medicinal Crop Science* 12, no. 4 (2004): 309–14.

Rousseau, B., Tateya, I., Lim, X., Munoz-del-Rio, A., Bless, D. M. "Investigation of Anti-hyaluronidase Treatment on Vocal Fold Wound Healing." *Journal of Voice* 20, no. 3 (September 2006): 443–51.

FEVERFEW

Curry, E. A. 3rd, Murry, D. J., Yoder, C., Fife, K., Armstrong, V., Nakshatri, H., O'Connell, M., Sweeney, C. J. "Phase I Dose Escalation Trial of Feverfew with Standardized Doses of Parthenolide in Patients with Cancer." *Investigative New Drugs* 22, no. 3 (August 2004): 299–305.

Czyz, M., Lesiak-Mieczkowska, K., Koprowska, K., Szulawska-Mroczek, A., Wozniak, M. "Cell Context-Dependent Activities of Parthenolide in Primary and Metastatic Melanoma Cells." *British Journal of Pharmacology* 160 (2010): 1144–57.

Dawood, M., Ooko, E., Efferth, T. "Collateral Sensitivity of Parthenolide via NF-κB and HIF-a Inhibition and Epigenetic Changes in Drug-Resistant Cancer Cell Lines." *Frontiers in Pharmaco*logy 10 (May 21, 2019): 542.

Jin, P., Madieh, S., Augsburger, L. L. "The Solution and Solid State Stability and Excipient Compatibility of Parthenolide in Feverfew." *American Association of Pharmaceutical Scientists* 8, no. 4 (2007): 200.

Loesche, W., Mazurov, A. V., Voyno-Yasenetskaya, T. A., Groenewegen, W. A., Heptinstall, S., Repin, V. S. "Feverfew—An Antithrombotic Drug?" *Folia Haematologica* 115, nos. 1–2 (1988): 181–84.

Pareek, A., Suthar, M., Rathore, G. S., Bansal, V. "Feverfew (*Tanacetum parthenium* L.): A Systemic Review." *Pharmacognosy Review* 5, no. 9 (2011). doi: 10.4103/0973-7847.79105.

Sztiller-Sikorska, M., Czyz, M. "Parthenolide as Cooperating Agent for Anti-cancer Treatment of Various Malignancies." *Pharmaceuticals* 13, no. 8 (2020): 194.

Xu, S., Li, X., Liu, Y., et al. "Inflammasome Inhibitors: Promising Therapeutic Approaches against Cancer." *Journal of Hematology and Oncology* 12, no. 64 (2019).

GARLIC

Agbana, Y. L., Ni, Y., Zhou, M., Zhang, Q., Kassegne, K., Karou, S. D., Kuang, Y., Zhu, Y. "Garlic-Derived Bioactive Compound S-allylcysteine Inhibits Cancer Progression through Diverse Molecular Mechanisms." *Nutrition Research* 73 (January 2020): 1–14.

Almatroodi, Saleh A., Mohammed A. Alsahli, Ahmad Almatroudi, and Arshad H. Rahmani. "Garlic and Its Active Compounds: A Potential Candidate in the Prevention of Cancer by Modulating Various Cell Signalling Pathways." *Anti-cancer Agents in Medicinal Chemistry* 19, no. 11 (2019): 1314–24.

Li, W. Q., Zhang, J. Y., Ma, J. L., Li, Z. X., Zhang, L., Zhang, Y., Guo, Y., Zhou, T., Li, J. Y., Shen, L., Liu, W. D., Han, Z. X., Blot, W. J., Gail, M. H., Pan, K. F., You, W. C. "Effects of Helicobacter pylori Treatment and Vitamin and Garlic Supplementation on Gastric Cancer Incidence and Mortality: Follow-up of a Randomized Intervention Trial." *British Medical Journal* 366 (September 11, 2019): l5016.

Miraghajani, Maryam, Rafie, Nahid, Hajianfar, Hossein, Larijani, Bagher, Azadbakht, Leila. "Aged Garlic and Cancer: A Systematic Review." *International Journal of Preventive Medicine* 9 (2018).

Mondal, Arijit, Banerjee, Sabyasachi, Bose, Sankhadip, Mazumder, Sujayita, Haber, Rebecca A., Farzaei, Mohammad Hosein, Bishayee, Anupam. "Garlic Constituents for Cancer Prevention and Therapy: From Phytochemistry to Novel Formulations." *Pharmacological Research* 175 (2022): 105837.

Özkan, İ., Koçak, P., Yıldırım, M., et al. "Garlic (Allium sativum)-Derived SEVs Inhibit Cancer Cell Proliferation and Induce Caspase Mediated Apoptosis." *Science Reports* 11, no. 1 (2021): 14773.

Yarnell, E. "Garlic (and Relatives), Platelets and Combination with Anticoagulant Drugs." Bot Med Rocks website. Accessed March 26, 2022. https://www.botmed.rocks/garlic-platelets-anticoagulants.html.

Zhang, Y., Liu, X., Ruan, J., Zhuang, X., Zhang, X., Li, X. "Phytochemicals of Garlic: Promising Candidates for Cancer Therapy." *Biomedicine & Pharmacotherapy* 123 (2020): 109730.

Zhou, X., Qian, H., Zhang, D., Zeng, L. "Garlic Intake and the Risk of Colorectal Cancer: A Meta-analysis." *Medicine* 99, no. 1 (2020): e18575.

GINGER

Bordia, A., Verma, S. K., Srivastava, K. C. "Effect of Ginger (*Zingiber officinale* Rosc.) and Fenugreek (*Trigonella foenumgraecum* L.) on Blood Lipids, Blood Sugar and Platelet Aggregation in Patients with Coronary Artery Disease." *Prostaglandins Leukotrienes and Essential Fatty Acids* 56, no. 5 (May 1997): 379–84.

Chang, W. P., Peng, Y. X. "Does the Oral Administration of Ginger Reduce Chemotherapy-Induced Nausea and Vomiting? A Meta-analysis of 10 Randomized Controlled Trials." *Cancer Nursing* 42, no. 6 (November–December 2019): E14–23.

De Lima, R. M. T., et al. "Protective and Therapeutic Potential of Ginger (*Zingiber officinale*) Extract and [6]-gingerol in Cancer: A Comprehensive Review." *Phytotherapy Research* 32, no. 10 (October 2018): 1885–907.

Hamza, A. A., et al. "Standardized Extract of Ginger Ameliorates Liver Cancer by Reducing Proliferation and Inducing Apoptosis through Inhibition Oxidative Stress/Inflammation Pathway." *Biomedicine & Pharmacotherapy* 134 (2021).

Marx, W., McKavanagh, D., McCarthy, A. L., Bird, R., Ried, K., Chan, A., Isenring, L. "The Effect of Ginger (*Zingiber officinale*) on Platelet Aggregation: A Systematic Literature Review." *PLOS One* 10, no. 10 (October 21, 2015): e0141119.

Memorial Sloan Kettering Cancer Center. "Ginger." https://www.mskcc.org/cancer-care/integrative-medicine/herbs/ginger.

Ryan, J. L., Morrow, G. R. "Ginger." *Oncology Nurse Edition* 24, no. 2 (2010) 46–49.

GOTU KOLA

Gohil, K. J., Patel, J. A., Gajjar, A. K. "Pharmacological Review on *Centella asiatica*: A Potential Herbal Cure-All." *Indian Journal of Pharmaceutical Science* 72, no. 5 (2010): 546–56.

Han, A. R., et al. "Triterpenoids from the Leaves of *Centella asiatica* Inhibit Ionizing Radiation-Induced Migration and Invasion of Human Lung Cancer Cells." *Evidence-Based Complementary and Alternative Medicine* (2020): article ID 3683460.

Lv, J., Sharma, A., Zhang, T., Wu, Y., Ding, X. "Pharmacological Review on Asiatic Acid and Its Derivatives: A Potential Compound." *SLAS Technology* 23 no. 2 (April 2018): 111–27.

Naidoo, D. B., et al. "*Centella asiatica* Fraction-3 Suppresses the Nuclear Factor Erythroid 2-Related Factor 2 Antioxidant Pathway and Enhances Reactive Oxygen Species-Mediated Cell Death in Cancerous Lung A549 Cells." *Journal of Medicinal Food* 20, no. 10 (2017).

Prakash, V., et al. "A Review on Medicinal Properties of Centella asiatica." *Asian Journal of Pharmaceutical and Clinical Research* 10, no. 10 (2017): 69–74.

Sun, B., et al. "Therapeutic Potential of *Centella asiatica* and Its Triterpenes: A Review." *Frontiers in Pharmacology* (September 4, 2020).

GREEN TEA

Dal, S., Sigrist, S. "The Protective Effect of Antioxidants Consumption on Diabetes and Vascular Complications." *Diseases* 4, no. 3 (2016): 24.

Das, S., et al. "Health Benefits of Epigallocatechin-3-gallate (EGCG)." *Journal of Biochemical and Pharmacological Research* 2 no. 3 (September 2014): 167–74.

Filippini, T., Malavolti, M., Borrelli, F., Izzo, A. A., Fairweather-Tait, S. J., Horneber, M., Vinceti, M. "Green Tea (*Camellia sinensis*) for the Prevention of Cancer." *Cochrane Database of Systematic Reviews* 3, no. 3 (accessed January 4, 2022): CD005004.

Fujiki, H., Watanabe, T., Sueoka, E., Rawangkan, A., Suganuma M. "Cancer Prevention with Green Tea and Its Principal Constituent, EGCG: From Early Investigations to Current Focus on Human Cancer Stem Cells." *Molecules and Cells* 41, no. 2 (2018): 73–82.

Puviani, M., Galluzzo, M., Talamonti, M., Mazzilli, S., Campione, E., Bianchi, L., Milani, M., Luppino, I., Micali G. "Efficacy of Sinecatechins 10% as Proactive Sequential Therapy of External Genital Warts after Laser CO2 Ablative Therapy: The PACT Study (Post-ablation Immunomodulator Treatment of Condylomata with Sinecatechins): A Randomized, Masked Outcome Assessment, Multicenter Trial." *International Journal of STD and AIDS* 30, no. 2 (February 2019): 131–36.

Shirakami, Y., Shimizu, M. "Possible Mechanisms of Green Tea and Its Constituents against Cancer." *Molecules* 23, no. 9 (2018): 2284.

HORSE CHESTNUT

Hadi, M., Hameed, I. H., Hussein, H. J. "Anti-microbial, Anti-inflammatory Effect and Cardiovascular Effects of Garlic: *Allium sativum*." *Research Journal of Pharmacy and Technology* 10, no. 11 (November 2017).

Miraghajani, M., Rafie, N., Hajianfar, H., Larijani, B., Azadbakht, L. "Aged Garlic and Cancer: A Systematic Review." *International Journal of Preventative Medicine* 9 (September 2018): 84.

Na, W. J., Kang, Y. E. "Aesculetin Inhibits Bone Resorption through Down-regulating Differentiation and Lysosomal Formation in Osteoclasts." *Current Developments in Nutrition* 4, suppl. 2 (June 2020): 442.

Petrovic, V., et al. "Anti-cancer Potential of Homemade Fresh Garlic Extract Is Related to Increased Endoplasmic Reticulum Stress." *Nutrients* 10, no. 4 (2018): 450.

Sharma, P., Shimura, T., Banwait, J. K., Goel, A., "Andrographis-Mediated Chemo-sensitization through Activation of Ferroptosis and Suppression of B-catenin/Wnt-Signaling Pathways in Colorectal Cancer." *Carcinogenesis* 41, no. 10 (October 2020): 1385–94.

Shimura, T., Sharma, P., Sharma, G. G., et al. "Enhanced Anti-cancer Activity of Andrographis with Oligomeric Proanthocyanidins through Activation of Metabolic and Ferroptosis Pathways in Colorectal Cancer." *Science Report* 11 (2021): 7548.

Zhang Y., et al. "Phytochemicals of Garlic: Promising Candidates for Cancer Therapy." *Biomedicine & Pharmacotherapy* 123 (2020): 109730.

Zhou, X. Y., Fu, F. H., Li, Z., Dong, Q. J., He, J., Wang, C. H. "Escin, a Natural Mixture of Triterpene Saponins, Exhibits Antitumor Activity against Hepatocellular Carcinoma." *Planta Medica* 75, no. 15 (December 2009): 1580–85.

INDIAN FRANKINCENSE

Poornima, B. N., Farah, D. "Activities of Cinnamaldehyde from *Boswellia serrata* on MCF-7 Breast Cancer Cell Line." *International Journal of Scientific Research in Biological Sciences* 7, no. 4 (August 2020): 35–43.

Yadav, V. R., Prasad, S., Sung, B., et al. "Boswellic Acid Inhibits Growth and Metastasis of Human Colorectal Cancer in Orthotopic Mouse Model by Downregulating Inflammatory, Proliferative, Invasive and Angiogenic Biomarkers." *International Journal of Cancer* 130, no. 9 (2012): 2176–84.

MAGNOLIA

Arora, S., Singh, S., Piazza, G. A., Contreas, C. M., Panyam, J., Singh, A. P. "Honokiol: A Novel Natural Agent for Cancer Prevention and Therapy." *Current Molecular Medicine* (July 23, 2012).

Garcia, A., et al. "Honokiol Suppresses Survival Signals Mediated by Ras-Dependent Phospholipase D Activity in Human Cancer Cells." *Clinical Cancer Research* 14, no. 13 (July 1, 2008): 4267–74.

Hou, W., et al. "Synergistic Antitumor Effects of Liposomal Honokiol Combined with Adriamycin in Breast Cancer Models." *Phytotherapy Research* 22, no. 8 (August 2008): 1125–32.

Hou, Y. C., Chao, P. D., Chen, S. Y. "Honokiol and Magnolol Increased Hippocampal Acetylcholine Release in Freely-Moving Rats." *American Journal of Chinese Medicine* 28, nos. 3, 4 (2000): 379–84.

Jiang, Q. Q., Fan, L. Y., Yang, G. L., Guo, W. H., Hou, W. L., Chen, L. J., Wei, Y. Q. "Improved Therapeutic Effectiveness by Combining Liposomal Honokiol with Cisplatin in Lung Cancer Model." *BMC Cancer* 8 (August 16, 2008): 242.

Kuribara, M., Kuribara, H. "Overview of the Pharmacological Features of Honokiol Yuji." *CNS Drug Reviews* 6, no. 1 (2000): 35–44.

Liou, K. T., Shen, Y. C., Chen, C. F., Tsao, C. M., Tsai, S. K. "Honokiol Protects Rat Brain from Focal Cerebral Ischemia-Reperfusion Injury by

Inhibiting Neutrophil Infiltration and Reactive Oxygen Species Production." *Brain Research* 992, no. 2 (December 5, 2003): 159–66.

Liu, H., et al. "Anti-tumor Effect of Honokiol Alone and in Combination with Other Anti-cancer Agents in Breast Cancer." *European Journal of Pharmacology* 591, nos. 1–3 (September 4, 2008): 43–51.

Park, E. J., Kim, S. Y., Zhao, Y. Z., Sohn, D. H. "Honokiol Reduces Oxidative Stress, c-Jun-NH2-Terminal Kinase Phosphorylation and Protects against Glycochenodeoxycholic Acid-Induced Apoptosis in Primary Cultured Rat Hepatocytes." *Planta Medica* 72, no. 7 (June 2006): 661–64.

Schühly, W., Khan, S. I., Fischer, N. H. "Neolignans from North American Magnolia Species with Cyclooxygenase 2 Inhibitory Activity." *Inflammo-pharmacology* 17, no. 2 (April 2009): 106–10.

Teng, Che-Ming, Chen, Chien-Chih, Ko, Feng-Nien, Lee, Lih-Gen, Huang, Tur-Fu, Chen, Yuh-Pan, Hsu, Hong-Yen. "Two Antiplatelet Agents from Magnolia officinalis." *Thrombosis Research* 50, no. 6 (1988): 757–65.

Tse, A. K., Wan, C. K., Zhu, G. Y., Shen, X. L., Cheung, H. Y., Yang, M., Fong, W. F. "Magnolol Suppresses NF-kappaB Activation and NF-KappaB Regulated Gene Expression through Inhibition of IkappaB kinase Activation." *Molecules and Immunology* 44, no. 10 (April 2007): 2647–58.

Wang, Y., Yang, Z., Zhao, X. "Honokiol Induces Paraptosis and Apoptosis and Exhibits Schedule-Dependent Synergy in Combination with Imatinib in Human Leukemia Cells." *Toxicology Mechanisms and Methods* 20, no. 5 (June 2010): 234–41.

Woodbury, A., Yu, S. P., Wei, L., García, P. "Neuro-modulating Effects of Honokiol: A Review." *Frontiers in Neurology* 4 (September 11, 2013): 130.

Xu, Q., et al. "Antidepressant-like Effects of the Mixture of Honokiol and Magnolol from the Barks of *Magnolia officinalis* in Stressed Rodents." *Progress in Neuropsychopharmacology and Biological Psychiatry* (November 28, 2007).

NIGELLA

Ahmad, A., Husain, A., Mujeeb, M., et al. "A Review on Therapeutic Potential of Nigella sativa: A Miracle Herb." *Asian Pacific Journal of Tropical Biomedicine* 3, no. 5 (2013): 337–52.

Arafa, E.-S. A., et al. "Thymoquinone Up-regulates PTEN Expression and Induces Apoptosis in Doxorubicin-Resistant Human Breast Cancer Cells." *Mutation Research* 706, nos. 1, 2 (January 10, 2011): 28–35.

Asgary, S., Sahebkar, A., Goli-malekabadi, N. "Ameliorative Effects of Nigella sativa on Dyslipidemia." *Journal of Endocrinology Investigation* 38 (2015): 1039–46.

Bamosa, A., Ali, B. A., Sowayan, S. "Effect of Oral Ingestion of Nigella sativa Seeds on Some Blood Parameters." *Saudi Pharmacology Journal* 5 (1997): 126–29.

Banerjee, S., et al. "Antitumor Activity of Gemcitabine and Oxaliplatin Is Augmented by Thymoquinone in Pancreatic Cancer." *Cancer Research* 69, no. 13 (July 1, 2009): 5575–83.

Demir, E., Taysi, S., Ulusal, H., Kaplan, D. S., Cinar, K., Tarakcioglu, M. "*Nigella sativa* Oil and Thymoquinone Reduce Oxidative Stress in the Brain Tissue of Rats Exposed to Total Head Irradiation." *International Journal of Radiation Biology* 96, no. 2 (February 2020): 228–35.

Effenberger-Neidnicht, K., Schobert, R. "Combinatorial Effects of Thymoquinone on the Anti-cancer Activity of Doxorubicin." *Cancer Chemotherapy and Pharmacology* 67, no. 4 (April 2011): 867–74.

Goyal, Sameer N., Prajapati, Chaitali P., Gore, Prashant R., Patil, Chandragouda R., Mahajan, Umesh B., Sharma, Charu, Talla, Sandhya P., Ojha, Shreesh K. "Therapeutic Potential and Pharmaceutical Development of Thymoquinone: A Multitargeted Molecule of Natural Origin." *Frontiers in Pharmacology* (2017).

Khader, M., Eckl, P. M. "Thymoquinone: An Emerging Natural Drug with a Wide Range of Medical Applications." *Iran Journal of Basic Medical Science* 17, no. 12 (2014): 950–57.

Kumar, G., Gupta, P. "Mutagenic Efficiency of Lower Doses of Gamma rays in Black Cumin (*Nigella sativa* L.)." *Cytologia* 72, no. 4 (2007).

Najmi, A., et al. "Therapeutic Effect of *Nigella sativa* in Patients of Poor Glycemic Control." *Asian Journal of Pharmaceutical and Clinical Research* 5, suppl. 3 (2012).

Sabzghabaee, Ali Mohammad, Dianatkhah, Mehrnoush, Sarrafzadegan, Nizal, Asgary, Sedigheh, Ghannadi, Alireza. "Clinical Evaluation of *Nigella sativa* Seeds for the Treatment of Hyperlipidemia: A Randomized, Placebo Controlled Clinical Trial." *Medical Archives* (Sarajevo) 66, no. 3 (2012): 198.

Sahebkar, Amirhossein, Beccuti, Guglielmo, Simental-Mendía, Luis E., Nobili, Valerio, Bo, Simona. "*Nigella sativa* (Black Seed) Effects on Plasma Lipid Concentrations in Humans: A Systematic Review and Meta-analysis of Randomized Placebo-Controlled Trials." *Pharmacological Research* 106 (2016): 37–50.

Salem, E. M., Yar, T., Bamosa, A. O., et al. "Comparative Study of *Nigella sativa* and Triple Therapy in Eradication of Helicobacter pylori on Patients with Non-ulcer Dyspepsia." *Saudi Journal of Gastroenterology* 16, no. 3 (2010): 207–14.

Zaoui, A., Cherrah, Y., Mahassini, N., Alaoui, K., Amarouch, H., Hassar, M. "Acute and Chronic Toxicity of Nigella sativa Fixed Oil." *Phytomedicine* 9, no. 1 (January 2002): 69–74.

POMEGRANATE

Adams, L. S., Seeram, N. P., Aggarwal, B. B., Takada, Y., Sand, D., Heber, D. "Pomegranate Juice, Total Pomegranate Ellagitannins and Punicalagin Suppress Inflammatory Cell Signalling in Colon Cancer Cells." *Journal of Agriculture and Food Chemistry* 54 (2006): 980–85.

Heber, D., et al. "Safety and Antioxidant Activity of a Pomegranate Ellagitannin-Enriched Polyphenol Dietary Supplement in Overweight Individuals with Increased Waist Size." *Journal of Agriculture and Food Chemistry* 55, no. 24 (November 28, 2007): 10050–54.

Jandari, S., Hatami, E., Ziaei, R., Ghavami, A., Yamchi, A. M. "The Effect of Pomegranate (*Punica granatum*) Supplementation on Metabolic Status in Patients with Type 2 Diabetes: A Systematic Review and Meta-analysis." *Complementary Therapies and Medicine* 52 (August 2020): 102478.

Jurenka, J. "Therapeutic Applications of Pomegranate (*Punica granatum* L.): A Review." *Alternative Medicine Review* 13, no. 2 (June 2008): 128–44.

Khwairakpam, A. D., et al. "Possible Use of *Punica granatum* (Pomegranate) in Cancer Therapy." *Pharmacological Research* 133 (2018): 53–64.

Pacheco-Palencia, L. A., Noratto, G., Hingorani, L., Talcott, S. T., Mertens-Talcott, S. U. "Protective Effects of Standardized Pomegranate (*Punica granatum* L.) Polyphenolic Extract in Ultraviolet-Irradiated Human Skin Fibroblasts." *Journal of Agriculture Food Chemistry* 56 (2008): 8434–41.

Seeram, N. P., et al. "*In vitro* Antiproliferative, Apoptotic and Antioxidant Activities of Punicalagin, Ellagic Acid and a Total Pomegranate Tannin Extract Are Enhanced in Combination with Other Polyphenols as Found in Pomegranate Juice." *Journal of Nutritional Biochemistry* 16, no. 6 (June 2005): 360–67.

Sharma, P., McClees, S. F., Afaq, F. "Pomegranate for Prevention and Treatment of Cancer: An Update." *Molecules* 22, no. 1 (2017): 177.

Syed, D. N., Malik, A., Hadi, N., Sarfaraz, S., Afaq, F., Mukhtar, H. "Photochemopreventive Effect of Pomegranate Fruit Extract on UVA-Mediated Activation of Cellular Pathways in Normal Human Epidermal Keratinocytes." *Photochemistry and Photobiology* 82, no. 2 (2006): 398–405.

Tanaka, T., Sugie, S. "Inhibition of Colon Carcinogenesis by Dietary Non-nutritive Compounds." *Journal of Toxicology and Patho*logy 20, no. 4 (2009): 215–35.

Viuda-Martos, M., Fernández-López, J., Pérez-Álvarez, J. A. "Pomegranate and Its Many Functional Components as Related to Human Health: A Review." *Comprehensive Reviews in Food Science and Food Safety* 9, no. 6 (November 2010): 635–54.

PROPOLIS

Akyol, S., et al. "Caffeic Acid Phenethyl Ester as a Protective Agent against Nephrotoxicity and/or Oxidative Kidney Damage: A Detailed Systematic Review." *Scientific World Journal* 2014, no. 16 (June 2014): art. ID 561971.

Chu, Joe Hing Kwok, ed. "Propolis." Complementary and Alternative Healing University Dictionary of Chinese Herbs (2016). http://alternativehealing.org/propolis.htm.

De Almeida, E. C., Menezes, H. "Anti-inflammatory Activity of Propolis Extracts: A Review." *Journal of Venomous Animals and Toxins* 8, no. 2 (2002).

Kabała-Dzik, A., et al. "Flavonoids, Bioactive Components of Propolis, Exhibit Cytotoxic Activity and Induce Cell Cycle Arrest and Apoptosis in Human Breast Cancer Cells MDA-MB-231 and MCF-7—A Comparative Study." *Cellular and Molecular Biology* 64, no. 8 (2018).

Kabała-Dzik, A., Rzepecka-Stojko, A., Kubina, R., Wojtyczka, R. D., Buszman, E., Stojko, J. "Caffeic Acid versus Caffeic Acid Phenethyl Ester in the Treatment of Breast Cancer MCF-7 Cells: Migration Rate Inhibition." *Integrative Cancer Therapies* 17, no. 4 (2018): 1247–59.

Król, W., et al. "Propolis: Properties, Application, and Its Potential." *Evidence-Based Complementary and Alternative Medicine* 2013 (2013): art. ID 807578.

Kuo, C. C., Wang, R. H., Wang, H. H., et al. "Meta-analysis of Randomized Controlled Trials of the Efficacy of Propolis Mouthwash in Cancer Therapy-Induced Oral Mucositis." *Supportive Care in Cancer* 26 (2018): 4001–9.

Muli, E. M., Maingi, J. M. "Antibacterial Activity of *Apis mellifera* L. Propolis Collected in Three Regions of Kenya." *Journal of Venomous Animals and Toxins including Tropical Diseases* 13, no. 3 (2007).

Murtaza, G., et al. "Caffeic Acid Phenethyl Ester and Therapeutic Potentials." *BioMedical Research International* 2014 (2014): art. ID 145342.

Salehi, B., Venditti, A., Sharifi-Rad, M., et al. "The Therapeutic Potential of Apigenin." *International Journal of Molecular Science* 20, no. 6 (March 15, 2019): 1305.

Sawaya, A.C.H.F., da Silva Cunha I, Barbosa, Marcucci, M. C. "Analytical Methods Applied to Diverse Types of Brazilian Propolis." *Chemistry Central Journal* 5, no. 27 (2011).

Wezgowiec, J., et al. "Polish Propolis—Chemical Composition and Biological Effects in Tongue Cancer Cells and Macrophages." *Molecules* 25, no. 10 (2020): 2426.

Yordanov, Y. "Caffeic Acid Phenethyl Ester (CAPE): Pharmacodynamics and Potential for Therapeutic Application." *Pharmacia* 66, no. 3 (2019): 107–14.

Zhou, X., Wang, F., Zhou, R., Song, X., Xie, M. "Apigenin: A Current Review on Its Beneficial Biological Activities." *Journal of Food Biochemistry* 41 (2017): e12376.

RED CLOVER

Akbaribazm, M., Khazaei, M. R., Khazaei, F., Khazaei, M. "Doxorubicin and Trifolium pratense L. (Red Clover) Extract Synergistically Inhibits Brain and Lung Metastases in 4T1 Tumor-Bearing BALB/c Mice." *Food Science and Nutrition* 8, no. 10 (September 1, 2020): 5557–70.

Budryn, G., Grzelczyk, J., Pérez-Sánchez, H. "Binding of Red Clover Isoflavones to Actin as a Potential Mechanism of Anti-metastatic Activity Restricting the Migration of Cancer Cells." *Molecules* 23, no. (2018): 2471.

Cassileth, B. R. "Red Clover (*Trifolium pratense*)." *Oncology* 24, no. 10 (September 21, 2010).

Kolodziejczyk-Czepas, J. "Trifolium species—The Latest Findings on Chemical Profile, Ethnomedicinal Use and Pharmacological Properties." *Journal of Pharmacy and Pharmacology* 68, no. 7 (July 2016): 845–61.

Krenn, L., Paper, D. H. "Inhibition of Angiogenesis and Inflammation by an Extract of Red Clover (*Trifolium pratense* L.)." *Phytomedicine* 16, no. 12 (December 2009): 1083–88.

Mannella, Paolo, et al. "Effects of Red Clover Extracts on Breast Cancer Cell Migration and Invasion." *Gynecological Endocrinology* 28, no. 1 (2012): 29–33.

Memorial Sloan Kettering Medical Education. "Red Clover." https://www.mskcc.org/cancer-care/integrative-medicine/herbs/red-clover.

Mu, H., Bai, Y. H., Wang, S. T., Zhu, Z. M., Zhang, Y. W. "Research on Antioxidant Effects and Estrogenic Effect of Formononetin from *Trifolium pratense* (Red Clover)." *Phytomedicine* 16, no. 4 (April 2009): 314–19.

Occhiuto, F. "Effects of Phytoestrogenic Isoflavones from Red Clover (*Trifolium pratense* L.) on Experimental Osteoporosis." *Phytotherapy Research* 21, no. 2 (February 2007): 130–34.

Powles, T. J., Howell, A., Evans, D. G., McCloskey, E. V., Ashley, S., Greenhalgh, R., Affen, J., Flook, L. A., Tidy, A. "Red Clover Isoflavones Are Safe and Well Tolerated in Women with a Family History of Breast Cancer." *Menopause International* 14, no. 1 (March 2008): 6–12.

Sivoňová, M. K., Kaplán, P., Tatarková, Z., Lichardusová, L., Dušenka, R., Jurečeková, J. "Androgen Receptor and Soy Isoflavones in Prostate Cancer (Review)." *Molecular and Clinical Oncology* 10, no. 2 (2019): 191–204.

Zhang, H. "Extraction, Purification, Hypoglycemic and Antioxidant Activities of Red Clover (*Trifolium pratense* L.) Polysaccharides." *International Journal of Biological Macromolecules* 148 (April 1, 2020): 750–60.

SEA BUCKTHORN

Hussain, S. Z., Naseer, B., Qadri, T., Fatima, T., Bhat, T. A. "Seabuckthorn (Hippophae tibetana)—Morphology, Taxonomy, Composition and Health Benefits." In *Fruits Grown in Highland Regions of the Himalayas.* Springer Cham, 2021. https://doi.org/10.1007/978-3-030-75502-7.

Ivanišová, E., Blašková, M., Terentjeva, M., Grygorieva, O., Vergun, O., Brindza, J., Kačániová, M. "Biological Properties of Sea Buckthorn (*Hippophae rhamnoides* L.) Derived Products." *Acta Scientiarum Pololonorum Technologia Alimentaria* 19, no. 2 (2020): 195–205.

Kuduban, Ozan, Mazlumoglu, Muhammed, Recai, Kuduban, Selma, Denktas, Erhan, Ertugrul, Kukula, Osman, Yarali, Oguzhan, Cimen, Ferda Keskin, Cankaya, Murat. "The Effect of Hippophae rhamnoides Extract on Oral Mucositis Induced in Rats with Methotrexate." *Journal of Applied Oral Science* 24, no. 5 (2016)): 423–30. https://doi.org/10.1590/1678-775720160139.

Ma, Xueying, Moilanen, Johanna, Laaksonen, Oskar, Yang, Wei, Tenhu, Elina, Yang, Baoru. "Phenolic Compounds and Antioxidant Activities of Tea-Type Infusions Processed from Sea Buckthorn (*Hippophaë rhamnoides*) Leaves." *Food Chemistry* 272 (2019): 1–11.

Pundir, Swati, Garg, Prakrati, Dviwedi, Ananya, Ali, Aaliya, Kapoor, V. K., Kapoor, Deepak, Kulshrestha, Saurabh, Lal, Uma Ranjan, Negi, Poonam. "Ethnomedicinal Uses, Phytochemistry and Dermatological Effects of Hippophae rhamnoides L.: A Review." *Journal of Ethnopharmacology* 266 (2021): 113434.

Rathor, R., Sharma, P., Suryakumar, G., et al. "A Pharmacological Investigation of Hippophae salicifolia (HS) and Hippophae rhamnoides turkestanica (HRT) against Multiple Stress (C-H-R): An Experimental Study Using Rat Model." *Cell Stress and Chaperones* 20 (2015): 821–31.

Saggu, S., Divekar, H. M., Gupta, V., Sawhney R. C., Banerjee, P. K., Kumar, R. "Adaptogenic and Safety Evaluation of Seabuckthorn (*Hippophae rhamnoides*) Leaf Extract: A Dose Dependent Study." *Journal of Food and Chemical Toxicology* 45, no. 4 (2007): 609–17.

Seo, D. Y., Lee, S. R., Heo, J. W., et al. "Ursolic Acid in Health and Disease." *Korean Journal of Physiology and Pharmacology* 22, no. 3 (2018): 235–48.

Solà Marsiñach, M., Cuenca, A. P. "The Impact of Sea Buckthorn Oil Fatty Acids on Human Health." *Lipids in Health and Disease* 18 (2019): 145.

Upadhyay, N., et al. "Safety and Healing Efficacy of Sea Buckthorn (*Hippophae rhamnoides* L.) Seed Oil on Burn Wounds in Rats." *Food and Chemical Toxicology* 47, no. 6 (2009): 1146–53.

Zielińska, A., Nowak, I. "Abundance of Active Ingredients in Sea-Buckthorn Oil." *Lipids in Health and Disease* 16, no. 1 (May 19, 2017): 95.

ST. JOHN'S WORT

Chrubasik-Hausmann, S., Vlachojannis, J., McLachlan, A. J. "Understanding Drug Interactions with St John's wort (*Hypericum perforatum* L.): Impact of Hyperforin Content." *Journal of Pharmacy and Pharmacology* 71, no. 1 (January 2019): 129–38.

Cohen, E. E., et al. "Phase I Studies of Sirolimus Alone or in Combination with Pharmacokinetic Modulators in Advanced Cancer Patients." *Clinical Cancer* 18, no. 17 (2012): 4785–93.

Hunt, E. J., Lester, C. E., Lester, E. A., Tackett, R. L. "Effect of St. John's Wort on Free Radical Production." *Life Sciences* 69, no. 2 (June 1, 2001): 181–90.

Kim, H., Kim, S. W., Seok, K. H., Hwang, C. W., Ahn, J. C., Jin, J. O., Kang, H. W. "Hypericin-Assisted Photodynamic Therapy against Anaplastic Thyroid Cancer." *Photodiagnosis and Photodynamic Therapies* 24 (December 2018): 15–21.

Matić, I. Z., Ergün, S., Đorđić Crnogorac, M., et al. "Cytotoxic Activities of *Hypericum perforatum* L. Extracts against 2D and 3D Cancer Cell Models." *Cytotechnology* 73 (2021): 373–89.

Menegazzi, M., Masiello, P., Novelli, M. "Anti-tumor Activity of *Hypericum perforatum* L. and Hyperforin through Modulation of Inflammatory Signaling, ROS Generation and Proton Dynamics." *Antioxidants* 10 (2021): 18.

Zhen, Ke, et al. "Naturally Available Hypericin Undergoes Electron Transfer for Type I Photodynamic and Photothermal Synergistic Therapy." *Biomaterials Science* 8 (2020): 2481–87.

TAHEEBO

Jimenez-Gonzalez, F. J., et al. "Antioxidant, Anti-inflammatory, and Antiproliferative Activity of Extracts Obtained from *Tabebuia rosea* (Bertol.) DC." *Pharmacognosy Magazine* 14, no. 55 (2018): 25–31.

Mukherjee, B., Telang, N., Wong, G. Y. C. "Growth Inhibition of Estrogen Receptor Positive Human Breast Cancer Cells by Taheebo from the Inner Bark of *Tabebuia avellanedae* tree." *International Journal of Molecular Medicine* 24, no. 2 (August 2009): 253–60.

Panda, S. P., Panigrahy, U. P., Panda, S., Jena, B. R. "Stem Extract of *Tabebuia chrysantha* Induces Apoptosis by Targeting sEGFR in Ehrlich Ascites Carcinoma." *Journal of Ethnopharmacology* 235 (May 10, 2019): 219–26.

Sandur, Santosh K., Ichikawa, Haruyo, Sethi, Gautam, Ahn, Kwang Seok, Aggarwal, Bharat B. "Plumbagin (5-hydroxy-2-methyl-1,4-naphthoquinone) Suppresses NF-κb Activation and NF-κb-Regulated Gene Products through Modulation of p65 and Iκbα Kinase Activation, Leading to Potentiation of Apoptosis Induced by Cytokine and Chemotherapeutic Agents." *Journal of Biological Chemistry* 281, no. 25 (June 23, 2006): P17023–33.

Zhang, J., Hunto, S. T., Yang, Y., Lee, J., Cho, J. Y. "*Tabebuia impetiginosa*: A Comprehensive Review on Traditional Uses, Phytochemistry, and Immunopharmacological Properties." *Molecules* 25, no. 18 (2020).

TULSI

Baliga, M. S., et al. "*Ocimum sanctum* L (Holy Basil or Tulsi) and Its Phytochemicals in the Prevention and Treatment of Cancer." *Nutrition and Cancer* 65, suppl. 1 (2013): 26–35.

Baliga, M. S., Rao, S., Rai, M. P., D'souza, P. "Radio Protective Effects of the Ayurvedic Medicinal Plant *Ocimum sanctum* Linn. (Holy Basil): A Memoir." *Journal of Cancer Research and Therapy* 12 (2016): 20–27.

Cohen, M. M. "Tulsi—*Ocimum sanctum*: A Herb for All Reasons." *Journal of Ayurveda and Integrative Medicine* 5, no. 4 (2014): 251–59.

Joseph, B., Nair, V. M. "*Ocimum sanctum* Linn. (Holy Basil): Pharmacology behind Its Anti-cancerous Effect." *International Journal of Pharma and Bio Sciences* 4, no. 2 (April 2013): 556–75.

Mishra, M. "Tulsi to Save Taj Mahal from Pollution Effects." *Times of India*, December 12, 2008.

Reshma, K., Rao, A. V., Dinesh, M., Vasudevan, D. M. "Radioprotective Effects of Ocimum Flavonoids on Leukocyte Oxidants and Antioxidants in Oral Cancer." *Indian Journal of Clinical Biochemistry* 23, no. 2 (April 2008): 171–75.

Sah, Ashok Kumar, Vijaysimha, M., Mahamood, M. "The Tulsi, Queen of Green Medicines: Biochemistry and Pathophysiology—A Review." *International Journal of Pharmaceutical Sciences Review and Research* 50, no. 2, art. no. 16 (May–June 2018): 106–14.

Shimizu, T., et al. "Holy Basil Leaf Extract Decreases Tumorigenicity and Metastasis of Aggressive Human Pancreatic Cancer Cells In Vitro and In Vivo: Potential Role in Therapy." *Cancer Letters* 336, no. 2 (2013): 270–80.

Shukla, S. T., et al. "Hepatoprotective and Antioxidant Activities of Crude Fractions of Endophytic Fungi of *Ocimum sanctum* Linn. in Rats." *Oriental Pharmacy and Experimental Medicine* 12 (2012): 81–91.

Singh, M. P. "Tulsi: A Herbal Remedy For Immunity Booster." *World Journal of Pharmaceutical Research* 10, no. 2 (2020): 801–6.

Thokchom, Sarda Dev, Gupta, Samta, Kapoor, Rupam. "Arbuscular Mycorrhiza Augments Essential Oil Composition and Antioxidant Properties of *Ocimum tenuiflorum* L.—A Popular Green Tea Additive." *Industrial Crops and Products* 153 (2020): 112418.

TURMERIC

Arpan, De, et al. "Anticancer Properties of Curcumin and Interactions with the Circadian Timing System." *Integrative Cancer Therapies* 18 (December 9, 2019).

Burgos-Moron, E., et al. "The Dark Side of Curcumin." *International Journal of Cancer* 126 (2020): 1771–75.

Carroll, R. E., Benya, R. V., Turgeon, D. K., et al. "Phase IIa Clinical Trial of Curcumin for the Prevention of Colorectal Neoplasia." *Cancer Prevention Research* (Philadelphia) 4, no. 3 (2011): 354–64.

Dharman, S., Maragathavalli, G., Shanmugasundaram, K., Sampath, R. K. "A Systematic Review and Meta-analysis on the Efficacy of Curcumin/Turmeric for the Prevention and Amelioration of Radiotherapy/Radiochemotherapy Induced Oral Mucositis in Head and Neck Cancer Patients." *Asian Pacific Journal of Cancer Prevention* 22, no. 6 (June 1, 2021): 1671–84.

Fabianowska-Majewska, K., et al. "Curcumin from Turmeric Rhizome: A Potential Modulator of DNA Methylation Machinery in Breast Cancer Inhibition." *Nutrients* 13, no. 2 (2021): 332.

Gupta, S. C., Patchva, S., Aggarwal, B. B. "Therapeutic Roles of Curcumin: Lessons Learned from Clinical Trials." *American Association of Pharmaceutical Scientists Journal* 15, no. 1 (2013): 195–218.

Mingyue, Li, et al. "Turmeric Is Therapeutic In Vivo on Patient-Derived Colorectal Cancer Xenografts: Inhibition of Growth, Metastasis, and Tumor Recurrence." *Frontiers in Oncology* (January 19, 2021).

Normando, A. G. C., de Menêses, A. G., de Toledo, I. P., Borges, G. Á., de Lima, C. L., Dos Reis, P. E. D., Guerra, E. N. S. "Effects of Turmeric and Curcumin on Oral Mucositis: A Systematic Review." *Phytotherapy Research* 33, no. 5 (May 2019): 1318–29.

Rao, Suresh, Dinkar, Chetana, Vaishnav, Lalit Kumar, Rao, Pratima, Rai, Manoj Ponadka, Fayad, Raja, Baliga, Manjeshwar Shrinath. "The Indian Spice Turmeric Delays and Mitigates Radiation-Induced Oral Mucositis in Patients Undergoing Treatment for Head and Neck Cancer: An Investigational Study." *Integrative Cancer Therapies* 13, no. 3 (2014): 201–10.

Shaikh, S., Shaikh, J., Naba, Y. S., Doke, K., Ahmed, K., Yusufi, M. "Curcumin: Reclaiming the Lost Ground against Cancer Resistance." *Cancer Drug Resistance* 4 (2021): 298–320.

Shen, L., Liu, C. C., An, C. Y., et al. "How Does Curcumin Work with Poor Bioavailability? Clues from Experimental and Theoretical Studies." *Science Reports* 6 (2016): 20872.

Smith, T. J., Ashar, B. H. "Iron Deficiency Anemia Due to High-dose Turmeric." *Cureus* 11, no. 1 (2019): e3858.

Somasundaram, S., et al. "Dietary Curcumin Inhibits Chemotherapy-Induced Apoptosis in Models of Human Breast Cancer." *Cancer Research* 62, no. 13 (2002): 3868–75.

Toden, S., Goel, A. "The Holy Grail of Curcumin and Its Efficacy in Various Diseases: Is Bioavailability Truly a Big Concern?" *Journal of Restorative Medicine* 6, no. 1 (2017): 27–36.

Zhang, L., Tang, G., Wei, Z. "Prophylactic and Therapeutic Effects of Curcumin on Treatment-Induced Oral Mucositis in Patients with Head and Neck Cancer: A Meta-analysis of Randomized Controlled Trials." *Nutrition and Cancer* 73, no. 5 (2021): 740–49.

MEDICINAL MUSHROOMS

Blagodatski, A., Yatsunskaya, M., Mikhailova, V., Tiasto, V., Kagansky, A., Katanaev, V. L. "Medicinal Mushrooms as an Attractive New Source of Natural Compounds for Future Cancer Therapy." *Oncotarget* 9, no. 49 (2018): 29259–74.

Borodina, I., Kenny, L., McCarthy, C., Paramasivan, K., Pretorius, E., Roberts, T., van der Hoek, K., Kell, D. "The Biology of Ergothioneine, an Antioxidant Nutraceutical." *Nutrition Research Reviews* 33, no. 2 (2020): 190–217.

Elkhateeb, W. A., Daba, G. M. "Review: The Endless Nutritional and Pharmaceutical Benefits of the Himalayan Gold, Cordyceps; Current Knowledge and Prospective Potentials." *Biofarmasi Journal of Natural Products Biochemistry* 18 (2020): 70–77.

Halliwell, B., Cheah, I. K., Tang, R. M. Y. "Ergothioneine—A Diet-Derived Antioxidant with Therapeutic Potential." *Federation of European Biochemical Societies Letters* 592 (2018): 3357–66.

Hassan, M. A., Rouf, R., Tiralongo, E., May, T. W., and Tiralongo, J. "Mushroom Lectins: Specificity, Structure and Bioactivity Relevant to Human Disease." *International Journal of Molecular Sciences* 16, no. 4 (2015): 7802–38. https://doi.org/10.3390/ijms16047802.

Hobbs, Christopher. *Medicinal Mushrooms: The Essential Guide.* Storey Publishing, 2021.

Rogers, Robert Dale. *Medicinal Mushrooms: The Human Clinical Trials.* Prairie Deva Press, 2020.

Zeb, M., Lee, C. H. "Medicinal Properties and Bioactive Compounds from Wild Mushrooms Native to North America." *Molecules* 26, no. 2 (2021): 251.

Chapter 7: Herbal Formulating for Cancer Care

Abotaleb, M., Samuel, S. M., Varghese, E., et al. "Flavonoids in Cancer and Apoptosis." *Cancers* (Basel) 11, no. 1 (2018): 28.

Alviano, C. S., et al. "Antimicrobial Activity of *Croton cajucara* Benth Linalool-Rich Essential Oil on Artificial Biofilms and Planktonic Microorganisms." *Molecular Oral Microbiology Journal* 20, no. 2 (April 2005): 101–5.

Association of Accredited Naturopathic Medical Colleges. "The Therapeutic Order." 2019. https://aanmc.org/featured-articles/therapeutic-order/.

Bone, K. M. "Potential Interaction of *Ginkgo biloba* Leaf with Antiplatelet or Anticoagulant Drugs: What Is the Evidence?" *Molecular Nutrition and Food Research* 52, no. 7 (2008): 764–71.

Boyle, P., et al. "Endogenous and Exogenous Testosterone and the Risk of Prostate Cancer and Increased Prostate-Specific Antigen (PSA) Level: A Meta-analysis." *British Journal of Urology International* 118, no. 5 (November 2016): 731–41.

Brahmbhatt, M., Gundala, S. R., Asif, G., et al. "Ginger Phytochemicals Exhibit Synergy to Inhibit Prostate Cancer Cell Proliferation." *Nutrition and Cancer* 65, no. 2 (2013): 263–72.

Caesar, L. K., Cech, N. B. "Synergy and Antagonism in Natural Product Extracts: When 1 + 1 Does Not Equal 2." *Natural Products Report* 36 (2019): 869–88.

Chen, M., May, B. H., Zhou, I. W., et al. "FOLFOX 4 Combined with Herbal Medicine for Advanced Colorectal Cancer: A Systematic Review." *Phytotherapy Research* 28, no. 7 (2014): 976–91.

Chen, M., May, B. H., Zhou, I. W., Sze, D. M., Xue, C. C., Zhang, A. L. "Oxaliplatin-Based Chemotherapy Combined with Traditional Medicines for Neutropenia in Colorectal Cancer: A Meta-analysis of the Contributions of Specific Plants." *Critical Reviews in Oncology and Hematology* 105 (September 2016): 18–34.

Chen, P., Ni, W., Xie, T., Sui, X. "Meta-analysis of 5-Fluorouracil-Based Chemotherapy Combined with Traditional Chinese Medicines for Colorectal Cancer Treatment." *Integrative Cancer Therapeutics* 18 (January–December 2019): 1534735419828824.

Chopra, B., Dhingra, A. K., Dhar, K. L., Nepali, K. "Emerging Role of Terpenoids for the Treatment of Cancer: A Review." *Mini Reviews of Medicinal Chemistry* 21, no. 16 (2021): 2300–36.

Costa, M. L., et al. "Hepatotoxicity Induced by Paclitaxel Interaction with Turmeric in Association with a Microcystin from a Contaminated Dietary Supplement." *Toxicon* 150 (August 2018): 207–11.

Cui, Y., Shu, X. O., Gao, Y. T., Cai, H., Tao, M. H., Zheng, W. "Association of Ginseng Use with Survival and Quality of Life among Breast Cancer Patients." *American Journal of Epidemiology* 163, no. 7 (April 1, 2006): 645–53.

Demiroglu-Zergeroglu, A., Basara-Cigerim, B., Kilic, E., Yanikkaya-Demirel, G. "The Investigation of Effects of Quercetin and Its Combination with Cisplatin on Malignant Mesothelioma Cells *In Vitro*." *Journal of Biomedicine and Biotechnology* (2010): 851589.

Dhandapani, K. M., Mahesh, V. B., Brann, D. W. "Curcumin Suppresses Growth and Chemoresistance of Human Glioblastoma Cells via AP-1 and NFkappaB Transcription Factors." *Journal of Neurochemistry* 102, no. 2 (July 2007): 522–38.

Du, B., Jiang, L., Xia, Q., Zhong, L. "Synergistic Inhibitory Effects of Curcumin and 5-Fluorouracil on the Growth of the Human Colon Cancer Cell Line HT-29." *Chemotherapy* 52, no. 1 (2006): 23–28.

Finnell, J. S., Snider, P., Myers, S. P., Zeff, J. "A Hierarchy of Healing: Origins of the Therapeutic Order and Implications for Research." *Integrative Medicine* 18, no. 3 (2019): 54–59.

Ganesan, K., Xu, B. "Telomerase Inhibitors from Natural Products and Their Anticancer Potential." *International Journal of Molecular Science* 19, no. 1 (2017): 13.

Gilbert, B., Alves, L. "Synergy in Plant Medicines." *Current Medicinal Chemistry* 10, no. 1 (2003): 13–20.

Hemalswarya, S., Doble, M. "Potential Synergism of Natural Products in the Treatment of Cancer." *Phytotherapy Research* 20, no. 4 (April 2006): 239–49.

Ide, H., et al. "Combined Inhibitory Effects of Soy Isoflavones and Curcumin on the Production of Prostate-Specific Antigen." *Prostate* 70, no. 10 (July 1, 2010): 1127–33.

Jian, B., Zhang, H., Han, C., Liu, J. "Anti-cancer Activities of Diterpenoids Derived from *Euphorbia fischeriana* Steud." *Molecules* 23, no. 2 (2018): 387.

Junio, H. A., et al. "Synergy Directed Fractionation of Botanical Medicines: A Case Study with Goldenseal (*Hydrastis canadensis*)." *Journal of Natural Products* 74, no. 7 (July 22, 2011): 1621–29.

Kapadia, G. J., Rao, G. S., Ramachandran, C., Iida, A., Suzuki, N., Tokuda, H. S. "Synergistic Cytotoxicity of Red Beetroot (*Beta vulgaris* L.) Extract with Doxorubicin in Human Pancreatic, Breast and Prostate Cancer Cell Lines." *Journal of Complementary and Integrative Medicine* (June 26, 2013).

Kim, J. M., White, R. H. "Effect of Vitamin E on the Anticoagulant Response to Warfarin." *American Journal of Cardiology* 77, no. 7 (March 1, 1996): 545–46.

Kuttan, G., Pratheeshkumar, P., Manu, K. A., Kuttan, R. "Inhibition of Tumor Progression by Naturally Occurring Terpenoids." *Pharmaceutical Biology* 49, no. 10 (October 2011): 995–1007.

Lee, G. Y., Lee, J. J., Lee, S. M. "Antioxidant and Anticoagulant Status Were Improved by Personalized Dietary Intervention Based on Biochemical and Clinical Parameters in Cancer Patients." *Nutrition & Cancer* 67, no. 7 (2015): 1083–92.

Liu, R. H. "Potential Synergy of Phytochemicals in Cancer Prevention: Mechanism of Action." *Journal of Nutrition* 134, no. 12 suppl. (December 2004): 3479S–85S.

Marshall, K. "Therapeutic Applications of Whey Protein." *Alternative Medicine Review* 9, no. 2 (2004).

McCulloch, M., See, C., Shu, X. J., et al. "Astragalus-Based Chinese Herbs and Platinum-Based Chemotherapy for Advanced Non-Small-Cell Lung Cancer: Meta-analysis of Randomized Trials." *Journal of Clinical Oncology* 24, no. 3 (2006): 419–30.

Mundy, L., Pendry, B., Rahman, M. "Antimicrobial Resistance and Synergy in Herbal Medicine." *Journal of Herbal Medicine* 6, no. 2 (2016): 53–58.

Owens, C., Baergen, R., Puckett, D. "Acute, Dose-Dependent Cognitive Effects of Ginkgo biloba, Panax ginseng and Their Combination in Healthy Young Volunteers: Online Sources of Herbal Product Information." *American Journal of Medicine* 127, no. 2 (February 2014): 109–15.

Pezzani, R., Salehi, B., Vitalini, S., et al. "Synergistic Effects of Plant Derivatives and Conventional Chemotherapeutic Agents: An Update on the Cancer Perspective." *Medicina* (Kaunas, Lithuania) 55, no. 4 (April 17, 2019): 110.

Scholey, A., Kennedy, D. O. "Differential Interactions with Cognitive Demand." *Human Psychopharmacology Clinical and Experimental* 17, no. 1 (December 2001): 35–44.

Selvakumar, K., Sunil Kumar, A., Aiswarya Gandhi, R., and Geetha, M. "Synergic Antioxidant Efficiency of Ginger and Green Tea Phytomolecular Complex." *Asian Journal of Plant Science and Research* 5, no. 11 (2015): 46–52.

Wagner, Hildebert. "Synergy Research: Approaching a New Generation of Phytopharmaceuticals." *Fitoterapia* 82 (2011): 34–37.

Williamson, E. M. "Synergy and Other Interactions in Phytomedicines." *Phytomedicine* 8, no. 5 (2001): 401–9.

Yang, Y., Zhang, Z., Li, S., Ye, X., Li, X., He, K. "Synergy Effects of Herb Extracts: Pharmacokinetics and Pharmacodynamic Basis." *Fitoterapia* 92 (January 2014): 133–47.

Yarnell, Eric. "Garlic (and Relatives), Platelets, and Combination with Anticoagulant Drugs." Bot Med Rocks website, May 28, 2022. https://www.botmed.rocks/garlic-platelets-anticoagulants.html.

Yarnell, Eric. "Synergy in Herbal Medicines." *Journal of Restorative Medicine* 4, no. 1 (December 1, 2015): 60–73.

Zhou, J. R., Li, L., Pan, W. "Dietary Soy and Tea Combinations for Prevention of Breast and Prostate Cancers by Targeting Metabolic Syndrome Elements in Mice." *American Journal of Clinical Nutrition* 86, no. 3 (2007): s882–88.

SAFETY OF SUPPLEMENTS AND HERBS WITH CHEMOTHERAPY

Akbari, S., Kariznavi, E., Jannati, M., Elyasi, S., Tayarani-Najaran, Z. "Curcumin as a Preventive or Therapeutic Measure for Chemotherapy and Radiotherapy Induced Adverse Reaction: A Comprehensive Review." *Food and Chemical Toxicology* 145 (November 2020): 111699.

Banerjee, S., et al. "Combinatorial Effect of Curcumin with Docetaxel Modulates Apoptotic and Cell Survival Molecules in Prostate Cancer." *Frontiers in Bioscience* 9 (2017): 235–45.

Biswal, B. M., Sulaiman, S. A., Ismail, H. C., Zakaria, H., Musa, K. I. "Effect of *Withania somnifera* (Ashwagandha) on the Development of Chemotherapy-Induced Fatigue and Quality of Life in Breast Cancer Patients." *Integrative Cancer Therapies* 12, no. 4 (July 2013): 312–22.

Block, K. I., Koch, A. C., Mead, M. N., Tothy, P. K., Newman, R. A., Gyllenhaal, C. "Impact of Antioxidant Supplementation on Chemotherapeutic Toxicity: A Systematic Review of the Evidence from Randomized Controlled Trials." *International Journal of Cancer* 123, no. 6 (September 15, 2008): 1227–39.

Cao, A., He, H., Wang, Q., Li, L., An, Y., Zhou, X. "Evidence of Astragalus Injection Combined Platinum-Based Chemotherapy in Advanced Non Small Cell Lung Cancer Patients: A Systematic Review and Meta-analysis." *Medicine* 98 (2019): e14798.

Cao, J., Han, J., Xiao, H., Qiao, J., Han, M. "Effect of Tea Polyphenol Compounds on Anticancer Drugs in Terms of Anti-tumor Activity, Toxicology, and Pharmacokinetics." *Nutrients* 8, no. 12 (2016): 762.

Di Minno, A., et al. "Old and New Oral Anticoagulants: Food, Herbal Medicines and Drug Interactions." *Blood Reviews* 31, no. 4 (2017): 193–203.

Duan, P., Wang, Z. M. "Clinical Study on Effect of Astragalus in Efficacy Enhancing and Toxicity Reducing of Chemotherapy in Patients of Malignant Tumor." *Chinese Journal of Integrated Traditional and Western Medicine* 22, no. 7 (July 2002): 515–17.

Funk, J. L., Frye, J. B., Oyarzo, J. N., Zhang, H., Timmermann, B. N. "Anti-arthritic Effects and Toxicity of the Essential Oils of Turmeric (*Curcuma longa* L.)." *Journal of Agriculture Food and Chemistry* 58 (2010): 842–49.

Ge, J., Tan, B. X., Chen, Y., et al. "Interaction of Green Tea Polyphenol Epigallocatechin-3-Gallate with Sunitinib: Potential Risk of Diminished Sunitinib Bioavailability." *Journal of Molecular Medicine* 89 (2011): 595–602.

Hudson, A., et al. "A Review of the Toxicity of Compounds Found in Herbal Dietary Supplements." *Planta Medica* 84, nos. 9, 10 (2018): 613–26.

Kalluru, H., Kondaveeti, S. S., Telapolu, S., Kalachaveedu, M. "Turmeric Supplementation Improves the Quality of Life and Hematological Parameters in Breast Cancer Patients on Paclitaxel Chemotherapy: A Case Series." *Complementary Therapies in Clinical Practice* 41 (November 2020): 101247.

Kang, Y., et al. "Curcumin Sensitizes Human Gastric Cancer Cells to 5-Fluorouracil through Inhibition of the Nfκb Survival-Signaling Pathway." *Oncology Targets and Therapeutics* 9 (2016): 7373–84.

Lin, N. H., Yang, H. W., Su, Y. J., Chang, C. W. "Herb Induced Liver Injury after Using Herbal Medicine: A Systematic Review and Case-Control Study." *Medicine* (Baltimore) 98, no. 13 (March 2019): e14992.

Lin, S., et al. "Meta-analysis of Astragalus-Containing Traditional Chinese Medicine Combined with Chemotherapy for Colorectal Cancer: Efficacy and Safety to Tumor Response." *Frontiers in Oncology* (August 13, 2019).

Simone, C. B., Simone, N. L., Simone, V., Simone, C. B. "Antioxidants and Other Nutrients Do Not Interfere with Chemotherapy or Radiation Therapy and Can Increase Kill and Increase Survival." Parts 1 and 2. *Alternative Therapies in Health and Medicine* 13, no. 1 (January–February 2007): 22–28, and 13, no. 2 (March–April 2007): 40–47.

Singh, K., Bhori, M., Kasu, Y. A., Bhat, G., Marar, T. "Antioxidants as Precision Weapons in War against Cancer Chemotherapy Induced Toxicity—Exploring the Armoury of Obscurity." *Saudi Pharmaceutical Journal* 26, no. 2 (2018): 177–90.

Singh, Narendra P., Lai, Henry C. "Synergistic Cytotoxicity of Artemisinin and Sodium Butyrate on Human Cancer Cells." *Anticancer Research* 25, no. 6B (November 2005): 4325–31.

Tan, B. L., Norhaizan, M. E. "Curcumin Combination Chemotherapy: The Implication and Efficacy in Cancer." *Molecules* 24, no. 14 (2019): 2527.

Wang, S. F., Wang, Q., Jiao, L. J., Huang, Y. L., Garfield, D., Zhang, J., Xu, L. "Astragalus-Containing Traditional Chinese Medicine, with and without Prescription Based on Syndrome Differentiation, Combined with Chemotherapy for Advanced Non-Small-Cell Lung Cancer: A Systemic Review and Meta-analysis." *Currents in Oncology* 23, no. 3 (June 2016): e188–95.

Yiannakopoulou, E. C. "Interaction of Green Tea Catechins with Breast Cancer Endocrine Treatment: A Systematic Review." *Pharmacology* 94 (2014): 245–48.

Zhang, P., et al. "Curcumin Synergizes with 5-Fluorouracil by Impairing AMPK/ULK1-Dependent Autophagy, AKT Activity and Enhancing Apoptosis in Colon Cancer Cells with Tumor Growth Inhibition in Xenograft Mice." *Journal of Experimental Clinical Cancer Research* 36 (2017): 190.

Chapter 8: Diagnosis and Treatment Planning in Collaborative Oncology

Abdullah, S. E., Haigentz, M. Jr., Piperdi, B. "Dermatologic Toxicities from Monoclonal Antibodies and Tyrosine Kinase Inhibitors against EGFR: Pathophysiology and Management." *Chemotherapy Research and Practice* (2012): 351210.

Adlard, J., et al. "Prediction of the Response of Colorectal Cancer to Systemic Therapy." *Lancet Oncology* 3 (2002): 75–82.

Ahmad, A., Biersack, B., Li, Y., Kong, D., Bao, B., Schobert, R., Padhye, S. B., Sarkar, F. H. "Targeted Regulation of PI3K/Akt/mTOR/NF-κB Signaling by Indole Compounds and Their Derivatives: Mechanistic Details and Biological Implications for Cancer Therapy." *Anticancer Agents and Medicinal Chemistry* 13, no. 7 (2013).

American Cancer Society. "Cancer Treatment and Survivorship." https://www.cancer.org/content/dam/cancer-org/research/cancer-facts-and-statistics/ 2019-2021.pdf.

Bachelder, R. E., et al. "Vascular Endothelial Growth Factor Is an Autocrine Survival Factor for Neuropilin-Expressing Breast Carcinoma Cells." *Cancer Research* 61, no. 15 (2001): 5736–40.

Blackwell, K., Haroon, Z., Broadwater, G., Berry, D., Harris, L., Iglehart, J. D., Dewhirst, M., Greenberg, C. "Plasma D-Dimer Levels in Operable Breast Cancer Patients Correlate with Clinical Stage and Axillary Lymph Node Status." *Journal of Clinical Oncology* 18, no. 3 (February 2000): 600–608.

Borst, P., et al. "A Family of Drug Transporters: The Multidrug Resistance-Associated Proteins." *Journal of the National Cancer Institute* 92 (2000): 1295–302.

Chappell, William H., et al. "Ras/Raf/MEK/ERK and PI3K/PTEN/Akt/mTOR Inhibitors: Rationale and Importance to Inhibiting These Pathways in Human Health." *Oncotarget* 2, no. 3 (March 2011): 135–64.

Chen, W., Lu, Y., Chen, G., Huang, S. "Molecular Evidence of Cryptotanshinone for Treatment and Prevention of Human Cancer." *Anticancer Agents in Medicinal Chemistry* 13, no. 7 (2013): 979–87.

Chen, X., Gole, J., Gore, A., et al. "Non-invasive Early Detection of Cancer Four Years before Conventional Diagnosis Using a Blood Test." *Nature Communications* 11, no. 1 (2020): 3475.

Chung, Y. M., et al. "Establishment and Characterization of 5-Fluorouracil-Resistant Gastric Cancer Cells." *Cancer Letters* 159, no. 1 (2000): 95–101.

Colomer, R., Menendez, J. A. "Mediterranean Diet, Olive Oil and Cancer." *Clinical and Translational Oncology* 8, no. 1 (January 2006): 15–21.

Dankort, D., et al. "Braf(V600E) Cooperates with Pten Loss to Induce Metastatic Melanoma." *Nature Genetics* 41, no. 5 (May 2009): 544–52.

Dashwood, R. H., Ho, E., "Dietary Histone Deacetylase Inhibitors: From Cells to Mice to Man." *Seminars in Cancer Biology* (May 2007).

Davidovich, S., Ben-Izhak, O., Shapira, M., Futerman, B., Hershko, D. D. "Overexpression of Skp2 Is Associated with Resistance to Preoperative Doxorubicin-Based Chemotherapy in Primary Breast Cancer." *Breast Cancer Research* 10, no. 4 (2008): R63.

Duggan, C., et al. "Associations of Sex Steroid Hormones with Mortality in Women with Breast Cancer." *Breast Cancer Research and Treatment* 155, no. 3 (2016): 559–67.

Efe, D. "Carbonic Anhydrase Enzyme Inhibition and Biological Activities of *Satureja hortensis* L. Essential Oil." *Industrial Crops and Products* 156 (2020): 112849.

Elimam, Diaaeldin M., et al. "Natural Inspired Piperine-Based Sulfonamides and Carboxylic Acids as Carbonic Anhydrase Inhibitors: Design, Synthesis and Biological Evaluation." *European Journal of Medicinal Chemistry* 225 (2021): 113800.

Hanhineva, K., et al. "Impact of Dietary Polyphenols on Carbohydrate Metabolism." *International Journal of Molecular Science* 11, no. 4 (2010).

Huang, S. "Inhibition of PI3K/Akt/mTOR Signaling by Natural Products." *Anticancer Agents in Medicinal Chemistry* 13, no. 7 (2013): 967–70.

Huang, T. H.-W., Kota, B. P., Razmovski, V., Roufogalis, B. D. "Herbal or Natural Medicines as Modulators of Peroxisome Proliferator-Activated Receptors and Related Nuclear Receptors for Therapy of Metabolic Syndrome." *Basic & Clinical Pharmacology & Toxicology* 96 (2005): 3–14.

Ichikawa, W., et al. "Combination of Dihydropyrimidine Dehydrogenase and Thymidylate Synthase Gene Expressions in Primary Tumors as Predictive Parameters for the Efficacy of Fluoropyrimidine-Based Chemotherapy for Metastatic Colorectal Cancer." *Clinical Cancer Research* 9, no. 2 (February 2003): 786–91.

Inoue-Narita, T., et al. "Pten Deficiency in Melanocytes Results in Resistance to Hair Graying and Susceptibility to Carcinogen-Induced Melanomagenesis." *Cancer Research Journal* 68, no. 14 (2008).

Kanzaki, A., et al. "Expression of Uridine and Thymidine Phosphorylase Genes in Human Breast Carcinoma." *International Journal of Cancer* 97, no. 5 (2002): 631–35.

Karakaya, Songul, et al. "Identification of Non-alkaloid Natural Compounds of *Angelica purpurascens* (Avé-Lall.) Gilli. (Apiaceae) with Cholinesterase and Carbonic Anhydrase Inhibition Potential." *Saudi Pharmaceutical Journal* 28, no. 1 (2020): 1–14.

Kartal, E., Schmidt, T. S. B., Molina-Montes, E., et al. "A Faecal Microbiota Signature with High Specificity for Pancreatic Cancer." *Gut* 71 (2022). doi: 10.1136/gutjnl-2021-324755.

Kim, T. W., Joh, E. H., Kim, B., Kim, D. H. "Ginsenoside Rg5 Ameliorates Lung Inflammation in Mice by Inhibiting the Binding of LPS to Toll-Like Receptor-4 on Macrophages." *International Immunopharmacology* 12, no. 1 (January 2012): 110–16.

Levine, M. A. H., et al. "Self-Reported Use of Natural Health Products: A Cross-Sectional Telephone Survey in Older Ontarians." *American Journal Geriatric Pharmacotherapy* 7, no. 6 (2009): 383–92.

Lo, Y. C., Cruz, T. F. "Involvement of Reactive Oxygen Species in Cytokine and Growth Factor Induction of c-fos Expression in Chondrocytes." *American Society for Biochemistry and Molecular Biology* 270, no. 20 (May 19, 1995): 11727–30.

Mansouri, A., Hachem, L. D., Mansouri, S., Nassiri, F., Laperriere, N. J., Xia, D., Lindeman, N. I., Wen, P. Y., Chakravarti, A., Mehta, M. P., Hegi, M. E., Stupp, R., Aldape, K. D., Zadeh, G. "MGMT Promoter Methylation Status Testing to Guide Therapy for Glioblastoma: Refining the Approach Based on Emerging Evidence and Current Challenges." *Neurological Oncology* 21, no. 2 (February 2019): 167–178.

Matsumoto, M., et al. "Toll-Like Receptor 3 Signal in Dendritic Cells Benefits Cancer Immunotherapy." *Frontiers in Immunology* 8 (December 2017).

Metzger, R. "High Basal Level Gene Expression of Thymidine Phosphorylase (Platelet-Derived Endothelial Cell Growth Factor) in Colorectal Tumors Is Associated with Nonresponse to 5-Fluorouracil." *Clinical Cancer Research* 4, no. 10 (October 1998): 2371–76.

Milhem, M., et al. "Abstract CT144: Intratumoral Toll-Like Receptor 9 (TLR9) Agonist, CMP-001, in Combination with Pembrolizumab Can Reverse Resistance to PD-1 Inhibition in a Phase Ib Trial in Subjects with Advanced Melanoma." *Cancer Research* 78, suppl. 13 (2018): CT144. https://doi.org/10.1158/1538-7445.AM2018-CT144.

Mocan, A., et al. "Bioactive Isoflavones from *Pueraria lobata* Root and Starch: Different Extraction Techniques and Carbonic Anhydrase Inhibition." *Food and Chemical Toxicology* 112 (2018): 441–47.

Molteni, M., Bosi, A., Rossetti, C. "Natural Products with Toll-Like Receptor 4 Antagonist Activity." *International Journal of Inflammation* (March 2018): 2859135.

Morgan, G., Ward, R., Barton, M. "The Contribution of Cytotoxic Chemotherapy to 5-Year Survival in Adult Malignancies." *Clinical Oncology* 16, no. 8 (December 2004): 549–60.

National Institutes of Health National Cancer Institute. "Cancer Statistics." Updated September 25, 2020. https://www.cancer.gov/about-cancer/understanding/statistics.

Ohara, S., Suda, K., Tomizawa, K., et al. "Prognostic Value of Plasma Fibrinogen and D-Dimer Levels in Patients with Surgically Resected Non-Small Cell Lung Cancer." *Surgery Today* 50 (2020): 1427–33.

Onodera, Y., Nam, J.-M., Bissell, M. "Increased Sugar Uptake Promotes Oncogenesis via EPAC/RAP1 and O-GlcNAc Pathways." *Journal of Clinical Investigation* (2013).

Park, S. J., et al. "Serum Concentration of Sex Hormone-Binding Globulin in Healthy Volunteers and Patients with Breast Cancer Stratified by Sex and Age." *Oncology Letters* (April 21, 2020): 364–72.

Phoenix, K. N., Vumbaca, F., Fox, M. M., Evans, R., Claffey, K. P. "Dietary Energy Availability Affects Primary and Metastatic Breast Cancer and Metformin Efficacy." *Breast Cancer Research and Treatment* (November 22, 2009).

Rice, S., Pellatt, L., Ramanathan, K., Whitehead, S. A., Mason, H. D. "Metformin Inhibits Aromatase via an Extracellular Signal-Regulated Kinase-Mediated Pathway." *Endocrinology* 150, no. 10 (2009): 4794–801.

Rigano, Daniela, Sirignano, Carmina, Taglialatela-Scafati, Orazio. "The Potential of Natural Products for Targeting PPARα." *Acta Pharmaceutica Sinica B* 7, no. 4 (2017): 427–38.

Robledinos-Antón, N., Fernández-Ginés, R., Manda, G., Cuadrado, A. "Activators and Inhibitors of NRF2: A Review of Their Potential for Clinical Development." *Oxidative Medicine and Cellular Longevity* (2019): art. ID 9372182.

Rogero, M. M., Calder, P. C. "Obesity, Inflammation, Toll-Like Receptor 4 and Fatty Acids." *Nutrients* 10 (2018): 432.

Rosell, R., et al. "Molecular Predictors of Response to Chemotherapy in Lung Cancer." *Seminars in Oncology* 31, no. 20-7 (2004).

Rozengurt, E., Sinnett-Smith, J., Kisfalvi, K. "Crosstalk between Insulin/Insulin-Like Growth Factor-1 Receptors and G Protein-Coupled Receptor Signaling Systems: A Novel Target for the Antidiabetic Drug Metformin in Pancreatic Cancer." *Clinical Cancer Research* 16, no. 9 (May 1, 2010): 2505–11.

Sahin, H. "Inhibition of Carbonic Anhydrase Isozymes I and II with Natural Products Extracted from Plants, Mushrooms and Honey." *Journal of Enzyme Inhibition and Medicinal Chemistry* 27, no. 3 (2012): 395–402.

Salonga, D., et al. "Colorectal Tumors Responding to 5-Fluorouracil Have Low Gene Expression Levels of Dihydropyrimidine Dehydrogenase, Thymidylate Synthase, and Thymidine Phosphorylase." *Clinical Cancer Research* 6 no. 4 (April 2000): 1322–27.

Secord, A., et al. "The Relationship between Serum Vascular Endothelial Growth Factor, Persistent Disease, and Survival at Second-Look Laparotomy in Ovarian Cancer." *Gynecology Oncology* 94, no. 1 (July 2004): 74–79.

Shirota, Y., et al. "ERCC1 and Thymidylate Synthase mRNA Levels Predict Survival for Colorectal Cancer Patients Receiving Combination Oxaliplatin and Fluoruracil Chemotherapy." *Journal of Clinical Oncology* 19 (2001): 4298–304.

Shojania, K. G., Dixon-Woods, M. "Estimating Deaths Due to Medical Error: The Ongoing Controversy and Why It Matters." *BMJ Quality & Safety* 26 (2017): 423–28.

Simó, R., Sáez-López, C., Barbosa-Desongles, A., Hernández, C., Selva, D. M. "Novel Insights in SHBG Regulation and Clinical Implications." *Trends in Endocrinology and Metabolism* 26, no. 7 (July 2015): 376–83.

Sledge, G. W. Jr. "Vascular Endothelial Growth Factor in Breast Cancer: Biologic and Therapeutic Aspects." *Seminars in Oncology* 29, no. 3, suppl. 11 (2002): 104–10.

Spear, B. B., Heath-Chiazzi, M., Huff, J. J. "Clinical Applications of Pharmacogenetics." *Trends in Molecular Medicine* 7 (2001): 201–4.

Sporn, M. B., Liby, K. T. "NRF2 and Cancer: The Good, the Bad and the Importance of Context." *Nature Reviews Cancer* 12, no. 8 (2012): 564–71.

Statistics Canada. "Cancer Incidence in Canada, 2017." January 29, 2020. https://www150.statcan.gc.ca/n1/daily-quotidien/200129/dq200129a-eng.htm?indid=4754-1&indgeo=0.

Syed, D. N., Adhami, V. M., Khan, M. I., Mukhtar, H. "Inhibition of Akt/mTOR Signaling by the Dietary Flavonoid Fisetin." *Anticancer Agents in Medicinal Chemistry* 13, no. 7 (September 2013): 995–1001.

Sznarkowska, A., et al. "Inhibition of Cancer Antioxidant Defense by Natural Compounds." *Oncotarget* 8 (2017): 15996–6016.

Tan, H. K., Moad, A. I. H., Tan, M. L. "The mTOR Signalling Pathway in Cancer and the Potential mTOR Inhibitory Activities of Natural Phytochemicals." *Asian Pacific Organization for Cancer Prevention* 15, no. 16 (2014): 6463–75.

Tong, X., Pelling, J. C. "Targeting the PI3K/Akt/mTOR Axis by Apigenin for Cancer Prevention." *Anticancer Agents in Medicinal Chemistry* 13, no. 7 (2013): 971–78.

Tsao, H., Goel, V., Wu, H., Yang, G., Haluska, F. G. "Genetic Interaction between NRAS and BRAF Mutations and PTEN/MMAC1 Inactivation in Melanoma." *Journal of Investigative Dermatology* 122, no. 2 (2004): 337–41.

Wallace, D. C. "Mitochondria and Cancer." *Nature Reviews Cancer* 12, no. 10 (2012): 685–98.

Welch, H. G., Passow, H. J. "Quantifying the Benefits and Harms of Screening Mammography." *JAMA Internal Medicine* 174, no. 3 (2014): 448–54.

Wong, A., et al. "Genomic and In Vivo Evidence of Synergy of a Herbal Extract Compared to Its Most Active Ingredient: Rabdosia rubescens vs. Oridonin." *Experimental and Therapeutic Medicine* 1, no. 6 (November–December 2010): 1013–17.

Woolf, S. H., Chapman, D. A., Lee, J. H. "COVID-19 as the Leading Cause of Death in the United States." *Journal of the American Medical Association* 325, no. 2 (2021): 123–24.

Xie, J., Wang, X., Proud, C. G. "mTOR Inhibitors in Cancer Therapy." F1000 Research. *F1000 Faculty Review* 5 (August 25, 2016): 2078.

Yiu, S., et al. "Cancer-Generated Lactic Acid: A Regulatory, Immunosuppressive Metabolite?" *Journal of Pathology* 230, no. 4 (2013): 350–55.

Yoshinare, K., et al. "Gene Expression in Colorectal Cancer and *In Vitro* Chemosensitivity to 5-Fluorouracil: A Study of 88 Surgical Specimens." *Cancer Science* 94, no. 7 (July 2003): 633–38.

Zienoldddiny, S., et al. "A Comprehensive Analysis of Phase I and Phase II Metabolism Gene Polymorphisms and Risk of Non-Small Cell Lung Cancer in Smokers." *Carcinogenesis* 29, no. 6 (June 2008): 1164–69.

Chapter 9: Materia Medica for Managing Cancer: The Cytotoxic Herbs

ARTEMISIA ANNUA

Bilia, A. R. "Essential Oil of *Artemisia annua* L.: An Extraordinary Component with Numerous Antimicrobial Properties." *Evidence-Based Complementary and Alternative Medicine* (2014): art. ID 159819.

Brisibe, E. A., et al. "Nutritional Characterisation and Antioxidant Capacity of Different Tissues of *Artemisia annua* L." *Food Chemistry* 115 (2009): 1240–46.

Efferth, T. "From Ancient Herb to Modern Drug: *Artemisia annua* and Artemisinin for Cancer Therapy." *Seminars in Cancer Biology* 46 (October 2017): 65–83.

Gordi, T., Huong, D. X., Hai, T. N., Nieu, N. T., Ashton, M. "Artemisinin Pharmacokinetics and Efficacy in Uncomplicated-Malaria Patients Treated with Two Different Dosage Regimens." *Antimicrobial Agents and Chemotherapy* 46, no. 4 (April 2002): 1026–31.

Klayman, D. L. "Qinghaosu (Artemisinin): An Antimalarial Drug from China." *Science* 228, no. 4703 (May 31, 1985): 1049–55.

Konstat-Korzenny, E., Ascencio-Aragón, J. A., Niezen-Lugo, S., Vázquez-López, R. "Artemisinin and Its Synthetic Derivatives as a Possible Therapy for Cancer." *Medical Sciences* 6, no. 1 (2018): 19.

Lam, N. S., et al. "Combination Therapy Enhanced the Antitumor Activity of Artemisinin-Iron in Lung Cancer Calu-6 Cells." *European Journal of Oncology* 22, no. 1 (2017): 31–37.

Langa, S. J., et al. "Antitumor Activity of an *Artemisia annua* Herbal Preparation and Identification of Active Ingredients." *Phytomedicine* 62 (September 2019): 152962.

Lichota, A., Gwozdzinsk, K. "Anticancer Activity of Natural Compounds from Plant and Marine Environment." *International Journal of Molecular Sciences* 19, no. 11 (November 9, 2018): 3533.

Mukhtar, E. "Targeting Microtubules by Natural Agents for Cancer Therapy." *Molecular Cancer Therapeutics* 13, no. 2 (February 2014): 275–84.

Rassiasa, D. J., Weathers, P. J. "Dried Leaf *Artemisia annua* Efficacy against Non-Small Cell Lung Cancer." *Phytomedicine* 52 (January 2019): 247–53.

Shahbazfàr, A. A., Zare, P., Mohammadpour, H. "Artemisinin and Its Derivatives: A Potential Treatment for Leukemia." *Anti-cancer Drugs* 30, no. 1 (January 2019): 1–18.

Singh, N. P., Lai, H. C. "Synergistic Cytotoxicity of Artemisinin and Sodium Butyrate on Human Cancer Cells." *Anticancer Research* 25, no. 6B (November 2005): 4325–31.

Zheng, G. Q. "Cytotoxic Terpenoids and Flavonoids from *Artemisia annua*." *Planta Medica* 60, no. 1 (February 1994): 54–57.

Zheng, W., Wang, S. Y. "Antioxidant Activity and Phenolic Compounds in Selected Herbs."

Journal of Agricultural and Food Chemistry 40, no. 11 (2001): 5165–70.

Zhu, X., et al. "Effects of Sesquiterpene, Flavonoid and Coumarin Types of Compounds from *Artemisia annua* L. on Production of Mediators of Angiogenesis." *Pharmacological Reports* 65, no. 2 (March–April 2013): 410–20.

ASIMINA TRILOBA

Horne, S. H. *The Power of Paw Paw* (audiotape). Tree of Light Publishing, 2003.

Lannuzel, A., et al. "The Mitochondrial Complex I Inhibitor Annonacin Is Toxic to Mesencephalic Dopaminergic Neurons by Impairment of Energy Metabolism." *Neuroscience* 121, no. 2 (2003): 287–96.

McLaughlin, J. L. "Paw Paw and Cancer: Annonaceous Acetogenins from Discovery to Commercial Product." *Journal of Natural Products* 71 (2008): 1311–21.

Nam, J. S., Jang, H. L., Rhee, Y. H. "Antioxidant Activities and Phenolic Compounds of Several Tissues of Pawpaw (*Asimina triloba* [L.] Dunal) Grown in Korea." *Journal of Food Sciences* 82, no. 8 (August 2017): 1827–33.

Nam, J. S., Park, S. Y., Lee, H. J., Lee, S. O., Jang, H. L., Rhee, Y. H. "Correlation between Acetogenin Content and Antiproliferative Activity of Pawpaw (*Asimina triloba* [L.] Dunal) Fruit Pulp Grown in Korea." *Journal of Food Sciences* 83, no. 5 (May 2018): 1430–35.

Potts, L. F., Luzzio, F. A., Smith, S. C., Hetman, M., Champy, P., Litvan, I. "Annonacin in *Asimina triloba* Fruit: Implication for Neurotoxicity." *Neurotoxicology* 33, no. 1 (January 2012): 53–58.

BUTYRATE

Banasiewicz, T., Domagalska, D., Borycka-Kiciak, K., Rydzewska, G. "Determination of Butyric Acid Dosage Based on Clinical and Experimental Studies—A Literature Review." *Przegląd Gastroenterologiczny* 15, no. 2 (2020): 119–25.

Borycka-Kiciak, K., Banasiewicz, T., Rydzewska, G. "Butyric Acid—A Well-Known Molecule Revisited." *Przegląd Gastroenterologiczny* 12, no. 2 (2017): 83–89.

Cleophas, M. C. P., Ratter, J. M., Bekkering, S., et al. "Effects of Oral Butyrate Supplementation on Inflammatory Potential of Circulating Peripheral Blood Mononuclear Cells in Healthy and Obese Males." *Science Reports* 9, no. 1 (2019): 775.

Donohoe, D. R., et al. "The Warburg Effect Dictates the Mechanism of Butyrate-Mediated Histone Acetylation and Cell Proliferation." *Molecular Cell* 48, no. 4 (2012): 612–26.

Guan, X., et al. "A Double Edged Sword: The Role of Butyrate in the Oral Cavity and the Gut." *Molecular Oral Microbiology* (2020): 1–11.

McOrist, A. L., et al. "Fecal Butyrate Levels Vary Widely Among Individuals but Are Usually Increased by a Diet High in Resistant Starch." *Journal of Nutrition* 141, no. 5 (May 2011): 883–89.

Nakagawa, H., Sasagawa, S., Itoh, K. "Sodium Butyrate Induces Senescence and Inhibits the Invasiveness of Glioblastoma Cells." *Oncology Letters* 15, no. 2 (2018): 1495–502.

Singh, V., Yeoh, B. S., Vijay-Kumar, M. "Feed Your Gut with Caution!" *Translational Cancer Research* 5, suppl. 3 (2016): S507–13.

Vernia, P., Monteleone, G., Grandinetti, G., et al. "Combined Oral Sodium Butyrate and Mesalazine Treatment Compared to Oral Mesalazine Alone in Ulcerative Colitis." *Digestive Diseases and Sciences* 45 (2000): 976–81.

CAMPTOTHECA ACUMINATA

He, H., Shang, X. Y., Liu, W. W., Zhang, Y., Song, S. J. "Triterpenes from the Fruit of *Camptotheca acuminata* Suppress Human Hepatocellular Carcinoma Cell Proliferation through Apoptosis Induction." *Natural Product Research* 33, no. 24 (December 2019): 3527–32.

Li, S., Yi, Y., Wang, Y., Zhang, Z., Beasley, R. S. "Camptothecin Accumulation and Variations in Camptotheca." *Planta Medica* 68, no. 11 (November 2002): 1010–16.

Li, S., Zhang, W., Northrup, K., and Zhang, D. "Distribution of Camptotheca Decaisne: Endangered Status." Pharmaceutical Crops 5, no. 1 (2014): 135–39.

Lin, C. H., et al. "Antitumor Effects and Biological Mechanism of Action of the Aqueous Extract of the *Camptotheca acuminata* Fruit in Human Endometrial Carcinoma Cells." *Evidence-Based Complementary and Alternative Medicine* (2014): art. ID 564810.

Lucas, Jeremy W. "Why Is This the 'Happy Tree?' (*Camptotheca acuminate*) (Xi Shu)." Dave's Garden (online horticulture forum). https://davesgarden.com/guides/articles/view/206.

Potmesil, M., Pinedo, H. *Camptothecins: New Anticancer Agents.* CRC Press, 1994.

Sun, H., Li, C., Ni, Y., Yao, L., Jiang, H., Ren, X., Fu, Y., Zhao, C. "Ultrasonic/Microwave-Assisted Extraction of Polysaccharides from *Camptotheca acuminata* Fruits and Its Antitumor Activity." *Carbohydrate Polymers* 206 (2019): 557–64.

CATHARANTHUS ROSEUS

Arora, R., et al. "Anticancer Alkaloids of *Catharanthus roseus*: Transition from Traditional to Modern Medicine." In *Herbal Medicine: A Cancer Chemopreventive and Therapeutic Perspective*. Jaypee Brothers Medical Publishing, 2009. https://www.researchgate.net/publication/312936839.

Asija, R., Samariya, S., Khanijau, R., Verma, T. "A Pharmacological Review on *Catharanthus roseus* Linn." *Chemistry Research Journal* 7, no. 3 (2022): 73–79.

Das, S., Sharangi, A. "Madagascar periwinkle (*Catharanthus roseus* L.): Diverse Medicinal and Therapeutic Benefits to Humankind." *Journal of Pharmacognosy and Phytochemistry* 6, no. 5 (2017): 1695–701.

Mishra, J., Verma, N. "A Brief Study on *Catharanthus roseus*: A Review." *International Journal of Research in Pharmacy and Pharmaceutical Sciences* 2, no. 2 (2017): 20–23.

Nisar, A., et al. "An Updated Review on *Catharanthus roseus*: Phytochemical and Pharmacological Analysis." *Indian Research Journal of Pharmacy and Science* 3, no. 2 (June 2016): 6.

Paarakh, M., et al. "*Catharanthus roseus* Linn—A Review." *Acta Scientific Pharmaceutical Sciences* 3, no. 10 (2019): 19–24.

Pereira, D., et al. "Exploiting *Catharanthus roseus* Roots: Source of Antioxidants." *Food Chemistry* 12, no. 1 (2010): 56–61.

CHELIDONIUM MAJUS

Biswas, S. J., Khuda-Bukhsh, A. R. "Effect of a Homeopathic Drug, Chelidonium, in Amelioration of p-DAB Induced Hepatocarcinogenesis in Mice." *BMC Complementary and Alternative Medicine* 2 (April 10, 2002): 4.

El-Readi, M. Z., Eid, S. F., Ashour, M. L., Tahrani, A., Wink, M. "Modulation of Multidrug Resistance in Cancer Cells by Chelidonine and *Chelidonium majus* Alkaloids." *Phytomedicine* 20, nos. 3–4 (2013): 282–94.

Ernst, E., Schmidt, K. "Ukrain—A New Cancer Cure? A Systematic Review of Randomised Clinical Trials." *BMC Cancer* 5, no. 69 (2005).

Gansauge, F., et al. "NSC-631570 Ukrain in the Palliative Treatment of Pancreatic Cancer. Results of a Phase II Trial." *Langenbecks Archives of Surgery* 386, no. 8 (March 2002): 570–74.

Lohninger, A., Hamler, F. "*Chelidonium majus* L. (Ukrain) in the Treatment of Cancer Patients." *Drugs under Experimental and Clinical Research* 18, suppl. (1992): 73–77.

Mazzanti, G., Di Sotto, A., Franchitto, A., Mammola, C. L., Mariani, P., Mastrangelo, S., et al. "*Chelidonium majus* Is Not Hepatotoxic in Wistar Rats, in a 4 Weeks Feeding Experiment." *Journal of Ethnopharmacology* 126 (2009): 518–24.

Memorial Sloan Kettering Cancer Center. "Ukrain." https://www.mskcc.org/cancer-care/integrative-medicine/herbs/ukrain.

Panzer, A., et al. "Chemical Analyses of Ukrain™, a Semi-Synthetic *Chelidonium majus* Alkaloid Derivative, Fail to Confirm Its Trimeric Structure." *Cancer Letters* 160, no. 2 (2000): 237–41.

Park, S., Kim, S. R., Kim, Y., Lee, J., Woo, H., Yoon, Y., Kim, Y. I. "*Chelidonium majus* L. Extract Induces Apoptosis through Caspase Activity via MAPK-Independent NF-κB Signaling in Human Epidermoid Carcinoma A431 Cells." *Oncology Reports* 33 (2015): 419–24.

Uglyanitsa, K. N., et al. "Ukrain–A Novel Antitumor Drug." *Drugs under Experimental and Clinical Research* 26, nos. 5–6 (2000): 341–56.

Zielińska, S. "Greater Celandine's Ups and Downs—21 Centuries of Medicinal Uses of *Chelidonium majus*." *Frontiers in Pharmacology* 9 (2018): 299.

LARREA DIVARICATA/ L. TRIDENTATA

Gnabre, J., Bates, R., Huang, R. C. "Creosote Bush Lignans for Human Disease Treatment and Prevention: Perspectives on Combination Therapy." *Journal of Traditional and Complementary Medicine* 5, no. 3 (March 2015): 119–26.

Heron, S., Yarnell, E. "The Safety of Low-Dose *Larrea tridentata* (DC) Coville (Creosote Bush or Chaparral): A Retrospective Clinical Study." *Journal of Alternative and Complementary Medicine* 7, no. 2 (April 2001): 175–85.

Lambert, J. D., Sang, S., Dougherty, A., Caldwell, C. G., Meyers, R. O., Dorr, R. T., Timmermann, B. N. "Cytotoxic Lignans from *Larrea tridentata*." *Phytochemistry* 66, no. 7 (April 2005): 811–15.

Martins, S., Aguilar, C. N., Teixeira, J. A., Mussatto, S. I., "Bioactive Compounds (Phytoestrogens) Recovery from *Larrea Tridentata* Leaves by Solvents Extraction." *Separation and Purification Technology* 88 (2012): 163–67.

Navarro, V. J., Barnhart, H., Bonkovsky, H. L., Davern, T., Fontana, R. J., Grant, L., Reddy,

K. R., Seeff, L. B., Serrano, J., Sherker, A. H., Stolz, A., Talwalkar, J., Vega, M., Vuppalanchi, R. "Liver Injury from Herbals and Dietary Supplements in the U.S. Drug-Induced Liver Injury Network." *Hepatology* 60, no. 4 (October 2014): 1399–408.

Seeff, L., Victor, J., Navarro, V. J. "Hepatotoxicity of Herbals and Dietary Supplements." In *Drug-Induced Liver Disease,* 3rd ed. Elsevier, 2013.

PHYTOLACCA DECANDRA, P. AMERICANA

Bailly, C. "Medicinal Properties and Anti-Inflammatory Components of *Phytolacca* (Shanglu)." *Digital Chinese Medicine* 4, no. 3 (2021): 159–169.

Cook, W. H. *The Physio-Medical Dispensatory.* (Wm. H. Cook, 1869): 519. Accessed at https://www.americanherbalistsguild.com/sites/americanherbalistsguild.com/files/1869-cook-physiomedical-dispensatory-combined.pdf.

Das, J., et al. "Strong Anticancer Potential of Nano-Triterpenoid from Phytolacca decandra against A549 Adenocarcinoma via a Ca2+-dependent Mitochondrial Apoptotic Pathway." *Journal of Acupuncture and Meridian Studies* 7, no. 3 (2014): 140-150.

Ghosh, S., et al. "Oleanolic Acid Isolated from Ethanolic Extract of Phytolacca decandra Induces Apoptosis in A375 Skin Melanoma Cells: Drug-DNA Interaction and Signaling Cascade." *Journal of Integrative Medicine* 12, no. 2 (2014): 102–114.

Ng, W. Y., et al. "Poisoning by Toxic Plants in Hong Kong: A 15-Year Review." *Hong Kong Medical Journal* 25, no. 2 (2019): 102.

PODOPHYLLUM PELTATUM

American Society for Horticultural Science. "Anticancer Compound Found in Common Plant: American Mayapple." *ScienceDaily,* September 8, 2009. www.sciencedaily.com/releases/2009/09/090904165243.htm.

Becker, H. "American Mayapple Yields Anti-cancer Extract." Agricultural Research Service, U.S. Department of Agriculture, 2000.

Brinker, F. "Podophyllum and Podophyllin." *Eclectic Medical Journals* II, no. 2. (April/May 1996).

Cook, W. H. *The Physio-Medical Dispensatory.* (Wm. H. Cook, 1869). 527. Accessed at https://www.americanherbalistsguild.com/sites/americanherbalistsguild.com/files/1869-cook-physiomedical-dispensatory-combined.pdf.

Felter, H. W., Lloyd, J. U. *King's American Dispensatory,* 1898. Reprinted by Eclectic Medical Publications, Oregon, 1985.

Gordaliza, M., Castro, M. A., del Corral, J. M., Feliciano, A. S. "Antitumor Properties of Podophyllotoxin and Related Compounds." *Current Pharmaceutical Design* 6, no. 18 (December 2000): 1811–39.

Hong, W. G., Cho, J. H., Hwang, S., Lee, E., Lee, J., Kim, J., Um, H., and Park, J. K. "Chemosensitizing Effect of Podophyllotoxin Acetate on Topoisomerase Inhibitors Leads to Synergistic Enhancement of Lung Cancer Cell Apoptosis." *International Journal of Oncology* 48 (2016): 2265–76.

Kandil, S., Wymant, J. M., Kariuki, B. M., Jones, A. T., McGuigan, C., Westwell, A. D. "Novel Cis-selective and Non-epimerisable C3 Hydroxy Azapodophyllotoxins Targeting Microtubules in Cancer Cells." *European Journal of Medicinal Chemistry* 110 (March 3, 2016).

Moura, Mariela Dutra Gontijo, Haddad, João Paulo Amaral, Senna, Maria Inês Barreiros, Ferreira e Ferreira, Efigênia, Mesquita, Ricardo Alves. "A New Topical Treatment Protocol for Oral Hairy Leukoplakia." *Oral Surgery, Oral Medicine, Oral Pathology, Oral Radiology, and Endodontology* 110, no. 5 (2010): 611–17.

SANGUINARIA CANADENSIS

Cook, W. H. *The Physio-Medical Dispensatory*. (Wm. H. Cook, 1869). 466–67. Accessed at https://www.americanherbalistsguild.com/sites/americanherbalistsguild.com/files/1869-cook-physiomedical-dispensatory-combined.pdf.

Croaker, A., King, G. J., Pyne, J. H., Anoopkumar-Dukie, S., Liu, L. "*Sanguinaria canadensis*: Traditional Medicine, Phytochemical Composition, Biological Activities and Current Uses." *International Journal of Molecular Sciences* 17, no. 9 (2016): 1414.

European Medicines Agency. Public assessment report (EPAR) from the Committee for Medicinal Products for Human Use (CHMP), Imiquimod Safety profile and EMA Summary of Product Characteristics. http://www.ema.europa.eu.

Gupta, M., Mahajan, V. K., Mehta, K. S., Chauhan, P. S. "Zinc Therapy in Dermatology: A Review." *Dermatology Research and Practice* 2014 (2014): 709152.

Senchina, D. S., Flinn, G. N., McCann, D. A., Kohut, M. L. Shearn, C. T. "Bloodroot (*Sanguinaria canadensis* L., Papaveraceae) Enhances Proliferation and Cytokine Production by Human Peripheral Blood

Mononuclear Cells in an *In Vitro* Model." *Journal of Herbs, Spices & Medicinal Plants* 15, no. 1 (2009): 45–65.

TAXUS BREVIFOLIA, T. BACCATA, T. WALLICHIANA

Amaral, R. G., et al. "Natural Products as Treatment against Cancer: A Historical and Current Vision." *Clinics in Oncology* 4 (2019): 15621.

Dai, J. "Chemo-Enzymatic Transformation of Taxanes and Their Reversal Activity towards MDR Tumor Cells." *Current Topics in Medicinal Chemistry* 9, no. 17 (December 31, 2008): 1625–35.

Gunther, E. *Ethnobotany of Western Washington.* University of Washington Press, 1973.

Hasegawa, T., Bai, J., Zhang, S., Wang, J., Matsubara, J., Kawakami, J., Tomida, A., Tsuruo, T., Hirose, K., Sakai, J., Kikuchi, M., Abe, M., Ando, M. "Structure-Activity Relationships of Some Taxoids as Multidrug Resistance Modulator." *Bioorganic and Medicinal Chemistry Letters* 17, no. 4 (February 15, 2007): 1122–26.

Juyal, D., Thawani, V., Thaledi, S., Joshi, M. "Ethnomedical Properties of *Taxus wallichiana* Zucc. (Himalayan Yew)." *Journal of Traditional and Complementary Medicine* 4, no. 3 (July 2014): 159–61.

Li, X., Choi, J. S. "Effect of Genistein on the Pharmacokinetics of Paclitaxel Administered Orally or Intravenously in Rats." *International Journal of Pharmacy* 337, nos. 1–2 (June 7, 2007): 188–93.

Nadeem, M., Rikhari, H. C., Kumar, A., Palni, L. M., Nandi, S. K. "Taxol Content in the Bark of Himalayan Yew in Relation to Tree Age and Sex." *Phytochemistry* 60, no. 6 (July 2002): 627–31.

Native American Ethnobotany Database. "*Taxus brevifolia* Nutt." http://naeb.brit.org.

Product Safety Labs. "Montana Yew Tip Powder Acute Oral Toxicity Test in Rats." Unpublished report. E90601-5D. 1999.

Sharma, H., Garg, M. "Neuropharmacological Activities of *Taxus wallichiana* Bark in Swiss Albino Mice." *Indian Journal of Pharmacology* 47, no. 3 (2015): 299–303.

Sharma, H., Garg, M. "A Review of Traditional Use, Phytoconstituents and Biological Activities of Himalayan Yew, *Taxus wallichiana*." *Journal of Integrated Medicine* 13, no. 2 (March 13, 2015): 80–90.

Tranca, S., Petrisor, C. L. "A Fatal Case of Taxus Poisoning." *Clinical Medicine* 86, no. 3 (2013): 279–81.

Wahab, Abdul, Khera R., et al. "A Review on Phytochemistry and Medicinal Uses of *Taxus wallichiana* L. (Himalayan Yew)." *International Journal of Chemical and Biochemical Sciences* 9 (2016): 116–20.

Wheeler, N. C., Jech, K., Masters, S., Brobst, S. W., Alvarado, A. B., Hoover, A. J., Snader, K. M. "Effects of Genetic, Epigenetic, and Environmental Factors on Taxol Content in *Taxus brevifolia* and Related Species." *Journal of Natural Products* 55, no. 4 (April 1992): 432–40.

THUJA OCCIDENTALIS

Biswas, R., Mandal, S. K., Dutta, S., Bhattacharyya, S. S., Boujedaini, N., Khuda-Bukhsh, A. R. "Thujone-Rich Fraction of *Thuja occidentalis* Demonstrates Major Anti-cancer Potentials: Evidences from *In Vitro* Studies on A375 Cells." *Evidence-Based Complementary Alternative Medicine* 2011 (2011): 568148.

Caruntu, S., Ciceu, A., Olah, N. K., Don, I., Hermenean, A., Cotoraci, C. "*Thuja occidentalis* L. (Cupressaceae): Ethnobotany, Phytochemistry and Biological Activity." *Molecules* 25, no. 22 (2020): 5416.

Durzan, D. J. "Arginine, Scurvy and Cartier's 'Tree of Life.'" *Journal of Ethnobiology and Ethnomedicine* 5 (February 2, 2009): 5.

Elsharkawy, E. M., Aljohar, H., Donia, A. E. L . "Comparative Study of Antioxidant and Anticancer Activity of *Thuja orientalis* Growing in Egypt and Saudi Arabia." *British Journal of Pharmaceutical Research* 15, no. 5 (January 2017): 1–9.

Kamdem, P. D., Hanover, J. W. "Inter-tree Variation of Essential Oil Composition of *Thuja occidentalis* L." *Journal of Essential Oil Research* 5, no. 3 (1993): 279–82.

Naser, B., Bodinet, C., Tegtmeier, M., Lindequist, U. "*Thuja occidentalis* (Arbor vitae): A Review of Its Pharmaceutical, Pharmacological and Clinical Properties." *Evidence-Based Complementary and Alternative Medicine* 2, no. 1 (2005): 69–78.

Offergeld, R., Reinecker, C., Gumz, E., Schrum, S., Treiber, R., Neth, R. D., Gohla, S. H. "Mitogenic Activity of High Molecular Polysaccharide Fractions Isolated from the Cuppressaceae *Thuja occidentalis* L. Enhanced Cytokine-Production by Thyapolysaccharide, G-Fraction (TPSg)." *Leukemia* 6, suppl. 3 (1992): 189S–91S.

Pelkonen, O., Abass, K., Wiesner, J. "Thujone and Thujone-Containing Herbal Medicinal and Botanical Products: Toxicological Assessment." *Regulatory Toxicology and Pharmacology* 65, no. 1 (February 2013): 100–107.

Sunila, E. S., Hamsa, T. P., Kuttan, G. "Effect of *Thuja occidentalis* and Its Polysaccharide on Cell-Mediated Immune Responses and Cytokine Levels of Metastatic Tumor-Bearing Animals." *Pharmaceutical Biology* 49, no. 10 (October 2011): 1065–73.

Torres, A., Vargas, Y., Uribe, D., Carrasco, C., Torres, C., Rocha, R., Oyarzún, C., San Martín, R., Quezada, C. "Pro-apoptotic and Anti-angiogenic Properties of the A /B-Thujone Fraction from *Thuja occidentalis* on Glioblastoma Cells." *Journal of Neurooncology* 128, no. 1 (May 2016): 9–19.

VISCUM ALBUM

Bar-Sela, G., Wollner, M., Hammer, L., Agbarya, A., Dudnik, E., Haim, N. "Mistletoe as Complementary Treatment in Patients with Advanced Non-Small-Cell Lung Cancer Treated with Carboplatin-Based Combinations: A Randomised Phase II Study." *European Journal of Cancer* 49, no. 5 (March 2013): 1058–64.

Freuding, M., Keinki, C., Micke, O., et al. "Mistletoe in Oncological Treatment: A Systematic Review." *Journal of Cancer Research and Clinical Oncology* 145 (2019): 695–707.

Huber, R., Schlodder, D., Effertz, C., et al. "Safety of Intravenously Applied Mistletoe Extract—Results from a Phase I Dose Escalation Study in Patients with Advanced Cancer." *British Medical Council Complementary and Alternative Medicine* 17 (2017): 465.

Kienle, G. S., Berrino, F., Büssing, A., Portalupi, E., Rosenzweig, S., Kiene, H. "Mistletoe in Cancer: A Systematic Review on Controlled Clinical Trials." *European Journal of Medical Research* 8, no. 3 (2003): 109–19.

Kienle, G. S., Kiene, H. "Review Article: Influence of *Viscum album* L (European Mistletoe) Extracts on Quality of Life in Cancer Patients: A Systematic Review of Controlled Clinical Studies." *Integrative Cancer Therapies* 9, no. 2 (June 2010): 142–57.

Loef, M., Walach, H. "Quality of Life in Cancer Patients Treated with Mistletoe: A Systematic Review and Meta-analysis." *BMC Complementary Medical Therapies* 20 (2020): 227.

Ostermann, T., Raak, C., Büssing, A. "Survival of Cancer Patients Treated with Mistletoe Extract (Iscador): A Systematic Literature Review." *British Medical Council Cancer* 9 (2009): 451.

Piao, B. K., Wang, Y.X., Xie, G. R., Mansmann, U., Matthes, H., Beuth, J., Lin, H. S. "Impact of Complementary Mistletoe Extract Treatment on Quality of Life in Breast, Ovarian and Non-Small Cell Lung Cancer Patients. A Prospective Randomized Controlled Clinical Trial." *Anticancer Research* 24, no. 1 (January–February 2004): 303–9.

Chapter 10: Case Histories

Au, J. L., Badalament, R. A., Wientjes, M. G., Young, D. C., Warner, J. A., Venema, P. L., Pollifrone, D. L., Harbrecht, J. D., Chin, J. L., Lerner, S. P., Miles, B. J. International Mitomycin C Consortium. "Methods to Improve Efficacy of Intravesical Mitomycin C: Results of a Randomized Phase III Trial." *Journal of the National Cancer Institute* 93, no. 8 (April 18, 2001): 597–604.

Ielciu, I., Frédérich, M., Hanganu, D., Angenot, L., Olah, N.-K., Ledoux, A., Crişan, G., Păltinean, R. "Flavonoid Analysis and Antioxidant Activities of the *Bryonia alba* L. Aerial Parts." *Antioxidants* 8, no. 4 (2019): 108.

Ilhan, Mert, Dereli, Fatma Tuğçe Gürağaç, Tümen, Ibrahim, Akkol, Esra Küpeli. "Anti-inflammatory and Antinociceptive Features of *Bryonia alba* L.: As a Possible Alternative in Treating Rheumatism." *Open Chemistry* 17, no. 1 (2019): 23–30.

Kujawska, M., Svanber, I. "From Medicinal Plant to Noxious Weed: *Bryonia alba* L. (Cucurbitaceae) in Northern and Eastern Europe." *Journal of Ethnobiology and Ethnomedicine* 15 (2019): 22.

Lamm, D. L., Stogdill, V. D., Stogdill, B. J., Crispen, R. G. "Complications of Bacillus Calmette-Guerin Immunotherapy in 1,278 Patients with Bladder Cancer." *Journal of Urology* 135, no. 2 (February 1986): 272–74.

Lokeshwar, V. B., Block, N. L. "HA-HAase Urine Test. A Sensitive and Specific Method for Detecting Bladder Cancer and Evaluating Its Grade." *Urology Clinics of North America* 27, no. 1 (February 2000): 53–61.

Pedersen, S. A., Gaist, D., Schmidt, S. A. J., Hölmich, L. R., Friis, S., Pottegård, A. "Hydrochlorothiazide Use and Risk of Nonmelanoma Skin Cancer: A Nationwide Case-Control Study from Denmark." *Journal of the American Academy of Dermatology* 78, no. 4 (April 2018): 673–81.e9.

Pirzada, M. T., Ghauri, R., Ahmed, M. J., et al. "Outcomes of BCG Induction in High-Risk Non-Muscle-Invasive Bladder Cancer Patients (NMIBC): A Retrospective Cohort Study." *Cureus* 9, no. 1 (2017): e957.

Glossary

Adaptogen. A normalizing and tonic herb for adrenal and other neuroendocrine functions. Rejuvenating, restorative.

Akt. A protein kinase B receptor/enzyme that plays a key role in multiple cellular processes, such as glucose metabolism, apoptosis, cell proliferation, transcription, and cell migration.

ALT. Alanine transaminase; a liver enzyme that is elevated if there is liver stress or damage.

Alterative. An herb used in detoxification programs to remove toxins; a blood cleanser.

Amphoteric. Balancing and stabilizing; a term from chemistry meaning to normalize.

Angiogenesis. New blood vessel formation.

Anthraquinone. A water-soluble laxative phenolic compound.

Anxiolytic. An herb that reduces anxiety.

AP-1. Activator protein 1; a transcription factor.

Aperient. A very mild bowel-stimulating herb.

Apoptosis. Programmed cell death; a normal healthy cell behavior.

AST. Aspartate aminotransferase; a liver enzyme that is elevated if there is liver stress or damage.

Astringent. Toning, tightening, and drying to tissues.

ATP. Adenosine triphosphate; the major energy currency in the cell; cleaving a phosphate group releases energy.

Bax. A tumor suppressor gene.

BCG. Bacillus Calmette-Guérin; an immunotherapy for bladder cancer.

Bcl-2. A gene that codes for a protein that induces and regulates apoptosis; mutates early to resist apoptosis.

BDNF. Brain-derived neurotrophic factor; regulates and supports tissue repair; antioxidant and anti-inflammatory in nerve cells.

β-FGF. Beta-fibroblast growth factor; involved in angiogenesis.

BRCA1 and BRCA2. Tumor-suppressor genes; mutations lead to increased occurrence of several cancers, including breast, ovarian, primary peritoneal, prostate, and pancreatic.

BUN. Blood urea nitrogen; a routine blood test that measures the ability of the kidneys to clear metabolic wastes.

CA9. Carbonic anhydrase 9; a transmembrane protein induced by hypoxia that contributes to angiogenesis, apoptosis inhibition, and disruption of cell-to-cell adhesion.

CA15-3. Cancer antigen in the blood; indicates active breast cancer.

CA19-9. Cancer antigen in the blood; indicates active pancreatic and other abdominal cancers.

CA27/29. Cancer antigen in the blood; indicates active breast cancer.

CA125. Cancer antigen in the blood; indicates ovarian and pelvic cancers.

CAMs. Cell adhesion molecules; glycoproteins that glue cells together and facilitate cell-to-cell communication.

Carminative. Coordinating and regulating contractions of circular and longitudinal muscle around the gut to promote proper peristalsis; a function of the volatile oils.

CDK. Cyclin-dependent kinases; enzymes required for cell cycling (cell division).

CDK 4/6 inhibitor drugs. Ribociclib (Kisqali) and palbociclib (Ibrance).

CDKI. Cyclin-dependent kinase inhibitors; proteins, including p21 and p27, that regulate CDKs.

CEA. Carcinoembryonic antigen; indicates breast, lung, pancreatic, stomach, liver, or ovarian cancer. Note that CEA can also be elevated in peptic ulcer, ulcerative colitis, rectal polyps, emphysema, benign breast disease, or an inflammation such as pancreatitis or cholecystitis and in smokers who do not have cancer.

Cholagogue. An herb that promotes bile release from the gallbladder.

Choleretic. An herb that promotes bile production.

C-myc. A cancer-promoting oncogene.

COX. Cyclooxygenase; an enzyme that drives inflammation.

CPT. Camptothecin; an anticancer alkaloid from the *Camptotheca acuminata* tree.

CRP. C-reactive protein; a protein made in the liver; level rises in the blood during the acute phase of an inflammatory/infectious process.

CTC. Circulating tumor cells; measures how many cells in a blood sample express a certain type of cell adhesion molecule that indicates metastasis.

Cx. Connexins; proteins that span gap junctions, directly connecting cells to cells, and the genes that code for them.

DCIS. Ductal carcinoma in situ; local and indolent breast cancer.

Demulcent. The action of mucilage that is soothing, cooling, healing, and moistening to mucous membranes when ingested.

Dendritic cells. Antigen-presenting cells located in epithelial tissues exposed to the external environment (skin and the inner lining of the nose, lungs, stomach, and intestines) that alert T cells in the lymph nodes of impending danger or threat.

DHA. Docosahexaenoic acid; omega-3 essential fatty acid from fish oil.

DHEA. Dehydroepiandrosterone; a steroid hormone precursor made by adrenal glands.

Diaphoretic. Promotes and induces a desirable fever, directs blood to the skin, opens the pores, allows free perspiration.

DIM. 3,3'-diindolylmethane; promotes phase I liver detox support.

DNA. Deoxyribonucleic acid; codes for amino acids to make proteins.

EBV. Epstein Barr virus; may contribute to lymphoma.

ECM. Extracellular matrix; the gel in which all cells are embedded.

EGCG. Epigallocatechin gallate; a flavonoid from green tea.

EGF. Epidermal growth factor.

EGFr. A family of EGF receptors.

eGFR. Estimated glomerular filtration rate; a routine blood test that measures the ability of the kidneys to clear metabolic wastes.

Emmenagogue. An herb that promotes easier, free-flowing menses.

Emollient. The action of mucilage that is soothing, cooling, healing, and moistening to skin.

EPA. Eicosapentaenoic acid; omega-3 essential fatty acid from fish oil.

ER+. Estrogen receptor–positive; cancer expresses or overexpresses receptor sites for estrogen.

ESR. Erythrocyte sedimentation rate; a marker in a blood test showing inflammation.

EtOH. Ethyl alcohol.

GABA. Gamma-aminobutyric acid; an inhibitory neurotransmitter.

GAGs. Glycosaminoglycans; structural units in the ECM.

GGT. Gamma-glutamyl transferase; a liver enzyme that is elevated if there is liver stress or damage.

GLUT3. Glucose transporter 3; facilitates entry of sugar into cells.

Glycolytic shift. Replacement of normal oxygen respiration (Krebs cycle) by glycolysis.

Gram-positive bacteria. A category of bacteria with a thick peptidoglycan (protein and sugar) cell wall layer that shows up with specific staining (e.g., *Staphylococcus* and *Streptococcus* species). If the peptidoglycan layer is thin, it's classified as gram negative (e.g., cholera, *E. coli*, and plague).

H2O2. Hydrogen peroxide.

HDAC. Histone deacetylase; an enzyme that helps unwind DNA for copying.

HER2/neu. Epidermal growth factor receptor; target of Herceptin drug.

HIF-1. Hypoxia-inducible factor 1.

HMGR. Hydroxymethylglutaryl coenzyme A reductase; a gatekeeper enzyme in fat metabolism.

HPA axis. Hypothalamic-pituitary-adrenal axis.

HPV. Human papilloma virus; the cause of genital warts.

I3C. Indole-3-carbinol; a supplement that converts to DIM to promote phase I liver detox.

ICAM. Intercellular adhesion molecule; part of the immunoglobulin superfamily that regulates and controls inflammation, immune responses, and intracellular signaling events.

IGF. Insulin-like growth factor.

IGFBP. Insulin-like growth factor binding protein.

IL. Interleukin.

Integrins. Transmembrane receptors/proteins that anchor cells into the extracellular matrix by binding with collagen, laminin, and fibronectin.

In vitro. "In glass," referring to research done in test tubes and on growth media.

In vivo. "In real life," referring to research performed on animals and humans.

IP6. Inositol hexaphosphate; a supplement that downregulates signal transduction.

Ki67. A nuclear protein measured on pathology slides that is associated with more proliferative cancer.

LDH. Lactate dehydrogenase; a blood marker of liver stress and of glycolytic cancer cell metabolism with excess lactic acid production.

Leukotrienes. Inflammatory products that induce white cell activity.

Ligand. A hormone, a cell-derived growth factor, or another trigger molecule that binds to a specific receptor site.

LOX. Lipoxygenase; a family of enzymes that drive inflammation.

Lymphagogue. An herb that promotes lymph flow and reduces stagnation or congestion in tissues.

MAPK. Mitogen-activated protein kinase—a signal transduction enzyme and the pathway of controls.

MCP. Modified (fractionated) citrus pectin; a supplement that inhibits signal transduction.

MDR. Multidrug resistance; a function of P-glycoprotein pumps.

MMP. Matrix metalloproteinase; a family of enzymes that degrade extracellular matrix.

MSI. Microsatellite instability; predisposition to gene mutations as a result of mutations in the DNA mismatch repair (MMR) gene. Abnormally functioning MMR cannot correct errors that occur during DNA replication, which causes the creation of novel microsatellite fragments that can be measured.

MTD. Maximum tolerated dose.

MTHFR. Methylenetetrahydrofolate reductase; mutation may lead to high levels of homocysteine in the blood.

mTOR. Mammalian target of rapamycin; an intracellular signal transduction receptor.

NAC. N-acetylcysteine; a supplement with antioxidant action in the liver (stop during chemotherapy).

NAD/NADH+. Nicotinamide adenine dinucleotide/hydrogen; an electron carrier and donor involved in cellular respiration in mitochondria.

NASH. Nonalcoholic steatohepatitis.

NASP. Nonalcoholic steatopancreatitis.

NDGA. Nor-dihydroguiairetic acid; a pharmacologically active lignan in chaparral.

NF-κB. Nuclear factor-kappa B; an oncogenic transcription factor.

NRF2. Nuclear factor erythroid 2-related factor 2; a transcription factor that regulates redox damage in injury and inflammation.

NSCLC. Non–small-cell lung cancer.

OPCs. Oligomeric proanthocyanidins; a supplement that provides polyphenolic redox regulators.

ORAC. Oxygen radical absorbance capacity; a method of measuring the antioxidant capacity of foods and herbs.

p21, p27, p53. Genes and the proteins they code for that control DNA copying, repair, and onward cell cycling.

PAF. Platelet-activating factor; involved in clotting.

PDGF. Platelet-derived growth factor.

Pgp. P-glycoprotein; a cellular efflux pump that contributes to multidrug resistance.

PIK. Phosphatidylinositol kinase; a family of enzymes involved in signal transduction and regulating cell cycling, proliferation, differentiation, motility, and survival.

PKC. Protein kinase C receptors.

PPE. Palmar-plantar erythrodysesthesia; hand-foot syndrome, as a result of certain cancer drugs.

PR+. Progesterone receptor–positive; cancer expresses or overexpresses receptor sites for progesterone.

PTEN. Phosphatase and tensin homologue; a tumor-suppressor protein.

PTK. Protein tyrosine kinase; a family of receptor sites on the cell membrane that trigger signal transduction.

Ras protein. Enzymes involved in signal transduction.

Redox. Reduction/oxidation reactions.

ROS. Reactive oxygen species (free radicals).

SAMe. S-adenosylmethionine; a methyl donor molecule.

Selectins. Cell-surface lectins that bind cancer cells together (cell adhesion molecules).

SERMs. Selective estrogen receptor modifiers; agonist/antagonist effect on estrogen receptors.

SHBG. Sex hormone–binding globulin; carries estrogen and testosterone in blood.

SNP. Single nucleotide polymorphism; unique gene mutations specific to a given person.

SOD. Superoxide dismutase; an intracellular redox regulator.

Stomachic. A tonic of the upper digestive system; promotes gastric functions and secretions.

TGF-α/β. Transforming growth factor alpha/beta; regulated cell cycling.

TLR. Toll-like receptors; immune-activating receptor sites usually expressed on macrophages and dendritic cells.

TMB. Tumor mutational burden; indicates how much gene mutation has occurred in the genome of a cancer cell.

TME. Tumor microenvironment; the condition of the interstitial fluid around a tumor, including blood vessels, immune cells, fibroblasts, signaling molecules, and the extracellular matrix.

TNF-α. Tumor necrosis factor-alpha; immunomodulating.

TNM. Tumor, node, metastases; a way to describe the spread of cancer.

Tomosynthesis. A type of digital x-ray mammogram that creates 2D and 3D-like pictures of the breasts.

TRP channels. Transient receptor potential channels (receptor sites); responsible for detection, integration, and initiation of pain signals in the peripheral nervous system (e.g., TRPA1 is a sensor for pain, cold, and itching and for environmental irritants causing tears, airway resistance, and cough).

uPA. Urokinase plasminogen activator; involved in blood clotting.

VCAM. Vascular cell adhesion molecule; mediates the adhesion of lymphocytes, monocytes, eosinophils, and basophils to vascular endothelium.

VDR. Vitamin D receptor.

VEGF. Vascular endothelial growth factor.

Vitamin D 25. Hydroxycholecalciferol, or 25-hydroxyvitamin D3.

Vulnerary. An herb that promotes granulation and wound healing.

Resources

Professional Herbal Associations with Referral Directories of Practitioners

American Herbalists Guild (USA)
https://americanherbalistsguild.com

British Columbia Herbalists Association (Canada)
https://bcherbalists.ca

The College of Practitioners of Phytotherapy (UK)
https://thecpp.uk

Guilde des Herboristes (Québec)
https://guildedesherboristes.org

Herbalist Association of Nova Scotia
https://herbalns.org

Irish Register of Herbalists
https://irh.ie

National Institute of Medical Herbalists (UK)
https://nimh.org.uk

Naturopaths & Herbalists Association of Australia
https://nhaa.org.au

New Zealand Association of Medical Herbalists
https://nzamh.org.nz

Ontario Herbalists Association
https://ontarioherbalists.ca

South African Association of Registered Phytotherapists
https://phytotherapists.co.za

Professional Naturopathic Associations with Referral Directories of Practitioners

American Association of Naturopathic Physicians
https://naturopathic.org

Association of Naturopathic Practitioners (UK)
https://theanp.co.uk

Canadian Association of Naturopathic Doctors
https://cand.ca

Naturopaths & Herbalists Association of Australia
https://nhaa.org.au

Oncology Association of Naturopathic Physicians (OncANP)
https://oncanp.org

Herb Suppliers

Look for shops run by herbalists and with herbalists on staff and offering clinical services. The quality and sourcing of good herbs is critically important, and clinical herbalists are trained to assess and evaluate their suppliers and supplies constantly, as a crop can change from season to season and from year to year. The businesses listed below are well established and personally known to me, and they consistently and reliably offer top-quality herbs and herbal products. There are many other wonderful regional herbal suppliers and independent herbal stores and apothecaries, and these also can be a great resource for some of the herbs.

An excellent resource listing for herbal suppliers around the world is available at Herbal Academy, https://theherbalacademy.com/purchase-herbs-and-supplies-world-wide.

Finlandia Pharmacy & Natural Health Centre (Canada)
https://finlandiahealthstore.com
A full-service herbal medicine and natural pharmacy with its own branded herbal formulas and custom dispensing available. Teas, tinctures, and much more. Mail order available.

Gaia Garden Herbal Dispensary (Canada)
https://gaiagarden.com
A full-service herbal medicine store with its own branded herbal formulas and custom dispensing available. Teas, tinctures, and much more. Mail order available.

G. Baldwin & Co. (London)
https://baldwins.co.uk
Herbal supplies and its own brand of remedies and skin care line. Teas, tinctures, and much more.

Harmonic Arts (Canada)
https://harmonicarts.ca
Online retail sales as well as wholesale. Mushroom extracts, elixirs, superfoods, and dried herbs. Top quality and a big range.

HerbNET (USA)
https://herbnet.com
HerbNET is sponsored by the Herb Growing and Marketing Network, with hundreds of sources and resources that link everybody herbal to everything herbal—an incredible rich resource.

Heron Botanicals (USA)
https://heronbotanicals.com/
Exceptional-quality herbal extracts made by Dr. Eric Yarnell, including hard-to-find and specialty herbs.

Mountain Rose Herbs (USA)
https://mountainroseherbs.com
This company supplies all sorts of herbs, herbal products, and herbal accoutrements—an amazing resource with a huge mail-order catalog. They also offer a whole lot of sponsorships and support in the herbal community.

Napiers the Herbalists Dispensary (Scotland)
https://napiers.net
A full-service herbal medicine shop and dispensary with its own branded herbal formulas and custom dispensing available. Teas, tinctures, and much more. Mail order available.

Neal's Yard Remedies (UK)
https://nealsyardremedies.com
Herbal supplies, its own brand of remedies and skin care line, and clinics. In towns across the UK.

The Rosemary House & Gardens (USA)
https://therosemaryhouse.com
Started in 1968 and still run by the same family of herbalists. A charming old-world herb store.

The Scarlet Sage Herb Co. (USA)
https://scarletsage.com
Small independent herb shop and teaching center.

Smile Herb Shop
https://smileherb.com
Small independent herb shop and teaching center. Started in 1975.

Packaging Supplies for Herbal Products

Cap M Qwik
This simple and cheap device can be purchased from your local health food store, or contact the manufacturer, Cap M Qwik, via email at capsulefillers@gmail.com or online at https://capmquikhome.com.

From Nature with Love (USA)
https://fromnaturewithlove.com/packaging

Voyageur Soap & Candle Co. (British Columbia)
https://voyageursoapandcandle.com

Wholesale Suppliers of Bulk Herbs and Extracts for Practitioners

Herbal Vitality (USA)
2810 Hopi Drive
Sedona, AZ 86336
928-204-6455

Heron Botanicals (USA)
https://heronbotanicals.com

Pacific Botanicals (USA)
https://pacificbotanicals.com

Panacea Health Limited (UK)
https://panaceahealthonline.com

Rutland Biodynamics (UK)
https://rutlandbio.com

Viriditas (Canada)
https://viriditasherbalproducts.com

Brands of Supplements and Herbal Capsules I Recommend

Products from a number of these companies are available only through practitioners because they are particularly potent mixes, and some are also available in retail stores.

Advanced Orthomolecular Research (AOR)
My main Canadian supplier, with a wide array of strong and effective nutritional supplements, including resveratrol, CoQ10, green tea, arjuna, MCHC calcium, and others.

Bioclinic Naturals
A really good all-around supplement and encapsulated herb company. I use a lot of their regular products, including vitamins and minerals. A couple of products I especially like are Mito AMP, with acetyl-L-carnitine, ginkgo extract (24% flavone glycosides, 6% terpene lactones), Japanese knotweed extract, Coenzyme Q10, R-Alpha-Lipoic Acid, grapeseed extract, and PQQ

(pyrroloquinoline quinone), and Somno-Pro, with Suntheanine L-theanine, 5-hydroxytryptophan (5-HTP), and melatonin.

Cyto-Matrix
This brand has a very high-potency liquid fish oil with vitamin D that is useful: with EPA 1,900 mg, DHA 900 mg, and vitamin D 1,000 IU in every teaspoon. They also make a good ACE&Z mix (vitamin A, vitamin C, mixed tocopherols, selenium, and zinc).

Designs for Health
One of my main suppliers in the United States. They have an extensive range of excellent, high-potency products originally designed by a nutritionist. In particular, the whey protein is excellent as an easily digested protein source and a source of lactoglobulins that are immune modulating. The zinc with molybdenum is particularly useful in inhibiting angiogenesis, and the B-Supreme blend is a potent B-vitamin complex mix.

INNATE Response
Highly potentized nutritional supplements. I use the Thyroid Response Formula, iron, and multivitamin blends in particular.

JHS Natural Products
The best brand for mushrooms. They have several different mushrooms and different blends so I choose reishi and turkey tail for all my cancer patients, chaga for the more advanced or severe cases, and cordyceps if there is lung compromise and oxygen deficiency. They also have a very good five-mushroom blend I use a lot.

MediHerb
Really good herbal capsule formulas, exceptional quality and potency. I use vitex, boswellia, andrographis, kava, and more from this company.

Natura Health Products
This company's product line was created by Donnie Yance, and they are some of the smartest and most elegant formulations available anywhere. Using extraordinarily potent extracts, blending herbs together for optimal synergy, using bioavailable nutritional supplements (vitamins and minerals), and formulated with the cancer patient in mind, these are some of the highest-quality formulations I can find. Some are sold retail or direct off the website; others are for practitioner use only.

Nordic Naturals
The best brand for fish oils and omega-3 fats. They are exceptionally pure and exceptionally powerful.

Pure Encapsulations
This brand is especially made with lower levels of fillers, binders, and excipients and is intended for the highly sensitive or very weak person. Hypoallergenic.

Renew Life
This brand makes excellent, comprehensive detox kits.

Xymogen
Some unusual formulas from this company. I use GlutAloeMine, which has L-glutamine, arabinogalactan (from *Larix laricina* wood), licorice (*Glycyrrhiza glabra* root and rhizome), and *Aloe vera* (leaf gel). They also supply diamine oxidase to treat histamine intolerance symptoms and Methyl Protect with betaine, riboflavin, vitamin B6, folate, and vitamin B12. They support botanical sanctuaries throughout North America and promote sustainable practices in herbal medicine cultivation and trade.

SPECIALTY LABS FOR CANCER TESTING

Sensitivity and Resistance Testing

Dr. Robert Nagourney
https://nagourneycancerinstitute.com

Weisenthal Cancer Group
www.weisenthalcancer.com

Genomic Testing

Caris Life Sciences
https://carislifesciences.com

FoundationOne CDx from Foundation Medicine
foundationmedicine.com

Oncotype Screening from Exact Sciences
oncotypeiq.com

Functional Medicine Testing

Evexia Diagnostics
https://evexiadiagnostics.com/home

Genova Diagnostics
https://gdx.net

Educational Organizations and Sites

Adult Post-treatment Cancer Survivorship Care Guidelines
https://cancer.org/health-care-professionals.html

Alternative Medicine Review
https://altmedrev.com/resources
High-quality research studies and clinical trials in natural medicine.

American Botanical Council
https://abc.herbalgram.org
A nonprofit herbal research and education organization established to inform and educate the public about beneficial herbs and plants. Excellent monographs on lots of plants. Lots of great educational offerings.

American Cancer Society
https://cancer.org
The major cancer patient support organization in the US. They also publish numerous resources for practitioners.

American Herbal Pharmacopoeia
https://herbal-ahp.org
Produces authoritative monographs on botanicals and on quality assurance issues in the supply chain.

American Herb Association
https://ahaherb.com
General-interest society of herb lovers and users. This organization publishes a useful journal of herbal knowledge.

Association for the Advancement of Restorative Medicine (AARM)
https://restorativemedicine.org
Education for practitioners and online references and resources; great monographs on herbs.

Beyond Conventional Cancer Therapies (BCCT)
https://bcct.ngo/integrative-cancer-care
This site gives a deep dive into collaborative oncology; detailed and explicit, technical and intelligible. One of my main reference sites; exceptionally helpful.

The Block Center for Integrative Cancer Treatment
https://blockmd.com/services/cancer-surgery
This is the website for Dr. Keith Block, one of the leading functional medicine oncologists in the US. He runs a busy consulting practice and integrates conventional and holistic strategies.

Breastcancer.org
https://breastcancer.org
Resources and supportive information for breast cancer patients.

Camphill Wellbeing Trust (anthroposophic medicine)
www.camphillwellbeing.org.uk/anthrohealth
https://mistletoetherapy.org.uk
Anthroposophic medicine may include hydrotherapy, physiotherapy, and rhythmical massage therapy, dietetics, eurythmy movement therapy, art and music therapy, psychotherapy, and lifestyle approaches. Camphill also supplies mistletoe therapy in the UK.

Cancer Research UK
https://cancerhelp.org.uk
The main cancer research and cancer support organization in the UK.

Caregiver Resource Guide
https://cancer.org/caregiverguide

Caregiver Support Video Series
https://cancer.org/caregivervideos

Christopher Hobbs
https://christopherhobbs.com
Herbalist, mushroom expert, teacher, and writer.

The Cochrane Collaboration
https://cochrane.org
A UK-based not-for-profit medical research group that conducts meta-analyses of research to achieve high-level overviews of conditions and efficacy of treatments.

David Winston's Center for Herbal Studies
https://herbalstudies.net
An incredible resource of herbal history and lots of great links to other herbal sites.

Eric Yarnell, ND, RH(AHG)
https://botmed.rocks
One of the most informative, interesting, insightful, and extensive sites for information on clinical phytotherapy.

Henriette's Herbal Homepage
https://henriettes-herb.com
One of the oldest and largest herbal information sites on the web. Packed full of user-friendly herbal lore, including books by the Eclectic doctors of the 1800s, botany, materia medica, and thousands of photographs.

Herbal Educational Services
https://botanicalmedicine.org
These folks have a 20+-year back catalog of recorded lectures from botanical medicine conferences hosted twice annually in the US. Some of the older stuff may be out of date (I know some of mine are by now), but you can search by teacher or by topic and it gives a very broad spread of contemporary herbal practice.

The Herb Society of America
https://herbsociety.org
General-interest society of herb lovers. Great resource for all things herbal.

Life after Treatment Guide
https://cancer.org/survivorshipguide

Lloyd Library and Museum
https://lloydlibrary.org
The largest pharmacognosy and plant sciences library in the United States. Open to the public by appointment if you are in Cincinnati.

Macmillan Cancer Support
https://macmillan.org.uk
The main palliative cancer support organization in UK.

MD Anderson Cancer Center Complementary Therapy Integrative Medicine Education Resources (University of Texas)
https://mdanderson.org/research/departments-labs-institutes/programs-centers/integrative-medicine-program.html
Cautious and conservative but good on clinical evidence and collaborative or integrative medicine.

Memorial Sloan Kettering Cancer Center
https://mskcc.org/cancer-care/diagnosis-treatment/symptom-management/integrative-medicine/herbs
A large site with user-friendly information for patients and more technical information for practitioners. Extensive listing of monographs on herbs and supplements.

Mrs. Grieve's A *Modern Herbal*
http://botanical.com
A classic text with traditional and folkloric uses of hundreds of plants.

Nalini Chilkov, L.Ac. OMD
https://integrativecanceranswers.com
Dr. Chilkov is a leading-edge authority on integrative cancer care, immune enhancement, optimal nutrition, and wellness medicine.

National Cancer Institute
https://cancer.gov
Vast site covering all sorts of information on diagnosis and treatment of cancer. Not about holistic medicine, but if you want to understand your diagnosis and treatment better, this is a great place to look.

National Center for Complementary and Integrative Health
https://nccih.nih.gov
US government research agency for natural medicines and best practices.

Natural Medicines Comprehensive Database
https://naturalmedicines.therapeuticresearch.com
This site offers both a free consumer (layperson's) version and a subscription professional version of this invaluable resource. The database allows you to cross-reference almost any natural product name, disease or condition, or drug and provides information on relative effectiveness, potential drug interactions, and nutrient-depletion issues caused by medications. Conservative but safe.

Naturopathic Medicine Network
https://pandamedicine.com
Promotes public awareness about naturopathic medicine and supports natural healthcare.

North American Institute of Medical Herbalism
https://naimh.com
An extraordinary wealth of information on all things herbal—this site has numerous books from the Eclectic herbal doctors of the 1800s, current herbal commentaries, links to MedLine, journals, and so much more.

Plants for a Future
https://pfaf.org
A US-based organization promoting native plants and sustainable commercialization practices.

Society for Integrative Oncology
https://integrativeonc.org
A not-for-profit organization that seeks to advance evidence-based, comprehensive, integrative healthcare and to promote communication, education, and research by practitioners from multiple disciplines focused on the care of cancer patients and survivors.

United Plant Savers
https://unitedplantsavers.org
A not-for-profit organization dedicated to the protection and preservation of native American medicinal plants. They support botanical sanctuaries throughout North America and promote sustainable practices in herbal medicine cultivation and trade.

Metric Conversions

Unless you have finely calibrated measuring equipment, conversions between US and metric measurements will be somewhat inexact. It's important to convert the measurements for all of the ingredients in a recipe to maintain the same proportions as the original.

WEIGHT		
To convert	**to**	**multiply**
ounces	grams	ounces by 28.35
pounds	grams	pounds by 453.5
pounds	kilograms	pounds by 0.45

US	Metric
0.035 ounce	1 gram
¼ ounce	7 grams
½ ounce	14 grams
1 ounce	28 grams
1¼ ounces	35 grams
1½ ounces	40 grams
1¾ ounces	50 grams
2½ ounces	70 grams
3½ ounces	100 grams
4 ounces	113 grams
5 ounces	140 grams
8 ounces	228 grams
8¾ ounces	250 grams
10 ounces	280 grams
15 ounces	425 grams
16 ounces (1 pound)	454 grams

TEMPERATURE		
To convert	**to**	
Fahrenheit	Celsius	subtract 32 from Fahrenheit temperature, multiply by 5, then divide by 9

US	Metric
1 teaspoon	5 milliliters
1 tablespoon	15 milliliters
¼ cup	60 milliliters
½ cup	120 milliliters
1 cup	240 milliliters
1¼ cups	300 milliliters
1½ cups	355 milliliters
2 cups	480 milliliters
2½ cups	600 milliliters
3 cups	710 milliliters
4 cups (1 quart)	0.95 liter
4 quarts (1 gallon)	3.8 liters

VOLUME		
To convert	**to**	**multiply**
teaspoons	milliliters	teaspoons by 4.93
tablespoons	milliliters	tablespoons by 14.79
fluid ounces	milliliters	fluid ounces by 29.57
cups	milliliters	cups by 236.59
cups	liters	cups by 0.24
pints	milliliters	pints by 473.18
pints	liters	pints by 0.473
quarts	milliliters	quarts by 946.36
quarts	liters	quarts by 0.946
gallons	liters	gallons by 3.785

List of Plants by Common Name

Common Name	Latin Name
Ajwan (a.k.a. ajwain)	*Carum copticum*
Alfalfa	*Medicago sativa*
Aloe	*Aloe vera*
Amalaki	*Emblica officinalis*
Amla	*Phyllanthus emblica*
Andrographis (a.k.a. chiretta)	*Andrographis paniculata*
Angelica	*Angelica archangelica*
Anise	*Pimpinella anisum*
Annual wormwood (a.k.a. Chinese wormwood or sweet Annie)	*Artemisia annua*
Argan	*Argania spinosa*
Arjuna	*Terminalia arjuna*
Arnica	*Arnica montana*
Artichoke leaf	*Cynara scolymus*
Ashwagandha	*Withania somnifera*
Astragalus (a.k.a. huang qi)	*Astragalus membranaceus*
Babassu	*Orbignya oleifera*
Baikal skullcap (a.k.a. Chinese skullcap)	*Scutellaria baicalensis*
Barberry	*Berberis vulgaris*
Basil	*Ocimum basilicum*
Bearberry (a.k.a. kinnikinnick)	*Arctostaphylos uva-ursi*
Belladonna (a.k.a. deadly nightshade)	*Atropa belladonna*
Bibhitaki	*Terminalia bellirica*
Bitter melon	*Momordica charantia*
Bitter orange	*Citrus aurantium*
Black alder	*Alnus glutinosa*
Black cohosh	*Actaea racemosa*
Black horehound	*Ballota nigra*
Black pepper	*Piper nigrum*
Bleeding heart	*Dicentra canadensis*
Bloodroot	*Sanguinaria canadensis*
Blue flag	*Iris versicolor*
Blue vervain	*Verbena officinalis, V. hastata*
Boldo	*Peumus boldus*
Brahmi	*Bacopa monnieri*
Bryony	*Bryonia dioica*
Bupleurum (a.k.a. bei chai hu or hare's ear)	*Bupleurum falcatum*
Burdock root	*Arctium lappa*
Butcher's broom	*Ruscus aculeatus*
Cacao	*Theobroma cacao*

Common Name	Latin Name
Calendula (a.k.a. pot marigold)	*Calendula officinalis*
California poppy	*Eschscholzia californica*
Cancer tree (a.k.a. happy tree or xi shu)	*Camptotheca acuminata*
Cannabis	*Cannabis sativa, C. indica*
Cape aloe	*Aloe barbadensis*
Caraway	*Carum carvi*
Cardamom	*Elettaria cardamomum*
Cascara (a.k.a. buckthorn)	*Rhamnus purshiana*
Castor	*Ricinus communis*
Catnip	*Nepeta cataria*
Cat's claw	*Uncaria tomentosa*
Cayenne	*Capsicum* species
Celery	*Apium graveolens*
Chaga	*Inonotus obliquus*
Chamomile	*Matricaria recutita, M. chamomilla*
Chaparral (a.k.a. creosote bush)	*Larrea divaricata, L. tridentata*
Chasteberry	*Vitex agnus-castus*
Chickweed	*Stellaria media*
Chinese indigo	*Isatis indigotica*
Chlorella	*Chlorella vulgaris, C. pyrenoidosa*
Cinnamon	*Cinnamomum zeylanicum*
Cleavers	*Galium aparine*
Clove bud	*Syzygium aromaticum*
Codonopsis (a.k.a. dangshen)	*Codonopsis pilosula*
Coffee	*Coffea arabica*
Coleus	*Coleus forskohlii*
Comfrey	*Symphytum officinale*
Condor vine	*Marsdenia condurango*
Cordyceps	*Cordyceps sinensis*
Coriander	*Coriandrum sativum*
Corn silk	*Zea mays*
Corydalis	*Corydalis ambigua, C. yanhusuo*
Couch grass	*Elymus repens*
Cramp bark	*Viburnum opulus*
Crataeva (a.k.a. varuna)	*Crataeva nurvala*
Cumin	*Cuminum cyminum*
Damiana	*Turnera diffusa*
Dandelion	*Taraxacum officinale*
Dan shen (a.k.a. Chinese red sage)	*Salvia miltiorrhiza*
Devil's claw	*Harpagophytum procumbens*
Devil's club	*Oplopanax horridus*

Common Name	Latin Name
Dill	*Anethum graveolens*
Dong quai (a.k.a. dang gui)	*Angelica sinensis*
Echinacea	*Echinacea purpurea, E. angustifolia, E. pallida*
Elderberry	*Sambucus nigra*
Eleuthero	*Eleutherococcus senticosus*
Evening primrose	*Oenothera biennis*
Fennel seed	*Foeniculum vulgare*
Fenugreek	*Trigonella foenum-graecum*
Feverfew	*Tanacetum parthenium*
Figwort	*Scrophularia nodosa*
Flax	*Linum usitatissimum*
Fringe tree	*Chionanthus virginicus*
Fumitory	*Fumaria officinalis*
Garlic	*Allium sativum*
Gentian	*Gentiana lutea*
Geranium (a.k.a. American cranesbill)	*Geranium maculatum*
Geum (a.k.a. avens)	*Geum urbanum*
Ginger	*Zingiber officinale*
Ginkgo	*Ginkgo biloba*
Ginseng	*Panax ginseng, P. quinquefolius*
Goat's rue	*Galega officinalis*
Goji berry	*Lycium barbarum*
Goldenrod	*Solidago virgaurea*
Goldenseal	*Hydrastis canadensis*
Gotu kola	*Centella asiatica*
Greater celandine	*Chelidonium majus*
Green tea	*Camellia sinensis*
Guaiac wood (a.k.a. lignum vitae)	*Guaiacum officinale*
Guarana	*Paullinia cupana*
Gurmar	*Gymnema sylvestre*
Haritaki	*Terminalia chebula*
Hawthorn	*Crataegus monogyna, C. oxyacantha, C. laevigata*
Henbane	*Hyoscyamus niger*
Hibiscus	*Hibiscus sabdariffa*
Hops	*Humulus lupulus*
Horehound	*Marrubium vulgare*
Horse chestnut	*Aesculus hippocastanum*
Horsetail	*Equisetum arvense*
Ho wood	*Cinnamomum camphora*
Huperzia (a.k.a. club moss)	*Huperzia serrata, Lycopodium serratum*

Common Name	Latin Name
Hydrangea	*Hydrangea arborescens, H. paniculata*
Indian frankincense (a.k.a. boswellia)	*Boswellia serrata*
Jamaican dogwood	*Piscidia piscipula*
Japanese knotweed	*Reynoutria japonica* (a.k.a. *Fallopia japonica* or *Polygonum cuspidatum*)
Jimson weed (a.k.a. thornapple)	*Datura stramonium*
Jujube	*Ziziphus jujuba*
Juniper	*Juniperus communis*
Kava	*Piper methysticum*
Kelp	*Fucus vesiculosus*
Kinnikinnick (a.k.a. bearberry)	*Arctostaphylos uva-ursi*
Kola	*Kola vera*
Kudzu	*Pueraria lobata*
Kutki	*Picrorhiza kurroa*
Larch	*Larix laricina*
Lavender	*Lavandula angustifolia*
Lemon balm	*Melissa officinalis*
Lemongrass	*Cymbopogon citratus*
Licorice	*Glycyrrhiza glabra*
Linden	*Tilia × europaea*
Lion's mane	*Hericium erinaceus*
Lobelia	*Lobelia inflata*
Leuzea (a.k.a. maral root)	*Rhaponticum carthamoides*
Maca	*Lepidium meyenii*
Madagascar periwinkle (a.k.a. rosy periwinkle)	*Catharanthus roseus*
Magnolia	*Magnolia* species
Marshmallow	*Althaea officinalis*
Mayapple	*Podophyllum peltatum*
Meadowsweet	*Filipendula ulmaria*
Milk thistle	*Silybum marianum*
Millettia	*Millettia* species
Mistletoe	*Viscum album*
Monkshood	*Aconitum napellus*
Motherwort	*Leonurus cardiaca*
Myrrh	*Commiphora molmol, C. myrrha*
Neem	*Azadirachta indica*
Nigella (a.k.a. black seed)	*Nigella sativa*
Nutmeg	*Myristica fragrans*
Oak	*Quercus alba, Q. rubra*
Oats (seed and straw)	*Avena sativa*
Orange	*Citrus × sinensis*

Common Name	Latin Name
Oregano	*Origanum vulgare*
Oregon grape	*Mahonia aquifolium, Berberis aquifolium*
Osha	*Ligusticum porteri*
Parsley piert	*Aphanes arvensis*
Passionflower	*Passiflora incarnata*
Pawpaw	*Asimina triloba*
Pellitory	*Parietaria diffusa, P. judaica, P. officinalis*
Peppermint	*Mentha × piperita*
Periwinkle	*Vinca major, V. minor*
Plantain	*Plantago lanceolata, P. major*
Pokeroot	*Phytolacca decandra, P. americana*
Pomegranate	*Punica granatum*
Pond lily (white or yellow)	*Nymphaea odorata*
Prickly ash	*Zanthoxylum clava-herculis*
Psyllium seed	*Plantago psyllium*
Red clover	*Trifolium pratense*
Red root	*Ceanothus americanus*
Rehmannia, prepared (a.k.a. Chinese foxglove or shēng dì huáng)	*Rehmannia glutinosa*
Reishi	*Ganoderma lucidum*
Rhodiola (a.k.a. Arctic rose)	*Rhodiola rosea*
Rhubarb	*Rheum officinale, R. palmatum*
Rooibos	*Aspalathus linearis*
Rose (hips and petals)	*Rosa* species
Rosemary	*Rosmarinus officinalis*
Sage	*Salvia officinalis, S. lavandulifolia*
Sarsaparilla	*Smilax ornata*
Sassafras	*Sassafras albidum*
Schisandra (a.k.a. wu wei zi)	*Schisandra chinensis*
Sea buckthorn	*Hippophae rhamnoides*
Self-heal	*Prunella vulgaris*
Senna	*Cassia* species
Shatavari	*Asparagus racemosus*
Sheep sorrel	*Rumex acetosella*
Shepherd's purse	*Capsella bursa-pastoris*
Shiitake	*Lentinula edodes*
Silk tree	*Albizia julibrissin*
Skullcap	*Scutellaria lateriflora*
Slippery elm	*Ulmus fulva, U. rubra*
Spearmint	*Mentha spicata*
St. John's wort	*Hypericum perforatum*
Star anise	*Illicium verum*

Common Name	Latin Name
Stillingia	*Stillingia sylvatica*
Stinging nettle	*Urtica dioica*
Sweet flag	*Acorus calamus*
Taheebo (a.k.a. pau d'arco or lapacho)	*Tabebuia impetiginosa, T. avellanedae, T. rosea, Handroanthus impetiginosus*
Thuja (a.k.a. eastern arborvitae or northern white cedar)	*Thuja occidentalis*
Thyme	*Thymus vulgaris*
Tulsi (a.k.a. holy basil)	*Ocimum sanctum, O. tenuiflorum*
Turkey tail	*Trametes versicolor*
Turmeric	*Curcuma longa*
Valerian	*Valeriana officinalis*
Violet	*Viola odorata*
White peony	*Paeonia lactiflora*
Wild indigo	*Baptisia tinctoria*
Wild lettuce	*Lactuca virosa*
Wild pansy	*Viola tricolor*
Wild yam	*Dioscorea villosa*
Willow	*Salix alba*
Wood betony	*Stachys betonica*
Wormwood	*Artemisia absinthium*
Yarrow	*Achillea millefolium*
Yellow dock	*Rumex crispus*
Yellow gentian	*Gentiana lutea*
Yellow jasmine	*Gelsemium sempervirens*
Yerba mate	*Ilex paraguariensis*
Yew	*Taxus brevifolia, T. baccata, T. wallichiana*
Yucca	*Yucca* species
Zhi mu	*Anemarrhena asphodeloides*

List of Plants by Latin Name

Latin Name	Common Name
Achillea millefolium	Yarrow
Aconitum napellus	Monkshood
Acorus calamus	Sweet flag
Actaea racemosa	Black cohosh
Aesculus hippocastanum	Horse chestnut
Albizia julibrissin	Silk tree
Allium sativum	Garlic
Alnus glutinosa	Black alder
Aloe barbadensis	Cape aloe
Aloe vera	Aloe
Althaea officinalis	Marshmallow
Andrographis paniculata	Andrographis (a.k.a. chiretta)
Anemarrhena asphodeloides	Zhi mu
Anethum graveolens	Dill
Angelica archangelica	Angelica
Angelica sinensis	Dong quai (a.k.a. dang gui)
Aphanes arvensis	Parsley piert
Apium graveolens	Celery
Arctium lappa	Burdock root
Arctostaphylos uva-ursi	Bearberry (a.k.a. kinnikinnick)
Argania spinosa	Argan
Arnica montana	Arnica
Artemisia absinthium	Wormwood
Artemisia annua	Annual wormwood (a.k.a. Chinese wormwood or sweet Annie)
Asimina triloba	Pawpaw
Aspalathus linearis	Rooibos
Asparagus racemosus	Shatavari
Astragalus membranaceus	Astragalus (a.k.a. huang qi)
Atropa belladonna	Belladonna (a.k.a. deadly nightshade)
Avena sativa	Oats (seed and straw)
Azadirachta indica	Neem
Bacopa monnieri	Brahmi
Ballota nigra	Black horehound
Baptisia tinctoria	Wild indigo
Berberis vulgaris	Barberry
Boswellia serrata	Indian frankincense (a.k.a. sabal guggul or boswellia)

Latin Name	Common Name
Bryonia dioica	Bryony
Bupleurum falcatum	Bupleurum (a.k.a. bei chai hu or hare's ear)
Calendula officinalis	Calendula (a.k.a. pot marigold)
Camellia sinensis	Green tea
Camptotheca acuminata	Cancer tree (a.k.a. happy tree or xi shu)
Cannabis sativa, C. indica	Cannabis
Capsella bursa-pastoris	Shepherd's purse
Capsicum species	Cayenne
Carum carvi	Caraway
Carum copticum	Ajwan (a.k.a. ajwain)
Cassia species	Senna
Catharanthus roseus	Madagascar periwinkle (a.k.a. rosy periwinkle)
Ceanothus americanus	Red root
Centella asiatica	Gotu kola
Chelidonium majus	Greater celandine
Chionanthus virginicus	Fringe tree
Chlorella vulgaris, C. pyrenoidosa	Chlorella
Cinnamomum camphora	Ho wood
Cinnamomum zeylanicum	Cinnamon
Citrus aurantium	Bitter orange
Citrus × sinensis	Orange
Codonopsis pilosula	Codonopsis (a.k.a. dangshen)
Coffea arabica	Coffee
Coleus forskholii	Coleus
Commiphora molmol, C. myrrha	Myrrh
Cordyceps sinensis	Cordyceps
Coriandrum sativum	Coriander
Corydalis ambigua, C. yanhusuo	Corydalis
Crataegus monogyna, C. oxyacantha, C. laevigata	Hawthorn
Crataeva nurvala	Crataeva (a.k.a. varuna)
Cuminum cyminum	Cumin
Curcuma longa	Turmeric
Cymbopogon citratus	Lemongrass
Cynara scolymus	Artichoke leaf
Datura stramonium	Jimson weed (a.k.a. thornapple)
Dicentra canadensis	Bleeding heart
Dioscorea villosa	Wild yam
Echinacea purpurea, E. angustifola, E. pallida	Echinacea

Latin Name	Common Name
Elettaria cardamomum	Cardamom
Eleutherococcus senticosus	Eleuthero
Elymus repens	Couch grass
Emblica officinalis	Amalaki
Equisetum arvense	Horsetail
Eschscholzia californica	California poppy
Filipendula ulmaria	Meadowsweet
Foeniculum vulgare	Fennel seed
Fucus vesiculosis	Kelp
Fumaria officinalis	Fumitory
Galega officinalis	Goat's rue
Galium aparine	Cleavers
Ganoderma lucidum	Reishi
Gelsemium sempervirens	Yellow jasmine
Gentiana lutea	Yellow gentian
Geranium maculatum	Geraniam (a.k.a. American cranesbill)
Geum urbanum	Geum (a.k.a. avens)
Ginkgo biloba	Ginkgo
Glycyrrhiza glabra	Licorice
Guaiacum officinale	Guaiac wood (a.k.a. lignum vitae)
Gymnema sylvestre	Gurmar
Harpagophytum procumbens	Devil's claw
Hericium erinaceus	Lion's mane
Hibiscus sabdariffa	Hibiscus
Hippophae rhamnoides	Sea buckthorn
Humulus lupulus	Hops
Huperzia serrata, Lycopodium serratum	Huperzia (a.k.a. club moss)
Hydrangea arborescens, H. paniculata	Hydrangea
Hydrastis canadensis	Goldenseal
Hyoscyamus niger	Henbane
Hypericum perforatum	St. John's wort
Ilex paraguariensis	Yerba mate
Illicium verum	Star anise
Inonotus obliquus	Chaga
Iris versicolor	Blue flag
Isatis indigotica	Chinese indigo
Juniperus communis	Juniper
Kola vera	Kola
Lactuca virosa	Wild lettuce

Latin Name	Common Name
Larix laricina	Larch
Larrea divaricata, L. tridentata	Chaparral (a.k.a. creosote bush)
Lavandula angustifolia	Lavender
Lentinula edodes	Shiitake
Leonurus cardiaca	Motherwort
Lepidium meyenii	Maca
Ligusticum porteri	Osha
Linum usitatissimum	Flax
Lobelia inflata	Lobelia
Lycium barbarum	Goji berry
Magnolia species	Magnolia
Mahonia aquifolium, Berberis aquifolium	Oregon grape
Marrubium vulgare	Horehound
Marsdenia condurango	Condor vine
Matricaria recutita, M. chamomilla	Chamomile
Medicago sativa	Alfalfa
Melissa officinalis	Lemon balm
Mentha × piperita	Peppermint
Mentha spicata	Spearmint
Millettia species	Millettia
Momordica charantia	Bitter melon
Myristica fragrans	Nutmeg
Nepeta cataria	Catnip
Nigella sativa	Nigella (a.k.a. black seed)
Nymphaea odorata	Pond lily (white or yellow)
Ocimum basilicum	Basil
Ocimum sanctum, O. tenuiflorum	Tulsi (a.k.a. holy basil)
Oenothera biennis	Evening primrose
Oplopanax horridus	Devil's club
Orbignya oleifera	Babassu
Origanum vulgare	Oregano
Paeonia lactiflora	White peony
Panax ginseng, P. quinquefolius	Ginseng
Parietaria diffusa, P. judaica, P. officinalis	Pellitory
Passiflora incarnata	Passionflower
Paullinia cupana	Guarana
Peumus boldus	Boldo
Phyllanthus emblica	Amla
Phytolacca decandra, P. americana	Pokeroot

Latin Name	Common Name
Picrorhiza kurroa	Kutki
Pimpinella anisum	Anise
Piper methysticum	Kava
Piper nigrum	Black pepper
Piscidia piscipula	Jamaican dogwood
Plantago lanceolata, P. major	Plantain
Plantago psyllium	Psyllium seed
Podophyllum peltatum	Mayapple
Prunella vulgaris	Self-heal
Pueraria lobata	Kudzu
Punica granatum	Pomegranate
Quercus alba, Q. rubra	Oak
Rehmannia glutinosa	Rehmannia, prepared (a.k.a. Chinese foxglove or shēng dì huáng)
Reynoutria japonica (a.k.a. *Fallopia japonica* or *Polygonum cuspidatum*)	Japanese knotweed
Rhamnus purshiana	Cascara (a.k.a. buckthorn)
Rhaponticum carthamoides	Luzea (a.k.a. maral root)
Rheum officinale, R. palmatum	Rhubarb
Rhodiola rosea	Rhodiola (a.k.a. Arctic rose)
Ricinus communis	Castor
Rosa species	Rose (hips and petals)
Rosmarinus officinalis	Rosemary
Rumex acetosella	Sheep sorrel
Rumex crispus	Yellow dock
Ruscus aculeatus	Butcher's broom
Salix alba	Willow
Salvia miltiorrhiza	Dan shen (a.k.a. Chinese red sage)
Salvia officinalis, S. lavandulifolia	Sage
Sambucus nigra	Elderberry
Sanguinaria canadensis	Bloodroot
Sassafras albidum	Sassafras
Schisandra chinensis	Schisandra (a.k.a. wu wei zi)
Scrophularia nodosa	Figwort
Scutellaria baicalensis	Baikal skullcap (a.k.a. Chinese skullcap)
Scutellaria lateriflora	Skullcap
Silybum marianum	Milk thistle
Smilax ornata	Sarsaparilla
Solidago virgaurea	Goldenrod

Latin Name	Common Name
Stachys betonica	Wood betony
Stellaria media	Chickweed
Stillingia sylvatica	Stillingia
Symphytum officinale	Comfrey
Syzygium aromaticum	Clove bud
Tabebuia impetiginosa, T. avellandae, T. rosea, Handroanthus impetiginosus	Taheebo (a.k.a. pau d'arco, lapacho)
Tanacetum parthenium	Feverfew
Taraxacum officinale	Dandelion
Taxus brevifolia, T. baccata, T. wallichiana	Yew
Terminalia arjuna	Arjuna
Terminalia bellirica	Bibhitaki
Terminalia chebula	Haritaki
Theobroma cacao	Cacao
Thuja occidentalis	Thuja (a.k.a. eastern arborvitae or northern white cedar)
Thymus vulgare	Thyme
Tilia × europea	Linden
Trametes versicolor	Turkey tail
Trifolium pratense	Red clover
Trigonella foenum-graecum	Fenugreek
Turnera diffusa	Damiana
Ulmus fulva, U. rubra	Slippery elm
Uncaria tomentosa	Cat's claw
Urtica dioica	Stinging nettle
Valeriana officinalis	Valerian
Verbena officinalis, V. hastata	Blue vervain
Viburnum opulus	Cramp bark
Vinca major, V. minor	Periwinkle
Viola odorata	Violet
Viola tricolor	Wild pansy
Viscum album	Mistletoe
Vitex agnus-castus	Chasteberry
Withania somnifera	Ashwagandha
Yucca species	Yucca
Zanthoxylum clava-herculis	Prickly ash
Zea mays	Corn silk
Zingiber officinale	Ginger
Ziziphus jujuba	Jujube

Index of Recipes and Formulas for Patient Care

Brighter Days Tea, page 33
Cardiotonic Hawthorn Tea, page 179
Carminative Chai Tea, page 201
Carob Drink to Stop Diarrhea, page 176
Diaphoretic Tea, page 229
Dong Quai and Millettia Formula, page 185
Essiac Formula, page 52
Golden Milk, page 303
Healing and Recuperation Tincture, page 124
Healing Lip Balm, page 216
Herbal Bitters Blend, page 200
Herbal Cream for Radiation Burn, page 235
Herbal Formula for Building Blood, page 185
Herbal Formula for Moving Lymph and Stimulating Lymphocytes, page 207
Herbal Formula for Nausea and Vomiting, page 217
Herbal Formula for Tonic Constipation, page 166
Herbal Formula to Calm the Nerves and Promote Appetite and Digestion, page 192
Herbal Lotion for Neuropathic Pain, page 224
Herbal Tea for Flaccid or Atonic Constipation, page 166
Herbal Tea for Rehydration, page 177
Herbal Tea Formula for Loose Stools, page 176
Immune Boot Camp Nutritional Breakfast Smoothie, page 60
Immunostimulating Tincture Formula, page 59
Let Go Liniment, page 105
Magnesium Lotion, page 224
Mineralizing Tea for Replenishing after Vomiting, page 216
Peppermint-Fennel Essential Oil Emulsion, page 218
Powdered Herb Formula to Soothe the Digestive System, page 192
Rooty Fruity Herbal Tea Frozen Pops, page 214
Scar Oil, page 120
Skin Lotion for Lymph Drainage, page 209
Skin Lotion for Lymph Node Stimulation, page 209
Soothing and Healing Mouthwash, page 214
Stomach Settler Seed Sprinkle, page 201
Super Moisturizing Skin Cream, page 196
Tumor Spray, page 115
"Weeding" Protocol, page 56
WHO Rehydration Formula, page 177
Wide Awake Tea, page 163

Index

Page numbers in **bold** indicate main subject entries.

A

Achillea millefolium. See yarrow
Aconitum napellus. See monkshood
actinic keratosis, using bloodroot for, 436
activator constituents in herbs, 326
activator herbs, incorporating, 325–27
activator protein 1 (AP-1), 382
adaptogen nervines, 143
adaptogens, **66–73**
    afternoon/evening use and, 73
    benefits of, 67–69
    choosing, 69
    morning use and, 73
    in oncology, 67–68
    for rejuvenation, 180–81
    restorative and balancing, 71–73
    stimulating, 69–71
    for stress, side effects and, 161
    target organs and, 68
adipose (fat) cells
    hormones and, 63
    obesity and, 367–68
adjuvant therapies, 146
adrenals, hormones and, 63
Aesculus hippocastanum. See horse chestnut
agents. *See* cytotoxic agents; natural agents
age of patient, 345
alder bark (*Alnus glutinosa*), 116
alfalfa (*Medicago sativa*), 181
alkaloids, specific actions of, 424
allostasis, 64
    states of, 317
Alnus glutinosa. See alder bark
aloe (*Aloe vera*), 117, 194–95, 235, **241–43**
    aloe emodin, 242
    caveats, 242–43
    dosing, 243
    as a laxative, 243
    medicinal properties of, 241–42
Aloe barbadensis. See Cape aloe
alternative medicine, 4
alteratives (herbs), 50–51
amplifying herbs, 322–23
anabolic/catabolic balance, 369–372
analgesics, toxic, 140–141
andrographis (*Andrographis paniculata*), **244–45**
    cancer care, benefits in, 244–245
    clinical pearls, 245
    dosing, 245
anesthesia, postoperative cognitive impairment and, 103
Angelica sinensis. See dong quai
angiogenesis
    assessing, 397
    blood tests and, 394
    copper and, 395
    hypoxia and, 395–96
    inhibiting, 394–97
    macrophages and, 396–97
    metabolic factors and, 395
    natural agents and, 397
    surgery-induced, 91, 124–25
    tumor suppressor gene p53 mutation and, 397
annual wormwood. *See Artemisia annua*
anorexia. *See* appetite loss
antiarthritic herbs for hands and feet, 482–83
antiasthma, 427
antibacterial action, honey and, 236
anticancer activity/actions
    herbs for, lung cancer and, 483
    honey and, 236
    mistletoe lectins, peptides, and polysaccharides, 447
    terpene compounds with, 326
anticancer compounds in foods, 45
anticancer constituents, mushrooms with, 305–7

anticancer diet, 34
anticancer drugs, tests for predicting responses, 354–55
anticancer effects, green tea and, 269–270
anticancer herbs, cytotoxic, 481
anticancer mechanisms of honey, 236
anticancer terpenes, metabolism of fats to, 380
anticancer treatments, other innovative, 156–57
  hyperthermia, 157
  photodynamic therapy (PDT), 157
anticoagulants
  as antithrombotic agents, 98
  herbal medicines and, 334–35
  supplements and herbs, caution when taking, 334–35
anti-inflammatory
  St. John's wort and, 290
  tulsi and, 297
antimetastatic natural agents, 394
antimicrobial, pomegranate and, 280
antioxidant interactions, 335–36
antiplatelets, 98
antithrombotic agents, 98
antithrombotic enzymes, 101–2
antiviral properties, herbs and, 29
anxiety, 30–31
anxiolytic herbs, 323
aperients, 169
apigenin, 282
apoptosis
  flavonoids that induce, 327
  inducing, 372–73
  natural agents and, 373–74
Appetite and Digestion, Herbal Formula to Calm the Nerves and Promote, 192
appetite loss, **197–202**
  cannabis, appetite promotion and, 202
  Carminative Chai Tea, 201
  factors contributing to, 197
  Herbal Bitters Blend, 200
  herbs to support appetite, 198–201
  holistic strategies for treating, 197–98
  meals and snacks, 197–98
  Stomach Settler Seed Sprinkle, 201
arginine, 213
arjuna (*Terminalia arjuna*), 179
arnica (*Arnica montana*), **138–140**
  dosing, topical application, 139–140
arrhythmia, 464
Artemisia annua (annual wormwood, Chinese wormwood, sweet Annie), **409–17**
  adverse reactions, 412
  clinical pearls, 412
  herb-drug interactions, 412–13
  molecular structure of, 410
  pulse dosing, 413–14
  synergists for, 414–17
  tissue targets for, specific, 407
arthritis
  acute, 481
  antiarthritic herbs for hands and feet, 482–83
  hand treatments, warm wax, 484–85
  Warm Wax Herbal Treatment, A, 485
ashwagandha (*Withania somnifera*), 72
  chemotherapy and, 340
Asian ginseng (*Panax ginseng*), 70
Asimina triloba (pawpaw), **417–20**
  adverse effects, 419
  clinical applications of, 418–19
  clinical pearls, 419–20
  dosing, 419
  tissue targets for, specific, 407
  what makes it medicinal, 418
aspirin, 101, 190, 262, 297, 393, 472, 486
asthma, 103, 249, 354
astragalus (*Astragalus membranaceus*), **62**
  anticancer actions of, 62
  benefits from, research on, 337
atonic or flaccid constipation, 165
Atropa belladonna. See belladonna
Avena sativa. See milky oat seed; oats; oat straw
Ayurvedic medicine
  brain tonic, gotu kola and, 266
  constitutional assessment and, 347
  crataeva and, 220
  Himalayan yew and, 439
  kapha excess in, 210
  triphala for bowel health, 172–73
  tulsi and, 295

B

Bach Flower Remedies, 76–77
  Bach Flower Remedy Mixture, 457
back stiffness/aching/tightness, 465–66
bacteria, gut microbiome and, 55
bacterial infections, 28–29
Baikal skullcap (*Scutellaria baicalensis*), **245–47**
  baicalin and, 246–47
  cancer care, benefits in, 246–47
  dosing, 247

Baikal skullcap (*Scutellaria baicalensis*), *continued*
indications in, traditional, 246
medicinal properties of, 246
balanced formula, creating, **314–19**
actions, supportive and directing, 315
allostasis, states of, 317
blending, questions prior to, 314–15
deep terrain support, 315
disease, addressing causes of, 316
pathological correction, 315–16, 317
physiological enhancement, 316–17
wellness, optimizing capacity for, 315
balancing herbs, 323
basal cell carcinoma, using bloodroot for, 436
base herbs. *See* foundation (herbs)
basil, essential oils and, 110
B-complex vitamins, 120–21
bedtime, supplements to take at, 123
bee resin. *See* propolis
belladonna (*Atropa belladonna*), 141–42
benign tumor, appearance and behavior of, 19
bereavement. *See* grief
beta-glucans, 182, 195, 303–4, 307
beta-glucans, immunomodulation and, 303–4
beta-sitosterol, 221
betulinic acid, 221
beverages. *See also* tea
Carob Drink to Stop Diarrhea, 176
Golden Milk, 303
Smoothie, Immune Boot Camp Nutritional Breakfast, 60
Smoothie Recipe, Daily, 458
biologicals, 147
biomarkers, 348
biopsies
diagnosis and, 87
pathology testing and, 353
patient-centered approach and, 6
sentinel node, 96, 103, 204, 453
start of treatment and, 7
types of, 89
bitter compounds from plants, 200
bitter herbs, 198–200
Herbal Bitters Blend, 200
secondary actions of, 200
black salve, 435
bladder
alteratives for, 51
frequent urination and, 476
bladder cancer case history, **463–476**
arrhythmia and, 464
back stiffness/aching/tightness, 465–66
blood work and, 466, 473
case summary, 463
case update/revised protocol, 472–75
Castor Oil Pack, Herbal, 472
Crohn's disease and, 464, 468
cytotoxic agents, specialty, 475
discussion, 475
goshajinkigan powder and, 473
health factors, additional, 463–66
Herbal Powder, Daily, 469
high blood pressure and, 464
kidney stones and, 465
liver detox support blends and, 473
Liver Tonic, 474
migraines and, 465
note from cancer patient, 475–76
prostate health recommendations, 465
prostate hyperplasia, benign, 465, 467
protocol analysis for patient, 470
specialty cytotoxic agents and, 471
supplements, 471, 473
Tea Blend, Daily, 470
Tincture, Daily, 474
Tincture Formula, Daily, 468
tincture formula, initial, 468
treatment options, 466–67
treatment planning, initial, 467
upper digestive aching, chronic, 464–65, 467
Urinary Tract Infection, Extra Strength Tea for Acute, 471
blood, thinning the
antithrombotic enzymes and, 101–2
blood-thinning herbs, 98
blood building
Dong Quai and Millettia Formula, 185
Herbal Formula for Building Blood, 185
herbs and nutrition for, 181–88
blood-cleansing herbs, 210
blood clots, prevention, 101–2
blood fats, pomegranate and, 280
blood-moving action, dan shen and, 256
bloodroot. *See Sanguinaria canadensis*
blood sugar, natural agents and, 368
blood sugar regulation
nigella and, 277–78
pomegranate and, 280
blood tests, 350–51
angiogenesis/metastatic progression, 394
lung cancer case history and, 477
blood work, treatment planning and, 348

bone broth, 182
bone density, soy and, 48
Boswellia serrata. *See* Indian frankincense
Boswellia spp. *See* frankincense
botanicals, mental sharpness and, 106
botanicals, pain management and, **126–142**
herbs, dosing to manage pain, 127–28
herbs, topical use, 138–142
mild to moderate pain, 129–137
supplements for pain, 128
where to begin, 127–28
bowel health. *See also* microbiome, gut
Essiac Formula, 51–52
restoration of, **54–57**, 96
triphala for, 172–73
brain/brain support. *See also* cognitive function
brain fog, 162–63
brain-repair effects, dan shen and, 256–57
brain tonic, gotu kola and, 266
cerebral circulatory stimulants, 163
"chemo brain," management of, 162
natural agents for functioning of, 163
neuroplasticity and, 133
useful agents for, 110–11
brain toxic herbs, 106
BRCA1, BRCA2
olaparib, test for predicting response, 355
pathology testing, excised tissue, 353
breast cancer
clinical strategies in managing, 398
dong quai and, 186
gene signature profiling, 355
mammograms and, 359
oncotype IQ genomic intelligence testing and, 355
Prosigna assay, 356
breast cancer case history, **452–62**
capsule formulas, proprietary, 458
case summary, 452–53
case update/revised protocol, 459–462
Castor Oil Pack, 461
clinical progression, 459
Daily Tincture Formula, Adjusted, 461
detoxification, 460
discussion, 462
extras, optional, 462
Flower Remedy Mixture, Bach, 457
Initial Tincture Formula, 454–55
lymphatic support, 460
pelvic decongestants and, 460
Poke Oil Breast Rub, 456–57
protocol analysis for patient, 456
supplements, 458, 459, 460, 462
Tea Formula, 455, 461
tissue cleansing, 460
treatment planning, 453–59
bromelain, 101
bryony, 483–84
bupleurum (*Bupleurum falcatum*), **247–48**
cancer care, benefits in, 248
dosing, 248
medicinal properties of, 247–48
resins, triterpenes and, 35
burdock root, 52
butcher's broom (*Ruscus aculeatus*), 208

C

cacao (*Theobroma cacao*), **249–251**
cancer care, benefits in, 250–51
dosing, 25
food of the gods, 250
medicinal properties of, 249–250
caffeic acid phenethyl ester (CAPE), 282
calcium-D-glucarate, estrogen removal and, 28
calendula (*Calendula officinalis*), 118, **208**, **251–53**
cancer care, benefits in, 252
dosing, 253
growing your own, 253
medicinal properties of, 252
California poppy (*Eschscholzia californica*), 127, **129**
calming herbs, 323
Camptotheca acuminata (cancer tree, happy tree, xi shu), **420–22**
dosing, 421–22
preservation, need for, 421
sourcing, importance of, 421
tissue targets for, specific, 407
what makes it medicinal, 420–21
cancer(s)
addressing directly, 361–403
bloodroot used in care for, 436–37
dosing guidelines, natural supplements, **399–403**
dysplasia compared to, 20
extent of, measuring, 20–22
inflammation and, 386, 387
mistletoe and, 447–48
obesity and, 367–68
physical effects of, 18

cancer(s), *continued*
- proliferation and progression of, 362–63
- promotion of, 361
- speed of growth and, 21
- staging and grading, 21

cancer care, introduction to holistic, 1–2
cancer cell(s). *See also* growth factors
- behaviors to target, 363
- gene testing, 353–54
- induce differentiation in, 372

cancer development, key processes in, 362
cancer-driven blood clots, blood tests and, 477
cancer drivers and inhibitors, blood tests and, 477
cancer herb directory. *See* materia medica
cancer markers, solid tumors and, 17
cancer prevention, soy and, 46
cancer-sugar connection, 366
cancer treatments. *See also* conventional cancer treatment
- curcumin in, studies of, 338–39
- strategies, implementation of, 330
- therapeutic intentions in, 324

cancer tree. *See Camptotheca acuminata*
cancer vaccines, 227–28
cancer virus therapy, 227
cannabis (*Cannabis* spp.), **131–35**
- appetite promotion and, 202
- cannabinoid receptors, 132–33
- CBD and THC content, 132
- dosage, 134–35
- endocannabinoids, 133, 137, 202
- endocannabinoid system, 132–33
- growing your own, 134
- hyperemesis and, 135
- medical, 134, 202, 223
- neuropathy and, 223, 225
- overdosing, 135
- which species to use, 133

Cape aloe (*Aloe barbadensis*), 169–70
Capsicum minimum. See cayenne
capsule-filling device, 134
capsule formulas, proprietary, 458
carbohydrate preloading, 99
carbonic anhydrase, 396
cardiac support, **176–79**
- Cardiotonic Hawthorn Tea, 179
- heart health, cacao and, 251
- herbs for, 178–79
- supplements for, 179

cardiotoxic drugs, 177–78, 179
cardiotoxic taxine alkaloids, 441, 442
cardiovascular health, blood tests and, 477
carminative herbs, 190–91
- Carminative Chai Tea, 201

Carob Drink to Stop Diarrhea, 176
case histories
- about, 450
- bladder cancer, 463–476
- breast cancer, 452–462
- lung cancer, 476–486

castor oil, pokeroot in, 431–32
castor oil packs, 118–19
- Castor Oil Pack, 461
- Herbal Castor Oil Pack, 472
- how to make and use, 119

catabolic/anabolic balance, 369–372
catechins, anticancer effects of, 269–270
Catharanthus roseus (Madagascar periwinkle, rosy periwinkle), **422–23**
- dosing, 423
- what makes it medicinal, 422–23

cathartics, 170
cayenne (*Capsicum minimum*), 140
CBD. *See* cannabis
Ceanothus americanus. See red root
cell(s). *See also* cancer cell(s)
- behaviors to target, cancer, 363
- mast cell degradation, 397
- natural killer, 393
- poor differentiation of, 22
- promoting cell-to-cell communication, 390–92

cell adhesion molecules (CAMs), 392
cell turnover/cycling
- controlling, 369–370
- natural agents and, 370

Centella asiatica. See gotu kola
cerebral circulatory stimulants, 163
chaga (mushroom), 305–6
chaparral. *See Larrea divaricata, L. tridentata*
chapped lips. *See* cracked lips
checkpoint inhibitors, 227
Chelidonium majus (greater celandine), **423–26**
- adverse reactions, 425
- alkaloids, specific actions of, 424
- clinical pearls, 425–26
- dosing, 426
- pharmaceuticals made from, 424–25
- specific indications and uses, 424
- tissue targets for, specific, 408
- toxicology, safety and, 426
- what makes it medicinal, 423–24

"chemo brain," management of, 162

chemotherapy
- about, 143
- adaptogens for stress, 161
- ashwagandha and, 340
- brain fog and, 162–63
- cardiotoxic drugs, 177–78, 179
- chronotherapy, 154
- considering, 147–48
- diarrhea caused by, 173–76
- dosing models, 153–56
- green tea and, 340–41
- healthy daily routine and, 160–61
- herbal medicine and, 335–37
- history of modern, 151–52
- hyperthermic intraperitoneal, 155–56
- hypothermic isolated limb perfusion, 154–55
- liposomal drug delivery, 155
- maximum tolerated dose (MTD), 153
- melatonin and, 84
- metronomic dosing, 153
- mouth sores and, 211
- nanoparticle drug delivery, 155
- patient who declines, managing, 360–61
- planning, key questions for, 349
- preventing, 211–12
- red clover, synergy with, 284
- redox regulators and, 338
- self-care daily routine example, 161
- side effects and, 148–49, 160–63
- "starving" cancer before, 149–150
- supplements and, 335–37
- synergy between plant compounds and, 321–22
- tolerating it better, 149–152
- toxicity and, 148–49
- tumor shrinkage and, 91–92
- turmeric and, 299–300, 338–39
- twentieth-century treatments, 151–52
- twenty-first-century treatments, 152

chemotherapy haze, 162–63
chickweed (*Stellaria media*), 194
chimeric antigen receptor T cell therapy, 228
Chinese wormwood. *See Artemisia annua*
chitin, 304
chlorella (*Chlorella* spp.), 122–23
chlorella growth factor (CGF), 123
chlorophyll, 183–84
- foods rich in, 184

chocolate. *See* cacao (*Theobroma cacao*)
cholagogues, 50
choleretics, 50, 322
choline, estrogen removal and, 28
chronic obstructive pulmonary disease (COPD), 103, 123
chronotherapy, 154
cicatrant herbs, wound cleansing and, 116–17
circadian rhythms, 81
circulatory stimulants, cerebral, 163
Clean and Green Detox Diet, **41–43**
- chemotherapy, radiation and, 143
- strictest days and, 41–42
- surgery and, 96
- vitality and, 40

cleavers (*Galium aparine*), 207–8
codonopsis, 61, 69, 180, 187
coexisting health conditions, 331
coffee enema, preparing, 172
cognitive function. *See also* brain/brain support
- huperzia and, 109
- natural agents for, 163
- tulsi and, 297

cognitive impairment. *See* postoperative cognitive impairment (POCI)
collaborative oncology, 342
collagenase, natural compounds and, 391
colloidal oatmeal, 195
colon cancer, gut microbiome and, 55
colorectal cancer, surgery-induced angiogenesis and, 91
combining herbs, key considerations, **323–24**
- person + purpose + potency = proportion, 324
- weighting formulas, goal and, 324

comfrey (*Symphytum officinale*), 117
comorbidities, 348
complementary and alternative medicine (CAM), 4
complementary herbs, 322
complementary medicine, 4
complement factor, 386
complications
- of healing, avoiding, 113–120
- wound healing and, 118

condiments
- seaweed as, 234
- Stomach Settler Seed Sprinkle, 201

connective tissue
- promoting and supporting, 116–18
- strengthening, 390
- tonic, gotu kola and, 266–67

consent, informed, 95–96
constipation, **164–173**
- causes of, 164

constipation, *continued*
- diet and, 165, 167
- enemas for pain and, 171
- flaccid or atonic, 165
- Herbal Formula for Tonic Constipation, 166
- Herbal Tea for Flaccid or Atonic Constipation, 166
- holistic treatment of, 165–172
- laxatives and, 168–171
- lifestyle and, 167–68
- reduction of, simple ways, 167
- tonic constipation, 165
- types of, 164–65

constituents. *See* herbal constituents

constitution, 347
- hot/cold assessment, 347–48

contributory factors, **23–26**
- anxiety, 30–32
- bacterial infections, 28–29
- dietary influences, 32–34
- hormones, 26–28
- inflammation, 34–36
- loneliness, 30–32
- stress/distress, 30–32
- toxins, exposure to, 24–26
- UV radiation exposure, 36–37
- viral infections, 28–29
- where you live, 23–24

conventional cancer treatment, 5–6, **146–152**
- best options, considering, 349
- local treatment, 146
- systemic treatment, 146
- therapies used in, 146–47

copper, angiogenesis and, 395

cordyceps (*Cordyceps* spp.), 220, **306–7**

corn silk (*Zea mays*), **117**, 219

cortisol
- adaptogens and, 68
- excess, 66

corydalis (*Corydalis* spp.), 127, 129, **130–31**, **253–55**
- actions and uses of, 130
- cancer care, benefits in, 254–55
- clinical pearls, 255
- dosing, 130--131, 255
- medicinal properties of, 254
- opioid drugs and, 131

COX-2 (cyclooxygenase-2)
- arthritis inflammation and, 149
- colorectal adenomas and tumors and, 354
- curcumin and, 321, 338, 339, 388
- prolonged activation of, 386–87
- prostaglandins and, 386
- protopine and, 437
- surgery and, 90
- tulsi and, 297
- turmeric and, 299

cracked lips, **215–16**
- holistic strategies for treating, 215
- Lip Balm, Healing, 216
- Replenishing after Vomiting, Mineralizing Tea for, 216

Crataegus spp. *See* hawthorn

crataeva (*Crataeva nurvala*), 220–21

cream(s)
- Moisturizing Skin Cream, Super, 196
- Radiation Burn, Herbal Cream for, 235

creosote bush. *See Larrea divaricata, L. tridentata*

Crohn's disease, 464, 468

CT scans, 231

Curcuma longa. *See* turmeric

curcumin
- in cancer treatment, studies on, 338–39
- risks of, 339–340

cyclins, 369

cyclooxygenase-2 (COX-2), 386–87

cytotoxic activity, calendula and, 252

cytotoxic agents, 147
- bladder cancer and, 471, 475

cytotoxic anticancer herbs, lung cancer and, 481

cytotoxic drugs, in combination, 148

cytotoxic effects, gotu kola and, 267

cytotoxic herbs, **405–6**. *See also specific herb*
- about, 404
- antiviral properties and, 29
- materia medica, 404–49
- prescribing, guidelines for, 406–9
- starting low, going slowly, 406
- taking the, 327, 329, 407–9
- tissue targets for, specific, 407–9
- when to avoid, 407

D

dan shen (*Salvia miltiorrhiza*), 255–57
- cancer care, benefits in, 256–57
- dosing, 257
- medicinal properties of, 256

Datura stramonium. *See* jimson weed

DCIS Score, 355

debility, 180–88

decoctions, 239

deep terrain support, 315
dehydration
 Rehydration Formula, WHO, 177
dental care and oral hygiene, bloodroot in, 436
depurative herbs, 210
detoxification
 breast cancer case history, 460
 Clean and Green Detox Diet, 41–43
 exposure to toxins and, 24–26
 liver detox support blends, 473
 liver in, role of, 48–52
detoxigenomic profile, 357
diagnosis of cancer
 about, 342
 classification of tissue by origin, 20
 dysplasia, cancer compared to, 20
 extent of cancer, measuring, 20–22
 first steps after, 6–9
 gathering information about, 348
 options, considering your, 7
 organization and empowerment, 8
 poor differentiation of cells, 22
 preparation plan and, 8–9
 tumors, classification of, 18–19, 20
 understanding your, **18–22**
Diaphoretic Tea, 229
diarrhea, **173–76**
 in cancer patients, 174
 Carob Drink to Stop Diarrhea, 176
 Herbal Tea Formula for Loose Stools, 176
 holistic treatment of, 174–175
 stopping, methods for, 175
 types of, 174
diet(s). *See also* fasting; food(s); nutrition
 anticancer diet, 34
 BRAT diet, 175
 Clean and Green Detox Diet, 41–43
 constipation and, 165, 167
 fiber-poor, 55
 FODMAP (restricted carbohydrate), 165
 how you eat matters, 191–93
 initiation of cancer and, 32–34
 nutrient-packed meals/snacks, 197–98
 resistant starch and, 57
dietary supplements. *See* supplements
differentiation
 in cancer cells, inducing, 372
 of cells, poor, 22
digestion. *See also* bowel health
 Appetite and Digestion, Herbal Formula to Calm the Nerves and Promote, 192
 bitter herbs and, 198
 Digestive System, A Powdered Herb Formula to Soothe the, 192
 promotion of good, 40–41
 upper digestive aching, chronic, 464–65, 467
 yellow gentian for, 199
diosgenin, 221
directing herbs, 323
directory, cancer herb. *See* materia medica
disease. *See also specific disease*
 causal chain of, 312–13
 excitatory or precipitating causes, 313
 predisposing causes, 312–13
 sustaining or perpetuating causes, 313
distress, 30–31
diuretic herbs, 206
DNA damage, 301, 354, 410
DNA repair, 233, 301, 371, 447
dong quai (*Angelica sinensis*), **186**
 breast cancer and, 186
 Dong Quai and Millettia Formula, 185
dosing/doses
 chemotherapy and, 153–156
 guidelines, natural supplements for cancer, **399–403**
 herbal teas, 239
 herbs, cancer care and, **239–241**
 maximum safe dose, 406
 threatened species and, 240–41
 timing of doses, 333
 tinctures, 241
drug(s). *See also* pharmaceuticals, off-label cancer-care uses for; platinum drugs; synergy of constituents in herbs/drugs
 predisposing causes and, 313
drug-induced respiratory depression (DIRD), 104
drug interactions, 331
drug responses, predictive testing for, 354–55
drug therapies, systemic, 147
dysbiosis, 55
dysplasia, cancer compared to, 20

E

early-warning signs, 17
eastern arborvitae. *See Thuja occidentalis, T. plicata*
eating. *See also* diet(s); food(s); nutrition
 healthy, ground rules for, 203

Eating Habits Questionnaire (EHQ), 202
echinacea (*Echinacea* spp.), 115–116, **257–59**
  cancer care, benefits in, 258–59
  dosing, 259
  medicinal properties of, 258
Eclectic physicians, 405, 424, 433
effector constituents in herbs, 326
effector herbs, incorporating, 325–27
eleuthero (*Eleutherococcus senticosus*), 71
emesis. *See* vomiting
emotions, essences for specific, 78–79
empowering yourself, 8
Emulsion, Peppermint-Fennel Essential Oil, 218
endocannabinoid receptor sites, 274
endocannabinoids, 133, 137, 202
endocannabinoid system, 132–33
endocrine/hormonal treatment, 147
enemas
  coffee or herbal, preparing, 172
  for constipation and pain, 171
Enhanced Recovery after Surgery (ERAS), 93
epidermal growth factor 1 (HER1), 375–76
epidermal growth factor 2 (HER2/neu), 376
Equisetum arvense. See horsetail
ER+ test, 353
ergothioneine, 304
escharotics, 435–36
Eschscholzia californica. See California poppy
essences, specific emotions and, 78–79
essential fatty acid pathways, 387
essential oils
  basil, peppermint, and rosemary, 110
  Peppermint-Fennel Essential Oil Emulsion, 218
Essiac Formula, 51–52
estrogenomic profile, 357
estrogen(s)
  as cell proliferant, 346
  environmental, avoiding, 27
  exposure to, increased, 26
  phytoestrogens, 27
  removal of, nutrients for, 27–28
  signaling, red clover and, 284
eugenol, 295
excised tissue, pathology testing on, 353
excitation, unresolved, 313
exercise, **85–86**
  cancer development and, 86
  constipation and, 167–168
extent of cancer, measuring, 20–22
extracellular matrix (ECM), 390–91
  natural compounds and, 391
exudative diarrhea, 174

F

fast-growing cancers, 21
fasting
  chemotherapy and, 149–150
  intermittent, 53–54, 203–4
  prechemotherapy, 143
  regimens, types of, 53–54
fatigue, 180–88
fats
  metabolism of, anticancer terpenes and, 380
  omega-3, immunomodulation and, 385–86
fatty acid pathways, essential, 387
fecal transplants, 54
fermentation, soy and, 47
fever
  immune response, encouraging, 229
  treatment, cautions and, 230
feverfew (*Tanacetum parthenium*), **259–261**
  dosing, 261
  medicinal properties of, 260
fibrin formation, 386
fibroblast growth factor (FGF), 391–92
Filipendula ulmaria. See meadowsweet
fish oil, **110–11**
  two main types of, 215
Fitzpatrick skin types, 36–37
5-fluorouracil (5-FU), tests for predicting responses, 354
5-LOX (5-lipoxygenase)
  chebulagic acid and, 172
  surgery and, 90
flaccid or atonic constipation, 165
flavones, 107. *See also* isoflavones
flavonoids, **326–27**
  as immunomodulating agents, 385
flower essences, 76–77
Flower Remedy Mixture, Bach, 457
folate, estrogen removal and, 28
food(s). *See also* diet(s); *specific food*
  anticancer compounds in, 45
  B vitamins and, 212
  fruits and vegetables, 40, 41–43
  rich in chlorophyll, 184
  soy, 45–48
forest bathing, 74–75

formula(s). *See also* herbal formulating
- Appetite and Digestion, Herbal Formula to Calm the Nerves and Promote, 192
- Building Blood, Herbal Formula for, 185
- Daily Tincture Formula, 482
- Daily Tincture Formula, Adjusted, 461
- Digestive System, A Powdered Herb Formula to Soothe the, 192
- Dong Quai and Millettia Formula, 185
- Essiac Formula, 52
- Initial Tincture Formula, 454–55
- logic of, developing, 311
- Moving Lymph and Stimulating Lymphocytes, Herbal Formula for, 207
- Nausea and Vomiting, Herbal Formula for, 217
- proprietary capsule, 458
- Rehydration Formula, WHO, 177
- Tea Formula, 455, 461, 479
- Tincture Formula, Daily, 468
- Tincture Formula, Initial, 478
- Tonic Constipation, Herbal Formula for, 166
- weighting toward a goal, 324

foundation (herbs), 318, 328
foundation interventions, 330
FoundationOne CDX (F1CDX) profiling, 356–57
frankincense (*Boswellia* spp.), 117
free radicals, addressing, 364–65

G

Galium aparine. See cleavers
gamma-aminobutyric acid (GABA)
- brain tonic and, 266
- hyperforin and, 290
- neuroreceptors and, 129
- terpenes and, 113

gap junctions, 392
garden, planting a memory, 77
garlic (*Allium sativum*), **261–63**
- cancer care, benefits in, 262
- caveats, 263
- dosing, 262–63
- medicinal properties of, 261–63
- roasting, 263

gastric ulcers, alleviating, 278
gastritis, **189–193**
- Appetite and Digestion, Herbal Formula to Calm the Nerves and Promote, 192
- Digestive System, A Powdered Herb Formula to Soothe the, 192
- holistic strategies for, 191
- how you eat and, 191–93

gastroesophageal disease (GERD), 108
Gelsemium sempervirens. See yellow jasmine
gender fluidity, 345
gender of patient, 345–46
gene(s)
- NM (nonmetastatic) 23 gene, 124–25
- proangiogenic, 394

gene expression
- mutated tumor suppressor BCL-2, natural agents, 373–74
- reduction of abnormal, 365–66

gene mutation, **12–15**
- causes of, 15
- cells that won't die, 14
- lack of contact inhibition, 14
- mutated oncogenes, 13–14
- mutated tumor suppressor genes, 13

general adaptation syndrome, stress and, 64–65
genetic instability, addressing, 364–65
genetics, 312, 346–47
genetic tests/testing
- in clinical practice, 354–55
- gene mutation and, 354
- gene testing, cancer cell, 353–54
- treatment planning and, 348

genomic testing, 353–54
Gentiana lutea. See yellow gentian
geographic location, 23–24
ginger (*Zingiber officinale*), **263–65**
- actions of, other, 265
- cancer care, benefits in, 264–65
- dosing, 265
- medicinal properties of, 264
- resins, triperpenes and, 35

ginkgo (*Ginkgo biloba*), **106–7**
- postoperative period and, 107
- surgery and, 98

ginseng. *See also* Asian ginseng (*Panax ginseng*)
- cancer-related fatigue and, 180–81

glucose metabolism, pathways of, 366
glutamine, 60
glycolitic shift, 366

Glycyrrhiza glabra. *See* licorice
goldenseal
  diarrhea and, 175
  local infection and, 114
  synergy within one plant and, 320–21
gonads, hormones and, 63
goshajinkigan, 225
gotu kola (*Centella asiatica*), **108**, 117–18, 223, **265–68**
  cancer care, benefits in, 267–68
  clinical pearls, 268
  dosing, 268
  medicinal properties of, 266–67
grade of cancer
  grading cancers, 21
  treatment planning and, 348
greater celandine. *See Chelidonium majus*
green tea (*Camellia sinensis*), **268–271**
  anticancer effects of, 269–270
  caffeine and, 270
  caveat, 270
  chemotherapy and, 340–41
  clinical pearls, 270–271
  dosing, 270
  medicinal properties of, 269
  surgery and, 98
grief, **75–77**
  herbs for, 76–77
  horticultural therapy activities for, 77
  stages of, 75
growth factors, **374–381**
  cancer promotion and, 374
  fibroblast growth factor (FGF), 391–92
  transforming growth factor-beta (TGF-ß), 376–77
gut peptides, 199

H

hallucinogens, healing journey and, 80
hand-foot syndrome, **193–96**
  grading scale for, 194
  herbs for skin, 194–96
  skin irritation, minimizing, 193–94
hand treatments, warm wax, 484–85
  Warm Wax Herbal Treatment, A, 485
happy tree. *See Camptotheca acuminata*
hawthorn (*Crataegus* spp.), 178
healing. *See also* wound healing
  avoiding complications of, **113–120**
  Healing and Recuperation Tincture, 124
health conditions, coexisting, 331
heart/heart disease. *See also* cardiac support
  arrhythmia, 464
  bloodroot and, 437
  irregular heartbeat, 481
henbane (*Hyoscyamus niger*), 141–42
hepatitis C, liver cancer and, 28, 29
hepatoprotective herbs, 322
hepatotoxicity, 331–32, 333
HER2/neu+ test, 353
herbal constituents. *See also* synergy of constituents in herbs/drugs
  radiosensitizing capacity and, 233
  radiotherapy and, 233
herbal enema, preparing, 172
herbal formulating, **309–41**. *See also* formula(s)
  about, 309
  balanced formula, creating, 314–19
  causal chain of disease and, 312–13
  pathological correction, formulating for, 325–29
  pyramid prescribing protocol, 318–19
  research, benefits from herbs, 337–341
  safety and toxicology with herbs, 331–37
  synergy of constituents in herbs/drugs, 319–324
  therapeutic order, 313–14
  timelines for herbal treatment, 329–331
herbal laxatives, four types of, 169–171
herbal medicine
  anticoagulants and, 334–35
  chemotherapy and, 335–37
Herbal Powder, Daily, 469
herbal teas, dosing and, 239
herbs. *See also* adaptogens; cytotoxic herbs; herbal constituents; materia medica; tinctures; *specific herb*
  activator constituents in, 326
  alteratives, 50–51
  amplifying, 322–23
  anticoagulants and, 334–35
  antiviral properties of, 29
  appetite support and, 198–201
  balancing, 323
  benefits from, research on, 337–341
  bitter, 198–200
  blood building and, 181–88
  blood-cleansing, 210
  blood-thinning, 98
  brain toxic, 106–11
  cardiac support and, 178–79

carminative, 190–191
cicatrant, wound cleansing and, 116–117
complementary, 322
cytotoxic anticancer, lung cancer and, 481
deep immune tonic, 61–63
directing, 323
diuretic, 206
dosing, cancer care and, 239–241
effector constituents in, 326
foundation, 318, 328
gastritis and, 189–191, 193
inflammation and, 35–36, 111–13
kidney function and, 219–221
liver and, 49–50
lymphedema and, 206–10
mouth sores and, 215
mucilaginous, 189–190
nervous system and, 112–13
neuropathy and, 222–25
pain, supplements for, 128
pain management, dosing, 127–28
pain management, moderate to severe, 140
pain management, topical use, 138–142
polyvalent, 450
post-surgery, recovery and, 106–13, 112–13
power of, 1–2
preparing for surgery and, 97, 99
primary or foundation, 318–19
radioprotective effects and, 233
radiotherapy and, 233
reflux and, 189–191, 193
safety and toxicology with, 331–37
secondary or supportive, 319
sleep and, 82–83
specifics, 318, 328
synergists, 318, 328
tertiary or targeted effectors/ activators, 319
threatened species and, 240–41
three levels of, 318–19
tonic, 112–13
topical, radiation burn and, 234–36
vulnerary, 117–18
hereditary risks. *See* genetics
herpes simplex, mouth sores and, 213
high blood pressure, 464
high-grade cancer, appearance and behavior of, 19
Himalayan yew. *See Taxus brevifolia, T. baccata, T. wallichiana*
Hippophae rhamnoides. See sea buckthorn
histamine, 386
histamine release, 397
histone deacetylase (HDAC), 371–72
natural agents and, 372
holistic practitioner, multifaceted role of, 311
honey, cancer care and, 235–36
skin healing and, 235
hormones, **26–28**. *See also* estrogen(s)
endocrine/hormonal treatment, 147
neuroendocrine system and, 63
phytoestrogens, 27
stress, 30
synthetic, 26–27
horse chestnut (*Aesculus hippocastanum*), 271–72
cancer care, benefits in, 271–72
clinical pearls, 272
dosing, 272
medicinal properties of, 271
horsetail (*Equisetum arvense*), 112, 219
horticultural therapy activities, 77
hot/cold constitution assessment, 347–48
HPA activity, sleep and, 80
humoral medicine, Western, 210, 289, 322, 347
huperzia (*Huperzia serrata*), **109**
historic use of, 110
hyaluronidase (HAase)
apigenin and, 282
echinacea and, 115–16, 259
TME and, 390–91
tumor growth and, 466
hydrangea (*Hydrangea* spp.), 220
Hyoscyamus niger. See henbane
hyperemesis, 135
hyperforin, 289–290
hypericin, 289
Hypericum perforatum. See St. John's wort
hyperthermia, 157
hyperthermic intraperitoneal chemotherapy, 155–56
hypothalamic-pituitary-adrenal (HPA) axis
adaptogens and, 67
cortisol and, 68
excess cortisol and, 66
general adaptation syndrome and, 65
licorice and, 73
stress and, 31

hypothalamic-pituitary-adrenal (HPA) pathway
    endocannabinoid system and, 132
    immunosuppression and, 105
hypothalamic-pituitary-thyroid (HPT) axis, adaptogens and, 30
hypothermic isolated limb perfusion, 154–55
hypoxia
    angiogenesis and, 395–96
    natural agents and, 397

I

immune boot camp, **58–61**
    Immune Boot Camp Nutritional Breakfast Smoothie, 60
immune dysregulation, 312
immune evasion, 389–390
immune function, boosting nonspecific, 96
immune responses
    cancer vaccines and, 227
    immune evasion and, 389
    sweating and fever, encouraging with, 229
    targeted therapies and, 147
immune system
    alteratives for, 51
    healing and, 115–16
    herbs, deep immune tonic, 61–63
    natural agents and, 385
    proteolytic enzymes and, 389–390
    support for, **58–63**, 385–86
    tincture formula for, 59
immunogenomic profile, 357
immunomodulation
    beta-glucans and, 303–4
    dark chocolate and, 250–51
    flavonoids and, 385
    omega-3 fats and, 385–86
immunostimulants, 322
Immunostimulating Tincture Formula, 59
immunosuppression
    counteracting, 105
    natural agents and, 389
immunotherapies, 152
immunotherapies, special considerations for, **226–230**
    managing immunotherapies, 228–230
    side effects, rare but high-risk, 229
    sweating, fever and, 229–230
Indian frankincense (*Boswellia serrata*), **272–73**
    resins, triterpenes and, 35
indolent cancer, appearance and behavior of, 19
industrial toxins, 25
infection(s)
    bloodroot and, 437
    local, controlling and treating, 114
    predisposing causes and, 313
    viral and bacterial, **28–29**
inflammation, **34–36**
    bloodroot and, 437
    cardinal symptoms of, 386
    chronic, 388–89
    herbs and, 35–36, 111–13
    initiation of cancer and, 34–36
    managing, 115–16
    natural agents, 387–88
    predisposing causes and, 313
    reduction of, 386–89
    Swelling and Inflammation, Herbal Tea for, 482
inflammatory exudate, 386
inflammatory pathways
    baicalin and, 246
    herbs and, 111
    surgery, cancer spread and, 90
informed consent, 95–96
infusions, 239
initiation of cancer. *See* contributory factors
insulin-like growth factor 1 (IGF-1)
    mTOR and, 379
    natural agents, 378
insulin-like growth factors (IGFs), 377–78
insulin resistance, obesity and, 368
integrative or integrated medicine, 4–5
interactions
    antioxidant, 335–36
    cross-reference to avoid, 406
    supplement, 336–37
intermittent fasting, 53–54
    reconsidering, 203–4
interventions, foundation, 330
intravenous vitamin C, 150–51
Irish yew. *See Taxus brevifolia, T. baccata, T. wallichiana*
isoflavones
    phytoestrogens and, 27
    red clover and, 284, 285
    soy and, 45–46
    synergy within one plant and, 320
isolation, social, 31–32

J

Jamaican dogwood (*Piscidia piscipula*), 135–36
jimson weed (*Datura stramonium*), 141–42

K

kelp, 182
key processes in cancer development, 362
kidneys
    alteratives for, 51
    damage to, 218–221
    herbs for improved function, 219–221
    kidney-repair effects, dan shen and, 257
kidney stones, 465
kinase enzymes, 12
Krebs cycle, 17, 149, 294, 366, 368, 417

L

lactic acid, natural agents and, 397
Lactuca virosa. *See* wild lettuce
Larrea divaricata, *L. tridentata* (chaparral, creosote bush), **426–29**
    actions of, 427
    caveats, 429
    clinical pearls, 429
    dosing, 429
    safety concerns, addressing, 428–29
    tissue targets for, specific, 408
    what makes it medicinal, 426–28
laxatives, **168–171**
    aloe as a, 243
    herbal, four types of, 169–171
    reducing use of, procedure for, 171
lectins, 304–5
Lepidium meyenii. *See* maca
leukotriene activity, normalization of, 386–89
leuzea (*Rhaponticum carthamoides*), 69–70
licorice (*Glycyrrhiza glabra*), **72–73**
    resins, triterpenes and, 35
lifestyle choices. *See also* diet(s); exercise
    about, 38
    constipation and, 167–68
    making changes, 342
Ligusticum porteri. *See* osha
liniments, 104
    Let Go Liniment, 105
liposomal drug delivery, 155
lips. *See* cracked lips
liver
    alteratives (herbs) and, 50–51
    detoxification and, 48–52
    Essiac Formula for, 51–52
    herbs and, 49–50
    Tonic, Liver, 474
liver cancer, hepatitis C and, 28, 29
liver detox support blends, 473
L-methionine, estrogen removal and, 28
lobelia (*Lobelia inflata*), **103–5**
    Let Go Liniment, 105
local physical effects, 18
loneliness, 30
    social isolation and, 31–32
longevity, increasing, 324
loss. *See* grief
lotion(s)
    Lymph Drainage, Skin Lotion for, 209
    Lymph Node Stimulation, Skin Lotion for, 209
    Magnesium Lotion, 224
    Neuropathic Pain, Herbal Lotion for, 224
low-grade malignant cancer, appearance and behavior of, 19
LOX enzymes. *See also* 5-LOX
    inflammatory prostaglandin production and, 35
    tulsi and, 297
lumbrokinase, 101, **102**, 415
lung cancer case history, **476–486**
    antiarthritic herbs for hands and feet, 482–83
    anticancer action, herbs for, 483
    arthritis, acute, 481
    blood testing, suggested schedule of, 477
    bryony, 483–84
    case update/revised protocol, 481–83
    cytotoxic anticancer herbs, 481
    discussion, 486
    hand treatments, warm wax, 484–85
    Herbal Tea for Swelling and Inflammation, 482
    lung tonics, 483
    medications, 486
    other health history of note, 476–77
    pleurisy root and, 483
    protocol analysis, 480
    Soup Blend, 479
    supplements, 480–481, 484
    Tea Formula, 479
    Tincture Formula, Daily, 482
    Tincture Formula, Initial, 478
    treatment planning, initial, 477
lymphatic support, breast cancer and, 460

lymphatic system, alteratives for, 51
lymphedema, **204–10**
Herbal Formula for Moving Lymph and Stimulating Lymphocytes, 207
herbal treatments for, 206–10
Lymph Drainage, Skin Lotion for, 209
Lymph Node Stimulation, Skin Lotion for, 209
moving lymph fluid and, 205
physical treatments for, 205–6
stages of, 205
symptoms of, 204
lysine, 213

M

maca (*Lepidium meyenii*), 183
macrophages
angiogenesis and, 396–97
natural agents and, 397
Madagascar periwinkle. *See Catharanthus roseus*
magnesium
estrogen removal and, 28
Lotion, Magnesium, 224
magnolia (*Magnolia* spp.), **273–76**
cancer care, benefits in, 275
caveats, 275–276
dosing, 275
medicinal properties of, 274
maintenance protocol, long-term, 330
malignant transformation, cellular and tissue changes associated with, 20
malignant tumor, appearance and behavior of, 19
maltodextrins, 99
mammalian target of rapamycin (mTOR), **378–79**
mTOR and IGF-1R, 379
natural agents, 379
MammaPrint test, 356
mammograms, 358–59
markers. *See* cancer markers; tumor markers
mast cell degradation, natural agents and, 397
materia medica
cytotoxic herbs, **404–49**
herbs for cancer, **237–307**
mayapple. *See Podophyllum peltatum*
meadowsweet (*Filipendula ulmaria*), **190**
salicylates and, 35
meals, supplements to take at, 123
measuring extent of cancer, 20–22
Medicago sativa. See alfalfa
medicinal mushrooms, **303–7**. *See also specific type*
active constituents of, 304–5
anticancer constituents and, 305–6
beta-glucans, immunomodulation and, 303–4
dosing, 307
foraging for, 307
Immune Boot Camp protocol and, 58
melanoma, UV radiation exposure and, 36–37
melatonin, **84–85**
cancer and, 84–85
supplementing with, 85
memory. *See also* brain/brain support; postoperative cognitive impairment (POCI); botanicals, mental sharpness and
memory garden, planting a, 77
mental health
emotions, essences for specific, 78–79
forest bathing, 74–75
grief and, 75–77
hallucinogens and, 80
nature therapy and, 74–80
mental outlook, 312
mental sharpness. *See* memory
mental stimulants, 106–11
metabolic factors, angiogenesis and, 395
metabolic functions, methylation and, 365
metabolic pathways, 16
metabolic syndrome
nigella and, 277–78
tulsi and, 297
metabolism of fats to anticancer terpenes, 380
metastasis
blood tests and, 394
inhibit invasion and, 393–94
melatonin and, 84–85
TNM classification and, 22
metastatic physical effects, 18
methylation
capacity, testing for, 365–66
metabolic functions and, 365
natural agents and, 366
metronomic dosing, 153
microbiome, gut
boosting, **54–57**, 96
fecal transplants and, 54
feeding, 57
functions of, 54–55

seeding, 56
sugary foods and, 44
weeding, 55–56
migraines, 465
milk thistle (*Silybum marianum*), **49**
surgery, supplement prior to, 96
milky oat seed (*Avena sativa*), 112–13
millettia (*Millettia* spp.), **188**
Dong Quai and Millettia Formula, 185
mindfulness meditation, 75
mitochondrial rescue, 368–69
mitotic index, 353
molecules, small, 226
monkshood (*Aconitum napellus*), 138
monoclonal antibodies (mAbs)
as immunotherapies, 152
managing therapy, 228–230
side effects, rare but high-risk, 229
special considerations, 226
sweating, fever and, 229–230
mood support, tulsi and, 297
mouth sores, **210–15**
chemotherapy and, 211
conventional treatment of, 212
herbs for, 215
herpes simplex and, 213
holistic strategies for treating, 212–15
Mouthwash, Soothing and Healing, 214
oral thrush and, 213
Pops, Rooty Fruity Herbal Tea Frozen, 214
mucilaginous herbs, 189–190
mushrooms. *See also* medicinal mushrooms; *specific type*
beta-glucans and, 61, 182, 303–4, 307
blood building and, 182–83
edible, 43, 61
immune system and, 61
lion's mane, 111, 161
mutated tumor suppressor Bcl-2 gene expression, natural agents and, 373–74
mutation. *See also* gene mutation, of regulatory proteins, 370–71
myrrh, 117

N

N-acetylcysteine (NAC), 28
nanoparticle drug delivery, 155
nattokinase, **101–2**, 389, 415
natural agents
angiogenesis and, 397
antimetastatic, 394
AP-1 or NF-κB, 382
blood sugar and, 368
carbonic anhydrase and, 396
cell cycling, downregulation and, 370
cell differentiation, 372
chelation of copper and, 395
epidermal growth factor 1 or 2, 376
histone protein deacetylation, 372
hypoxia, lactic acid and, 397
immune support, nonspecific, 385
immunosuppression, 389
inflammation, 387–388
insulin-like growth factors (IGFs), 378
mast cell degradation, 397
methylation and, 366
mitochondrial rescue, 368–69
mutated tumor suppressor Bcl-2 gene expression, 373–74
NRF2, induction of, 383–84
NRF2, inhibition of, 384
PPARs, 385
PTK or PKC receptors and, 375
redox regulating, 364–65
regulatory proteins and, 371
TLR4 antagonist activity and, 389
transforming growth factor-beta (TGF-ß), 376–77
vascular permeability and, 397
natural killer cells, 393
natural supplements for cancer, dosing guidelines, 399–403
nature therapy, mental health and, 74–80
nausea, **217–18**
Herbal Formula for Nausea and Vomiting, 217
Peppermint-Fennel Essential Oil Emulsion, 218
NDGA, pharmacology of, 427
neoadjuvant therapy, 146
nephritis, 218–221
nerves. *See also* stress
Herbal Formula to Calm the Nerves and Promote Appetite and Digestion, 192
restoratives and, 143
nervous system, herbs for post-surgery, 112–13
nettles. *See* stinging nettle
neuroendocrine system, 63
neuropathic pain, supplements for, 225–26
neuropathy, **222–26**
herbs for, 222–25
Lotion, Magnesium, 224

neuropathy, *continued*
- Lotion for Neuropathic Pain, Herbal, 224
- reducing, strategies for, 222

neuroplasticity, 133
neurotoxicity
- Asimina triloba and, 419
- CAPE and, 282
- cumulative dose and, 222
- *Thuja occidentalis* and, 444

neurotoxins, 135, 162, 383
nigella (*Nigella sativa*), **276–77**
- cancer care, benefits in, 276–78
- dosing, 278
- medicinal properties of, 276
- safety of, 278

NM (nonmetastatic) 23 gene, 124–25
node, TNM classification and, 22
northern white cedar. *See Thuja occidentalis*
nuclear factor erythroid 2-related factor 2 (NRF2), 382–83, 383–84
nuclear factor-kappa B (NF-κB), 382
nutrients, estrogen removal and, 27–28
nutrition. *See also* diet
- about, 38
- blood building and, 181–88
- eating for maximum, 43
- healthy eating, vitality and, **40–48**
- predisposing causes and, 312
- preparing for surgery and, 97

O

oatmeal, colloidal, 195
oatmeal bath, making a, 196
oats (*Avena sativa*), **196**
- green milky oats, 195
- other uses for, 195–196

oat straw (*Avena sativa*), 112, **195–96**
obesity
- cancer and, 367–368
- insulin resistance and, 368
- TLRs, obesity and, 388–89

Ocimum sanctum. See tulsi
off-label cancer-care uses for pharmaceuticals, 158–59
oil(s). *See also* castor oil; castor oil packs; essential oils; fish oil
- in diet, choosing good, 42
- Poke Oil Breast Rub, 456–57
- Scar Oil, 120
- sea buckthorn oil, 111
- St. John's wort–infused oil, making, 290–21

olaparib, test for predicting responses, 355
omega-3 fats, immunomodulation and, 385–86
oncogenes, mutated, 13–14
oncology
- adaptogens in, 67–68
- conventional cancer care vs. holistic, 5–6
- holistic, 5

oncotype IQ genomic intelligence testing, 355
opioid drugs
- botanicals and, 126
- corydalis and, 131
- pain management and, 127

oral carbohydrate preloading, 99
oral care, turmeric and, 300
oral hygiene and dental care, bloodroot in, 436
oral thrush, 213
organization and empowerment, 8
organs
- adaptogens and, 68
- hormones made by, 63

osha (*Ligusticum porteri*), 323
osmotic diarrhea, 174
orthorexia, **202–4**
- holistic strategies for treating, 203–4

ovarian cancer, chemotherapy and, 155–56
ovaries, alteratives for, 50
oxidative stress
- adaptogens and, 66
- addressing, 325
- andrographis and, 244
- antioxidant interactions and, 335–36
- arachidonic acid pro-inflammatory pathways and, 379
- arjuna, heart and, 179
- artemisinin and, 410, 411
- calendula and, 251
- *Chelidonium majus* and, 426
- chlorella and, 123
- chronic diseases and, 383
- curcumin and, 301
- detoxification and, 48
- DHA, EPA and, 415
- free radicals and, 364
- genetic mutations and, 15
- glycolitic shift and, 366
- gotu kola and, 267
- honey and, 236
- hypericin and, 289
- magnolia and, 274
- milk thistle and, 49

plant polyphenols and, 232
PPARs and, 385
propolis and, 282
proteins and, 32
redox regulation and, 335
rosemary and, 36
SIRT1 and, 257
thymoquinone and, 277
turmeric and, 299
vitamin C, K3 and, 414
wogonin and, 246

P

Pacific yew. *See Taxus brevifolia, T. baccata, T. wallichiana*
Paeonia lactiflora. See white peony root
paeoniflorin, 187
pain management. *See also* botanicals, pain management and; neuropathy
acute pain, 128
post surgery, 100
palliative therapies, 146
palmar-plantar erythrodysesthesia (PPE). *See* hand-foot syndrome
Palmitoylethanolamide (PEA), 137
Panax ginseng. See Asian ginseng
pancreas, hormones and, 63
papain, 101
parasympathetic nervous system, 40, 103, 104, 109, 132, 142
Parietaria spp. *See* pellitory
pathological correction, formulating for, **325–29**
cytotoxics, taking the, 327, 329
effector herbs, incorporating, 325–27
oxidative stress and, 325
pyramid prescribing model, 328
targeted activator herbs, incorporating, 325–27
pathological correction strategies/protocols, 317
pathology testing, excised tissue, 353
patient-centered approach, 6
pawpaw. *See Asimina triloba*
pellitory (*Parietaria* spp.), 219
pelvic decongestants, 460
peppermint
Essential Oil Emulsion, Peppermint-Fennel, 218
essential oils and, 110
perioperative immunonutrition, 105
peritoneum, alteratives for, 50
periwinkle (*Vinca major, Vinca minor*), 108–9
person + purpose + potency = proportion, 324
PET scans, 231
phagocyte migration, 386
pharmaceuticals, off-label cancer-care uses for, 158–59
phenolic acids, 139, 223, 236, 367, 411
phosphatidyl choline, **110**, 163
photodynamic therapy (PDT), 157, 289
physical effects of cancer, 18
physiological enhancement, 316–17
Physiomedical principles, 323, 347
phytoestrogens, 27
Phytolacca decandra, P. americana (pokeroot), **429–432**
actions and uses of, 430–31
caveats, 431
dosing, 431
making pokeroot preparations, 431–32
pokeroot in castor oil, 432
specific indications and uses, 430
therapeutic actions, 430–31
tissue targets for, specific, 408
phytotherapy, 311
pineal gland, hormones and, 63
Piscidia piscipula. See Jamaican dogwood
pituitary gland, hormones and, 63
Plantago spp. *See* plantain
plantain (*Plantago* spp.), 118, 194, 219, 223
plant compounds, telomerase and, 370
platelets, 98
platinum drugs
acute toxicity and, 148
chronic toxicity and, 148–49
DNA unwinding and copying, 149
goshajinkigan and, 225
kidney damage and, 218
synergy between plant compounds and, 321–22
pleurisy root, 483
Podophyllum peltatum (mayapple), **432–34**
caveats, 434
clinical pearls, 433
dosing, 433–34
tissue targets for, specific, 408
what makes it medicinal, 433
Poke Oil Breast Rub, 456–57
pokeroot. *See Phytolacca decandra, P. americana*
polypharmacy, 140
polyphenols
glycemic responses and, 367
herbs with high levels of, 35–36

pomegranate (*Punica granatum*), **278–281**
- cancer care, benefits in, 279–280
- dosing, 280–281
- medicinal properties of, 278–79

poor differentiation of cells, 22
poppies. *See* California poppy; corydalis
posology, 309
postoperative cognitive impairment (POCI), 102–5
- anesthesia and, 103
- lobelia and, 103–5

postoperative recovery, useful agents for, 124
Powder, Daily Herbal, 469
PPARs (peroxisome proliferator-activated receptors), 384–85
- natural agents, 385

PR+ test, 353
predictive testing for drug responses, 354
predisposing causes of disease, 312–13
preexisting conditions, 348
"prehabilitation," 93
preparation plan, starting, 8–9
prescription drugs, 126
proangiogenic genes, 394
proliferation and progression of cancer, 362–63
promotion of cancer, 361
- growth factors and, 374

propolis, 117, **281–83**
- cancer care, benefits in, 281–82
- dosing, 282–83
- medicinal properties of, 281
- safety of, 283
- sustainability of, 283

proprietary capsule formulas, 458
Prosigna assay, 356
prostaglandins, 386–87
prostaglandin activity, normalization of, 386–89
prostate
- alteratives for, 51
- health recommendations, general, 465
- hyperplasia, benign, 465, 467

prostate cancer
- apoptosis in, red clover and, 284
- growth and treatment of, 355
- testosterone and, 346
- "watchful waiting" and, 21

protein, whey, 183
proteins. *See also* transcription factors, stabilization of
- mutation of regulatory, 370–71
- Ras proteins, 379–381

proteolytic enzymes
- antacid drugs and, 191
- as antithrombotic agent, 98
- blood clots and, 101
- immune system and, 389–390
- as synergist for artemisia, 415

protocol analysis
- bladder cancer patient and, 470
- breast cancer patient and, 456
- lung cancer patient, 480

Prunella vulgaris. *See* self-heal
psychological stress. *See* stress
Punica granatum. *See* pomegranate
purgatives, 170
pus, 386
pyramid prescribing protocol, 318–19, 328

Q

quality of life, 324

R

radiation
- about, 143
- adaptogens for stress, 161
- calendula and, 252
- consequences of, 234
- diarrhea caused by, 173–76
- gotu kola and, 267–268
- healthy daily routine and, 160–61
- managing, 230–236
- predisposing causes and, 313
- removal from body, natural agents for, 234
- scans, x-rays and, 231
- seaweed for removal of, 234
- side effects, managing, 160–63
- sun, safety and, 37
- UV radiation exposure, 36–37

radiation burns
- Herbal Cream for Radiation Burn, 235
- topical herbs for, 234–36

radio protection, 232
- radioprotective effects, herbs and, 233

radioprotective effects, herbs and, 233
radio sensitizing, 232
- herbal constituents and, 233

radiotherapy, 231–32
- herbs and constituents for, 233

Ras proteins, 379–381
- natural agents, 381

reactive oxygen species (ROS), 155, 321, 335, 338, 383, 385, 414
Recurrence Score, 355
red clover (*Trifolium pratense*), **283–85**
    benefits of, other, 285
    cancer care, benefits in, 284
    dosing, 285
    safety of, 285
    salve, traditional, 285
redox regulators/regulation
    benefits from, research on, 338
    flavonoids and, 327
    natural agents and, 364–65
red root (*Ceanothus americanus*), 210
reflux, **189–193**
    Appetite and Digestion, Herbal Formula to Calm the Nerves and Promote, 192
    Digestive System, A Powdered Herb Formula to Soothe the, 192
    holistic strategies for, 191
    how you eat and, 191–193
regulatory proteins, mutation of, 370–71
rehmannia (*Rehmannia glutinosa*), 187
rehydration
    Rehydration, Herbal Tea for, 177
    Rehydration Formula, WHO, 177
reishi (mushroom), 305
rejuvenation, adaptogens for stress, 180–81
relaxants, 83
remedy
    Flower Remedy Mixture, Bach, 457
    Smoothie Recipe, Daily, 458
research, benefits from herbs, 337–341
resins, herbs with high levels of, 35
resistant starch, 57
respiratory deficiencies, 103
Rhaponticum carthamoides. See leuzea
rhodiola (*Rhodiola rosea*), 70–71, 110
rhubarb, 52
rose (herb of the heart), 77
rosemary (*Rosmarinus officinalis*), **108**
    essential oils, 110
    polyphenols and, 36
rosy periwinkle. *See Catharanthus roseus*
rubefacient, 322
Ruscus aculeatus. See butcher's broom

S

S-adenosylmethionine (SAMe), estrogen removal and, 28
sadness, herbs for, 76–77
safety with herbs, 331–37
    anticoagulants, herbal medicines and, 334–35
    chemotherapy and, 335–37
    determining herb safety, 332–33
    isolated constituents versus whole herbs, 331–32
    variability in herbal products, 332
sage (*Salvia* spp.), 113
salicylates, herbs with high levels of, 35
saliva/buccal swab testing, 357
salve, traditional red clover, 285
Salvia miltiorrhiza. See dan shen
salvianolic acid B, 257
Sanguinaria canadensis (bloodroot), **434–39**
    actinic keratosis and basal cell carcinoma, using for, 436
    black salve, 435
    cancer care and, 437
    caveats, 439
    dental care and oral hygiene, using for, 436
    dosing, 438
    escharotics, 435–36
    heart disease and, 437
    infections and, 438
    inflammation and, 437–38
    tissue targets for, specific, 408–9
sarsaparilla, 35
scans, 231
scarring
    castor oil packs, 118–19
    Scar Oil, 120
    topical treatments to reduce, 118–120
schisandra (*Schisandra chinensis*), 49–50
screening mammograms, 359
Scutellaria baicalensis. See Baikal skullcap
sea buckthorn (*Hippophae rhamnoides*), **285–87**
    dosing, 288
    medicinal properties of, 286
    oil, 111
seaweed, 182, 234
secretory diarrhea, 174
sedatives, 83
selective estrogen receptor modifiers (SERMs)
    estrogen signaling and, 284
    phytoestrogens and, 27
selenium, 28
self-care
    daily routine example, chemotherapy and, 161
    oatmeal bath, making a, 196
self-heal (*Prunella vulgaris*), 118

senescence, 313
sensitivity and resistance testing/functional profiling, 357–58
sentinel node assessment, 146
sentinel node biopsies, 96, 103, 204, 453
serrapeptase, 101–102
SHBG (sex hormone binding globulin) level, 367
sheep sorrel root, 52
Shinrin Yoku (forest bathing therapy), **74–75**
- grief, sadness and, 76

side effects
- associated drugs and, 148
- cytotoxic herbs and, 406
- high-risk, 229

signal transduction/transcription, 374–75
Silybum marianum. See milk thistle
skin
- alteratives for, 50
- damage, radiation and, 252
- healing, honey and, 235

skin cancer, UV radiation exposure to, 36–37
skin cream. *See* cream(s)
skin phototyping, 36–37
skin rashes, **193–96**
- herbs for, 194–96
- skin irritation, minimizing, 193–94

sleep, **80–85**
- bedtime, supplements to take at, 123
- circadian rhythms and, 81
- herbs and supplements for, 82–83
- sleep hygiene, good, 81–82

slippery elm, 52
slow-growing cancers, 21
small intestine bacterial overgrowth (SIBO), 108
small molecules, 226
Smoothie, Immune Boot Camp Nutritional Breakfast, 60
social isolation, 31–32
Soup Blend, 479
soy, **45–48**
- bone density and, 48
- cancer prevention and, 46–47
- case against, 47
- fermentation and, 47
- isoflavones and, 45–46
- as SERM, 46
- using, or not, 47–48

specialty blood tests, 351
specialty testing for cancer, 353–54
specifics (herbs), 328
Spray, Tumor, 115
stage of cancer
- staging cancers, 21
- treatment planning and, 348

starch, resistant, 57
statins, 305
Stellaria media. See chickweed
stimulants
- cerebral circulatory, 163, 322
- mental, 106–11
- peripheral circulatory, 322
- systemic relaxant and circulatory, 322

stinging nettle (*Urtica dioica*), 181–82, 220
St. John's wort (*Hypericum perforatum*), **112**, 223, **288–292**
- anti-inflammatory, 290
- cancer care, benefits in, 290–91
- clinical pearl, 291
- contraindications, 291
- dosing, 291
- drug interactions and, 291–92
- hyperforin, 289–290
- hypericin, 289
- medicinal properties of, 288–29
- St. John's wort–infused oil, making, 290–91

stomachics, 190
Stomach Settler Seed Sprinkle, 201
stress, **30–31**. *See also* nerves; oxidative stress
- adaptogens for stress, 161
- chronic, systemic effects of, 64
- general adaptation syndrome, 64–66
- managing, **63–66**
- mental outlook and, 312
- social isolation and, 31–32
- trauma and, 30–31
- unresolved, effects of, 66

stress management, poor, 476
stress response, 64
- bitter herbs, 198–99

sugar, progression of cancer and, 44
sugar-cancer connection, 366
sun
- safety and, 37
- UV radiation exposure and, 36–37

supplement interactions, 336–37
supplements. *See also* vitamins
- anticoagulants and, 334–35
- bladder cancer and, 471, 473
- breast cancer and, 458, 460, 462
- for cancer, dosing guidelines, **399–403**
- for cardiac protection, 179
- chemotherapy and, 335–37
- inflammation and, 35

lung cancer and, 480–81, 484
for meals and bedtime, 123
for pain, 128
for pain, neuropathic, 225–26
post-surgery, healing and, 120–24
preparing for surgery and, 99
sleep and, 82–83
supportive therapies, 146–47
surgery
about, 87, 146
better recovery starts before, 93
cancer spread and, 90–91
complications of, 89–90
herbal strategies prior to, 97, 99
nutritional strategies prior to, 97
preparing for, 94–100
recovering from, 100–105
risks, consideration of, 89–92
tumor shrinkage and, 91–92
surgery-induced angiogenesis, 91
sweating
Diaphoretic Tea, 229
fever and, 229–230
sweet Annie. *See Artemisia annua*
sympathetic nervous system, 40, 63, 102, 142, 199
Symphytum officinale. See comfrey
synergists, 318, 328
synergy of constituents in herbs/drugs, **319–324**
amplifying herbs, 322–23
balancing herbs, 323
clinical studies on synergy, 320–22
combining herbs, key considerations, 323–24
complementary herbs, 322
between different plants, 321
directing herbs, 323
formulation for synergy, 322–23
within one plant, 320–321
between plant compounds/ chemotherapy, 321–22
systemic disease, cancer as, **15–18**
metabolic pathways, 16
normal cell to malignant tumor, 16–17
physical effects, 18
warning signs, 17–18
systemic drug therapies, 147
systemic physical effects, 18

T

taheebo (*Tabebuia* spp.), **292–94**
cancer care, benefits in, 293–94
dosing, 294
medicinal properties of, 293
species to use, 294
targeted therapies, 147, 152, 226. *See also* immunotherapies, special considerations for
Taxus brevifolia, T. baccata, T. wallichiana (Pacific yew, a.k.a. Western yew); Irish yew; Himalayan yew, **439–443**
clinical pearls, 442
differences among species, 439–40
dosing, 441–42
metaphysical meaning of yew, 442–43
symbol of death and rebirth, 440
tissue targets for, specific, 408–9
toxicity, 440
what makes it medicinal, 440–41
T cell therapy, chimeric antigen receptor, 228
TCM. *See* Traditional Chinese Medicine
tea. *See also* green tea
Brighter Days Tea, 33
Cardiotonic Hawthorn Tea, 179
Carminative Chai Tea, 201
Constipation, Herbal Tea for Flaccid or Atonic, 166
Daily Tea Blend, 470
Diaphoretic Tea, 229
Formula, Tea, 455, 461, 479
herbal, dosing and, 239
Herbal Bitters Blend, 200
Loose Stools, Herbal Tea Formula for, 176
Rehydration, Herbal Tea for, 177
Replenishing after Vomiting, Mineralizing Tea for, 216
Swelling and Inflammation, Herbal Tea for, 482
Urinary Tract Infection, Extra Strength Tea for Acute, 471
Wide Awake Tea, 163
telomerase inhibition, 370
Terminalia arjuna. See arjuna
terminally ill, hallucinogens and, 80
terpene compounds, anticancer activity and, 326
terpenes, 305, 326
metabolism of fats to anticancer, 380

terrain
- blood work to assess, 348
- foundation interventions and, 330
- gathering information about, 348

testosterone, prostate cancer and, 346
tests/testing, **349–360**
- additional tests, 358–59
- in advance of therapy, 350
- blood tests to order, 350–351
- conclusions about, 360
- genetic, 348, 354–59
- importance of, 349–360
- methylation capacity, 365–66
- pathology testing, excised tissue, 353
- prioritizing additional tests, 359–360
- specialty testing for cancer, 353–54
- tumor markers, 351–52

TGF-ß (transforming growth factor-beta)
- natural agents and, 376–77

THC. *See* cannabis
therapeutic order, 313–14
thermographic imaging, 358
3,3'-diindolylmethane (DIM), estrogen removal and, 28
thrush, oral, 213
thuja (*Thuja* spp.), 116–17
Thuja occidentalis, T. plicata (Eastern arborvitae, a.k.a. northern white cedar; western red cedar), **443–46**
- clinical pearls, 446
- dosing, 445–46
- grandmother of the forest, 443
- modern research, 445
- therapeutic actions, 444
- tissue targets for, specific, 409
- toxicity, 446
- uses, traditional, 444
- what makes it medicinal, 444–45

thymus, hormones and, 63
thyroid, hormones and, 63
timelines for herbal treatment, 329–331
- treatment planning, summary of, 330

tinctures
- bladder cancer and, 468
- Daily Tincture, 474
- Daily Tincture Formula, 482
- Daily Tincture Formula, Adjusted, 461
- dosing herbs and, 240
- Formula, Daily Tincture, 468
- Healing and Recuperation Tincture, 124
- Herbal Bitters Blend, 200
- Immunostimulating Tincture Formula, 59
- Initial Tincture Formula, 454–55, 478

tissue
- changes, malignant transformation and, 20
- cleansing, breast cancer and, 460

tissue of origin, classification by, 20
tissue targets, cytotoxic herbs, 407–9
TNM classification, **22**
- treatment planning and, 348

toll-like receptors (TLRs), 388–89
- natural agents, 389

tonic(s)
- Liver Tonic, 474
- lung, 483

tonic constipation, 165
tonic herbs, 112–113
toxicology with herbs, **331–37**
- anticoagulants, herbal medicines and, 334–35
- chemotherapy and, 335–37
- hepatotoxicity, 331–32, 333
- isolated constituents versus whole herbs, 331–32
- variability in herbal products, 332

toxins
- detoxification and, 24–26
- exposure to, **24–26**, 313
- industrial, cancers and, 25

Traditional Chinese Medicine (TCM), 62, 69, 102, 107, 109, 130, 138, 180, 185, 186, 187, 188, 210, 225, 245, 255, 257, 264, 274, 275, 337, 347
transcription factors, stabilization of, 381–85
transcription pathways, flavonoids and, 327
transduction pathways, flavonoids and, 327
trastuzumab, synergists and potentiators of, 376
trauma
- predisposing causes and, 313
- stress and, 30–31

treatment options, considering your, 7
treatment plan. *See also* whole-person treatment planning
- developing, 8
- stages in treatment planning, 348–49
- summary of, 330

Trifolium pratense. *See* red clover
triphala, bowel health and, 172–73
tulsi (*Ocimum* spp.), **73**, **294–98**
- cancer care, benefits in, 296
- caveats, 298
- dosing, 297–98
- medicinal properties of, 295–96
- metabolic syndrome and, 297
- uses of, other, 297

umor(s)
appearance and behavior of, 19
classification of, 18–20, 22
shrinkage, chemotherapy response and, 91–92
tissue of origin and, 20
TNM classification, 22
umor-centered approach, 6
umor markers, 351–52
umor microenvironment (TME), extracellular matrix (ECM) and, 390–91
umor node metastases (TNM), 348
TNM classification, 22
umor Spray, 115
umor suppressor Bcl-2 gene expression, mutated, 373–74
umor suppressor gene p53 mutation, angiogenesis and, 397
urkey tail (mushroom), 306
urmeric (*Curcuma longa*), 235, **298–303**
absorption and, 301
benefits from, research on, 338–39
cancer care, benefits in, 299–300
caveats, 301–2
chemotherapy and, 299–300
clinical pearls, 302
dosing, 300
Golden Milk, 303
medicinal properties of, 299
oral care and, 300
polyphenols and, 35–36

U

Unani medicine, 136, 439
Urinary Tract Infection, Extra Strength Tea for Acute, 471
Urtica dioica. See stinging nettle
UV radiation exposure, 36–37

V

vaccines, cancer, 227–28
valerian, herbs to pair with, 323
varuna. *See* crataeva (*Crataeva nurvala*)
vascular endothelial growth factor (VEGF), 124
natural agents, 377
social isolation and, 31
vascular permeability
decreasing, 394–97
natural agents and, 397
Vinca spp. *See* periwinkle
viral infections, **28–29**
herbs and, 29
viral load, testing, 353
virus therapy, cancer, 227
Viscum album (mistletoe), **446–49**
cancer and, 448–49
Christmas, mistletoe at, 447
clinical applications of, traditional, 447
clinical pearls, 449
dosing, 449
indications, traditional, 447
modern research, 447
tissue targets for, specific, 409
vital force, adaptogens and, 66–73
vitality
healthy eating to restore, 40–48
restoration of, 316–317
vitamins. *See also* natural agents
B-complex, 120–21
B vitamins, 28, 121, 211–12
C, 122
C, intravenous, 150–51
D2, 305
E, anticoagulants and, 335
vomiting (emesis), **217–18**
counteracting, strategies for, 217
hyperemesis, 135
hyperemesis, cannabis and, 135
lobelia and, 104
Mineralizing Tea for Replenishing after Vomiting, 216
Nausea and Vomiting, Herbal Formula for, 217
vulnerary herbs, **117–18**
described, 116

W

warning signs of cancer, **17–18**
"watchful waiting," cancer growth and, 21
western red cedar. *See Thuja occidentalis, T. plicata*
Western yew. *See Taxus brevifolia, T. baccata, T. wallichiana*
where you live, 23–24
whey protein, 60, 183
white peony root (*Paeonia lactiflora*), 186–87
whole-person treatment planning, **344–48**
age of patient, 345
constitution, 347
gender of patient, 345–46
genetics, 346–347
who has the disease, 344–45

wild lettuce (*Lactuca virosa*), 136–37
wild yam, 35
willow, 35
Withania somnifera. See ashwagandha
wound cleansing, cicatrant herbs and, 116–17
"wound contraction," 113
wound healing
    complications of, 118
    phases of, 113–14
    tulsi and, 297

X

xi shu. *See Camptotheca acuminata*
x-rays, 231

Y

yarrow (*Achillea millefolium*), 117
yeast infections, oral thrush and, 213
yellow gentian (*Gentiana lutea*), 199
yellow jasmine (*Gelsemium sempervirens*), 141
yucca, 35

Z

Zea mays. See corn silk
zinc, 121